Illustrated Guide to Equine Diseases

Illustrated Guide to Equine Diseases

Sameeh M. Abutarbush
BVSc, MVetSc, Diplomate ABVP, Diplomate ACVIM
Assistant Professor, Large Animal Internal Medicine
Department of Veterinary Clinical Sciences
Faculty of Veterinary Medicine
Jordan University of Science and Technology
Irbid, Jordan

WILEY-BLACKWELL
A John Wiley & Sons, Inc., Publication

Edition first published 2009

Blackwell Publishing was acquired by John Wiley & Sons in February 2007. Blackwell's publishing program has been merged with Wiley's global Scientific, Technical, and Medical business to form Wiley-Blackwell.

Editorial Office
2121 State Avenue, Ames, Iowa 50014-8300, USA

For details of our global editorial offices, for customer services, and for information about how to apply for permission to reuse the copyright material in this book, please see our website at www.wiley.com/wiley-blackwell.

Library of Congress Cataloging-in-Publication Data

Illustrated guide to equine diseases / [edited by] Sameeh M. Abutarbush.
p. ; cm.
Includes bibliographical references and index.
ISBN-13: 978-0-8138-1071-3 (alk. paper)
ISBN-10: 0-8138-1071-X (alk. paper)
1. Horses–Diseases. I. Abutarbush, Sameeh M.
[DNLM: 1. Horse Diseases–diagnosis–Atlases. 2. Diagnostic Techniques and Procedures–veterinary–Atlases. SF 951 C7194 2009]
SF951.I45 2009
636.1′089–dc22

2008051624

A catalog record for this book is available from the U.S. Library of Congress.

Set in 9 on 11.5 pt Sabon by SNP Best-set Typesetter Ltd., Hong Kong
Printed in Singapore

1 2009

Dedication

To my father Mohammad who passed away after a long battle with cancer while I was writing this book. He was a man of principles and had a strong belief in science and pursuing higher degrees. He nurtured my ambitions, supported my aspirations, and had a strong belief in me. This book is also dedicated to my dearest mother Fatima, my beloved brothers and sisters, Nidal, Reem, Khalid, Mai, Omar, and Mahmoud, and to my loving wife Marah. They are outstanding people who have worked hard, made sacrifices, guided me, and lent their unending support to allow me the opportunity to pursue the career of my dreams. Their patience and support throughout my personal and professional life is immeasurable. Professor Otto M. Radostits had a great influence on my life and career. He was my mentor during my internship and residency at The Western College of Veterinary Medicine, University of Saskatchewan. He guided me through my higher education and ongoing professional training. I hope that this book meets your expectations.

You will make more mistakes not looking than not knowing.

Professor Otto M. Radostits

Contents

Preface ix

Contributors xi

Chapter 1 Diseases of the Gastrointestinal Tract and Liver 3
Author: *Sameeh M. Abutarbush*
Contributors: *Mary S. Delory, Montague N. Saulez, Ben Buchanan, Janice E. Sojka*

Chapter 2 Diseases of the Cardiovascular System 119
Author: *JoAnn Slack*
Contributors: *Sameeh M. Abutarbush, Susan J. Ashburner, Janice E. Sojka*

Chapter 3 Diseases of the Respiratory System 175
Author: *Laurent L. Couëtil*
Contributors: *Sameeh M. Abutarbush, Montague N. Saulez, Ben Buchanan*

Chapter 4 Diseases of the Nervous System 211
Author: *Sameeh M. Abutarbush*
Contributors: *Montague N. Saulez, Wendy Marlene Duckett*

Chapter 5 Diseases of the Integumentary System 255
Authors: *Susan J. Ashburner, James L. Carmalt, Wendy Marlene Duckett*
Contributors: *Sameeh M. Abutarbush, Montague N. Saulez, Janice E. Sojka*

Chapter 6 Diseases of the Muscles 343
Author: *Sameeh M. Abutarbush*
Contributor: *Ben Buchanan*

Chapter 7 Diseases of the Bones, Joints, and Connective Tissues 353
Author: *Patricia L. Rose*

Chapter 8	Diseases of the Reproductive System Author: *Rob Löfstedt*	445
Chapter 9	Diseases of the Endocrine System Author: *Janice E. Sojka* Contributors: *Sameeh M. Abutarbush, Ben Buchanan*	507
Chapter 10	Diseases of the Eye Author: *Bruce Grahn*	529
Chapter 11	Diseases of the Urinary System Author: *Sameeh M. Abutarbush* Contributor: *Ben Buchanan*	559
Chapter 12	Diseases of the Neonates Author: *Jane Elizabeth Axon* Contributors: *Patricia L. Rose, Sameeh M. Abutarbush*	579
Index		663

Preface

It has been said that "a picture is worth a thousand words." It is the fundamental idea behind this illustrated guide. One cannot study veterinary medicine and be a good clinician without seeing clinical cases. Knowledge is likely to be retained for a longer period of time when given a contextual basis (i.e., when connected to photographic data). In addition, some diseases are rare and one may not see them more than once in a professional lifetime.

The aim of this illustrated guide is to provide the reader with the clinical picture of a disease or syndrome, presenting signs, diagnostic procedures, and a brief synopsis. There are 12 chapters, 11 of which are based on the different body systems. The twelfth chapter embraces diseases and conditions of the neonate, which are not shared with the adult horse.

Although it is impossible to include all diseases of the horse in one volume, this illustrated guide covers hundreds of internationally recognized diseases and conditions, some of which prevail in specific geographic areas. Moreover, it not only approaches disease from a clinical point of view, but also embraces additional diagnostic modalities, where applicable, such as radiology, nuclear scintigraphy, CAT scan, cytology, histopathology, and postmortem findings. Chapter 7, Diseases of the Bones, Joints, and Connective Tissues, focuses mainly on diagnostic imaging that is available for most of the diseases, since clinical signs alone are of limited value in the diagnosis of the different lesions associated with these structures. Presentation of such options is one of the features of this illustrated guide. Each chapter is followed by a list of readings that are believed to be helpful to the reader.

The illustrated guide is not intended to be heavily texted. It contains over a thousand educational photographs, singular and compound. The photographs used on these pages are highly informative and of excellent quality and resolution.

The contributors to this volume are experts in their disciplines and well-known authors. Their efforts contribute to the high quality of the material presented here. To see, diagnose, and treat a condition is one thing; to document a condition photographically is entirely another.

This book is intended to be helpful to veterinary medicine students, technicians, clinicians, and specialists, as well as horse lovers.

Finally, I would like to pass on the advice that I have taken from my phenomenal mentor, Professor Otto M. Radostits, who advised me to have a camera handy and carry it around whenever I practice veterinary medicine. I never knew how valuable that advice was until I began work on this project.

Sameeh M. Abutarbush

Contributors

Sameeh M. Abutarbush, BVSc, MVetSc, Diplomate ABVP, Diplomate ACVIM; Assistant Professor, Large Animal Internal Medicine; Department of Veterinary Clinical Sciences, Faculty of Veterinary Medicine, Jordan University of Science and Technology, Irbid, Jordan

Susan J. Ashburner, DVM; Clinical Associate, File Service; Department of Large Animal Clinical Sciences, Western College of Veterinary Medicine, University of Saskatchewan, Saskatoon, SK, Canada

Jane Elizabeth Axon, BVSc (hons), Diplomate ACVIM; Director, Scone Veterinary Hospital, Clovelly Intesive Care Unit, Scone, NSW, Australia

Ben Buchanan, DVM, Diplomate ACVIM, Diplomate ACVECC; Clinician, Intensive Care, Internal Medicine; Brazos Valley Equine Hospital, Navasota, TX, USA

James L. Carmalt, MA, VetMB, MVetSc, MRCVS, Diplomate ABVP, Diplomate ACVS; Associate Professor, Large Animal Surgery, Department of Large Animal Clinical Sciences, Western College of Veterinary Medicine, University of Saskatchewan, Saskatoon, SK, Canada

Laurent L. Couëtil, DVM, PhD, Diplomate ACVIM; Professor, Department of Veterinary Clinical Sciences, School of Veterinary Medicine, Purdue University, West Lafayette, IN, USA

Mary S. Delory, DVM; President, Northwest Equine Dentistry, Inc., Kettle Falls, WA, USA

Wendy Marlene Duckett, DVM, MSc, Diplomate ACVIM; Associate Professor, Department of Health Management, Atlantic Veterinary College, University of Prince Edward Island, Charlottetown, PEI, Canada

Bruce Grahn, DVM, Diplomate ACVO, Diplomate ABVP; Professor, Department of Small Animal Clinical Sciences, Western College of Veterinary Medicine, University of Saskatchewan, Saskatoon, SK, Canada

Rob Löfstedt, BVSc, MSc, Diplomate ACT; Professor, Theriogenology; Department of Health Management, Atlantic Veterinary College, University of Prince Edward Island, Charlottetown, PEI, Canada

Patricia L. Rose, DVM, MS, Diplomate ACVS, Diplomate ACVR; Assistant Professor, Department of Companion Animals, Atlantic Veterinary College, University of Prince Edward Island, Charlottetown, PEI, Canada

Montague N. Saulez, MS, PhD, BVSc, Diplomate ACVIM; Section Head, Equine; Onderstepoort Veterinary Hospital, Faculty of Veterinary Science, University of Pretoria, Onderstepoort, South Africa

JoAnn Slack, DVM, MS, Diplomate ACVIM; Assistant Professor, Large Animal Cardiology & Ultrasound, Department of Sports Medicine and Imaging, School of Veterinary Medicine, University of Pennsylvania, Philadelphia, PA, USA

Janice E. Sojka, VMD, MS, Diplomate ACVIM; Associate Professor, Department of Veterinary Clinical Sciences, Purdue University; West Lafayette, IN, USA

Illustrated Guide to Equine Diseases

1 Diseases of the Gastrointestinal Tract and Liver

Diseases of Teeth
- Wave Malocclusion
- Rostral Hook
- Caudal Hooks or Ramps
- Stepped Tooth
- Step Mouth
- Hooks or Ramps
- Shear Mouth
- Overlong Distal Portion of the Third Incisor
- Diagonal Incisor Malocclusion
- Incisor Curvature
- Irregular Incisor Malocclusion
- Supernumerary Incisor
- Overbite (Parrot Mouth)
- Underbite (Sow or Monkey Mouth)
- Periodontal Disease, Diastema, and Enamel and Cemental Decay
- Geriatric Wear
- Teeth Eruption and Retained Deciduous Teeth "Cap"
- Wolf Teeth
- Deviation of the Maxilla
- Asynchronous Teeth Eruption
- Fractured Tooth
- Lingual and Buccal Laceration and Bit Pressure (Injury)
- Gingival and Lingual Ulceration of Systemic Origin
- Supernumerary Canine Tooth
- Polydontia
- Dysplastic Teeth
- Abnormal Tooth Wear

Diseases of the Mouth
- Squamous Cell Carcinoma
- Oral Foreign Body
- Glossitis

Diseases of the Esophagus
- Esophageal Obstruction (Choke), Primary
- Esophageal Obstruction (Choke), Secondary

Diseases of the Abdominal Region
- Abdominal Pain (Colic)
- Diseases of the Stomach
  - Gastric Dilatation
  - Gastric Impaction
  - Gastric Ulcers
- Diseases of the Small Intestine

1

Simple Obstruction of the Small Intestine
Ileal Impaction
Ileal Hypertrophy
Ascarid Impaction
Meckel's Diverticulum
Strangulating Obstruction
Mesodiverticular Band
Small Intestinal Volvulus (Mesenteric Torsion)
Small Intestinal Strangulation Caused by a Pedunculated Lipoma
Epiploic Foramen Entrapment of the Small Intestines
Diaphragmatic Hernia
Incarceration of the Small Intestine Through the Gastrosplenic Ligament
Intussusception
Functional Obstruction of the Small Intestine
Duodenitis-Proximal Jejunitis (DPJ) (Anterior or Proximal Enteritis)
Proliferative Enteropathy (*Lawsonia Intracellularis*)
Diseases of the Large Intestine
Large Colon Volvulus (LCV)
Large Colon Displacement (LCD)
Right Displacement of the (Left) Large Colon (RDLC)
Left Dorsal Displacement of the Large Colon (LDLC)
Large Colon Impaction (LCI)
Large Intestinal Intussusception
Salmonellosis
Strongylosis
Cyathostomiasis
Nonsteroidal Anti-Inflammatory Drugs (NSAIDs) Toxicity
Grain (Carbohydrate) Overload
Small Colon Impaction
Intralumenal Obstruction of the Small Colon with Enteroliths, Fecaliths, or Foreign Bodies
Idiopathic Inflammatory Bowel Disease
Antibiotic Induced Colitis
Miscellaneous
Abdominal Abscessation
Abdominal Adhesions
Peritonitis
Enterocutaneous Fistula and Parietal (Richter's) Hernia
Omental Hernia
Grass Sickness (Equine Dysautonomia)
Hyperlipemia and Hyperlipidemia

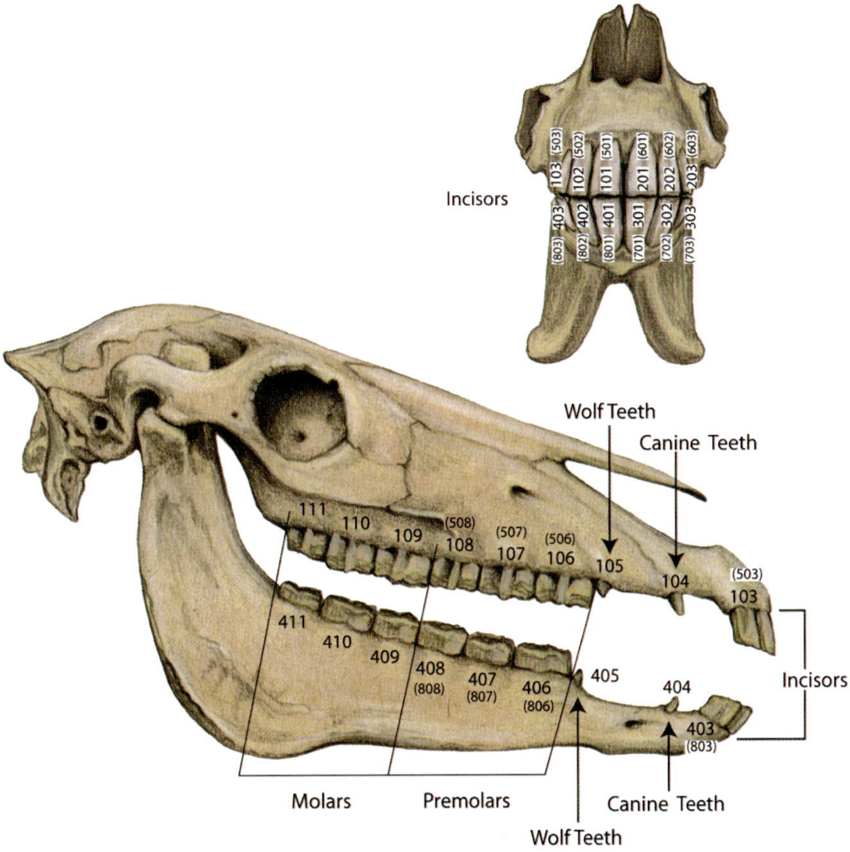

Figure 1.1 Illustration for the Triadan numbering system for equine dentition. The permanent dentition is described by 1–400s while the deciduous dentition is described by the 5–800s.

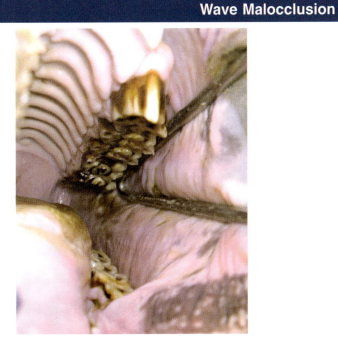

Wave Malocclusion

Figure 1.2a Wave malocclusion involving the 200 and 300 arcades in a middle-aged patient. The 206 is overlong. The 207 and 208 exhibit progressively shorter clinical crown to the 208/9 junction. Note that the gingival margin is displaced dorsally at this point and dips ventrally again at the 209/10 junction where the 210 is overlong. This involvement of the gingival margin is an indicator of chronicity and signals probable bony remodeling. Patient age and amount of clinical crown and gingival margin/bony changes collectively determine the amount of correction possible at a single session. Some wave malocclusions cannot be normalized but are best maintained to minimize progression and deterioration.

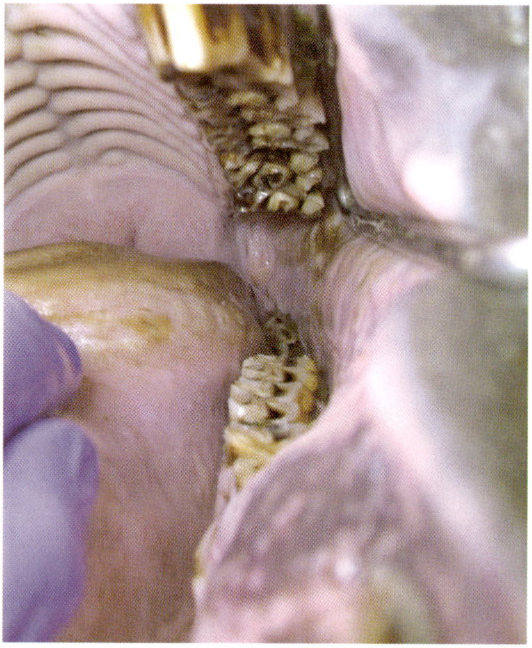

Figure 1.2b Same patient in fig. 1.2a. View of 300 arcade "wave" abnormality. Note that the distal 308 is the tallest point in the 300 arcade and the 309 is not visible at all.

Rostral Hook

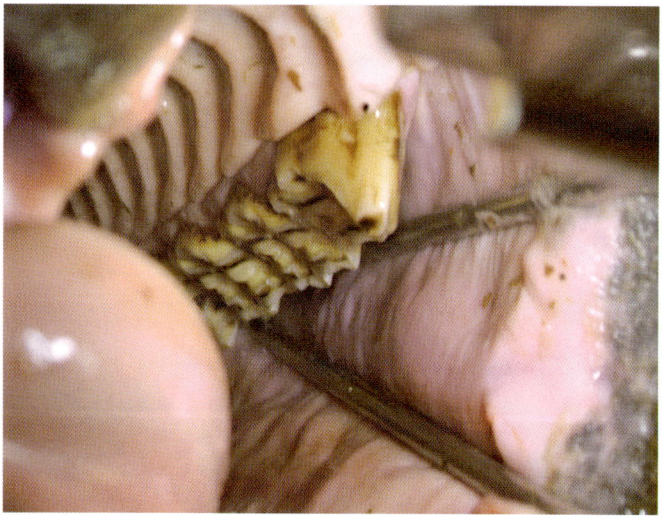

Figure 1.3 Mesial portion of 206 is overlong due to malocclusion with 306. Commonly referred to as a "rostral hook," this abnormality is often seen in class 2 malocclusions commonly known as "parrot mouth." Early recognition and reduction of the excessive crown is recommended to avoid large or staged reductions.

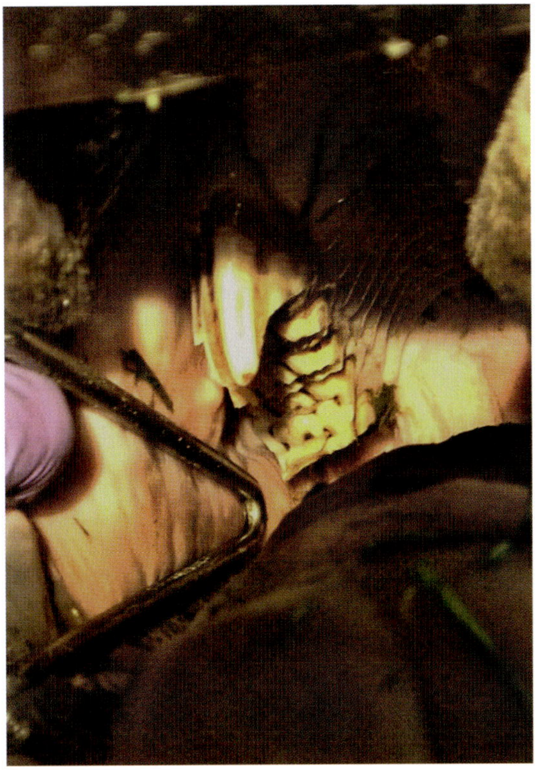

Figure 1.4 Large amount of excessive crown at the mesial portion of 106 in a 10-year-old quarter horse stallion. This abnormality is common in class 2 malocclusions (parrot mouth) although this patient has normal incisor occlusion. Commonly referred to as a “rostral hook,” it is progressive, can traumatize soft tissue, may exacerbate malocclusions elsewhere in the mouth, and may interfere with normal masticatory function. Overlong crown of this magnitude requires staged reductions to avoid pulpar exposure or thermal injury.

Caudal Hooks or Ramps

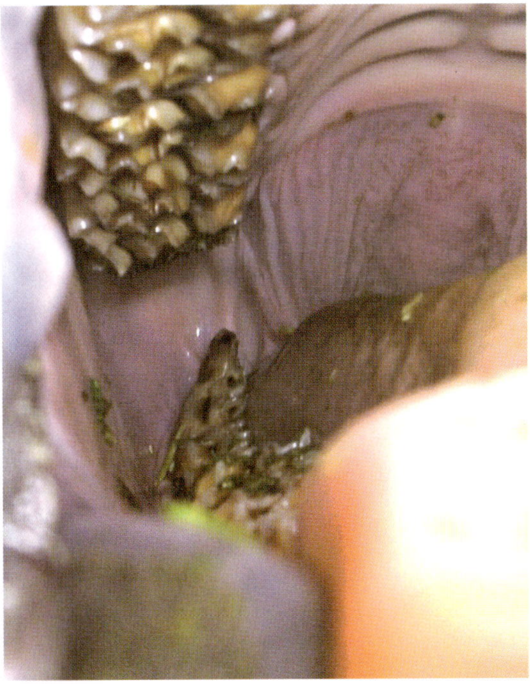

Figure 1.5 Overlong crown at distal 311 due to malocclusion with 211. Commonly known as “caudal hooks or ramps,” these abnormalities are progressive, can injure soft tissue, predispose to other malocclusions and periodontal disease, and may interfere with normal masticatory motion. Commonly, though not exclusively, seen in class 2 malocclusions (parrot mouth).

Stepped Tooth

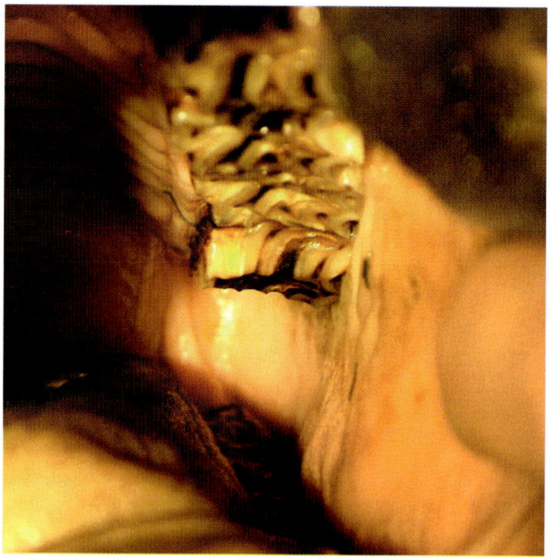

Figure 1.6 Overlong 209 due to missing 309. Commonly referred to as a "stepped tooth." Regular crown reductions may be necessary to maintain normal rostral/caudal mandibular movement.

Step Mouth

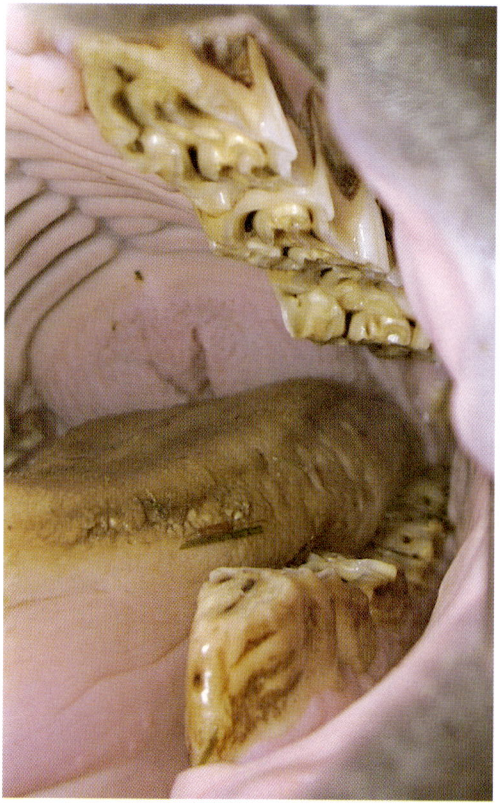

Figure 1.7 Abrupt, severe changes in crown height along an entire arcade pair is commonly known as a "step mouth." Normal mastication is significantly compromised with such malocclusions. Severe cases require serial crown reductions for safe correction.

Hooks or Ramps

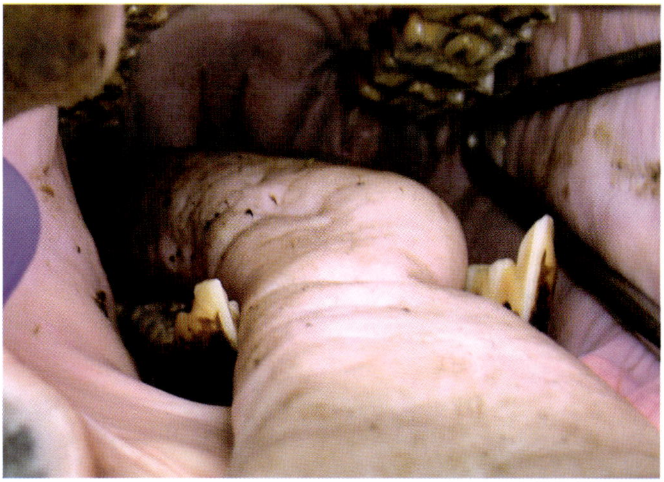

Figure 1.8 The 306 and 406 with excessive mesial crown commonly referred to as hooks or ramps. They are caused by malocclusion with the maxillary 6s. They are progressive and can cause soft tissue injury, biting pain, periodontal disease, and abnormal mastication.

Shear Mouth

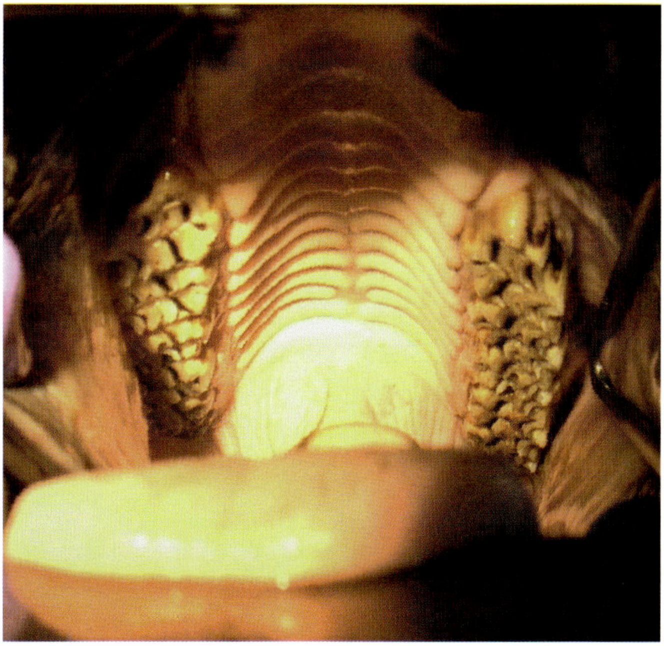

Figure 1.9 "Shear mouth" in an 8-year-old quarter horse mare. Note the slightly steeper table angle of the 200 arcade in comparison to the 100 arcade. Gradual reduction of the steep table angle can be helpful. If left unchecked, many cases will worsen to the point of abnormal mastication.

Overlong Distal Portion of the Third Incisor

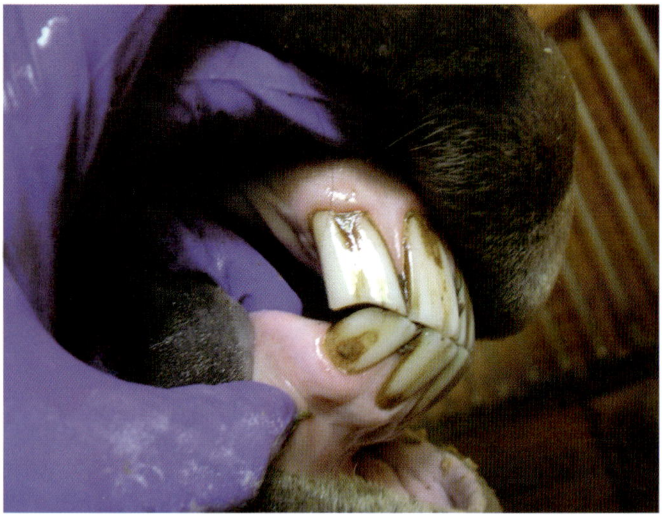

Figure 1.10a Distal portion of 103 is overlong caused by a malocclusion with 403. Such areas of excessive crown are progressive and can cause interference with normal lateral excursion of the mandible and thereby affect functional occlusion of the cheek teeth.

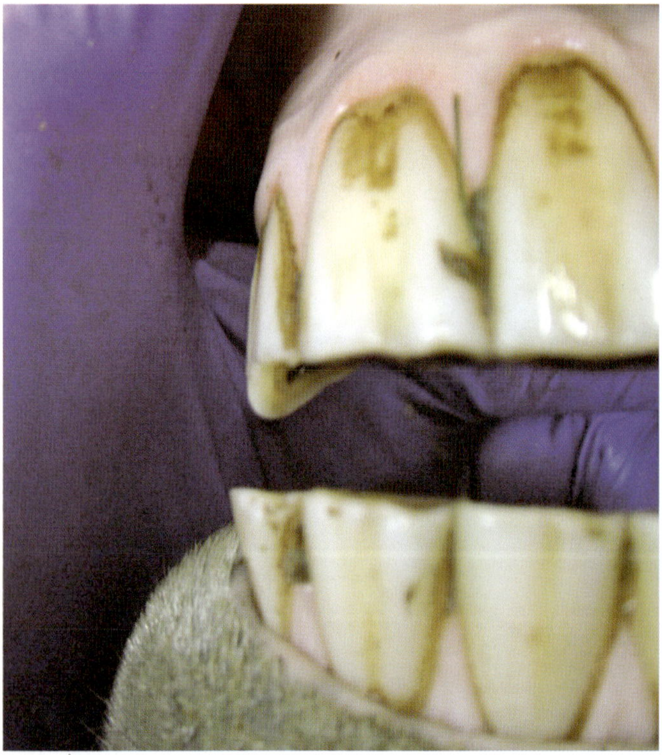

Figure 1.10b Rostral view of overlong distal 103. Same horse in fig. 1.10a

Diagonal Incisor Malocclusion

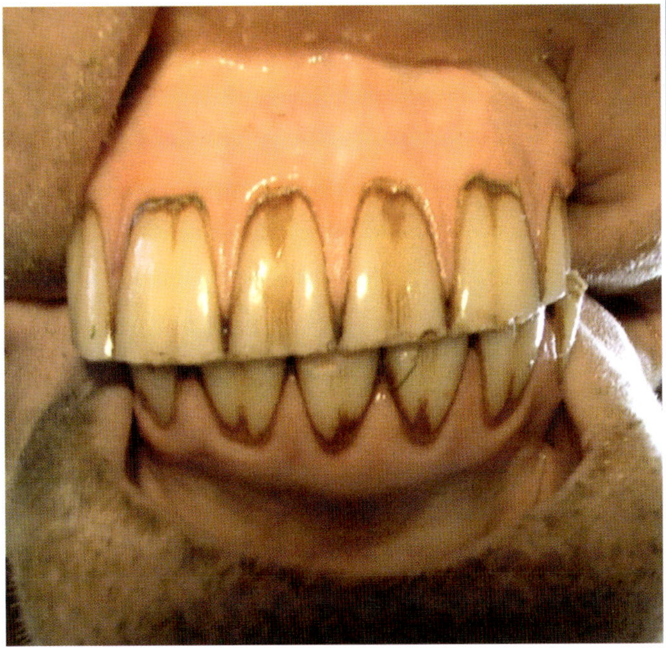

Figure 1.11 Diagonal incisor malocclusion (DGL3) in an aged horse. Note the progressively increasing length of clinical crown from the 203 right to the 103 and from the 403 left to the 303. There is also a mandibular offset to the horse's left. Etiology can be difficult to determine and may be multifactorial. This malocclusion is progressive and early detection and correction are beneficial. Correction in some cases can be harmful. A thorough understanding of equine mastication biomechanics is critical for successful correction and maintenance.

Incisor Curvature

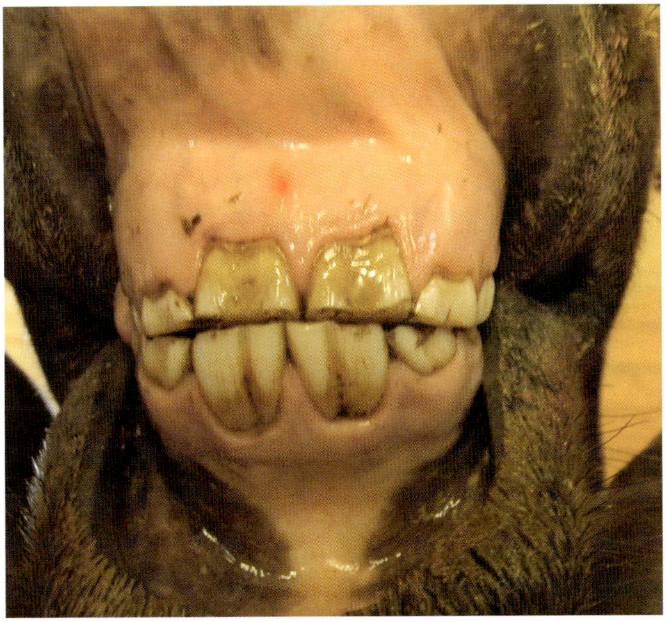

Figure 1.12 Dorsal incisor curvature in a juvenile. Etiology may be asynchronous eruption of the 1s or a cribbing/rubbing habit that is causing selective wear to 101 and 102.

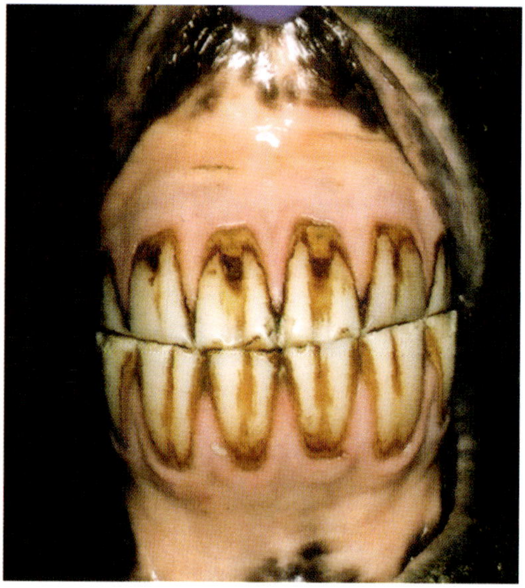

Figure 1.13 Ventral incisor curvature in an aged horse. This malocclusion is usually progressive and can cause abnormal lateral excursion. Overlong incisors should be reduced as necessary to maintain normal lateral excursion and to prevent progression of the malocclusion.

Irregular Incisor Malocclusion

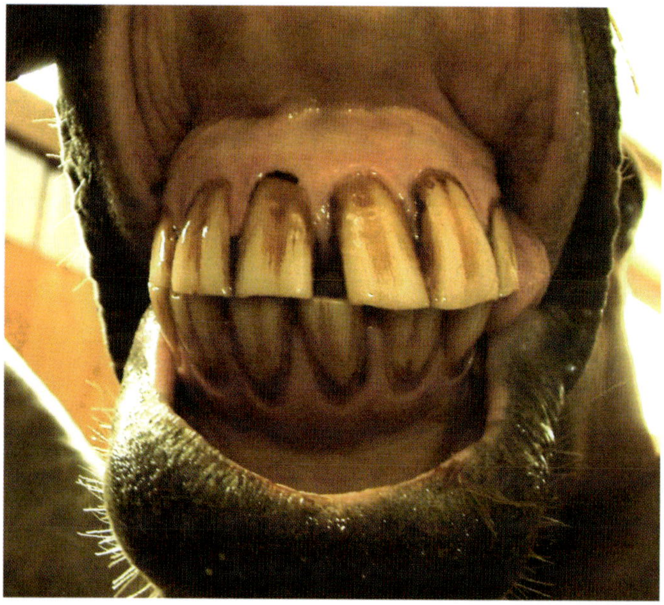

Figure 1.14 Irregular incisor malocclusion in which the occlusal plane undulates in a wave pattern. In this case, probably initiated by the abnormal positions of 101/201. As with any incisor malocclusion, lateral excursion and therefore efficient mastication may be affected.

Supernumerary Incisor

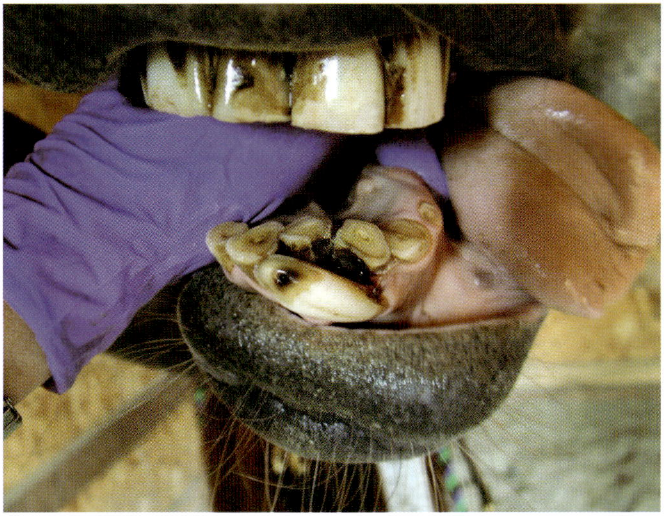

Figure 1.15 A 14-year-old Peruvian Paso mare with supernumerary and displaced incisors. Feed was collecting between the grossly displaced incisor and the ones lingual to it causing periodontal disease and dental decay. Extraction of the displaced incisor and reduction of other overlong incisor crowns to restore normal lateral excursion was beneficial.

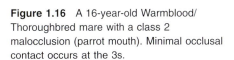

Overbite (Parrot Mouth)

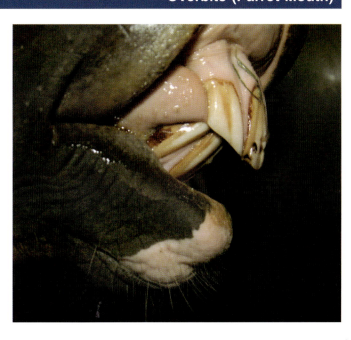

Figure 1.16 A 16-year-old Warmblood/ Thoroughbred mare with a class 2 malocclusion (parrot mouth). Minimal occlusal contact occurs at the 3s.

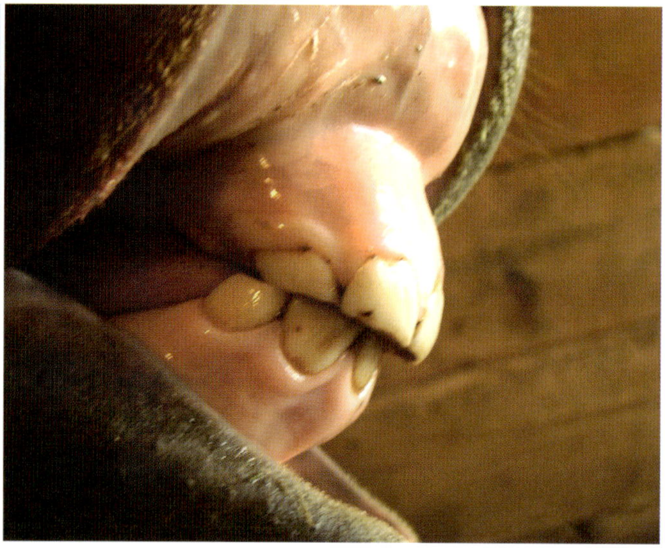

Figure 1.17a Class 2 malocclusion in a yearling. Commonly referred to as "parrot mouth" or "overbite." Early detection and removal of resultant overlong clinical crowns can be curative in mild to moderate cases. More severe cases may require orthodontic treatment.

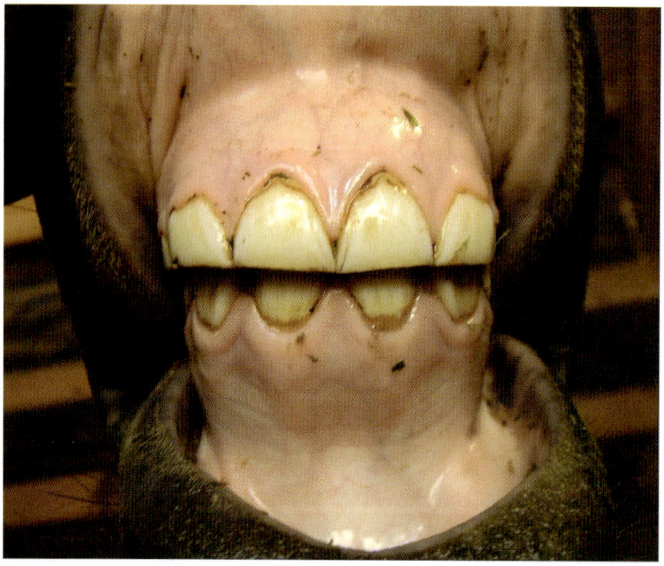

Figure 1.17b Same horse in 1.17a, rostral view of class 2 malocclusion.

Underbite (Sow or Monkey Mouth)

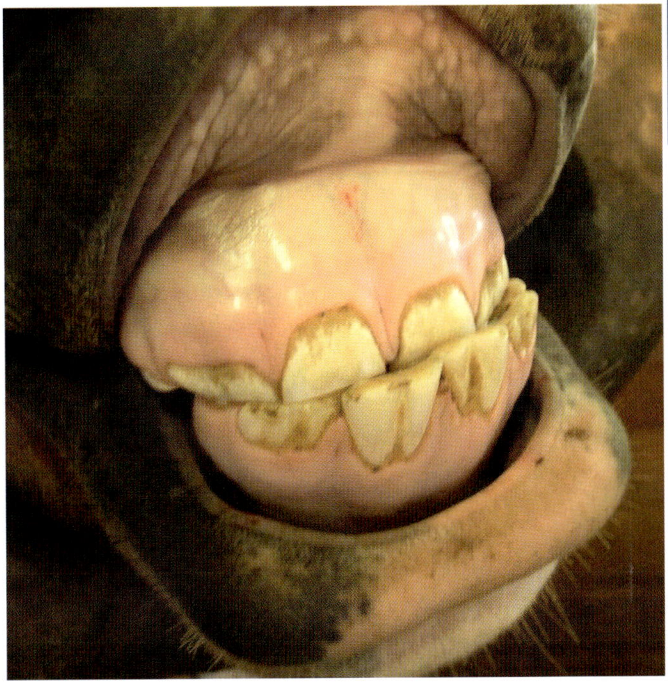

Figure 1.18 Class 3 malocclusion (sow mouth or monkey mouth) in a 2 1/2-year-old. Early recognition and treatment to release the promaxilla from behind the mandible may allow for normal growth and resolution. Advanced cases may not be correctable but benefit greatly from regular reduction of overlong crowns and restoration of normal mastication biomechanics.

Periodontal Disease, Diastema, and Enamel and Cemental Decay

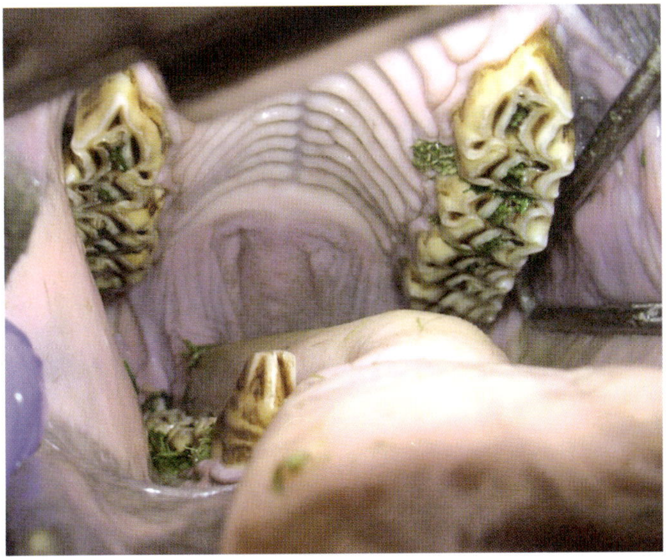

Figure 1.19a A 2-year-old Thoroughbred with feed packed between 506 and 507 and between 806, 807, and 808. This presentation is a strong indicator of periodontal disease and should prompt further examination. The 806 is also overlong due to a missing opposing tooth in the upper right arcade. The overlong crown may be contributing to the feed packing distal to it due to abnormal occlusal forces.

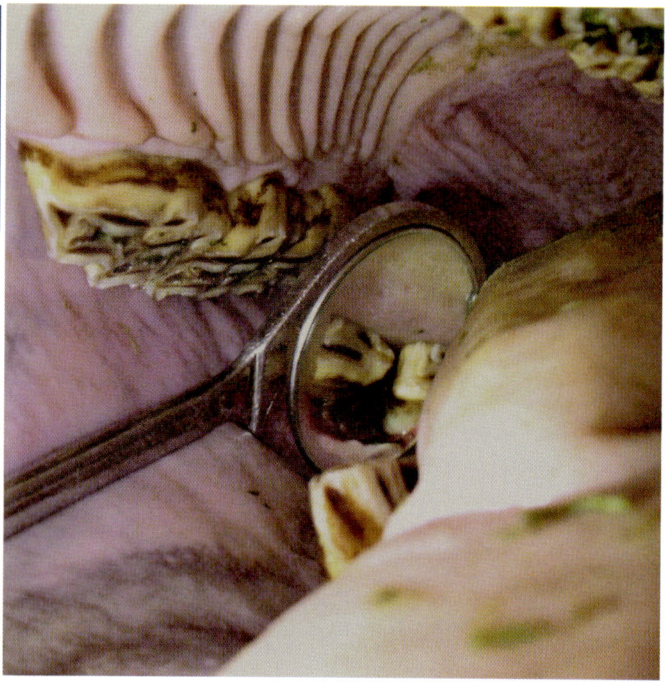

Figure 1.19b Same horse in fig. 1.19a; large periodontal pocket after cleaning trapped feed from interproximal space. Pockets of this size likely indicate bony involvement and radiography is warranted to assess the severity of the disease.

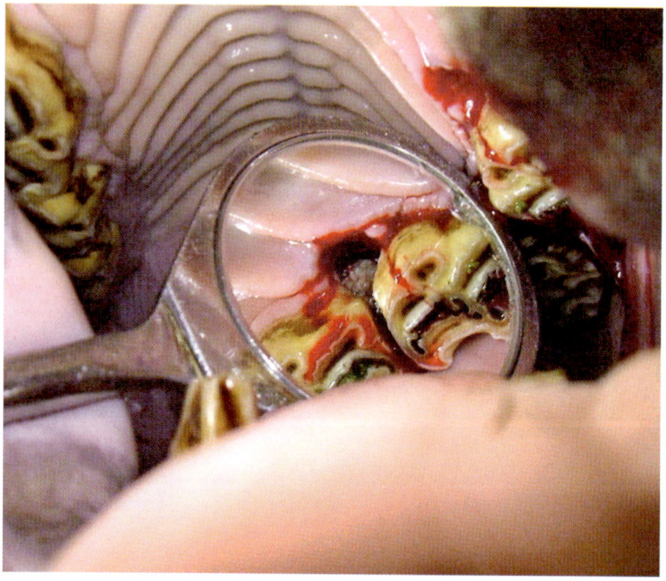

Figure 1.19c Same horse in fig. 1.19a; diastema and periodontal pocket between 506 and 507 after feed material was cleaned out. The grey tissue deep within the pocket is actually a free-floating "foreign body." Histological examination revealed that it was bone.

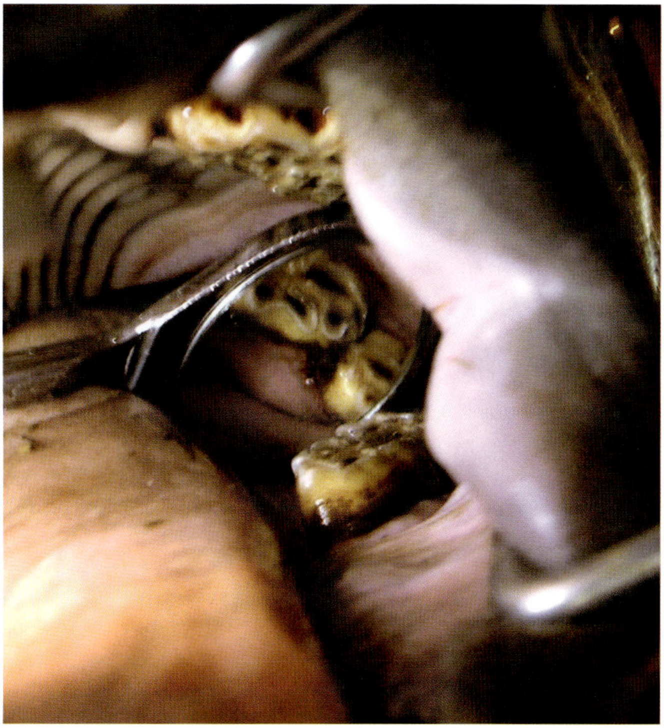

Figure 1.20 A 5-year-old paint mare with lingually displaced 308. The mirror is placed between 307 and 308. Feed is trapped at the lingual aspect of that interproximal space causing periodontal disease.

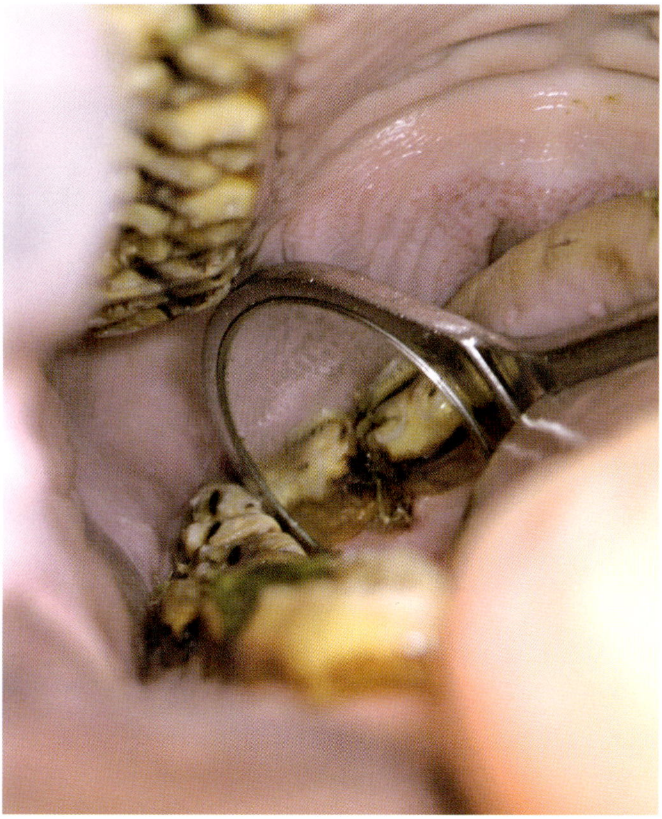

Figure 1.21 A 9-year-old Warmblood mare with lingual periodontal pocket at 410/11. Packed feed is visible in both views: the lingual (mirror) and the buccal aspect view. An overlong distal 411 has already been reduced. Excessive crown at the distal 311 or 411 may predispose to interproximal small diastema formation due to abnormal occlusal forces. Correction of malocclusions is sometimes curative. In other cases, primary treatment of the periodontal disease is also necessary.

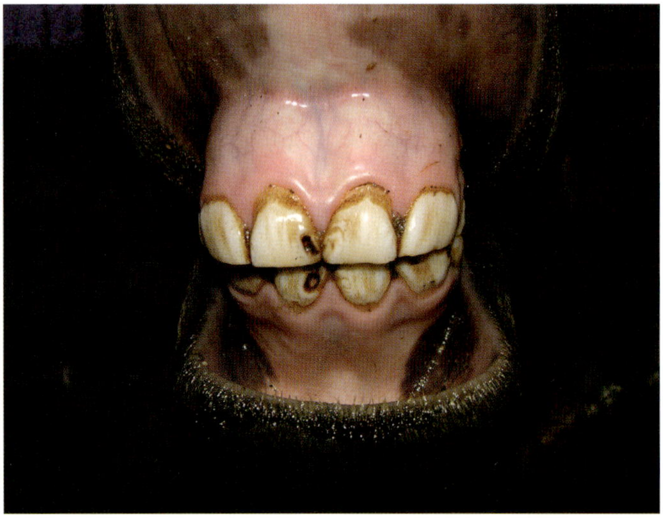

Figure 1.22a Focal areas of enamel decay at 501 and 801. The focal nature of the lesion involving deciduous teeth necessitates no treatment.

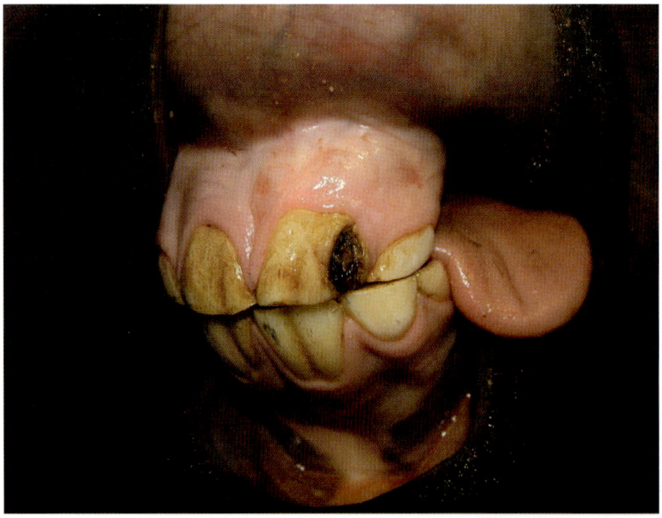

Figure 1.22b Large area of enamel decay involving a permanent incisor. This incisor quadrant is also oligodontic. Radiographic examination is warranted to fully explore the dental pathology. Debridement and/or endodontic or restorative procedures may be indicated pending deep structure evaluation via radiography.

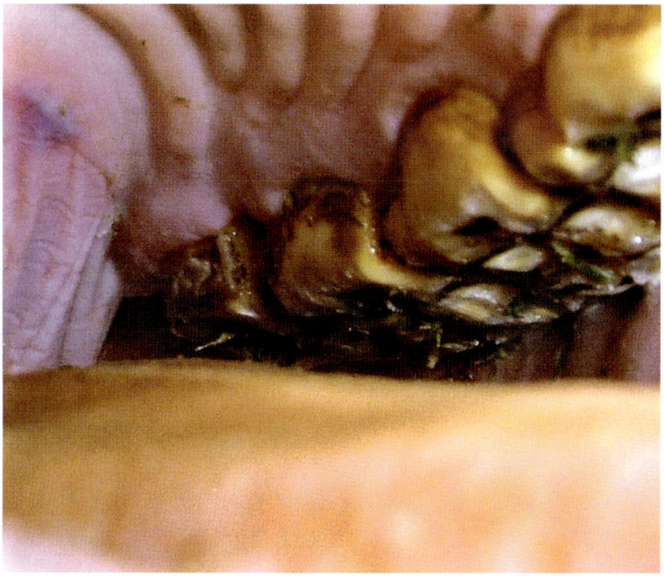

Figure 1.23 Peripheral cemental decay at the palatal aspect of 210 and 211. Note the normal yellow cementum on the palatal surfaces of 208 and 209. At 210 see darker staining roughened edge of a cemental "crescent" and a grey coating of "plaque" at the gingival margin marking early stage decay. At 211 see the underlying white enamel "skeleton," denuded of its cemental covering. Feed stasis is a common cause of this condition. Underlying causes for feed stasis should be identified and corrected.

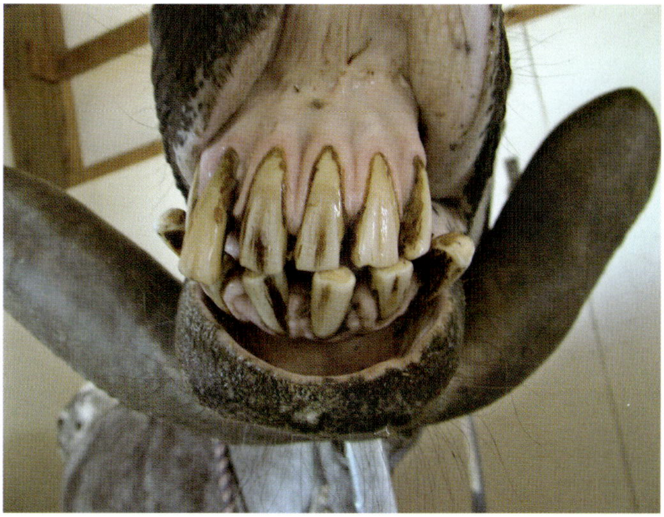

Figure 1.24a A 29-year-old Appaloosa gelding presented with dysphagia and acutely decreased water intake and loss of body condition. Diagnosis was chronic incisor periodontal disease with cemental hypoplasia. Radiographs showed predominantly cemental hypoplasia. The 102, 303, and 403 were grade 3 loose and were extracted. Water intake and feed consumption immediately returned to normal.

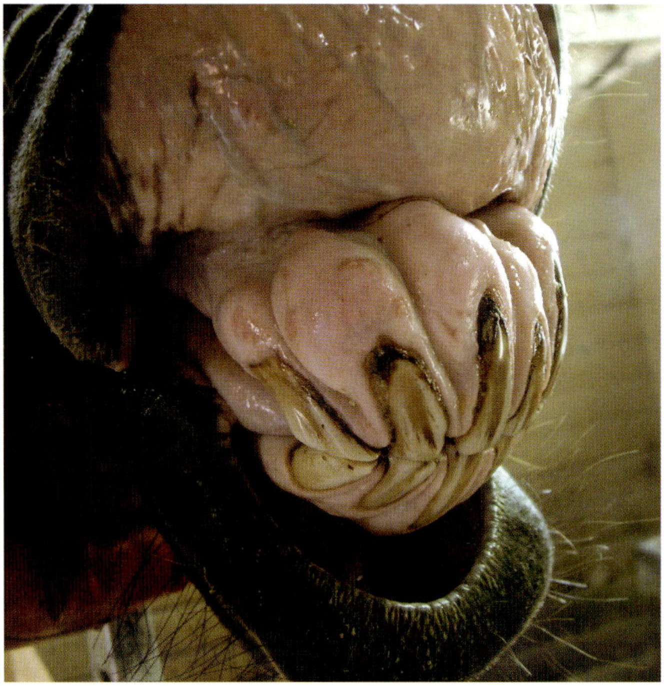

Figure 1.24b A 29-year-old Warmblood with chronic incisor periodontal disease. This disease is characterized by a concurrent cemental hyperplasia. This case displays predominantly cemental hyperplasia. None of the incisors are loose. Regular examination and periodic radiographs are recommended to monitor progress.

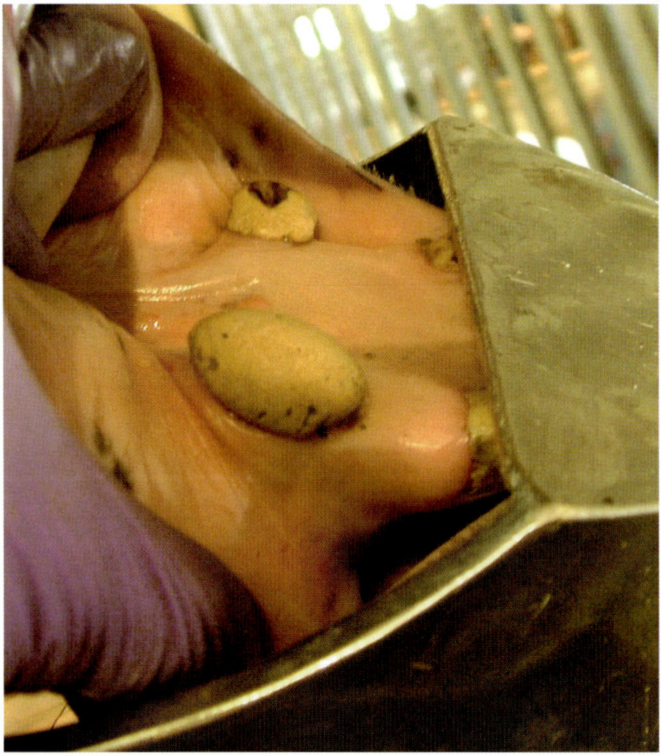

Figure 1.25 Severe calculus accumulation over and around 404. The 304 is also affected although to a lesser extent. Canine calculus can be a symptom of more severe periodontal disease. Careful examination of the affected tooth and its periodontal tissues is warranted in all cases of calculus formation.

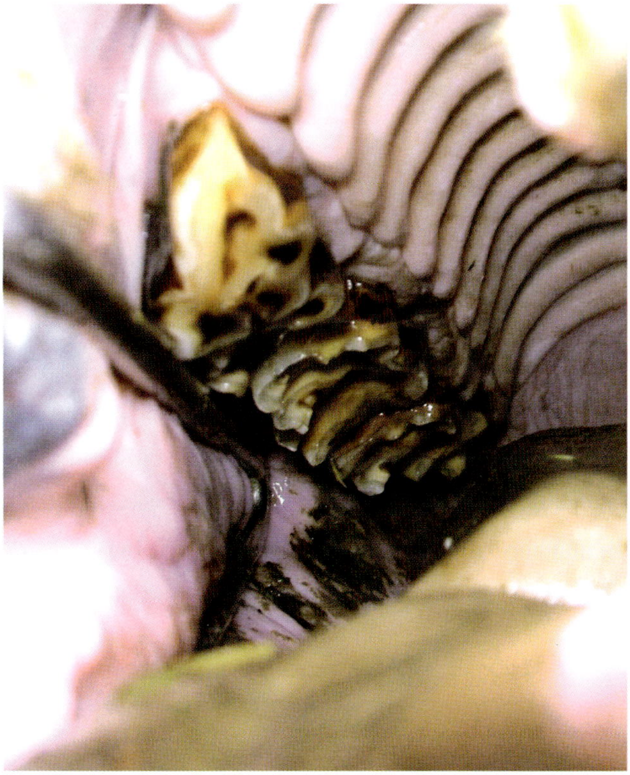

Figure 1.26a Geriatric wear in an older horse, approximately 27 years old. Note the loss of transverse ridges on occlusal surfaces. Much of the enamel is worn away leaving smooth dentin and cementum. Commonly referred to as "cupped," these occlusal surfaces have significantly reduced grinding ability. Dietary management may be necessary to meet this older horse's nutritional needs.

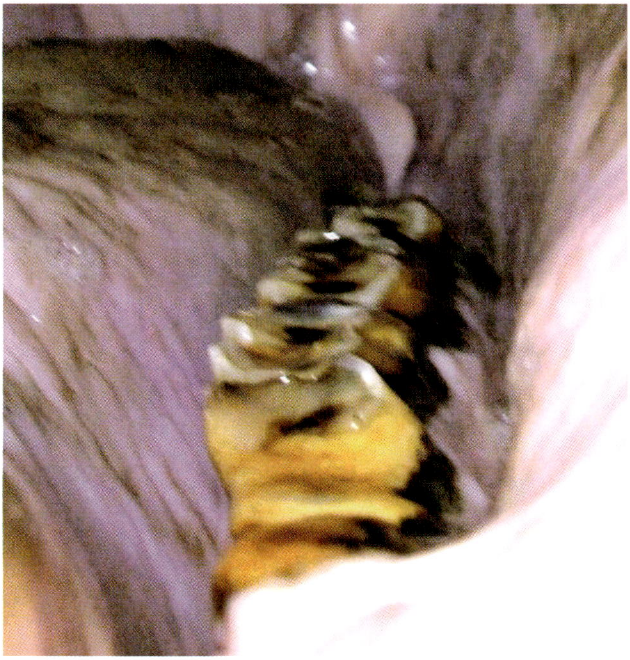

Figure 1.26b Geriatric wear involving mandibular cheek teeth in same horse in 1.26a. Note extreme wear at 306 and mesial 307. These teeth are often referred to as "smooth."

Teeth Eruption and Retained Deciduous Teeth "Cap"

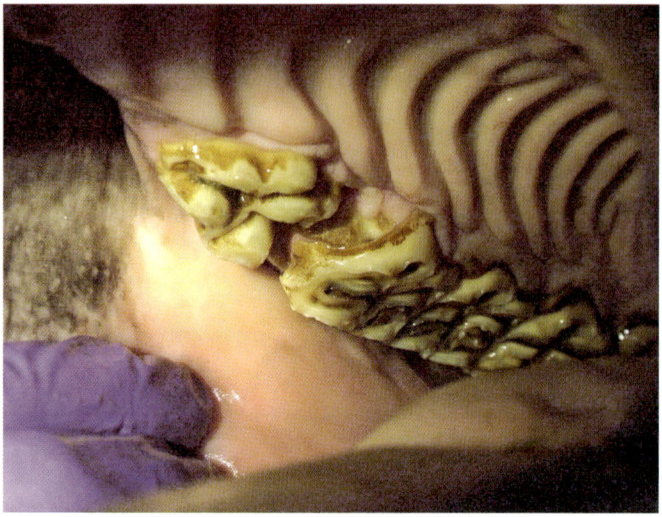

Figure 1.27 Typical appearance of erupting teeth in a 3-year-old patient. The 106 is erupted and very recently in wear. Tooth 107 is visible beneath its deciduous predecessor (507). The 507 in this stage is commonly referred to as a "cap." Deciduous teeth normally exfoliate spontaneously but if encountered during dental examination, it is safer to remove them if they are loose and the permanent tooth is visible beneath them. Premature removal of deciduous caps may result in damage to the permanent tooth.

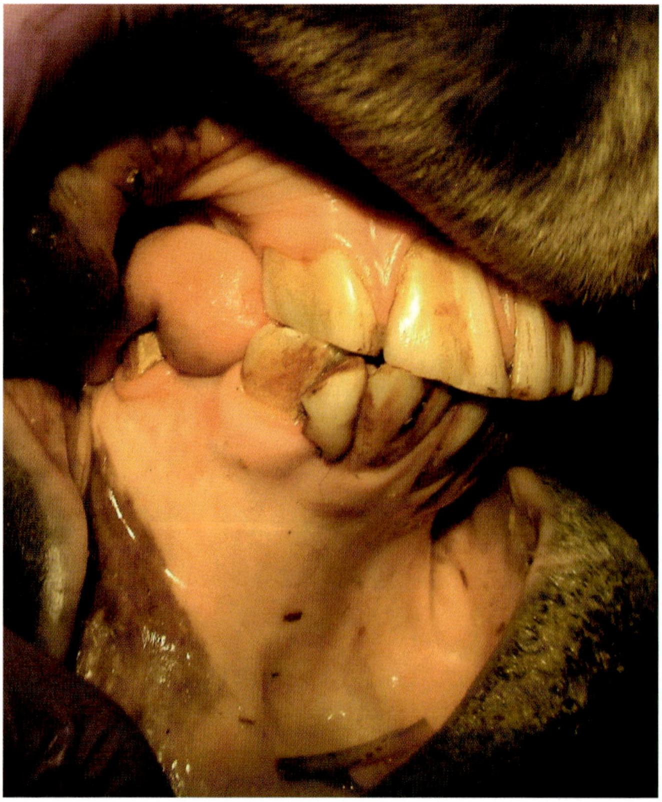

Figure 1.28 Retained 803 in a 5 1/2-year-old. Extraction is necessary to allow proper positioning of 403 and to avoid feed accumulation between teeth. Presence of even small root fragments from deciduous teeth can inhibit proper positioning of permanent teeth.

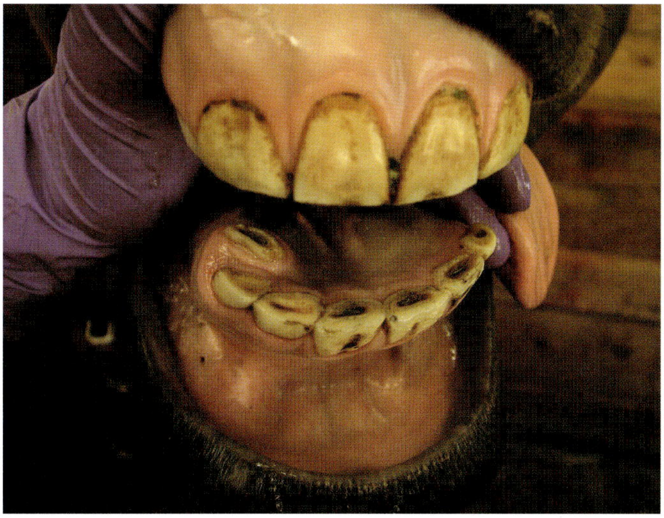

Figure 1.29a Retained tooth 802 in a 4-year-old Thoroughbred gelding. Note that tooth 302 is in normal position and in wear. Tooth 703 is still present. Tooth 803 is still present, and normally located. The right mandibular intermediate incisor is deciduous (802) and there is a permanent incisor erupted out of position distal to the rest of the arcade. Tooth 802 should be extracted.

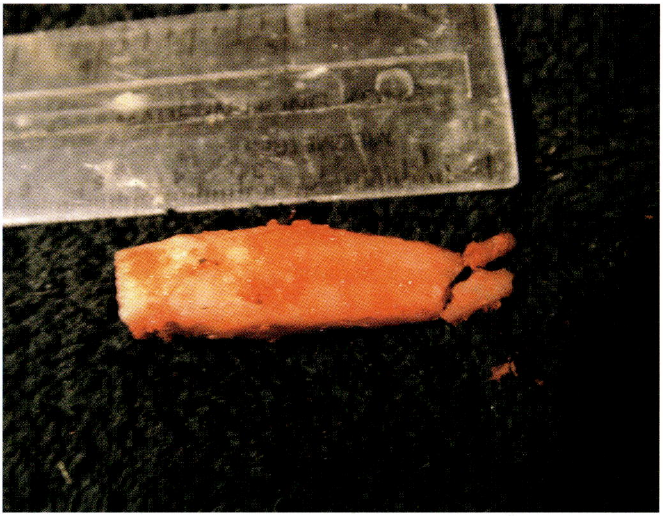

Figure 1.29b Same horse in fig. 1.29a. Retained tooth 802 was extracted. Note no evidence of radicular resorption.

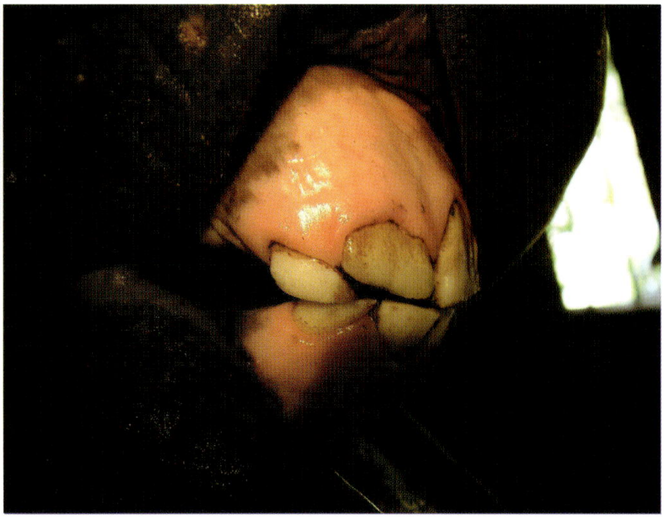

Figure 1.30 Crowding of 102 in a 3 year old. The 503 is preventing the 102 from full eruption into its normal position. Early detection and treatment may prevent permanent incisor malocclusions or periodontal disease.

Wolf Teeth

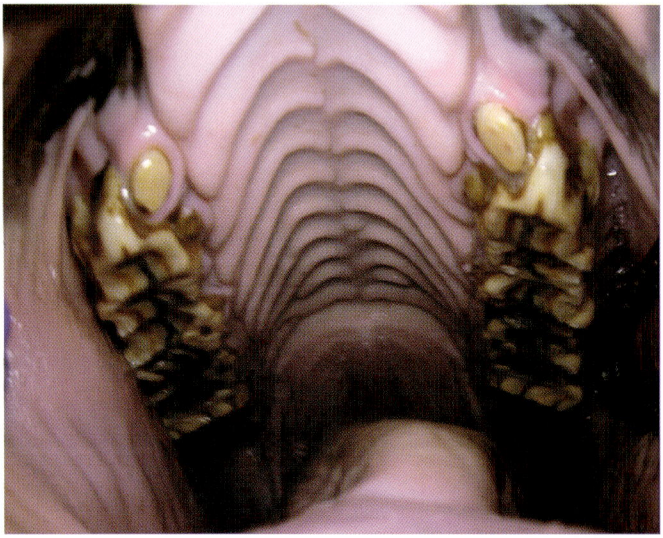

Figure 1.31 Very large wolf teeth in a 2-year-old Thoroughbred. Note that the mesial and buccal surfaces of the 506 and 606 have been previously rounded into a "bit seat" and wolf teeth have been reduced but not extracted. Large wolf tooth crown does not necessarily indicate a large root or a difficult extraction. Current recommendations are that wolf teeth be extracted before training to the bit. This is done to avoid "bit" discomfort. Excessive transverse ridges at the 109 and 209 are also present.

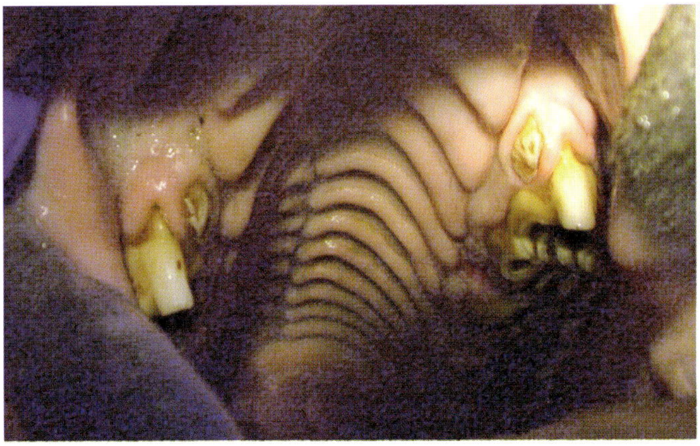

Figure 1.32 Atypical palatal location of wolf teeth in a yearling. Care should be taken when extracted to avoid the palatine artery.

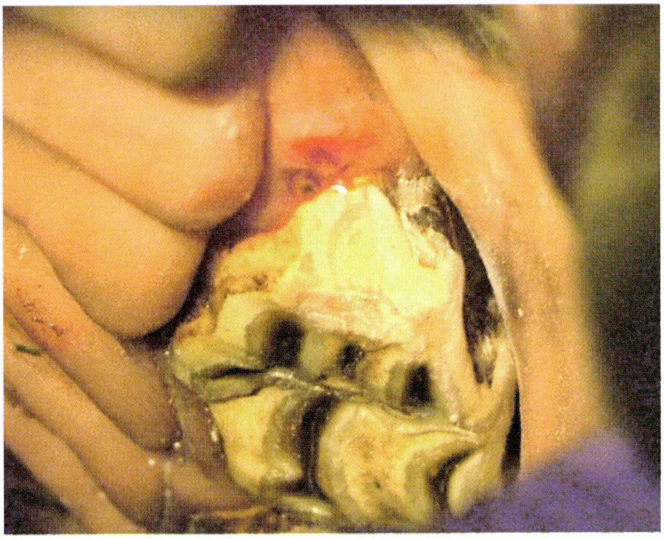

Figure 1.33 Iatrogenic soft tissue injury to the gingiva making a small wolf tooth fragment visible just palatal to 206. Wolf tooth fragments can cause biting discomfort and should be removed when identified. They can result from fracture at the time of initial extraction or may be rudimentary or polydontic and not visible at earlier examinations.

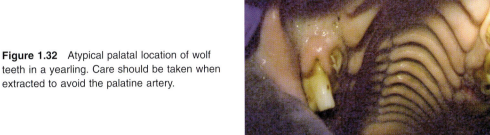

Deviation of the Maxilla

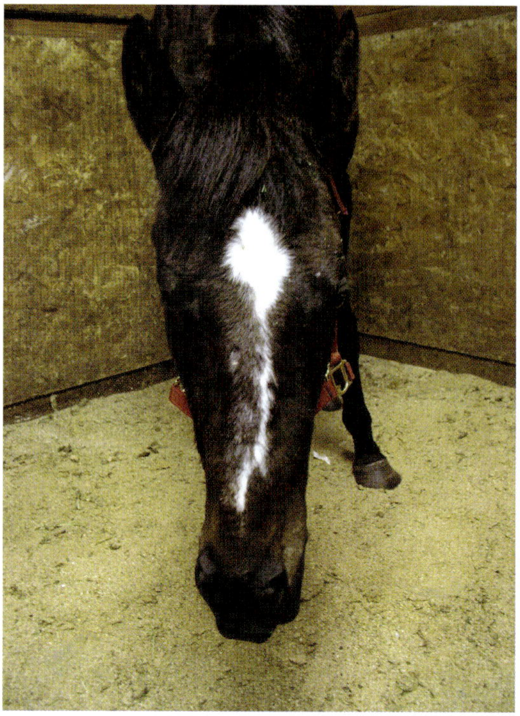

Figure 1.34 "Wry nose" in a 2-year-old Thoroughbred colt. His maxilla deviates to the right.

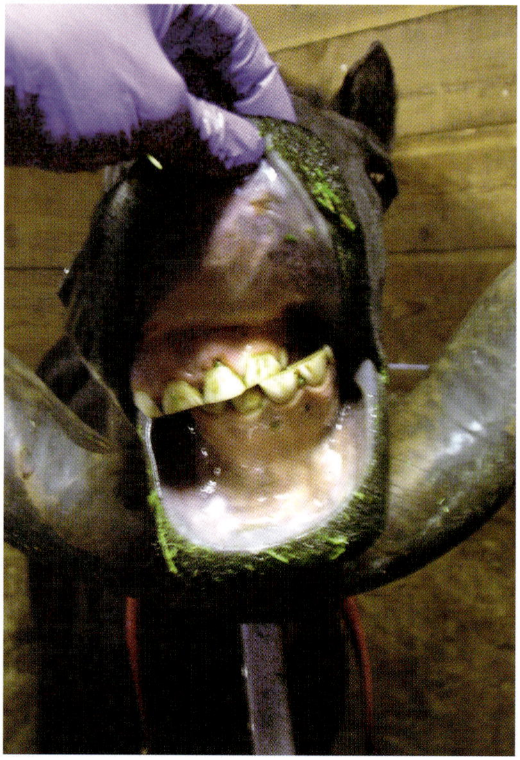

Figure 1.35 Same horse in fig. 1.34. Note the diagonal incisor malocclusion (DGL3) as a result of the deviation of the maxilla. This is a marked mandibular offset. Such malocclusions cannot be "corrected" but should be treated regularly to minimize overlong crown to maintain functional cheek teeth occlusion. If left unchecked as in this horse, it may progress to functional failure. This case exhibited other abnormalities including oligodontia, multiple diastemae, periodontal disease, and enophthalmos. See Diseases of the Respiratory System (Chapter 3) and Diseases of the Neonates (Chapter 12).

Asynchronous Teeth Eruption

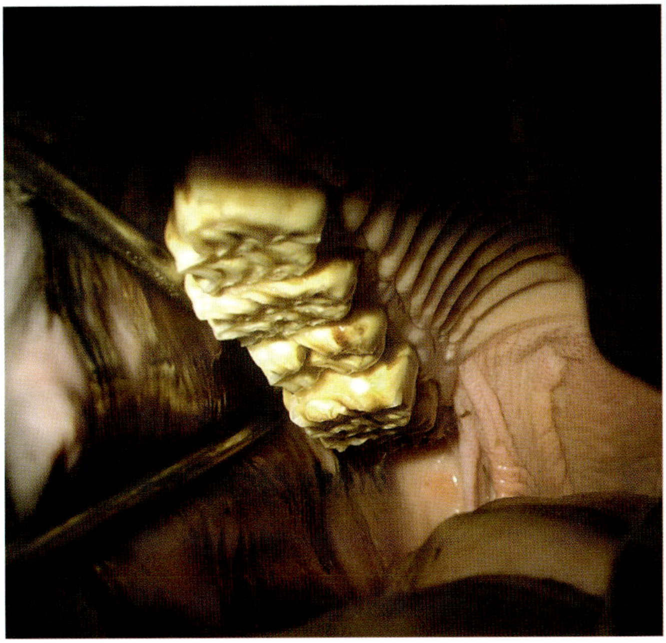

Figure 1.36 A 4-year-old horse with an overlong tooth 109. Note the difference in crown height when compared to tooth 110. Probable cause is asynchronous eruption. Tooth 109 likely erupted slightly before the 409. Failure to address this condition in the young horse can result in "wave" malocclusion.

Fractured Tooth

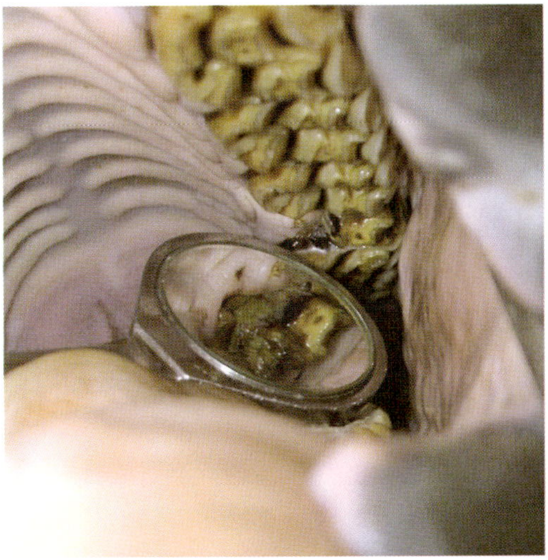

Figure 1.37a Cursory examination of the 200 teeth arcade reveals abnormality at the occlusal surface of tooth 209. When viewed with a dental mirror, a missing portion of the palatal crown was noted. Mirror also showed two small dental fragments embedded in the gingiva and mild superficial decay due to feed impaction.

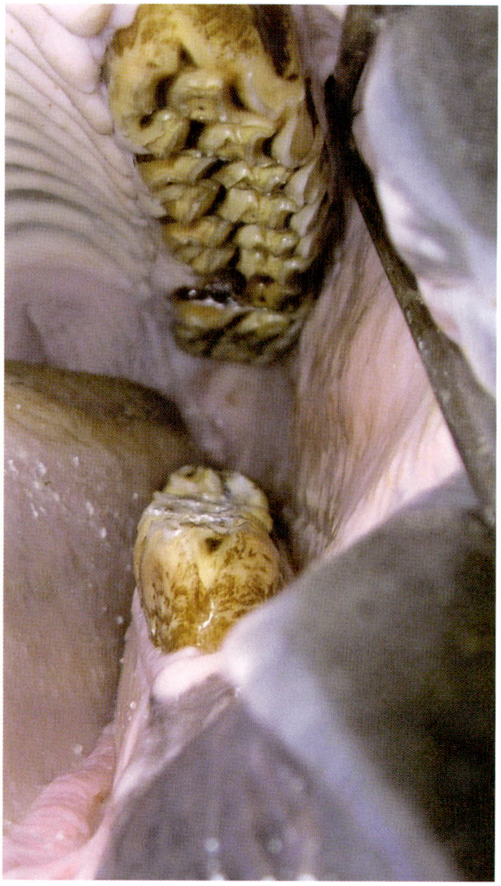

Figure 1.37b Same horse in fig. 1.37a. Overlong tooth 309 due to fractured tooth 209. Incomplete occlusion between the two teeth allows excessive crown overgrowth of the mandibular tooth. Commonly referred to as a "stepped tooth."

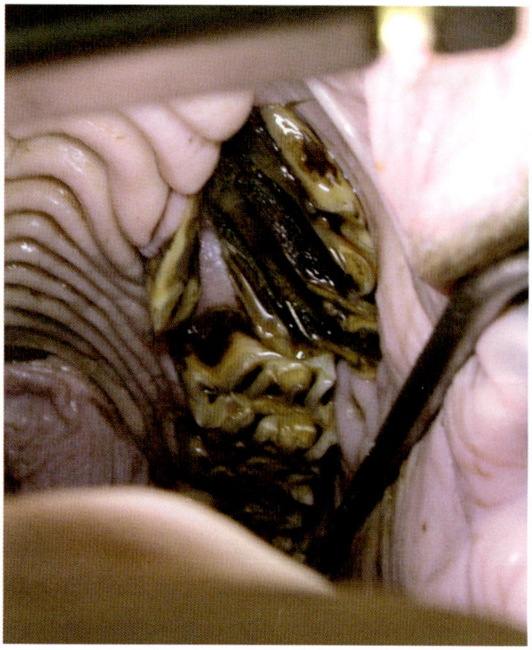

Figure 1.38a Sagittal fracture of tooth 206 in a middle-aged quarter horse mare. Fragments are displaced laterally and dorsally.

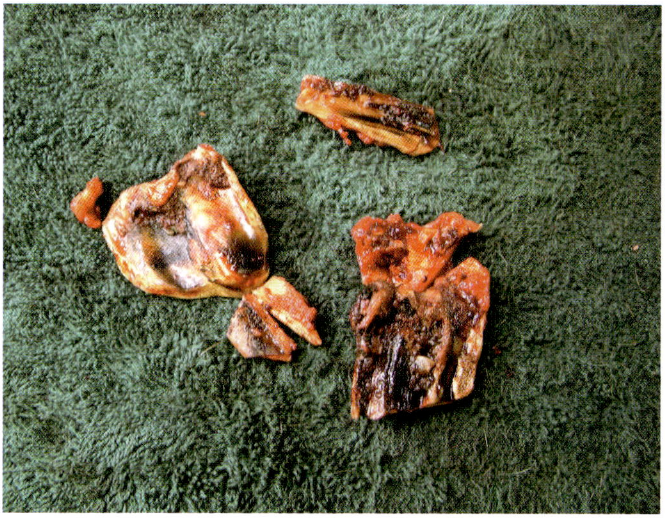

Figure 1.38b Extraction of the fractured tooth in fig. 1.38a. Multiple fragments were retrieved. Postprocedure radiographs are necessary to confirm that all fragments are removed.

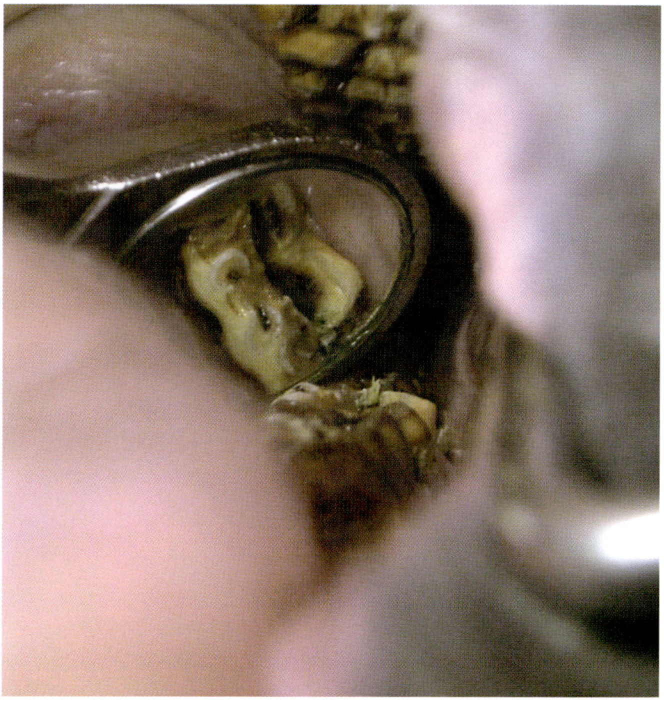

Figure 1.39a An 8-year-old Warmblood gelding with sagittal fracture of tooth 308. Fracture line is through the 4th and 5th pulp chambers. Buccal fragment is loose but nondisplaced.

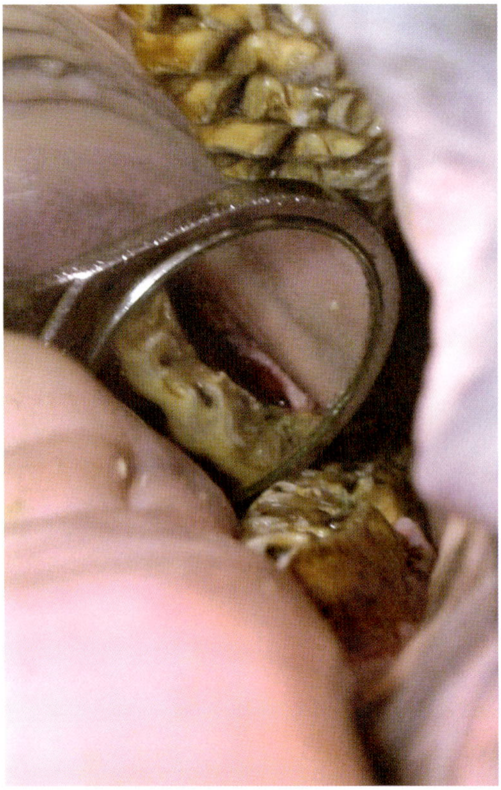

Figure 1.39b Same horse in fig. 1.39a. Appearance of tooth 308 following removal of buccal fragment. Radiographs showed no pulpar disease. Remaining tooth 308 was left in situ.

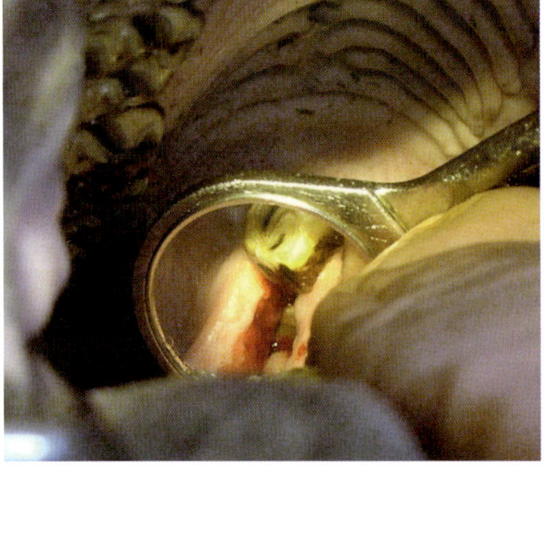

Figure 1.40a Tan object visible within the alveolus 8 weeks postextraction of fractured tooth 408. This is sequestrum of the alveolar wall. Pink mound distal to it is healthy granulation tissue. Subsequent extraction of sequestrae was curative.

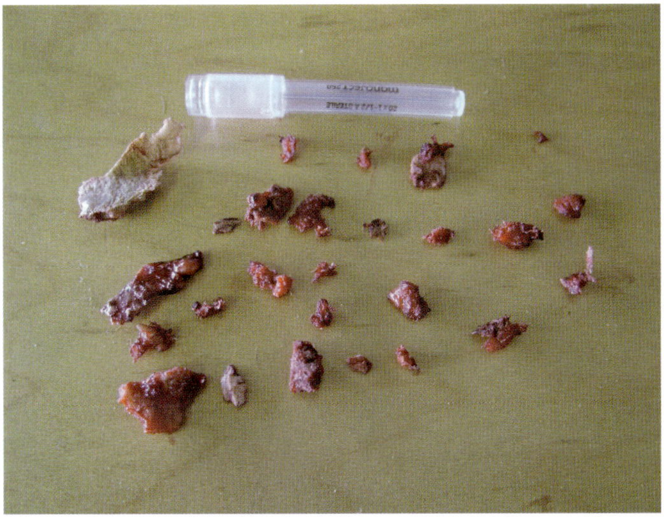

Figure 1.40b Same horse in fig. 1.40a. Multiple sequestrae fragments were removed from tooth 408 alveolus.

Lingual and Buccal Laceration and Bit Pressure (Injury)

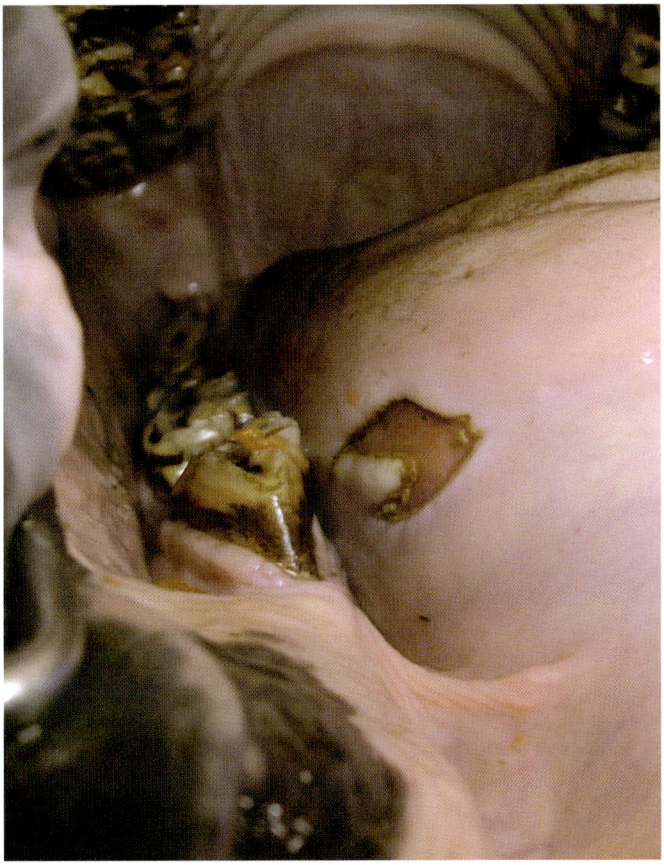

Figure 1.41 Lingual laceration in a 13-year-old Thoroughbred gelding presented with sudden reluctance to eat and increased salivation. Tooth 407 was fractured leaving a sharp shard of the tooth, which lacerated his tongue. Smoothing of the remaining portion of tooth 407 was curative. Fractured teeth can often be managed without extraction provided pulpar disease is not present.

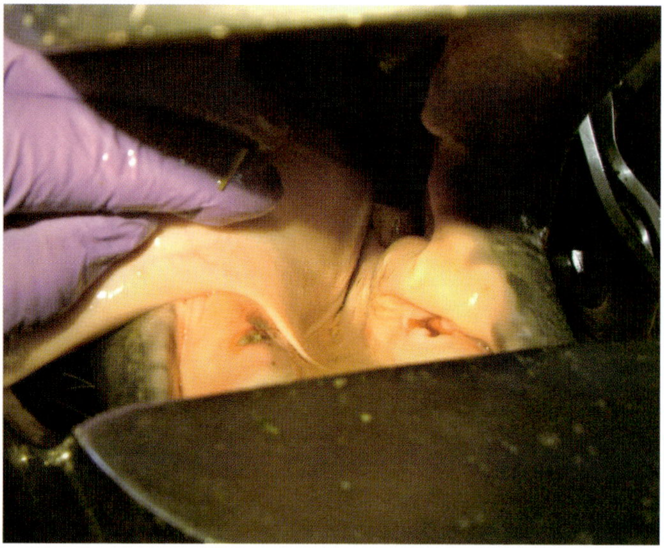

Figure 1.42a Bilateral soft tissue damage to the interdental spaces of a young quarter horse. Such injury is usually due to bit pressure, but autoinduced trauma using objects available in the horse's environment (i.e., edges and lips on feeders or water buckets) should be investigated. Radiographs may be indicated to rule out bony involvement.

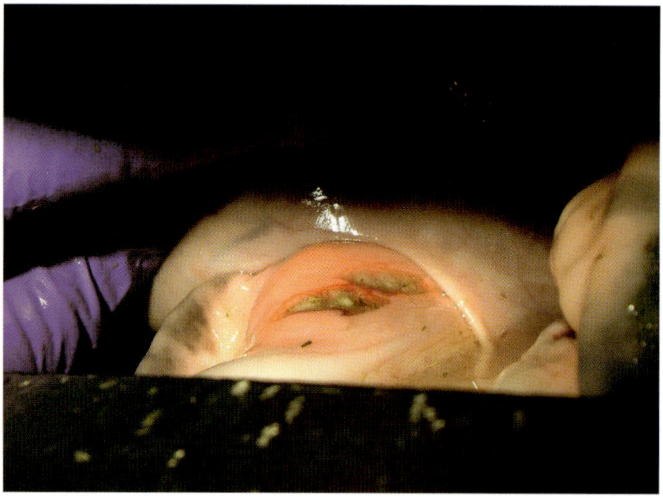

Figure 1.42b Close-up view of same horse in fig. 1.42a.

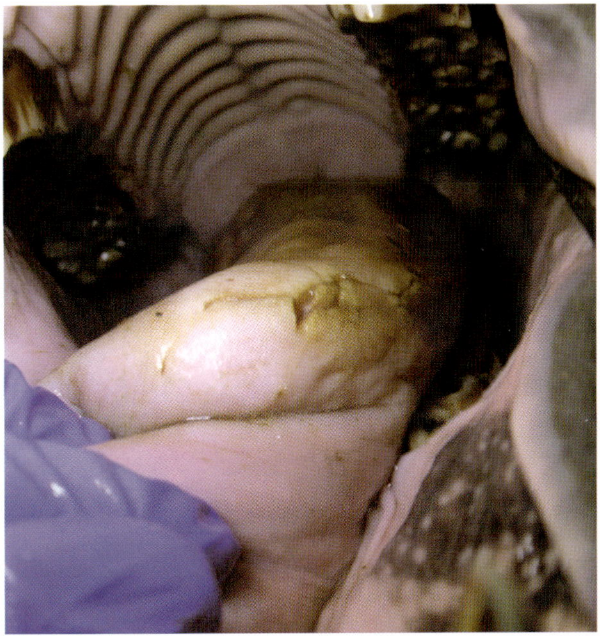

Figure 1.43 Chronic lingual laceration or ulceration due to sharp enamel points on the lingual aspects of the mandibular cheek teeth. Sharp points from fractured teeth or foreign bodies also cause similar soft tissue injuries.

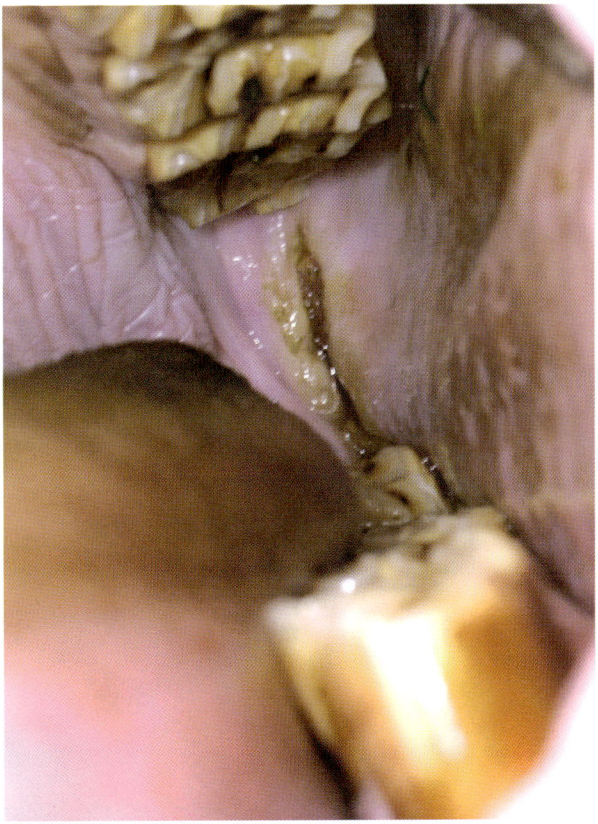

Figure 1.44 Severe laceration or ulceration of the oral mucosa caused by sharp enamel point on the distal aspect of 211 as it occludes with 311. Lacerations of this type illustrate the need for thorough oral examination with a full mouth speculum and powerful light source. This lesion heals spontaneously following removal of offending enamel point. Recurrence is likely if point is created due to persistent malocclusion and can be prevented by intervention at appropriate intervals.

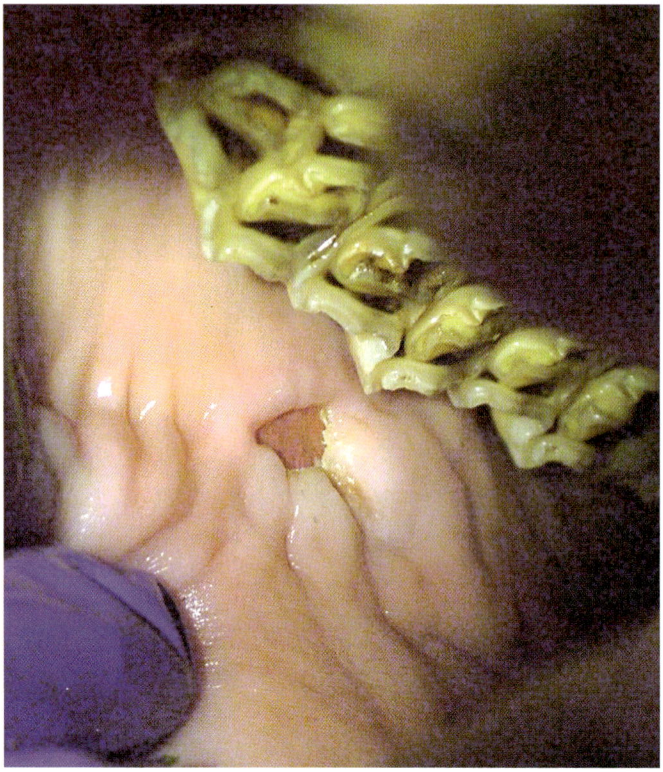

Figure 1.45 Buccal mucosal ulcer associated with sharp enamel point at the level of tooth 107. Such ulceration can cause performance impedance, abnormal mastication, or inappetence. Horses under the age of 8 years can develop sharp enamel points faster than mature horses. Some juveniles require routine care every 6 months to prevent such injury.

Gingival and Lingual Ulceration of Systemic Origin

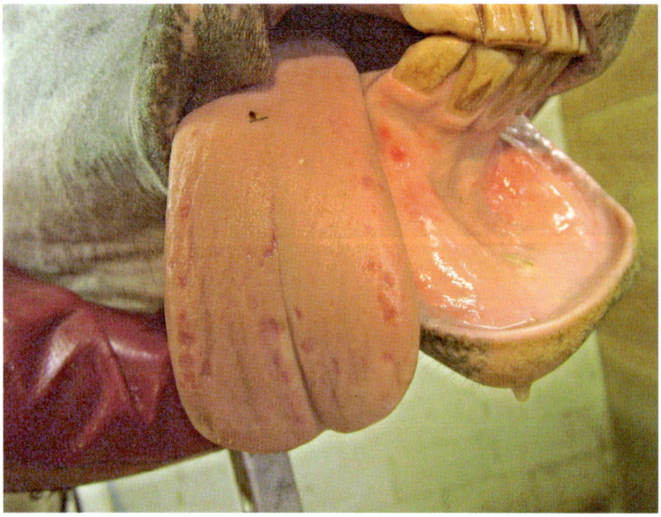

Figure 1.46 Multifocal gingival and lingual ulcerations that were found during routine oral examination of this middle-aged Thoroughbred mare. No other clinical signs were noted. No significant dental pathology was present. A thorough history, physical examination, and blood work are necessary to rule out significant viral pathogens. It is the veterinarian's responsibility to maintain adequate hygienic practices and disinfect instruments between patients and facilities to prevent disease spread.

Supernumerary Canine Tooth

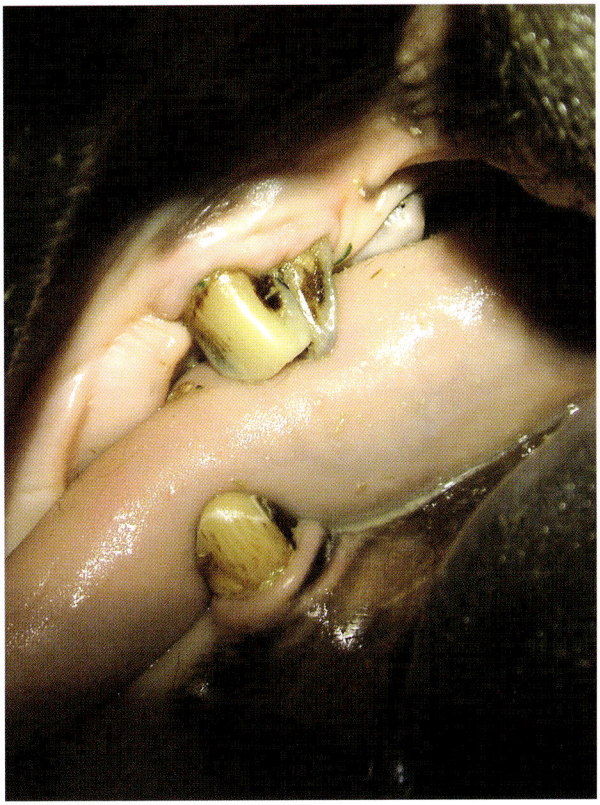

Figure 1.47 Aged horse with supernumerary maxillary canine tooth. No treatment was necessary since no periodontal disease was present. Conservative shaping of clinical crown is recommended to prevent soft tissue trauma.

Polydontia

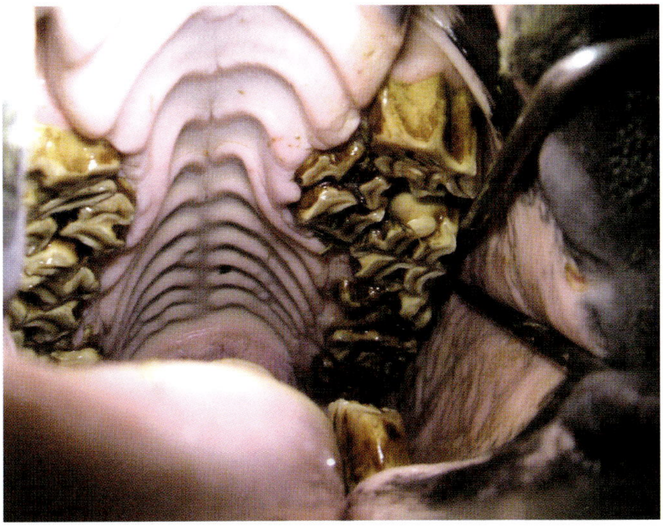

Figure 1.48 A 5-year-old draft mare with polydontia in maxillary teeth arcades. Supernumerary tooth is medial to apparent tooth 207. Feed was impacted between the supernumerary tooth and adjacent teeth resulting in periodontal disease. Some "extra teeth" may not be true supernumerary teeth and are retained deciduous teeth. Radiograph is warranted to find out if the supernumerary tooth is deciduous. Extraction of the displaced tooth is necessary to resolve periodontal disease.

Dysplastic Teeth

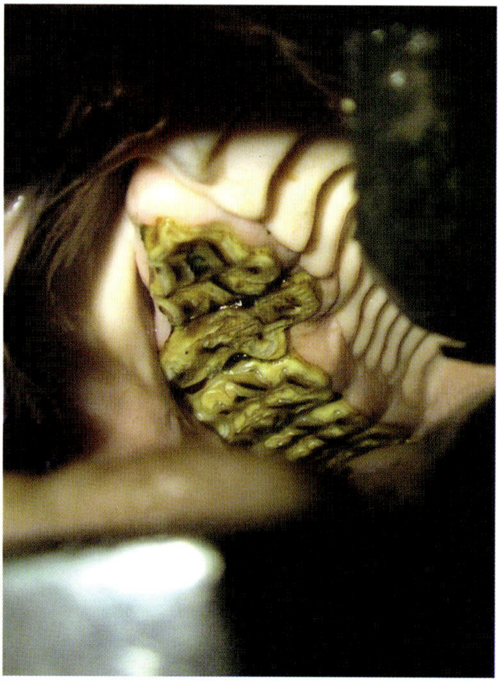

Figure 1.49 Dysplastic tooth 107 in an aged miniature horse with abnormal mastication. Note the abnormal architecture at the occlusal surface and the location of the gingival margin at the level of teeth 107/8 junction. This indicates bony remodeling due to chronic malocclusion. There is a small periodontal pocket at the level of teeth 106/7 and tooth 107 is loose. Radiographs showed evidence of chronic disease. The tooth was extracted and symptoms resolved.

Abnormal Tooth Wear

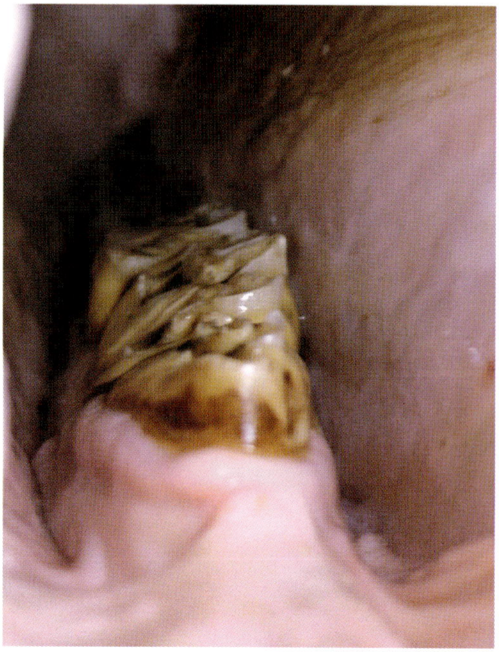

Figure 1.50 Abnormal wear at buccal aspect of tooth 406 and 407 in a 10-year-old paint gelding. Note the difference in appearance of the buccal aspect of 408. Suspected etiology is abnormal enamel formation of 406 and 407 allowing increased focal wear.

Figure 1.51 Severe atypical wear of mandibular incisors. This middle-aged horse is a known "cribber." His new stall door has a metal cap with an exposed edge that he was able to grasp causing extreme grooving on his mandibular incisors. Immediate removal of the metal cap arrested this wear. Pulpar exposure or fracture is possible if the situation were to continue unchecked.

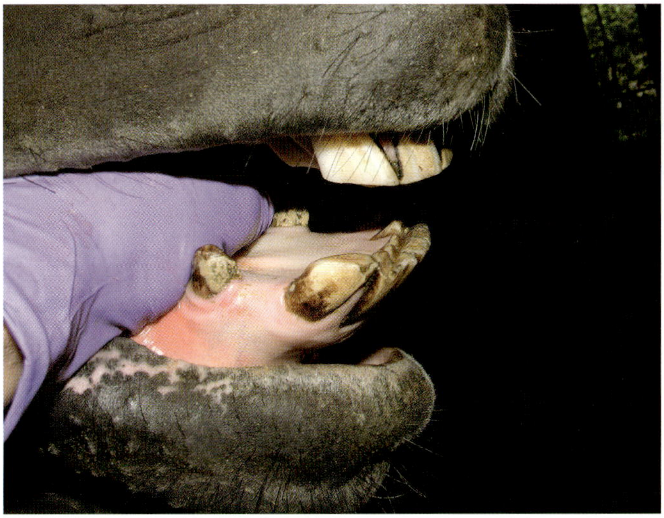

Squamous Cell Carcinoma

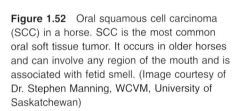

Figure 1.52 Oral squamous cell carcinoma (SCC) in a horse. SCC is the most common oral soft tissue tumor. It occurs in older horses and can involve any region of the mouth and is associated with fetid smell. (Image courtesy of Dr. Stephen Manning, WCVM, University of Saskatchewan)

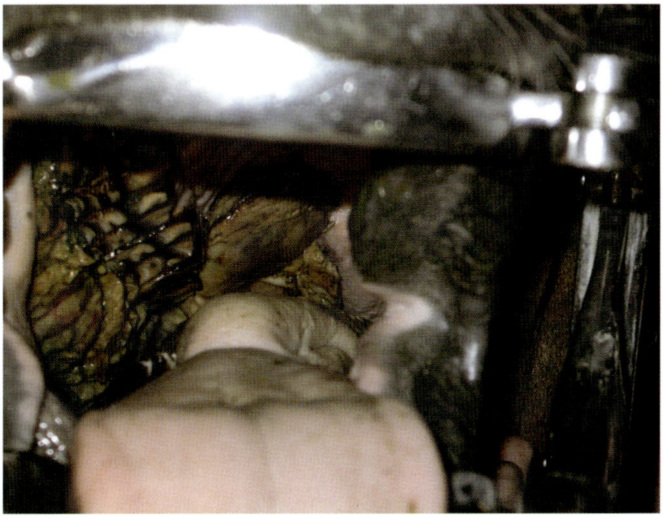

Oral Foreign Body

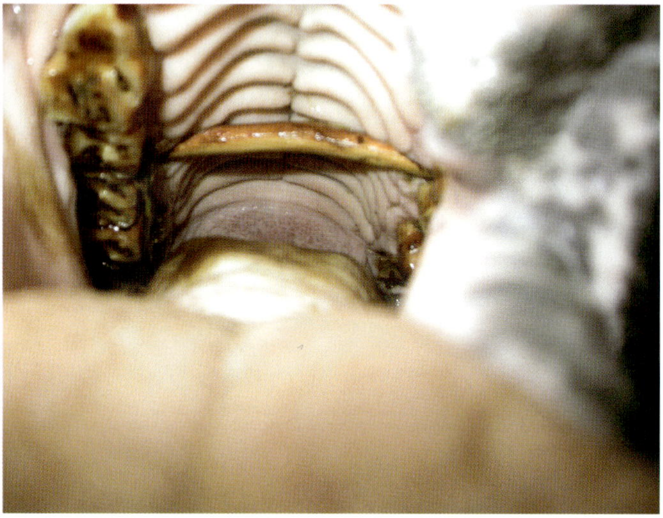

Figure 1.53 Oral foreign body in a horse. In this case there was a wooden stick lodged between the upper arcade of teeth. Affected horse may present with signs of dysphagia. Wooden sticks may also penetrate oral soft tissues and cause cellulitis. Wooden stick is the most common foreign body found in the oral cavity. (Image courtesy of Dr. Stephen Manning, WCVM, University of Saskatchewan)

Glossitis

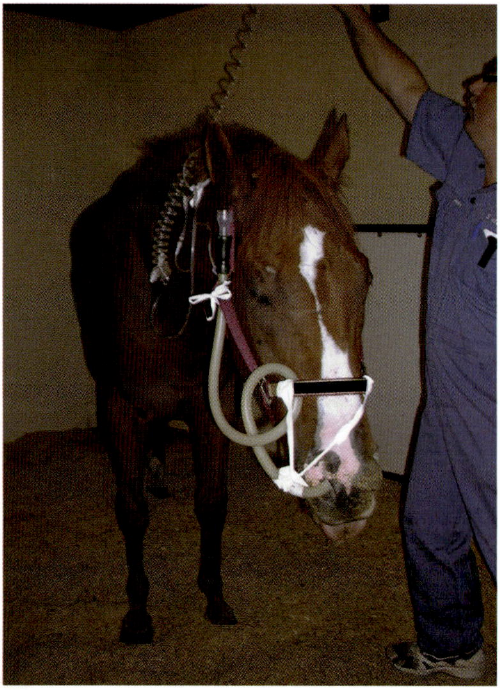

Figure 1.54 An adult horse affected with severe traumatic glossitis (trauma while oral dosing). The tongue was swollen and protruded from the mouth. The site of trauma can be seen in fig. 1.55. A nasogastric tube was used to feed the horse because the horse was severely dysphagic.

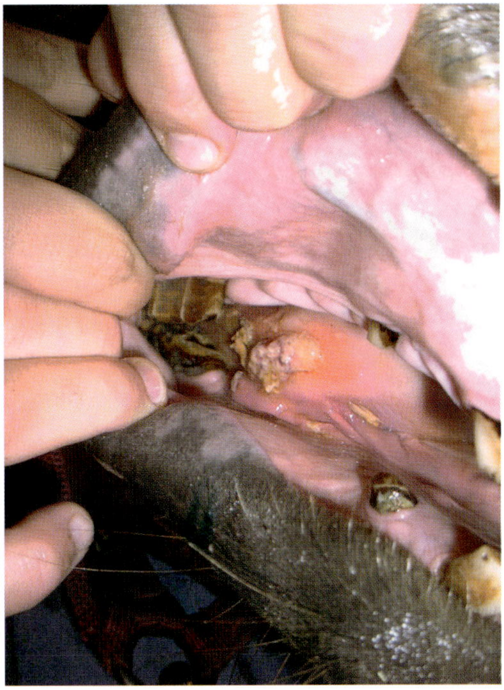

Figure 1.55 The site of trauma (penetrating) that has led to severe glossitis in fig. 1.54.

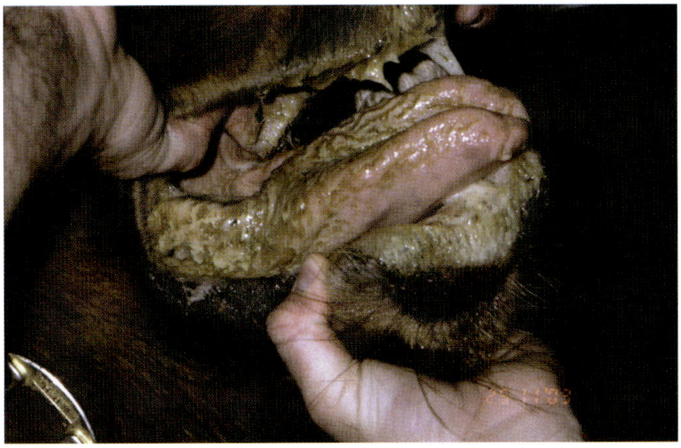

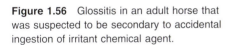

Figure 1.56 Glossitis in an adult horse that was suspected to be secondary to accidental ingestion of irritant chemical agent.

Esophageal Obstruction (Choke), Primary

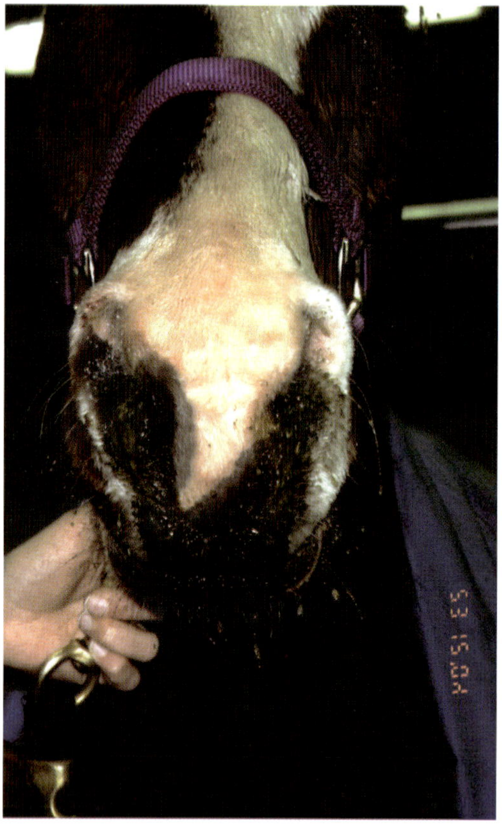

Figure 1.57 Choke in an adult horse; note the green nasal discharge. Choke or esophageal obstruction is the most common esophageal disorder seen in horses. Primary choke is usually caused by feed or foreign bodies (e.g., stones, bedding, medicinal boluses, carrot, potato, or wood fragments).

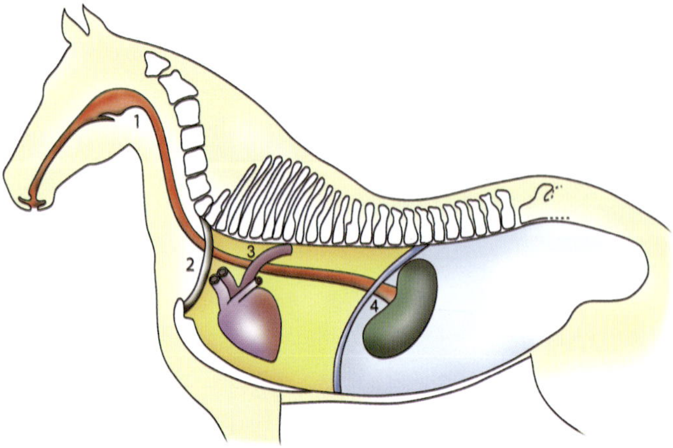

Figure 1.58 There are four common anatomical areas of natural narrowing where primary choke usually occurs; these are (1)the postpharyngeal area, (2)thoracic inlet, (3)base of the heart, and (4)cardia of the stomach (terminal esophagus). (Drawing by Dr. Juliane Deubner, WCVM, University of Saskatchewan)

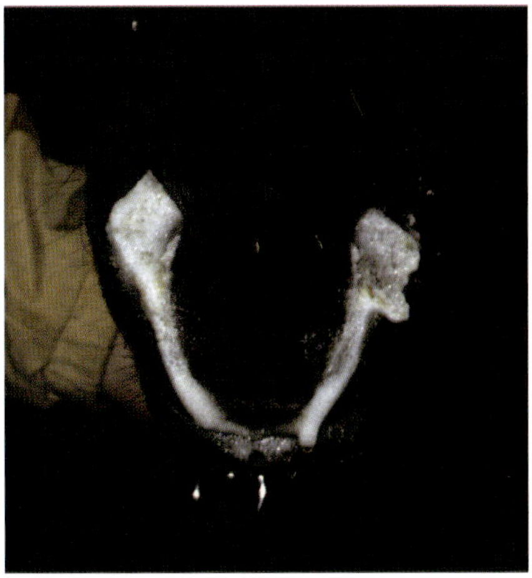

Figure 1.59 Clinical signs are usually acute and include anxiety, coughing, standing with the head and neck extended, gagging or retching, painful and repeated attempts at swallowing, bilateral white frothy nasal discharge, as in this photograph, or green and containing feed material. (Image from Abutarbush SM and Carmalt JL, Endoscopy and arthroscopy for the equine practitioner. Made Easy Series. Jackson, WY: Teton NewMedia, 2008)

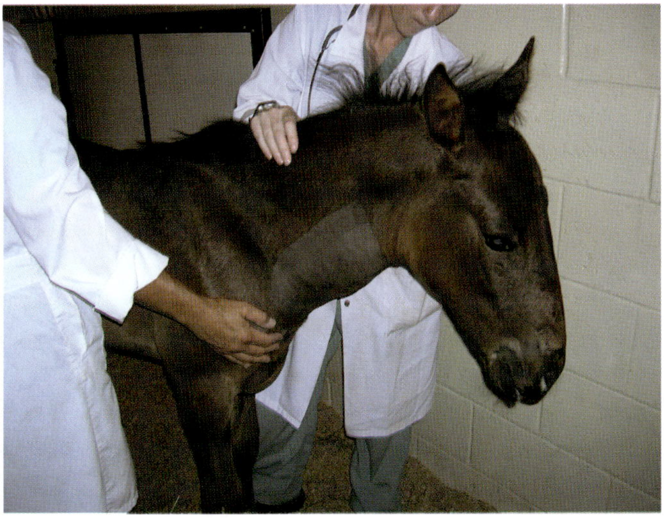

a

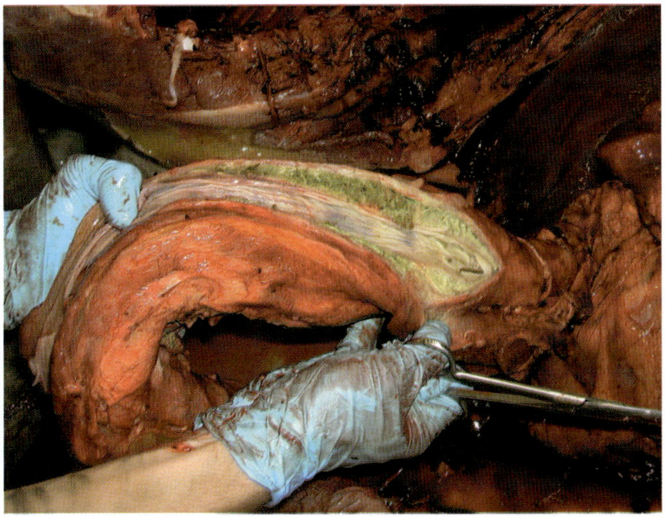

b

Figures 1.60a,b Esophageal laceration and peri-esophageal cellulitis in a foal secondary to esophageal obstruction. Note the cervical swelling (fig. 1.60a) and the peri-esophageal inflammation and feed accumulation in the postmortem photograph (fig. 1.60b). The esophagus can rupture secondary to esophageal obstruction. This will lead to cellulitis or crepitus, and a palpable or visible mass on the left lateroventral aspect of the neck, if the obstruction is in the cervical area of the esophagus. (Image 1.59a from Abutarbush SM and Carmalt JL, Endoscopy and arthroscopy for the equine practitioner. Made Easy Series. Jackson, WY: Teton NewMedia, 2008)

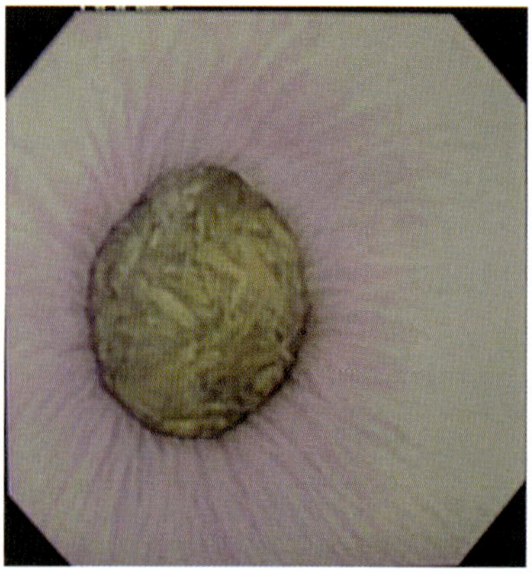

Figure 1.61 An endoscopic image of esophageal obstruction. Diagnosis of primary choke is based on a history, physical examination findings, inability or difficulty in passing a nasogastric tube to the stomach, ultrasonography, endoscopy, or radiography. (Image from Abutarbush SM and Carmalt JL, Endoscopy and arthroscopy for the equine practitioner. Made Easy Series. Jackson, WY: Teton NewMedia, 2008)

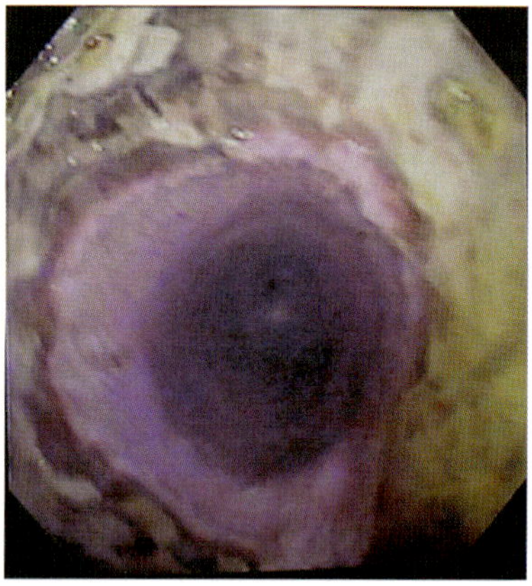

Figure 1.62 Endoscopic image of an esophagus after resolution of esophageal obstruction. Following resolution of choke, endoscopy can also be used to determine if ulceration, as in this photograph, perforation, masses, or strictures are present, which helps guide therapy and determine the prognosis. (Image from Abutarbush SM and Carmalt JL, Endoscopy and arthroscopy for the equine practitioner. Made Easy Series. Jackson, WY: Teton NewMedia, 2008)

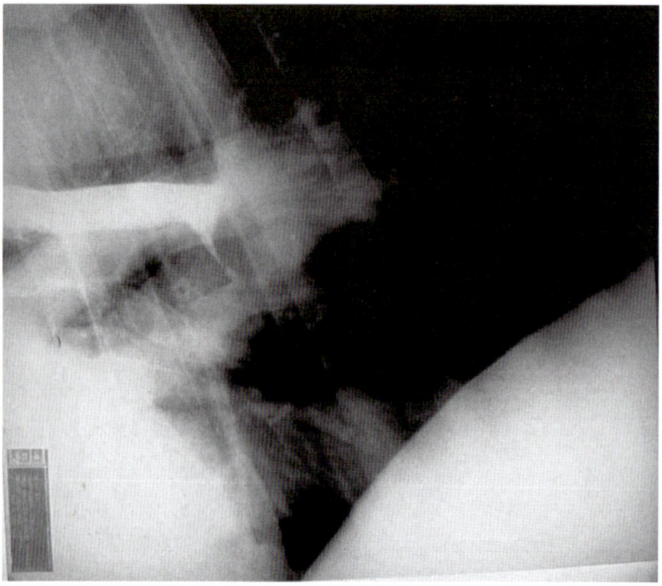

Figure 1.63 Radiological examination of the cervical and thoracic esophagus can be performed with portable equipment, but high-powered equipment and a grid are required to view the esophagus at the level of the shoulder and thoracic inlet. Plain films may be helpful but in most cases contrast radiography is more informative, as in this case.

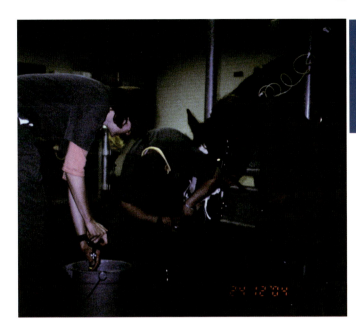

Figure 1.64 To treat the esophageal obstruction, esophageal lavage can be performed in standing horses under profound sedation in order to keep the head low and prevent aspiration. Warm water can be pumped gently using a stomach pump through a cuffed or uncuffed tube into the esophagus cranial to the obstruction, while the tube is gently manipulated against the obstruction. The returning water and impacted material often comes out of the nose or the mouth of the horse and should be examined to determine the cause and nature of the impaction.

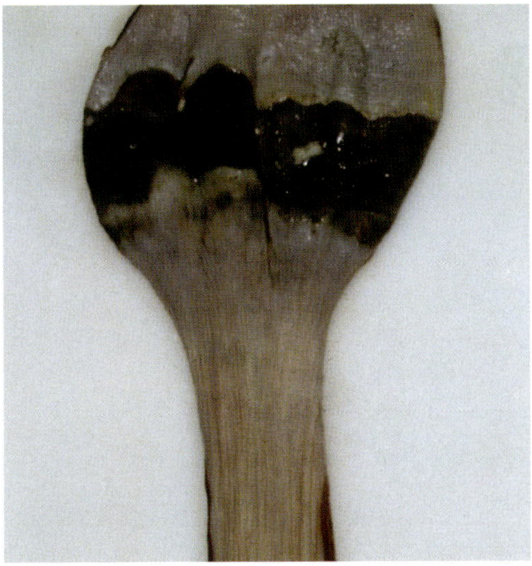

Figure 1.65 Postmortem image of circumferential esophageal ulceration in a horse secondary to long-standing esophageal obstruction. This type of ulceration is the one that is likely to result in esophageal stricture and narrowing. Other complications of esophageal obstruction that can be seen include stricture, perforation, megaesophagus (fig. 1.66), reobstruction, and aspiration pneumonia (fig. 1.67). (Image from Abutarbush SM and Carmalt JL, Endoscopy and arthroscopy for the equine practitioner. Made Easy Series. Jackson, WY: Teton NewMedia, 2008)

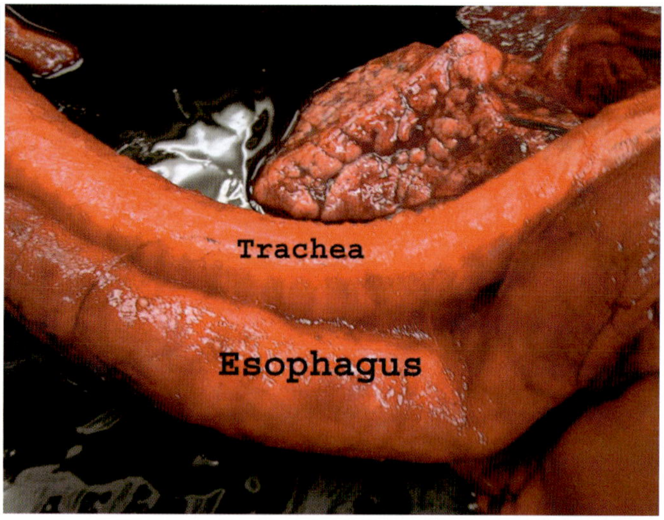

Figure 1.66 Postmortem photograph of megaesophagus in a foal secondary to esophageal obstruction.

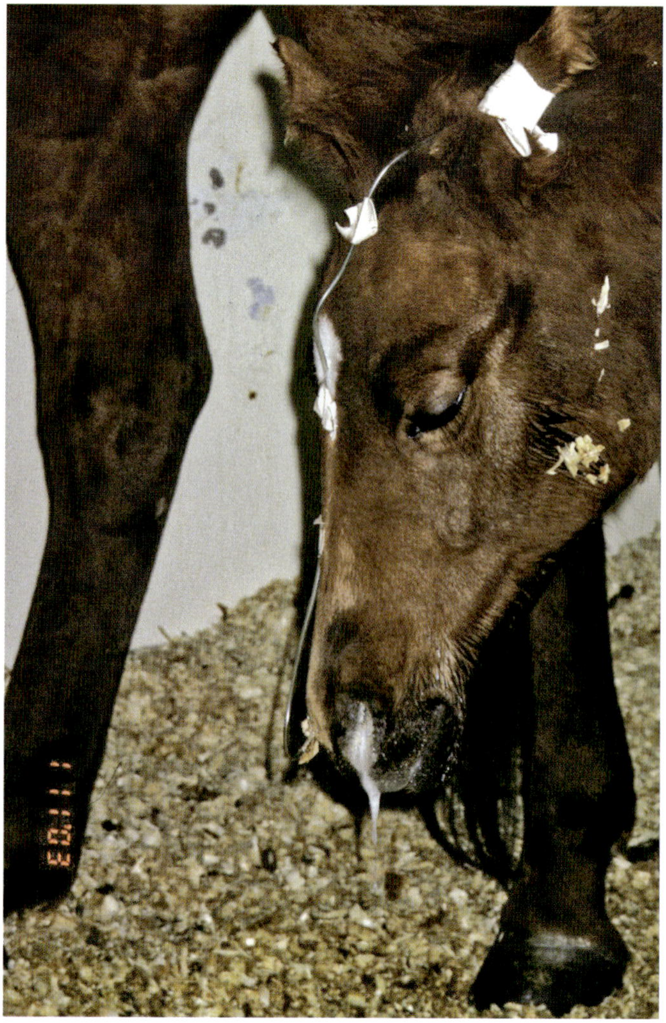

Figure 1.67 Aspiration pneumonia secondary to esophageal obstruction in a foal. Note the severe depression and nasal discharge.

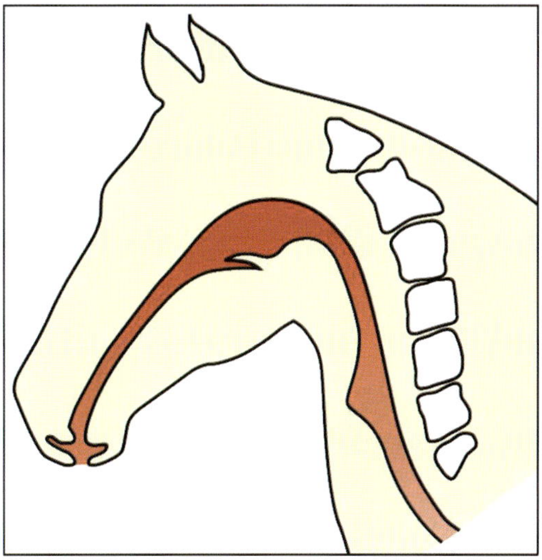

a

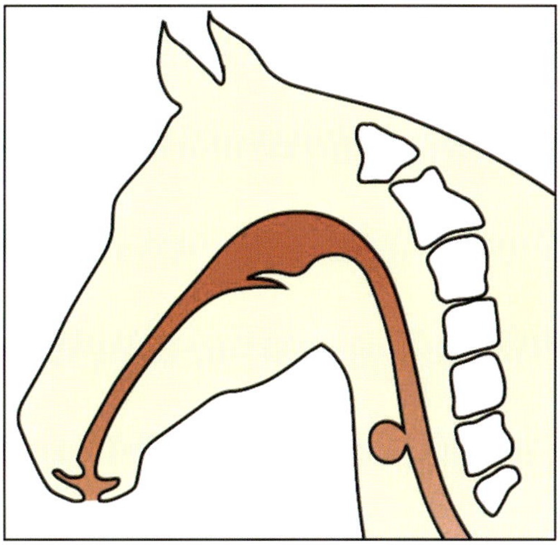

b

Figures 1.68a,b Drawings of esophageal diverticulae. Secondary choke is caused by intralumenal or extralumenal abnormalities that mechanically impede feed passage. Intralumenal abnormalities include esophageal stricture, diverticula, cysts, and tumors. Horses usually have recurrent choke episodes. A diverticulum is a focal outpouching of the esophagus with an intact mucosa. There are two types of diverticulae: traction and pulsion diverticulum. In a traction diverticulum, the neck of the sac is much wider than the bottom (fig. 1.68a). In a pulsion diverticulum, the neck of the sac is narrower than the bottom (fig. 1.68b). Contrast radiography can be used to diagnose the presence of esophageal diverticula (fig. 1.69). Mediastinal and cervical masses (tumor or abscess), and vascular ring anomalies may cause extralumenal obstruction by impinging on the esophagus. (Images from Abutarbush SM and Carmalt JL, Endoscopy and arthroscopy for the equine practitioner. Made Easy Series. Jackson, WY, Teton NewMedia, 2008)

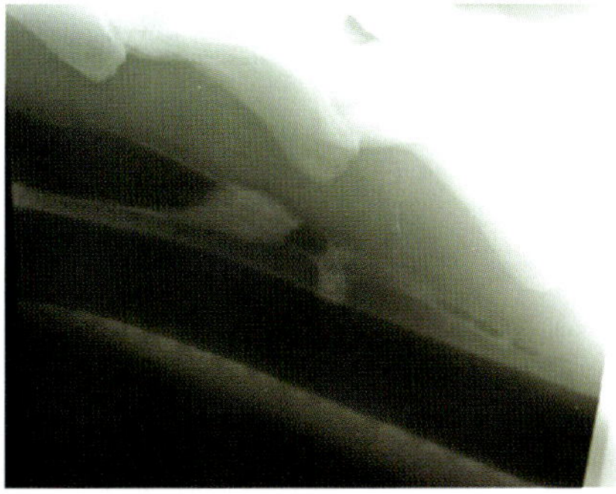

Figure 1.69 Radiographic image with contrast of a pulsion diverticulum in a horse.

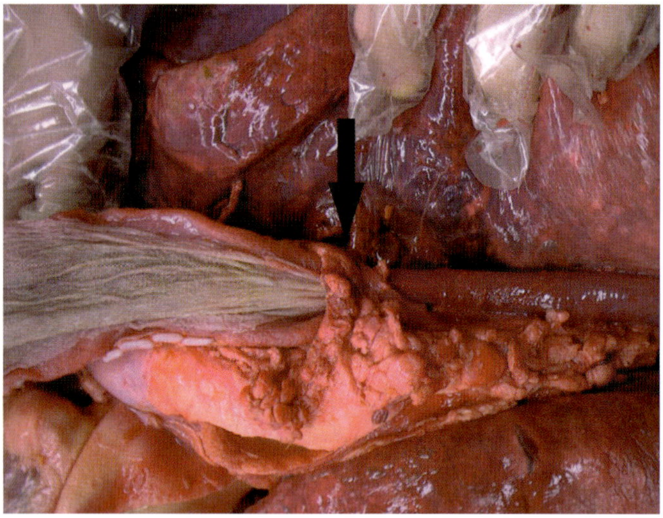

Figure 1.70 Postmortem photograph of vascular ring anomalies in a foal. It is a congenital anomaly of the aortic arch and its branches. These vessels may form a ring around the esophagus, which can lead to secondary esophageal obstruction. In foals, clinical signs start when the foal begins to eat solid feed. (Image from Abutarbush SM and Carmalt JL, Endoscopy and arthroscopy for the equine practitioner. Made Easy Series. Jackson, WY: Teton NewMedia, 2008)

Diseases of the Abdominal Region

Abdominal Pain (Colic)

Colic is one of the most common problems in equine practice. Colic in horses can be divided into two major categories: gastrointestinal and nongastrointestinal. Nongastrointestinal colic cases are those showing signs of abdominal pain due to causes related to urinary, reproductive, nervous, respiratory, or musculoskeletal system disorders. Gastrointestinal colic is usually caused by gut distension, tension on the root of mesentery, ischemia, deep ulceration of the gastrointestinal tract, or peritoneal pain. Strangulating and nonstrangulating obstruction of the small and large intestines causes different degrees of abdominal pain.

Clinical signs of colic include agitation, flank watching (figs. 1.71–1.74), pawing (fig. 1.75), stretching (figs. 1.76 and 1.77), kicking at the abdomen, frequent lying down (figs. 1.78–1.80), and rolling (figs. 1.81–1.84).

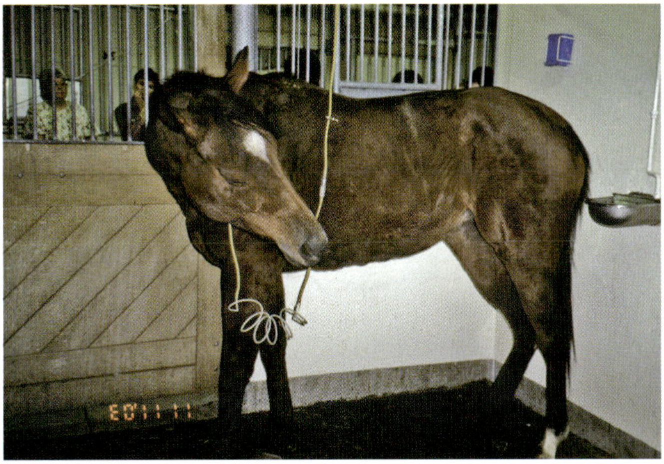

1.71

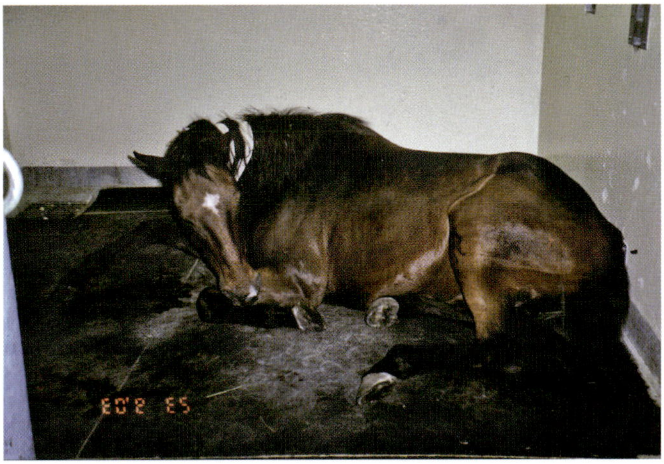

1.72

Figures 1.71–1.74 Clinical signs of colic include agitation and flank watching.

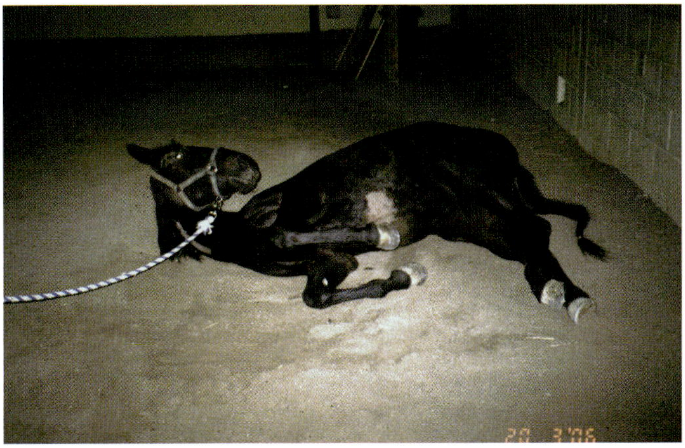

1.73

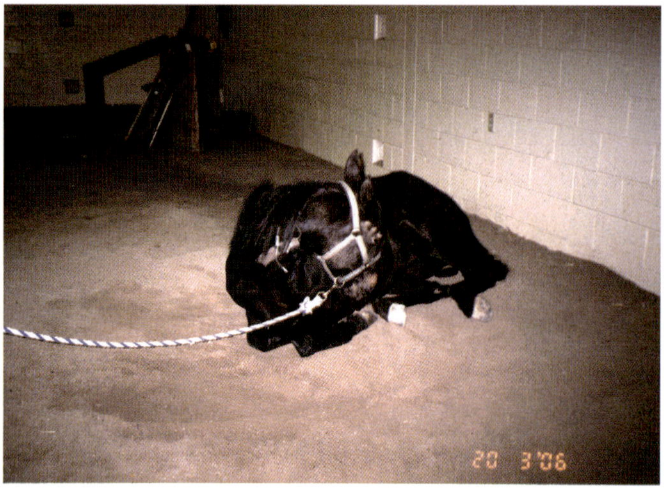

Figures 1.71–1.74 *Continued*

1.74

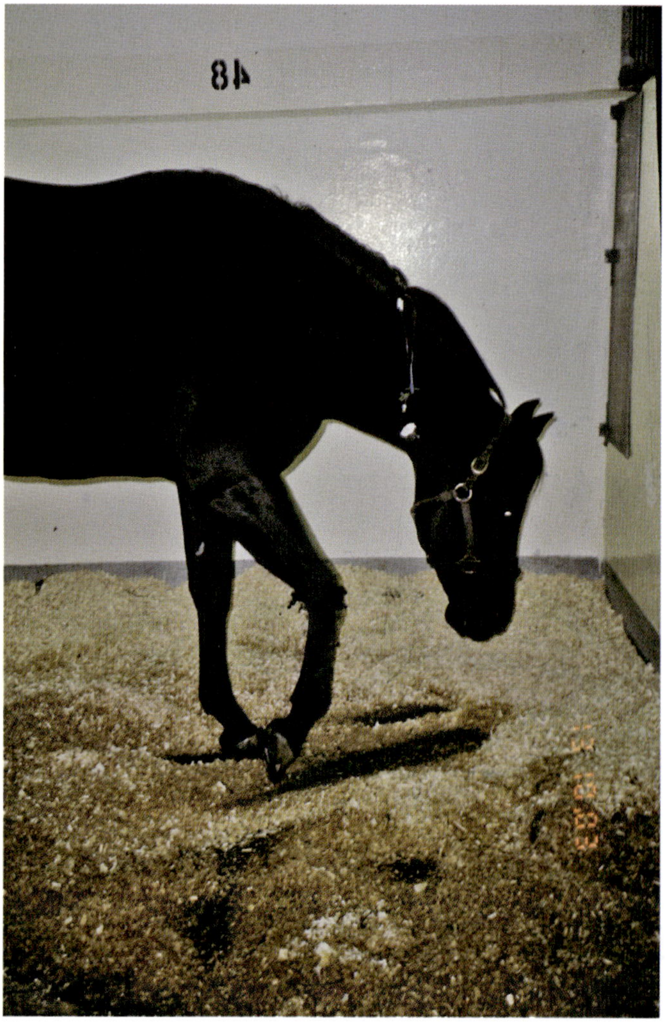

Figure 1.75 Pawing is another clinical sign of colic in horses.

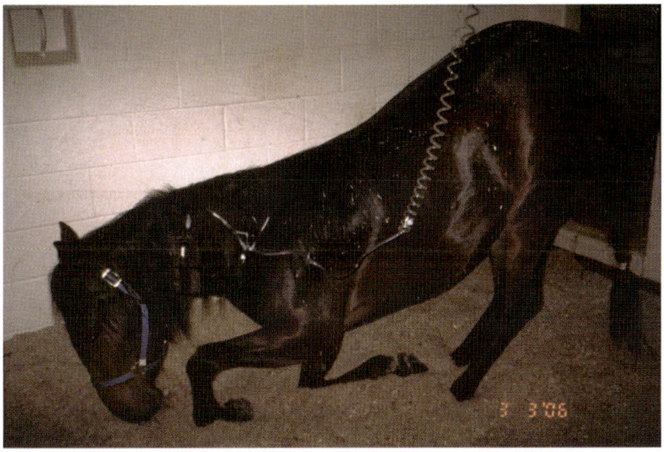

1.76

Figures 1.76–1.77 Colicky horses may stretch as in these figures.

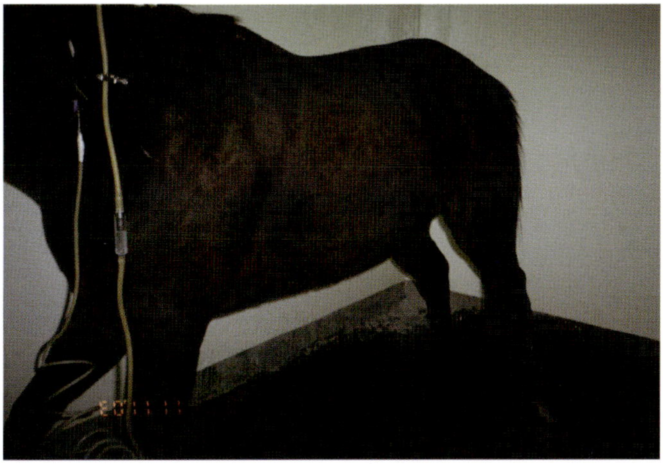

1.77

Figures 1.78–1.80 Colicky horses may kick at their abdomen and lie down frequently.

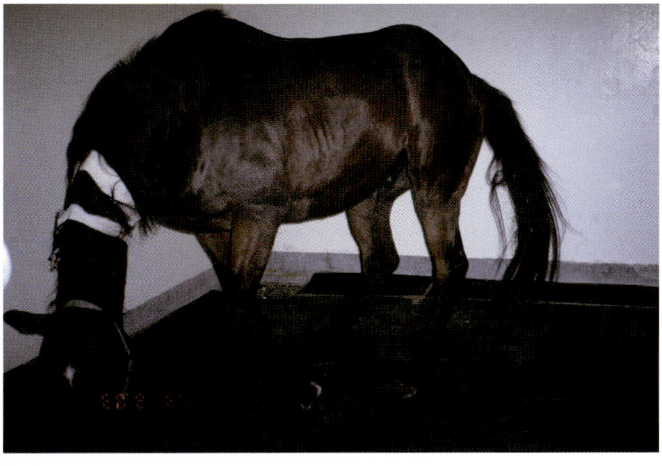

1.78

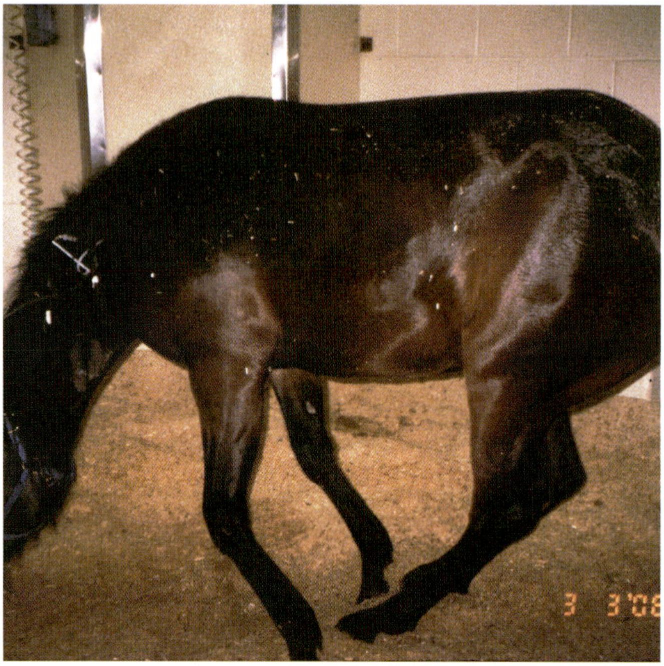

1.79

Figures 1.78–1.80 *Continued*

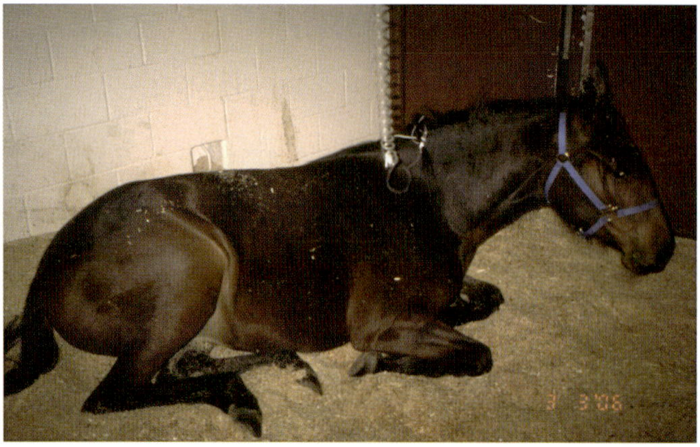

1.80

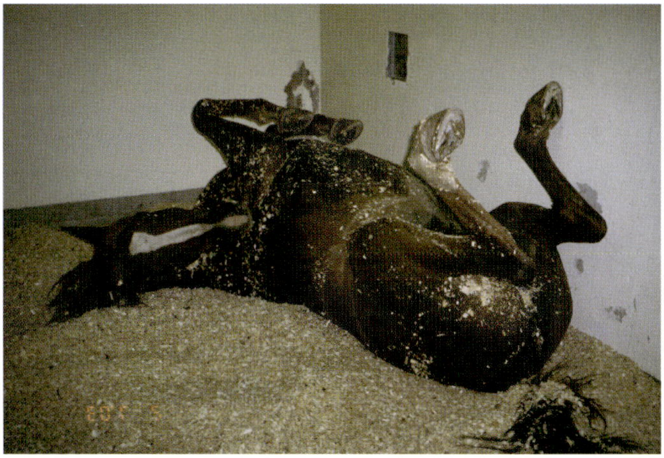

1.81

Figures 1.81–1.84 Rolling is a sign of severe colic in horses.

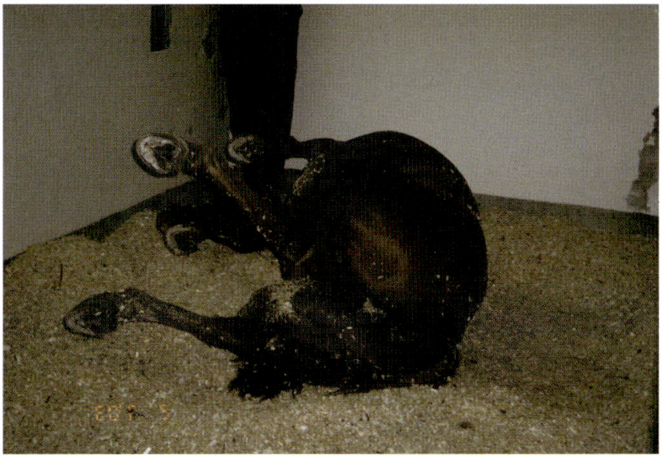

1.82

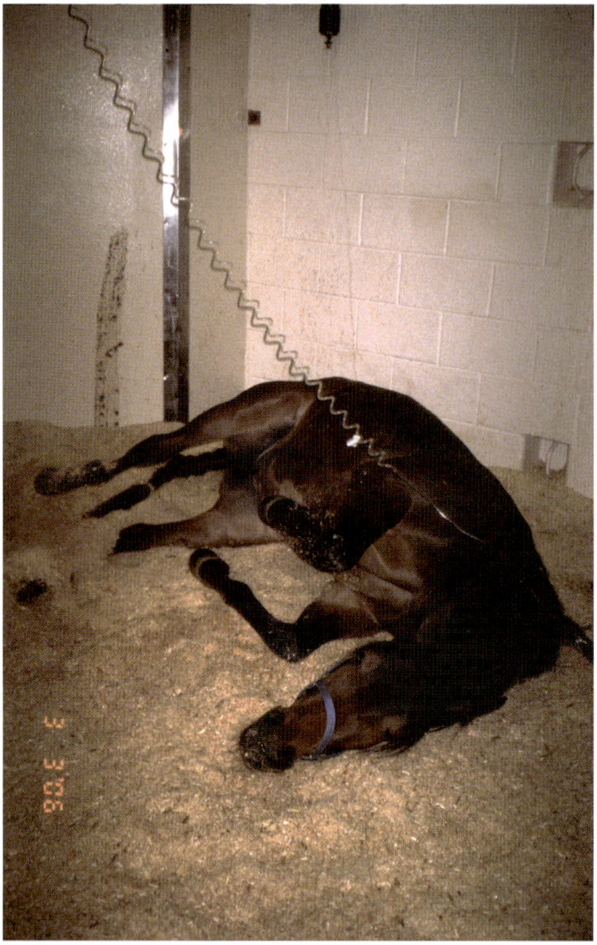

1.83

Figures 1.81–1.84 *Continued*

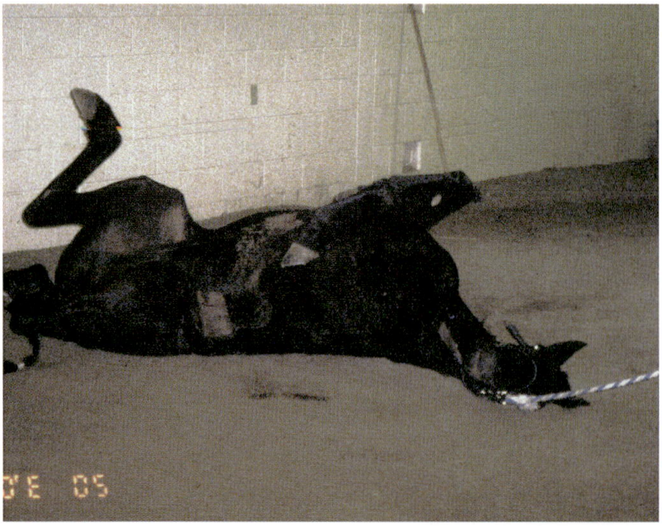

1.84

Diseases of the Stomach

Gastric Dilatation

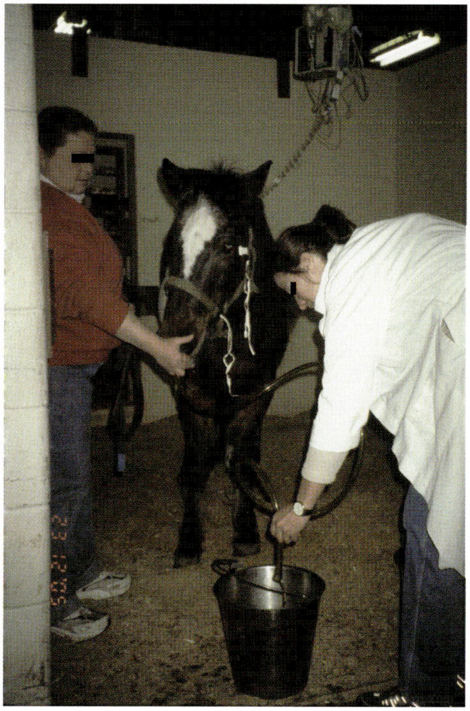

Figure 1.85 Gastric dilatation in a horse with small intestinal obstruction. Note the nasogastric reflux. Gastric dilatation is caused by gastric outflow obstruction (pyloric stenosis), intestinal contents reflux secondary to small intestinal obstruction, grain overload, gastric dilatation with air (aerophagea). So usually it is a secondary event to another disease, although it can be idiopathic. Clinical signs are not specific and are mainly abdominal pain in addition to other signs related to the associated condition. Some horses may regurgitate or vomit, which usually causes stomach rupture and is usually a terminal event. Passing a nasogastric tube is usually a lifesaving procedure and should be left in place to avoid rupture of the stomach (fig. 1.86). Stomach rupture and septic peritonitis can be the result of long-standing dilatation of the stomach (fig. 1.87).

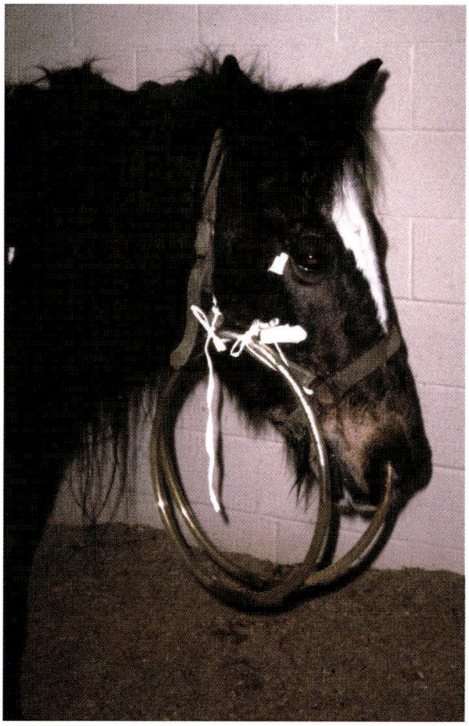

Figure 1.86 The nasogastric tube is left in place to avoid rupture of the stomach in a horse with gastric dilatation and large volume of nasogastric reflux.

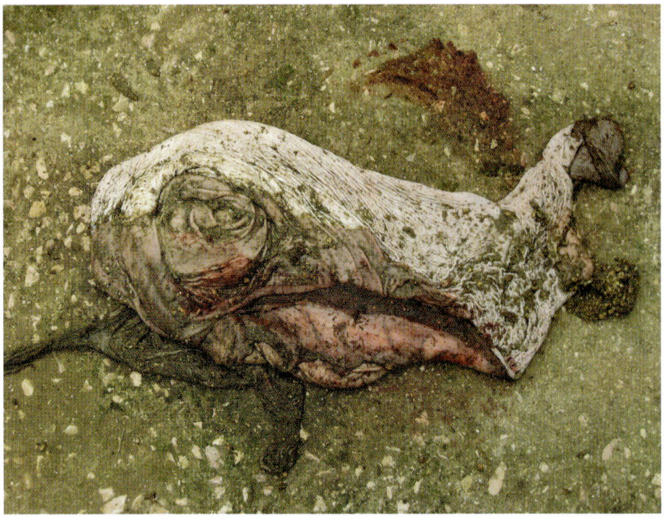

Figure 1.87 Postmortem photograph of a stomach rupture in a horse secondary to gastric dilatation.

Gastric Impaction

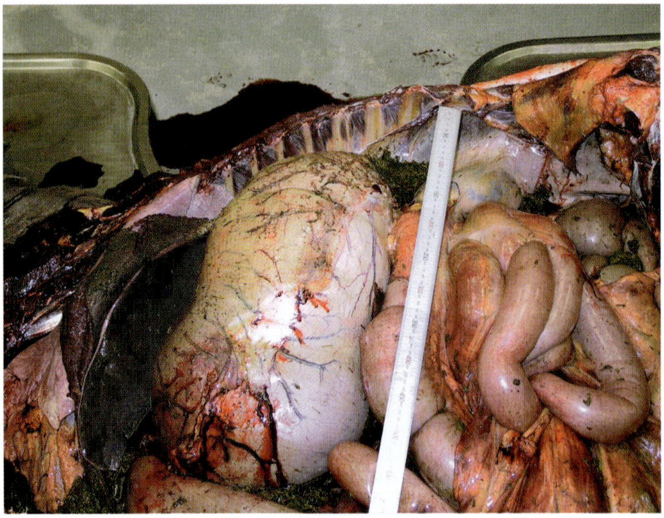

1.88

Figures 1.88–1.89 Postmortem photographs of gastric impaction in a horse. Gastric impaction can be caused by insufficient access to water, poor teeth, and atony in old horses. Affected horses are presented with abdominal pain and regurgitation of ingesta and fluids through the nostrils may be seen. Stomach may rupture in some horses (fig. 1.90).

Figures 1.88–1.89 *Continued*

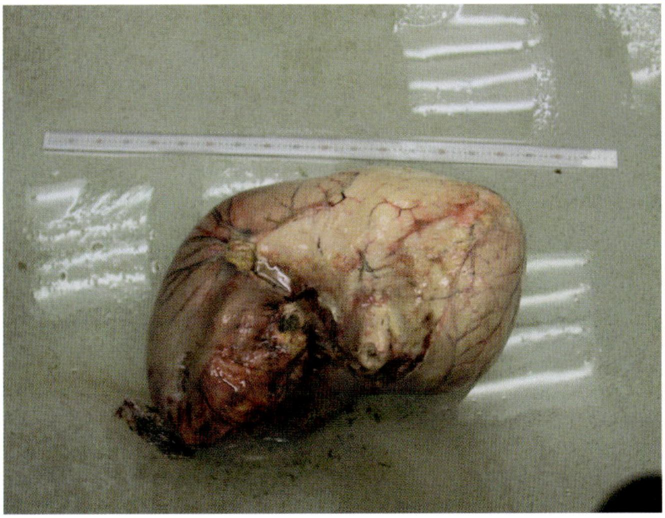

1.89

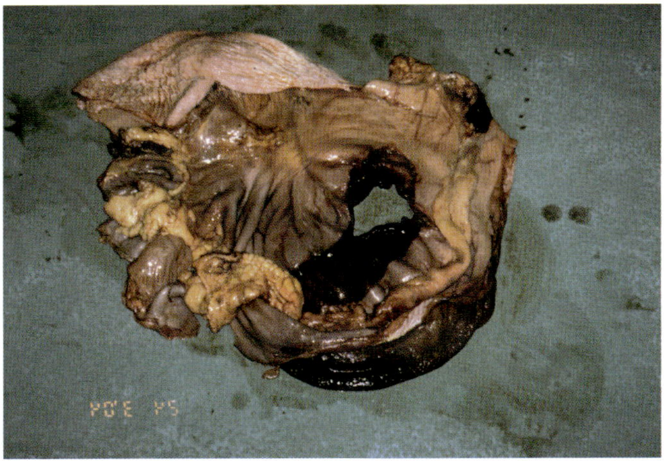

Figure 1.90 Postmortem photograph of gastric (stomach) rupture in a horse secondary to gastric impaction.

Gastric Ulcers

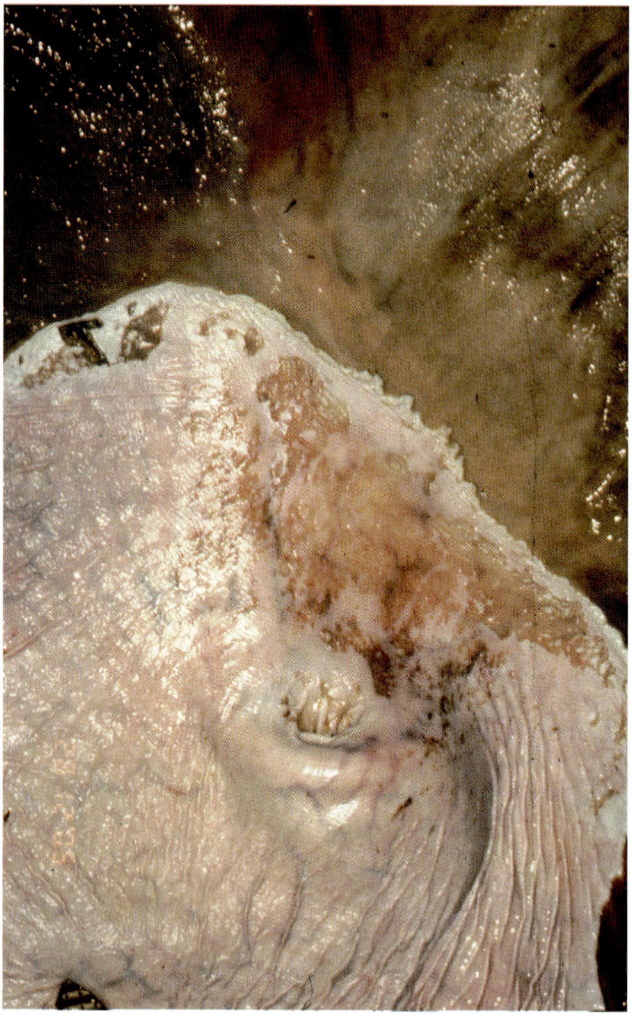

Figure 1.91 A postmortem photograph of gastric ulceration of the nonglandular part of the stomach. Gastric ulcers can be seen in foals and adult horses. Except for nonsteroidal anti-inflammatory drug toxicity, the exact cause is unknown. It can occur on the glandular (fig. 1.92) part of the stomach, nonglandular part of the stomach, or along the margo plicatus (fig. 1.93). Gastric ulcers are not clinical in most affected animals. Affected foals may show bruxism, ptyalism, froth at the mouth (fig. 1.94), colic signs (fig. 1.95), and dorsal recumbency (fig. 1.96). Please see Chapter 12, Diseases of the Neonates. Weanlings affected by chronic gastric ulceration are usually presented with intermittent colic and diarrhea and poor growth and hair coat. In adult horses, signs are mostly inapparent and vague. Affected horses may show mild intermittent colic, poor appetite and performance, and poor body condition. Endoscopic examination of the stomach provides a definitive diagnosis (fig. 1.97).

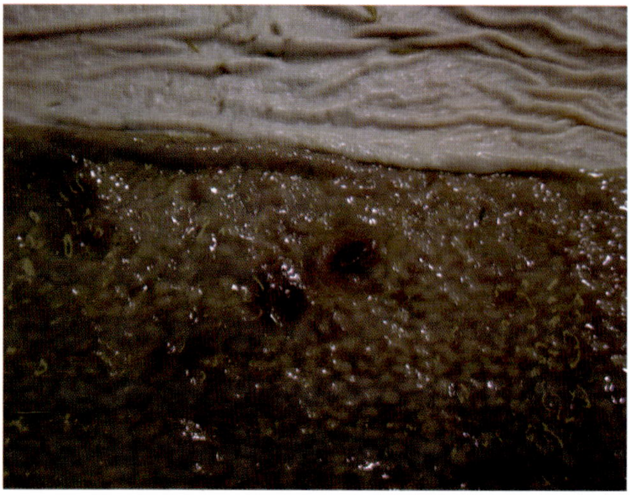

Figure 1.92 A postmortem photograph of gastric ulceration of the glandular part of the stomach.

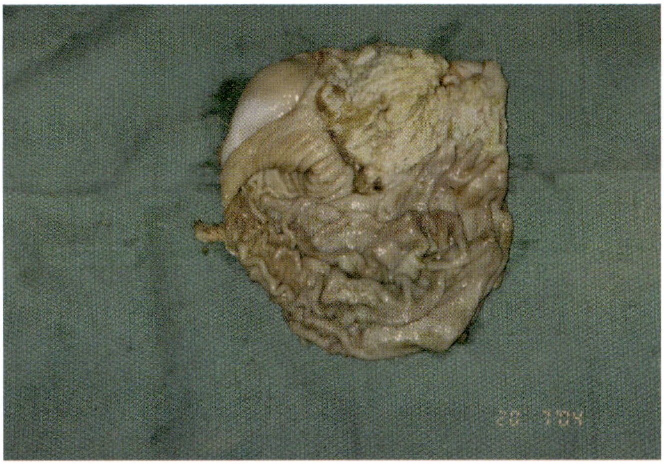

Figure 1.93 A postmortem photograph of gastric ulceration along the margo plicatus in a foal.

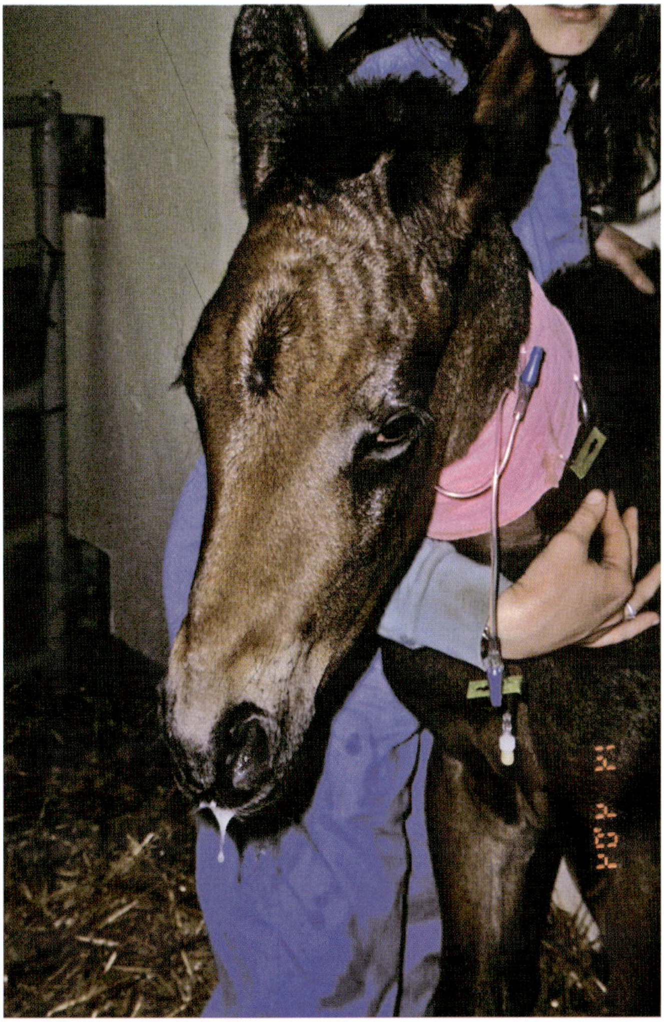

Figure 1.94 Foal affected with gastric ulcers. Note the presence of a froth at the mouth.

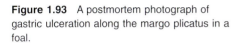

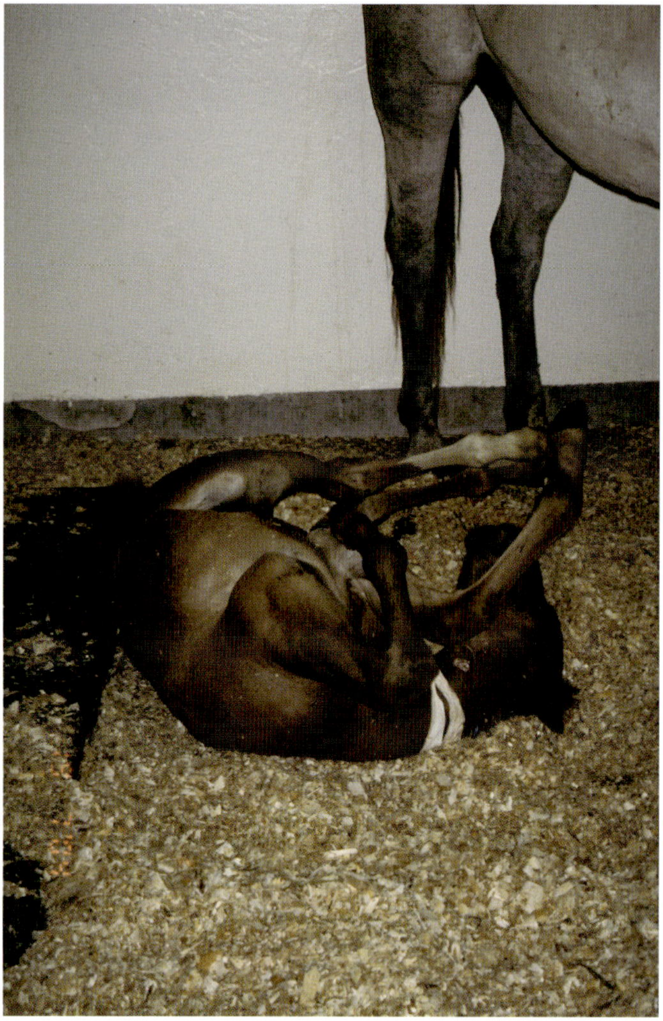

Figure 1.95 Foal affected with gastric ulcers showing signs of colic (rolling).

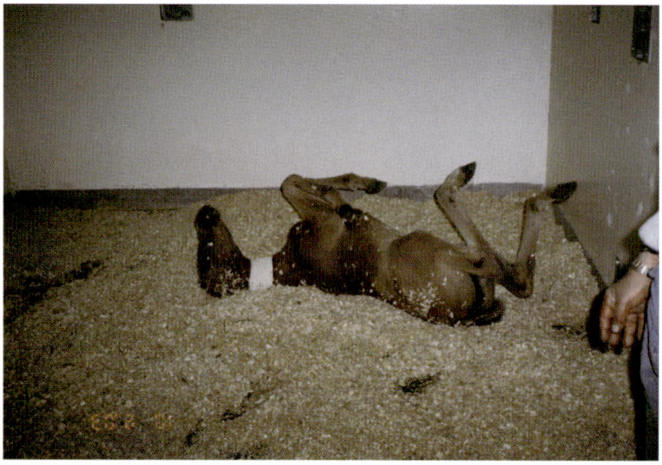

Figure 1.96 Foal affected with gastric ulcers. Note the dorsal recumbency.

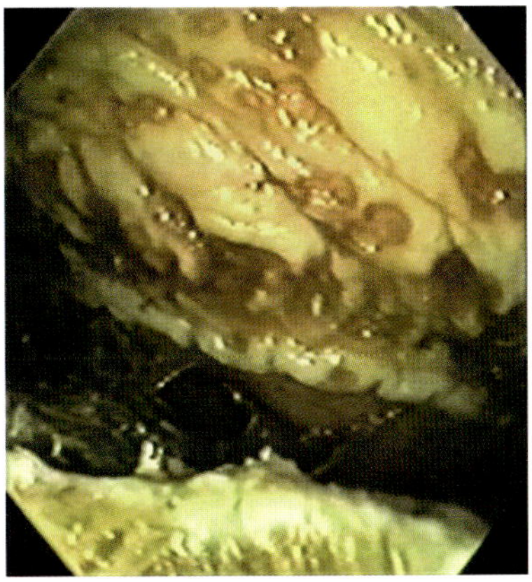

Figure 1.97 Endoscopic image of gastric ulcers of the nonglandular part of the stomach.

Diseases of the Small Intestine

Simple Obstruction of the Small Intestine

It is manifested by obstruction of the intestinal lumen only. Simple obstruction of the small intestine is usually associated with various degrees of abdominal pain. The presence of a nasogastric reflux and abnormal peritoneal fluid will depend on the stage of the disease and its location, the latter especially important or absence of nasogastric reflux.

Ileal Impaction

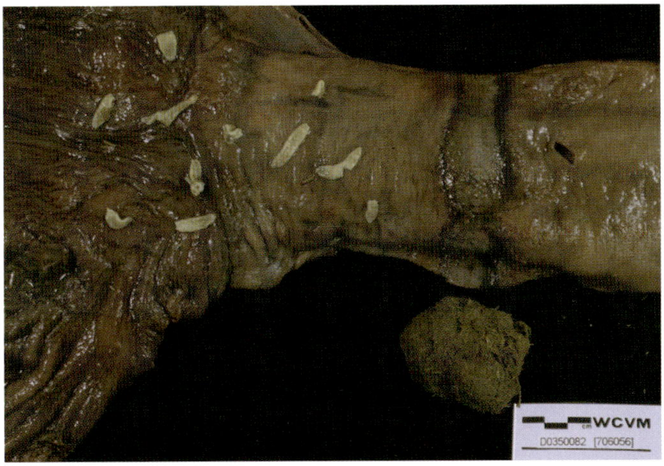

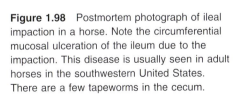

Figure 1.98 Postmortem photograph of ileal impaction in a horse. Note the circumferential mucosal ulceration of the ileum due to the impaction. This disease is usually seen in adult horses in the southwestern United States. There are a few tapeworms in the cecum.

Ileal Hypertrophy

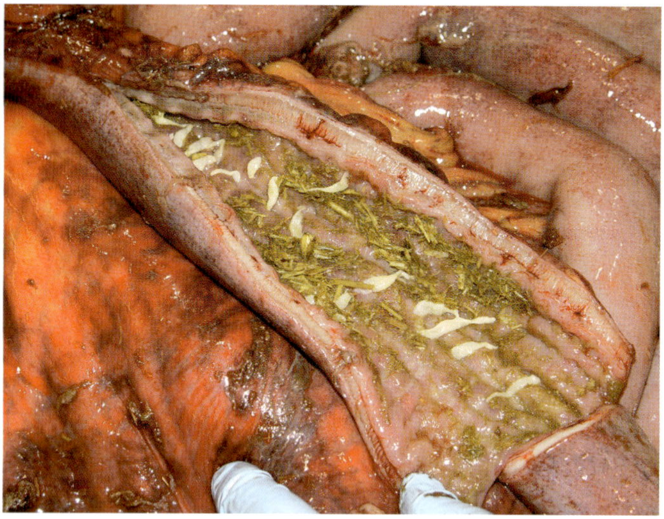

Figure 1.99 Postmortem photograph of ileal hypertrophy in an adult horse. There are also a few tapeworms present in the ileum. Hypertrophy of the muscular layer of the ileum is of unknown etiology. Initially affected horses have a history of recurrent colic.

Ascarid Impaction

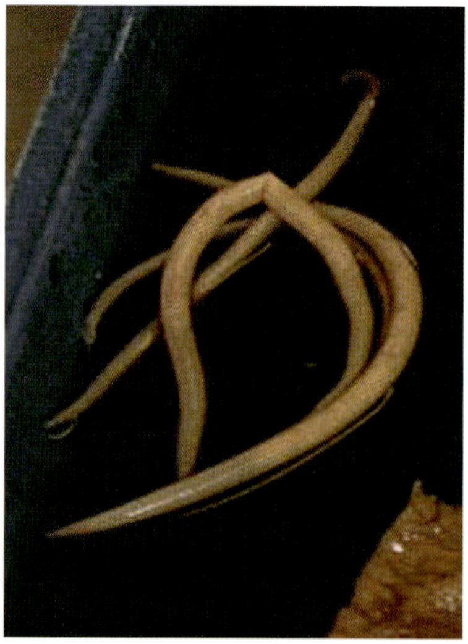

Figure 1.100 *Parascaris equorum*. Impaction with this parasite is usually seen in weanlings and yearlings and is caused by complete lumenal obstruction by *Parascaris equorum*. Anthelmintics that cause sudden paralysis of the ascarid worms are implicated. Affected horses usually show signs of colic within 5 days of anthelmintic administration.

Meckel's Diverticulum

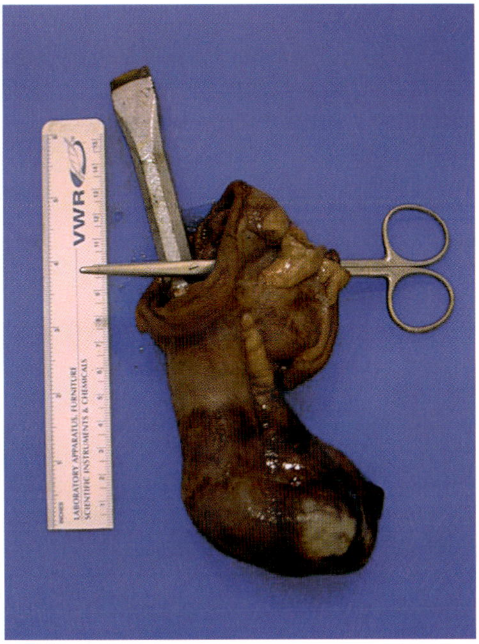

Figure 1.101 Postmortem photograph of Meckel's diverticulum. It is an embryonic remnant that can be found in the mid-jejunum area. It can become impacted and cause recurrent colic or serve as a point where intestines could twist.

Strangulating Obstruction

It is manifested by obstruction of both the intestinal lumen and blood supply. Strangulating obstruction is usually associated with severe abdominal pain, nasogastric reflux, and abnormal peritoneal fluid (serosanguinous).

Mesodiverticular Band

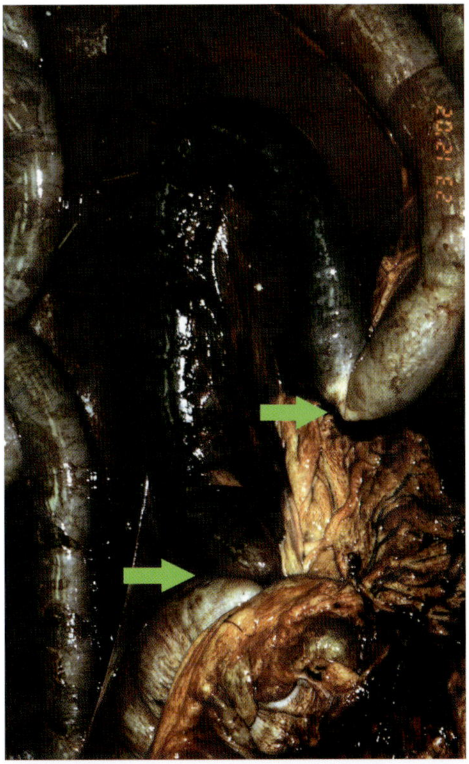

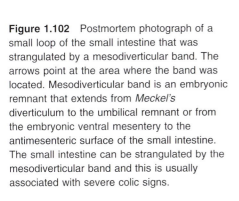

Figure 1.102 Postmortem photograph of a small loop of the small intestine that was strangulated by a mesodiverticular band. The arrows point at the area where the band was located. Mesodiverticular band is an embryonic remnant that extends from *Meckel's* diverticulum to the umbilical remnant or from the embryonic ventral mesentery to the antimesenteric surface of the small intestine. The small intestine can be strangulated by the mesodiverticular band and this is usually associated with severe colic signs.

Small Intestinal Volvulus (Mesenteric Torsion)

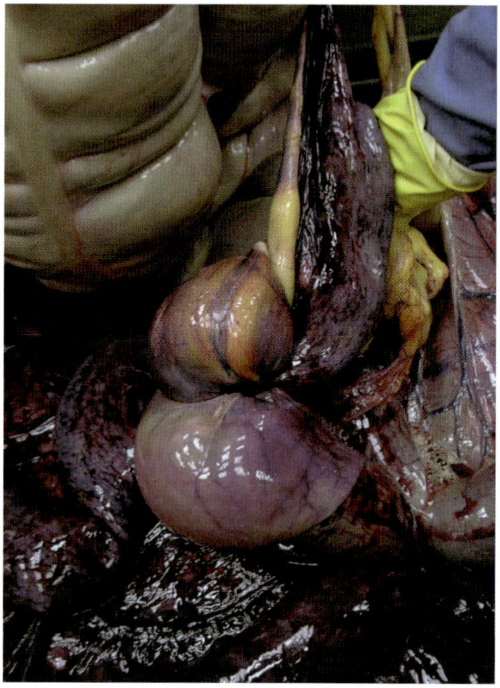

Figure 1.103 Postmortem photograph of mesenteric torsion in an adult horse. It can be partial or complete (involving all the small intestine). It appears to be more common in foals than adult horses. Mesenteric torsion causes severe colic signs and is one of the most serious causes of colic in horses. Affected horses are usually unresponsive to sedatives.

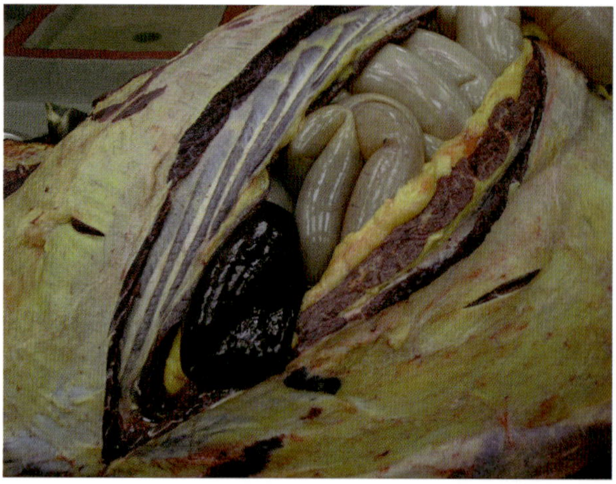

a

Figures 1.104a–c Postmortem photographs of partial mesenteric torsion in an adult horse. Note that not all the small intestines are involved. Also note the sharp demarcation between normal and abnormal small intestines.

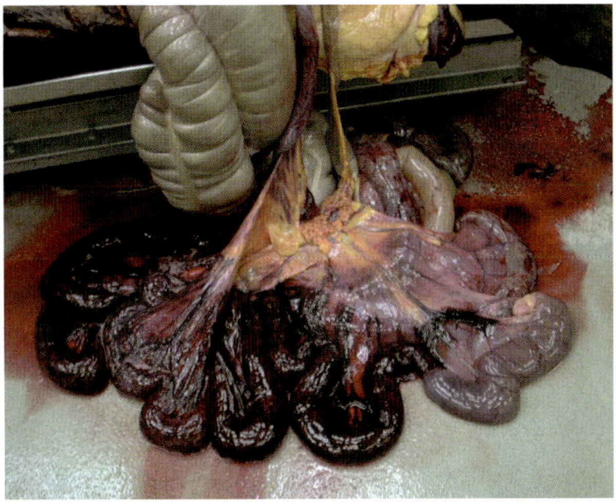

b

Figures 1.104a–c *Continued*

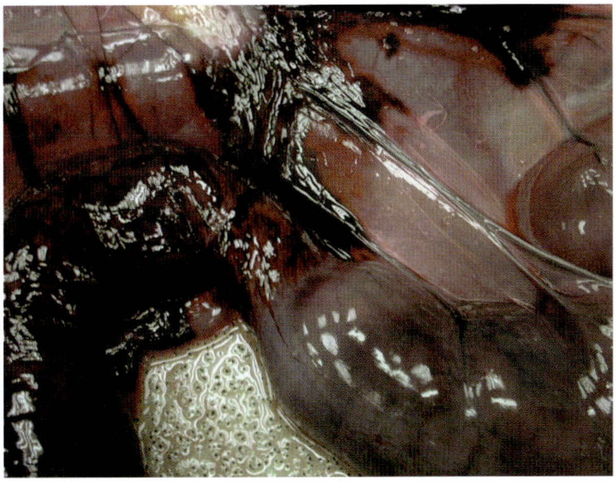

c

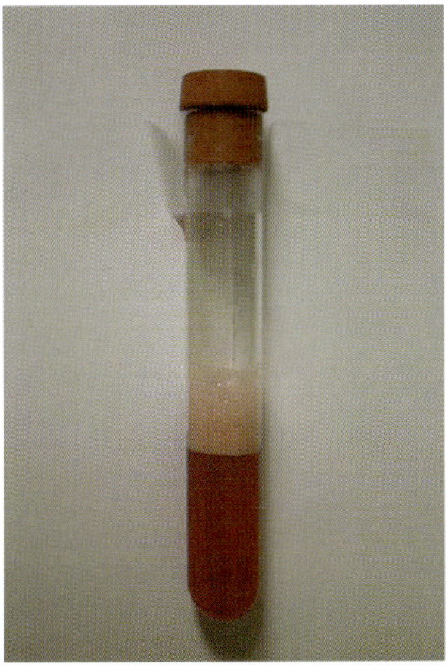

Figure 1.105 Peritoneal fluid from a horse affected with mesenteric torsion. Note the red color and the foam on the top of the fluid. The red color is mainly due to the presence of red blood cells while the foam is due to high protein content.

Small Intestinal Strangulation Caused by a Pedunculated Lipoma

a

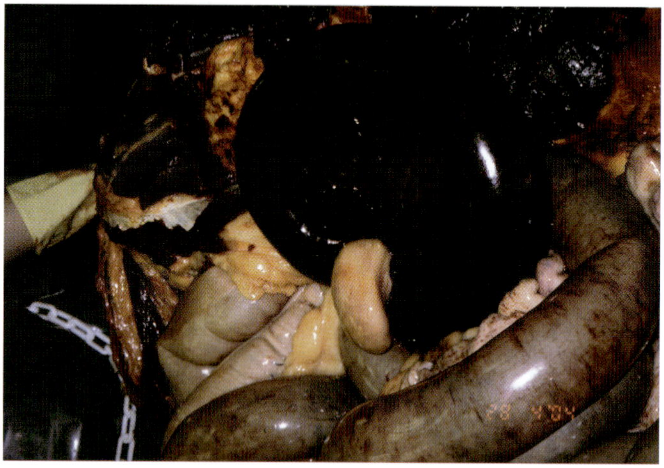

b

Figures 1.106a–e Figures a to d are postmortem photographs and e is an intraoperative photograph of small intestinal strangulation caused by pedunculated lipoma. Lipoma is a benign tumor in the horse and is usually spherical in shape (fig. 1.107). Pony horses and geldings are more predisposed to the disease. Also it is a disease of the older horse. It is usually located on the mesentery and it may or may not have a long stalk (fig. 1.108). Lipoma with a long stalk can strangle loop(s) of the small intestines (fig. 1.106 and 1.109) or serve as a point where intestines may rotate (fig. 1.110).

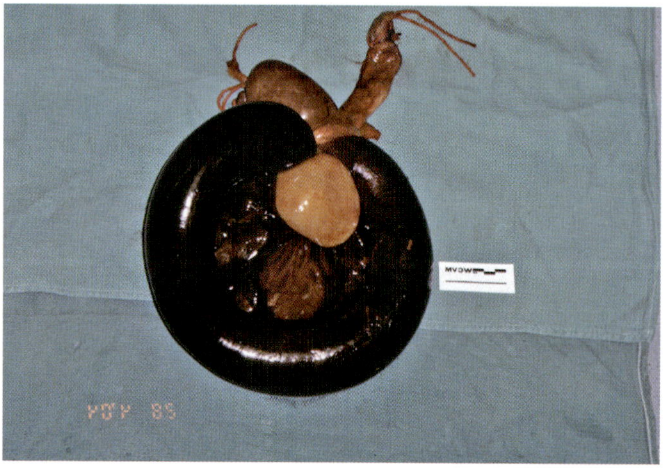

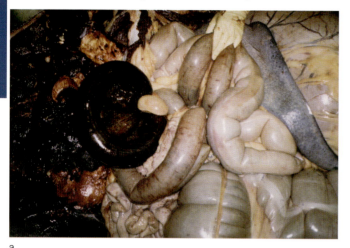

c

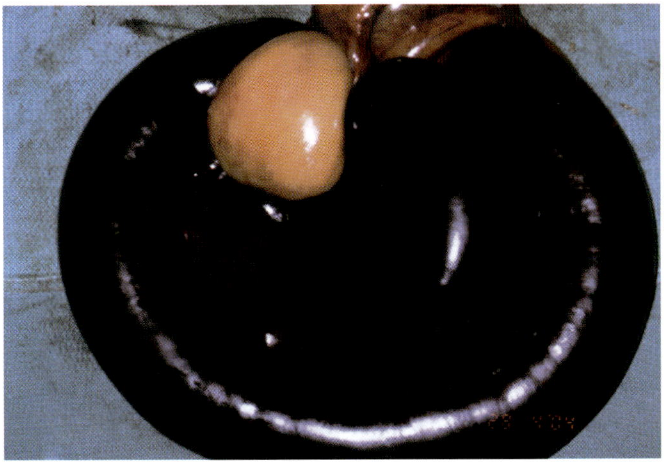

d

Figures 1.106a–e *Continued*

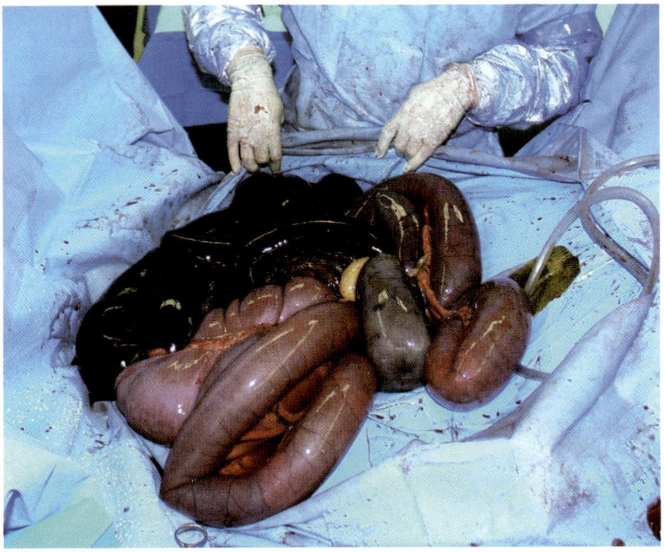

e

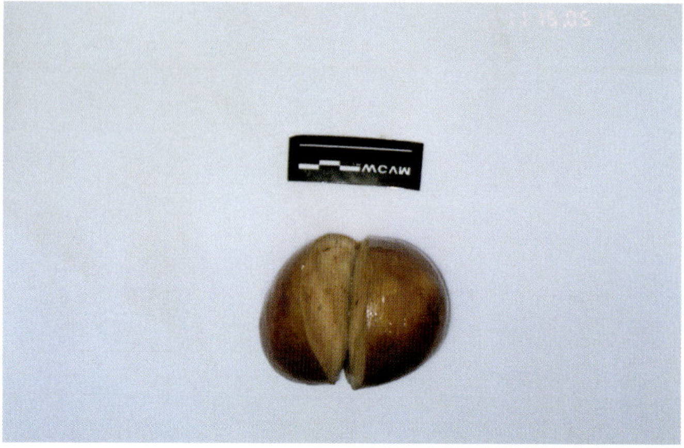

a

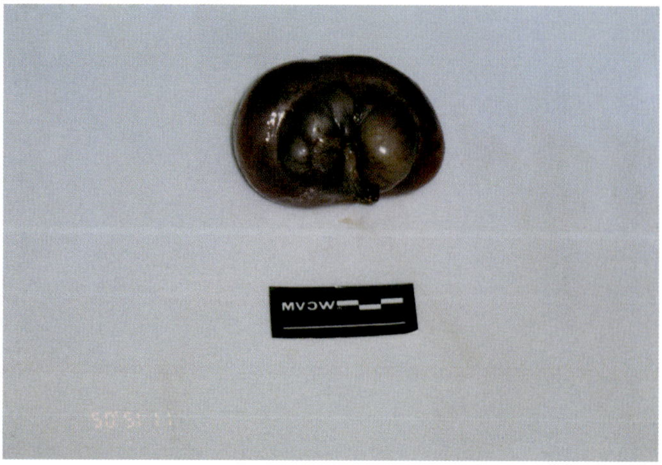

b

Figures 1.107a,b Postmortem photograph of a lipoma. It is a spherical benign tumor that is fatty in nature (cross section in fig. 1.107a).

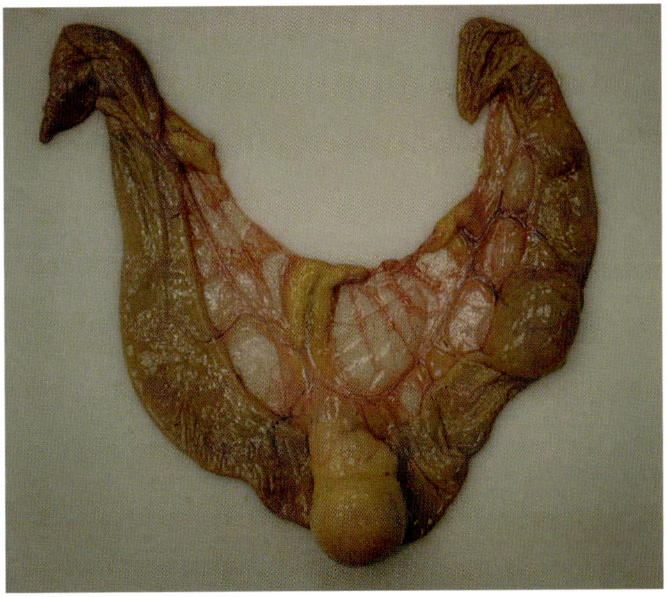

a

Figures 1.108a,b Short-stalk lipoma. Lipoma is usually located on the mesentery and may be found as an incidental finding.

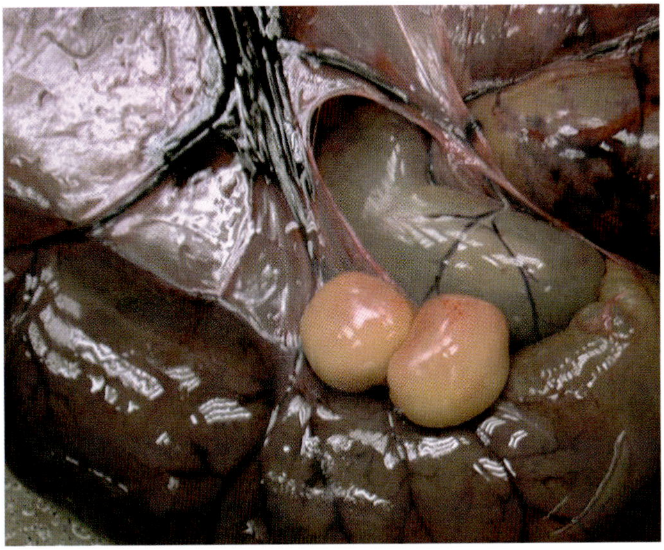

b

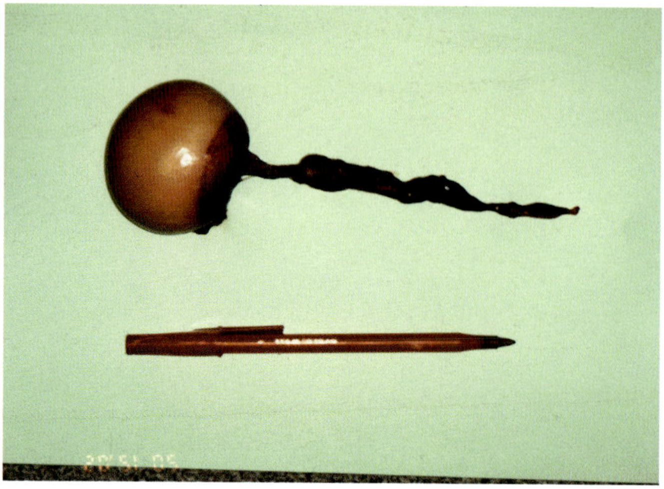

Figure 1.109 Long-stalk lipoma.

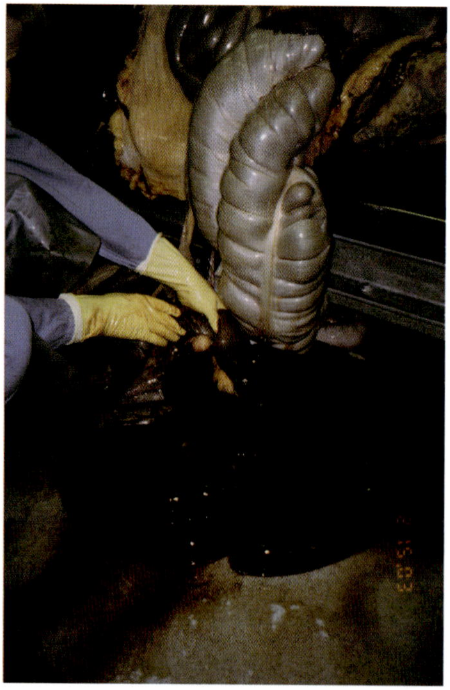

Figure 1.110 Postmortem photograph of a lipoma that served as a point where intestines rotated.

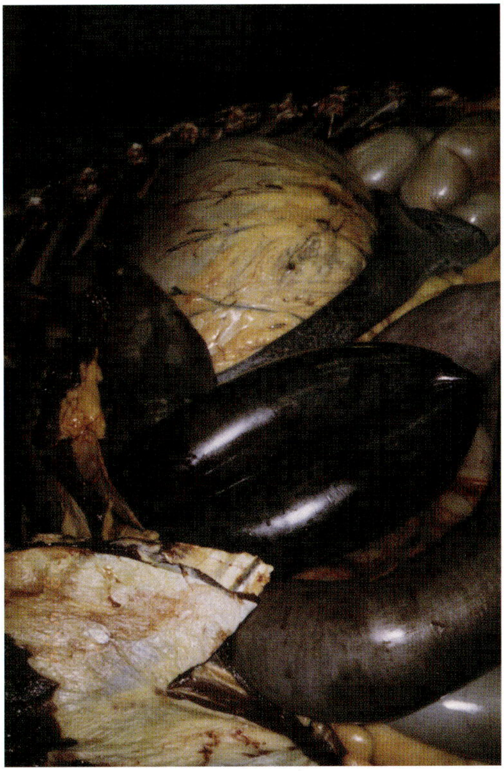

a

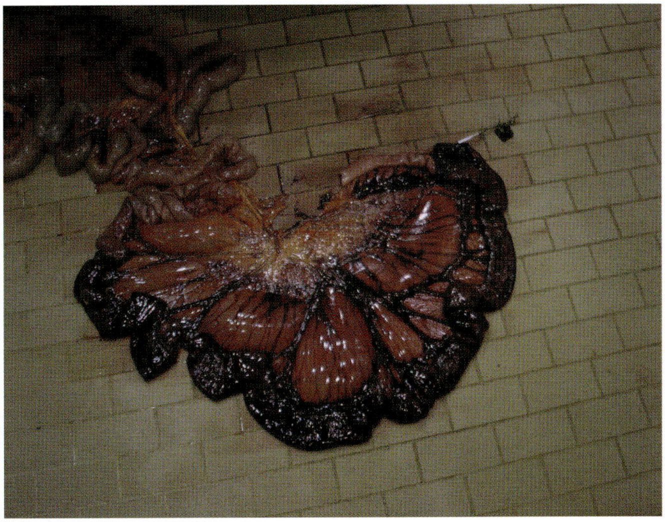

b

Figures 1.111a,b Postmortem photograph of epiploic foramen entrapment of the small intestines. Note the devitalized long loop of small intestines (fig. 1.111b). Strangulated small intestines are usually present in the cranial part of the abdomen (fig. 1.111a). It used to be considered a disease of the old horse only, but this assumption is no longer valid. Small intestines are the part of the bowel that is usually entrapped, but the large bowel can get entrapped too.

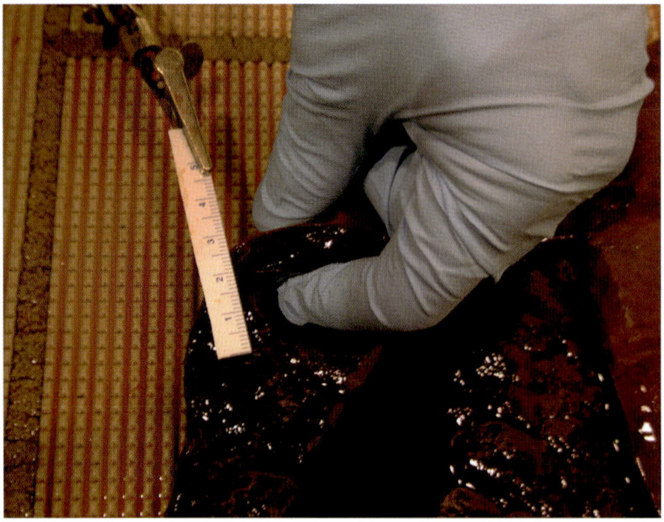

Figure 1.112 Postmortem photograph of epiploic foramen entrapment of the small intestines. Note the thickened small intestines.

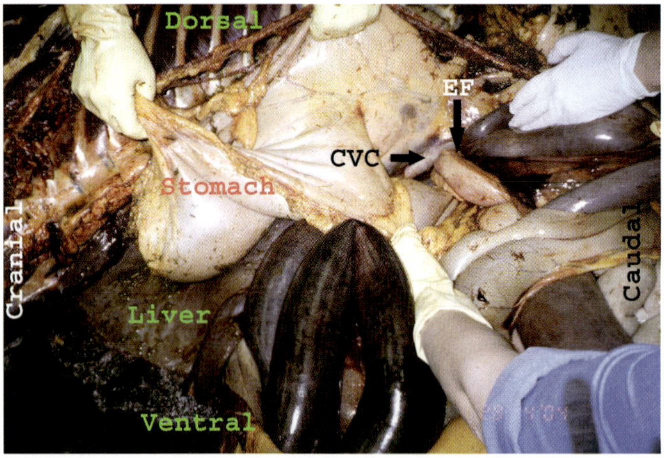

a

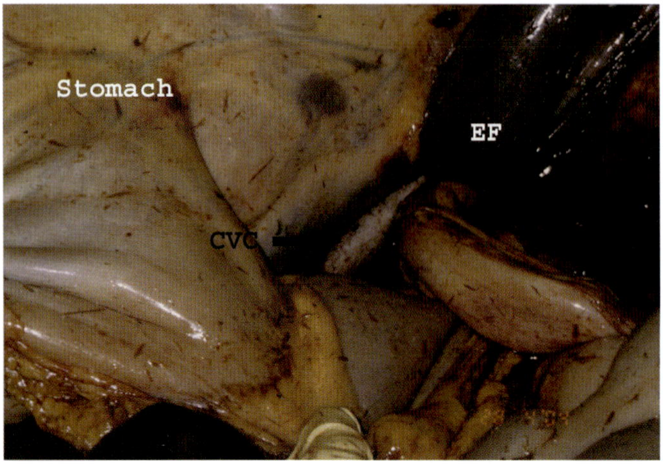

b

Figures 1.113a,b Postmortem photograph of epiploic foramen entrapment (EF) of the small intestines. Epiploic foramen is a natural opening in the abdomen to the omental bursa. It is bounded dorsally by the caudal vena cava (CVC) and caudate process of the liver, and ventrally by the portal vein and pancreas (figs. 1.114a,b). Fig. 1.113b is a close-up view of fig. 1.113a.

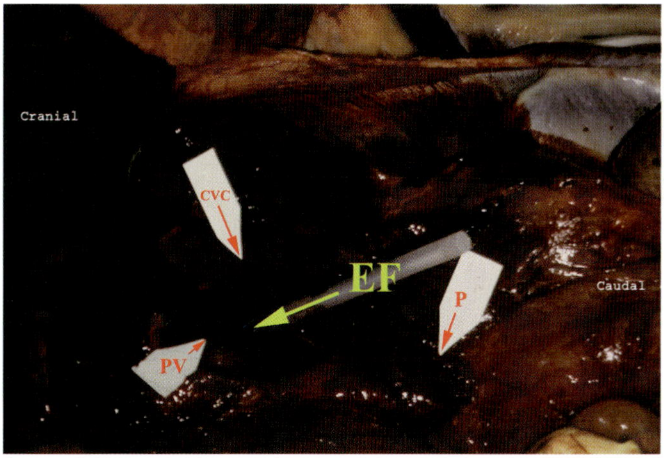

a

Figures 1.114a,b Postmortem photograph of a normal abdomen in a horse showing the normal boundaries of epiploic foramen (EF). Caudal vena cava (CVC), portal vein (PV), and pancreas (P). Fig. 1.114a and b are the same, but in fig. 1.114b, CVC and PV are outlined.

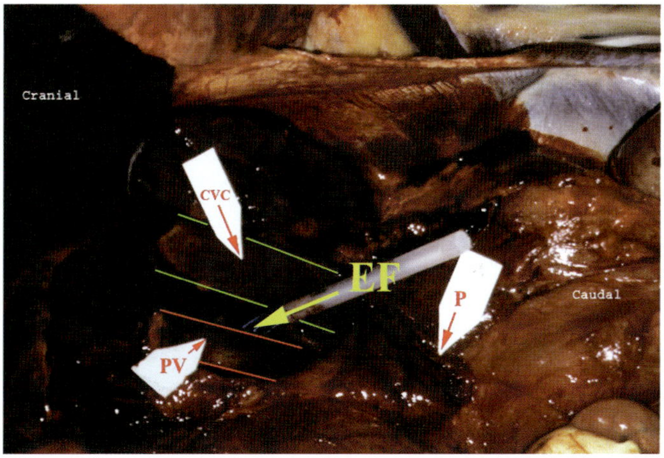

b

Diaphragmatic Hernia

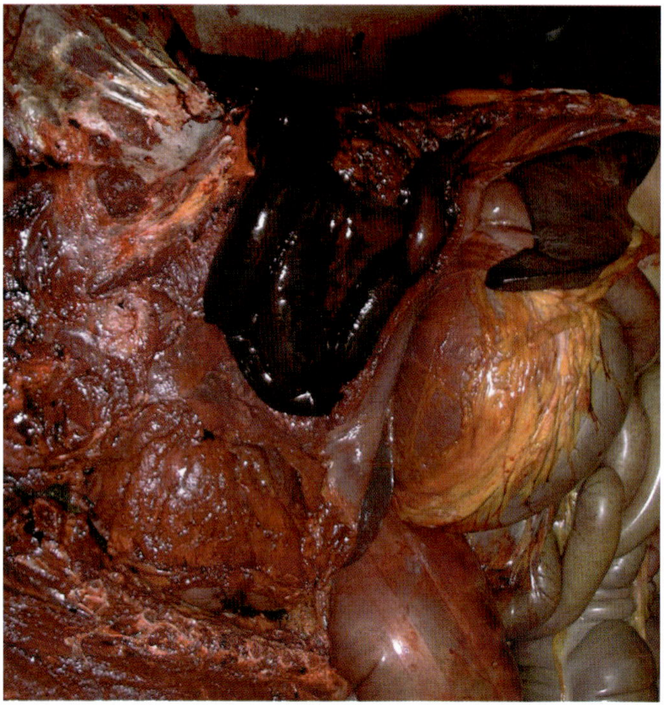

Figure 1.115 Postmortem photograph of diaphragmatic hernia and small intestinal strangulation. Note the presence of small intestines cranial to the diaphragm and in the thoracic cavity. It can be congenital or acquired and can be seen in all ages. Congenital diaphragmatic hernia is caused by incomplete fusion of the embryonic component of the diaphragm. Also, foals can develop diaphragmatic hernia because of the abdominal compression during birth. Acquired diaphragmatic hernia is assumed to be caused by trauma.

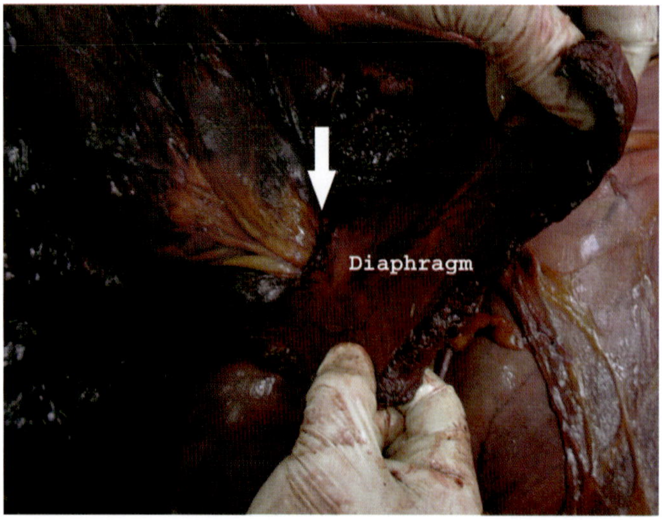

Figure 1.116 Point of herniation (arrow) in the diaphragm of the horse in fig. 1.115.

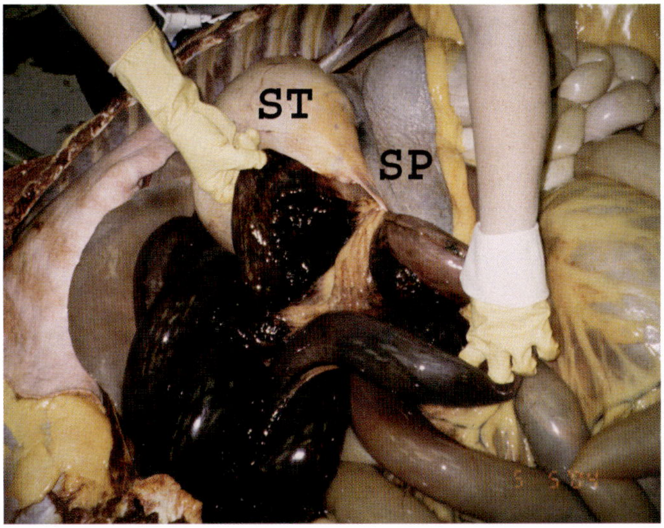

a

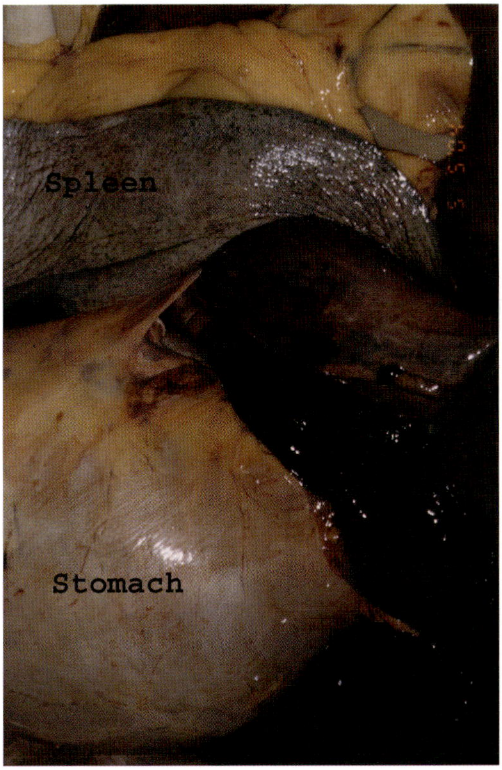

b

Figures 1.117a,b Postmortem photograph of incarceration of the small intestine through the gastrosplenic ligament. There is a congenital or traumatic rent in the gastrosplenic ligament through which the small intestine gets strangulated (fig. 1.118). Gastrosplenic ligament is located between the greater curvature of the stomach (ST) and spleen (SP). Fig. 1.117b is a close-up view of fig. 1.117a.

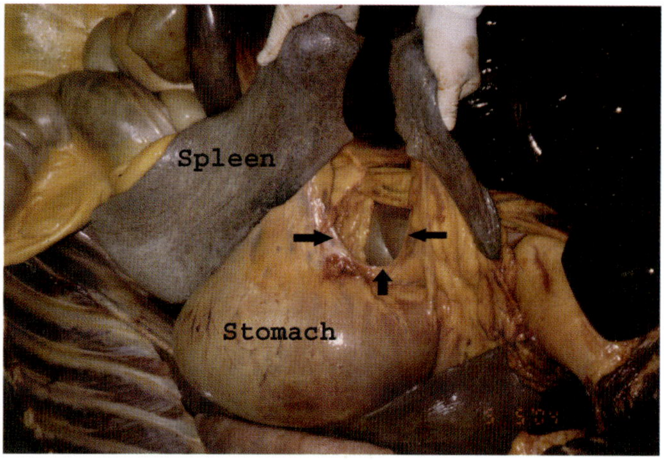

Figure 1.118 Postmortem photograph of a rent in the gastrosplenic ligament (arrows) through which the small intestines have gotten strangulated (fig. 1.117).

Intussusception

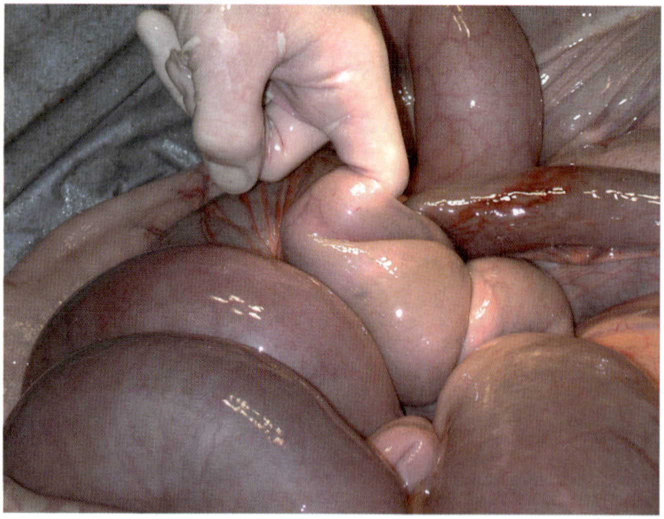

Figure 1.119 A photograph of small intestinal intussusception that was taken during exploratory laparotomy in an adult horse. Intussusception is seen more commonly in young horses. It is an invagination of a segment of the intestine into the adjacent segment. Tapeworms have been implicated to predispose the disease. Ileocecal intussusception is the most common.

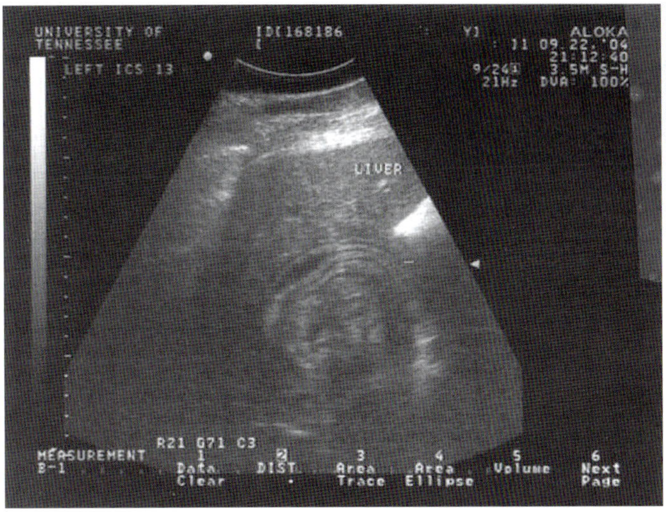

Figure 1.120 Ultrasonographic image of the right 13 intercostal space showing a classic target lesion of the duodenum in a horse presenting for chronic colic and weight loss. Target lesion (bull's-eye) seen on ultrasonography is diagnostic for the presence of intussusception.

Functional Obstruction of the Small Intestine

It is manifested by various degrees of abdominal pain and nasogastric reflux.

Duodenitis-Proximal Jejunitis (DPJ) (Anterior or Proximal Enteritis)

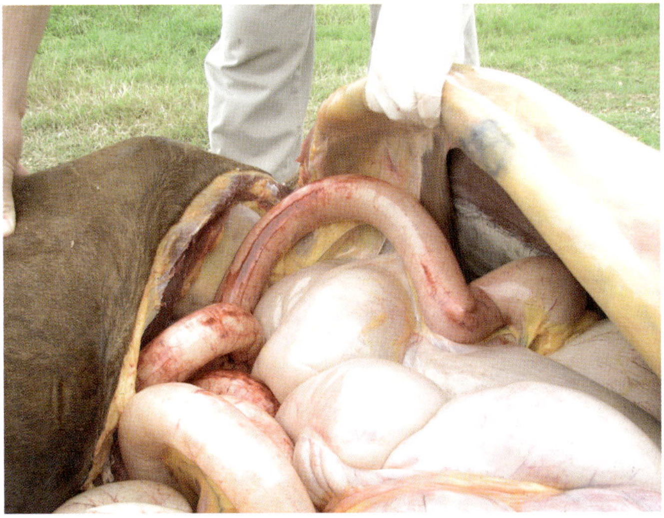

Figure 1.121a Postmortem photograph of duodenitis-proximal jejunitis (DPJ). Note the inflamed duodenum and distended jejunum. DPJ is a relatively new syndrome of unknown etiology. It is characterized by fever, abdominal discomfort, large volumes of nasogastric reflux (brownish orange with fetid odor), depression, and dehydration. Transrectal examination reveals distended loops of the small intestine. These signs are caused by a severe inflammation and edema of the duodenum and part of the jejunum. It is extremely important to differentiate DPJ from cases of small intestinal strangulating obstruction. The major difference is that in DPJ cases, colic signs are replaced by severe depression after the gastric decompression; this is not the case usually in strangulating lesions of the small intestines.

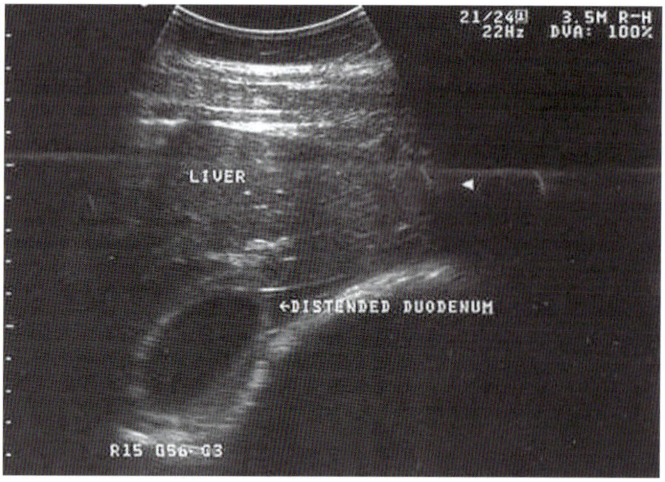

Figure 1.121b Ultrasonographic image of the right caudal abdomen showing distension and thickening of the duodenum (dorsal is to the left) in a case of duodenitis-proximal jejunitis.

Proliferative Enteropathy (*Lawsonia intracellularis*)

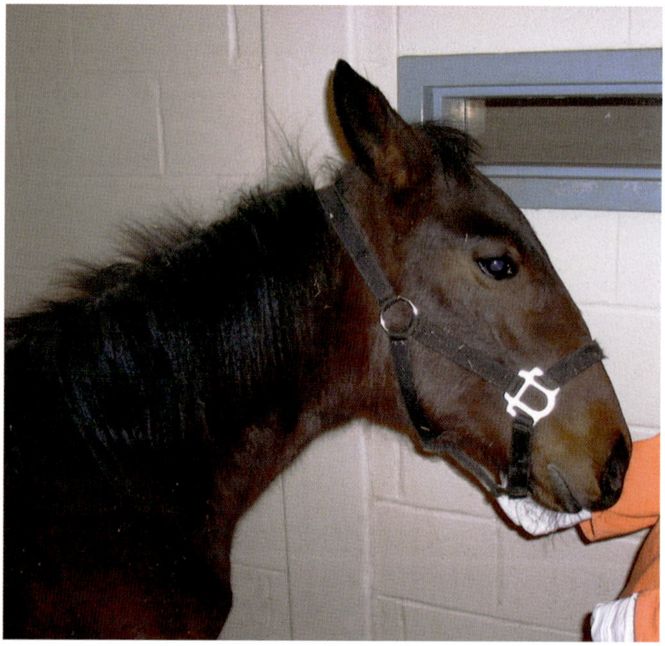

Figure 1.122a A foal affected with proliferative enteropathy. Note the intermandibular edema. Proliferative enteropathy is associated with *Lawsonia intracellularis*. Affected foals are 3 to 13 months old. Clinical signs include depression, weight loss, colic, diarrhea, and sometimes death in 2 to 3 days (fig. 1.122b). Affected horses are hypoproteinemic and usually develop ventral and intermandibular edema (fig. 1.122c). Thickening and irregular corrugation of the small intestines is usually seen on postmortem examination (fig. 1.122d).

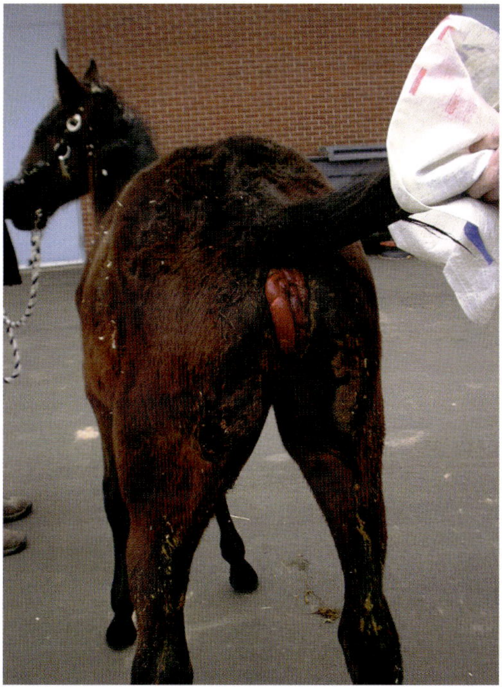

Figure 1.122b A foal affected with proliferative enteropathy. Note the diarrhea. In addition, the foal had a rectal prolapse.

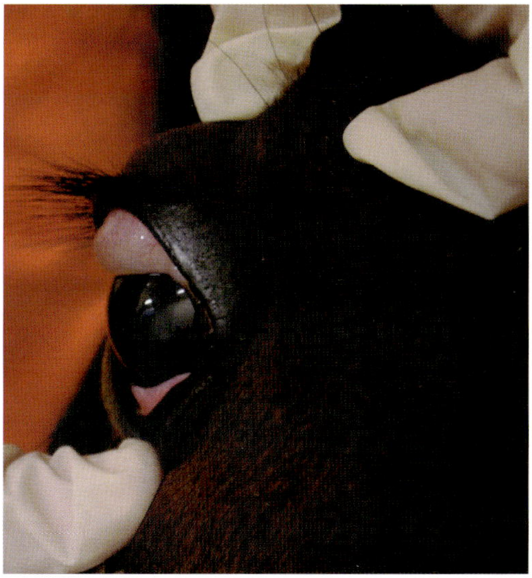

Figure 1.122c A foal affected with proliferative enteropathy. Note the chemosis that had developed secondary to severe hypoproteinemia.

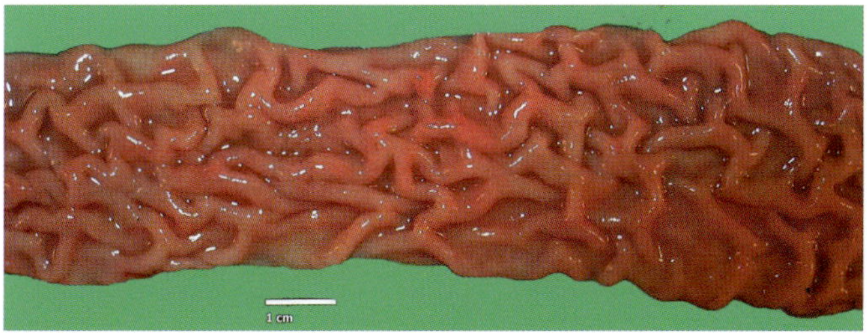

Figure 1.122d A postmortem photograph of the intestine of a foal affected with proliferative enteropathy. Note the thickened and irregular corrugation of the small intestines.

Diseases of the Large Intestine

Large Colon Volvulus (LCV)

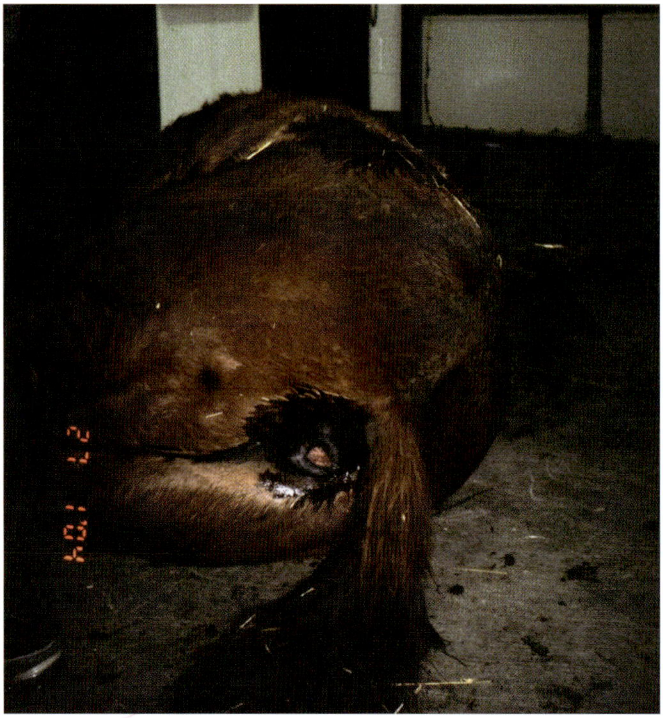

Figure 1.123 A horse with large colon volvulus. Note the abdominal distention that progresses very fast. Large colon volvulus is serious and often fatal. Horses with LCV usually have an acute onset of severe, unrelenting, abdominal pain, high heart rate, abdominal distention and are in a state of shock. Postpartum mares may be overrepresented. Diagnosis is usually based on clinical signs, severely distended large colon on transrectal examination and, recently, by using ultrasonography.

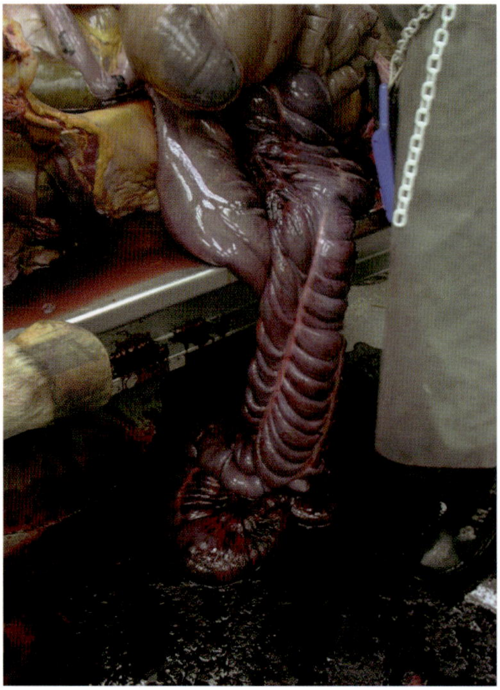

Figure 1.124 Postmortem photograph of large colon volvulus in a horse. Note the devitalized large colon and bloody intestinal content.

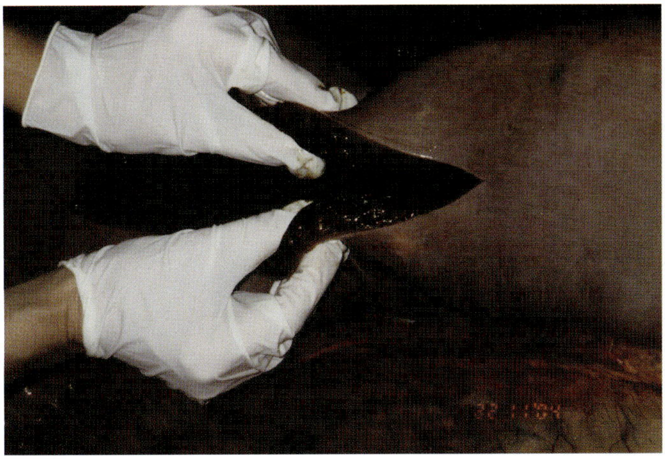

Figure 1.125 Postmortem photograph of large colon volvulus in a horse. Note the severely thickened large colon.

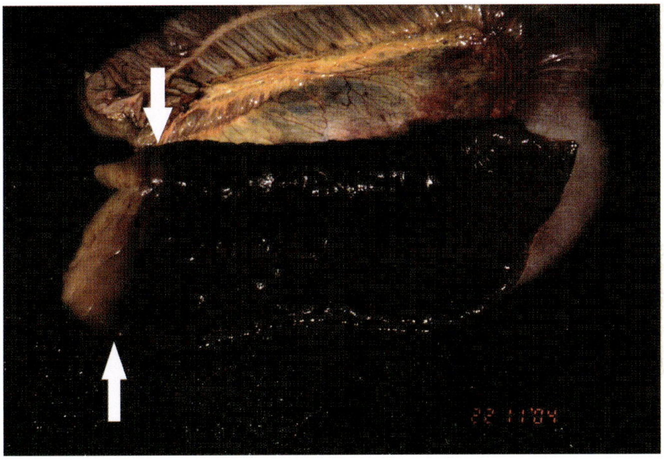

Figure 1.126 Postmortem photograph of large colon volvulus in a horse. Note the sharp demarcation at the site of rotation between the strangulated and nonstrangulated parts of the large colon (arrows).

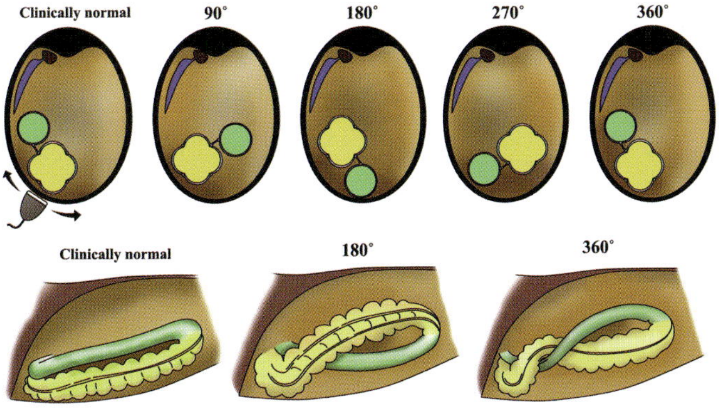

Figure 1.127 Cross and sagittal section diagram of the location of the left large colon in normal horses and horses with different degrees of large colon volvulus. There are different degrees of rotation of the large colon (80°–720°), the higher the degree the more severe the cases. There are two levels at which the LCV usually occurs – at the base of the cecum or at the level of the diaphragmatic and sternal flexures. (Used with permission from Abutarbush SM, Use of ultrasonography to diagnose large colon volvulus in horses, Journal of the American Veterinary Medical Association, 2006; 228[3] 409–13)

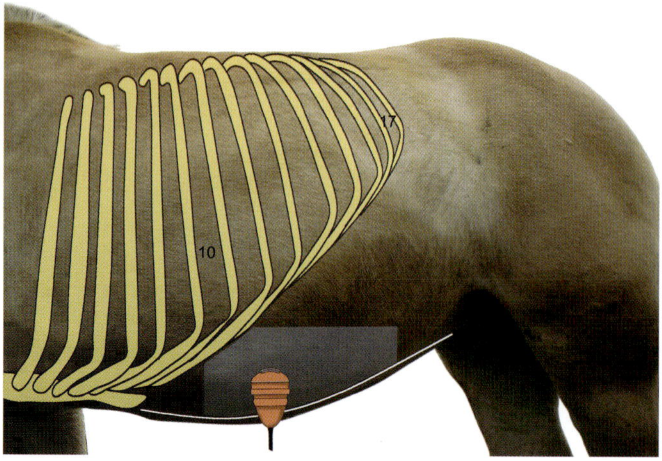

Figure 1.128 Ultrasonography can be used to diagnose LCV. This figure illustrates the landmarks that are used to ultrasound the left ventral colon (shaded area), which is used to diagnose large colon volvulus in horses based on the anatomical features of the left ventral and dorsal colon. The boundaries of the shaded area are midline, two vertical lines at the level of the 10th and 17th intercostal spaces, and a horizontal line between the two vertical lines at the level of the costal arch of the 10th intercostal area. (Used with permission from Abutarbush SM, Use of ultrasonography to diagnose large colon volvulus in horses, Journal of the American Veterinary Medical Association, 2006; 228[3] 409–13)

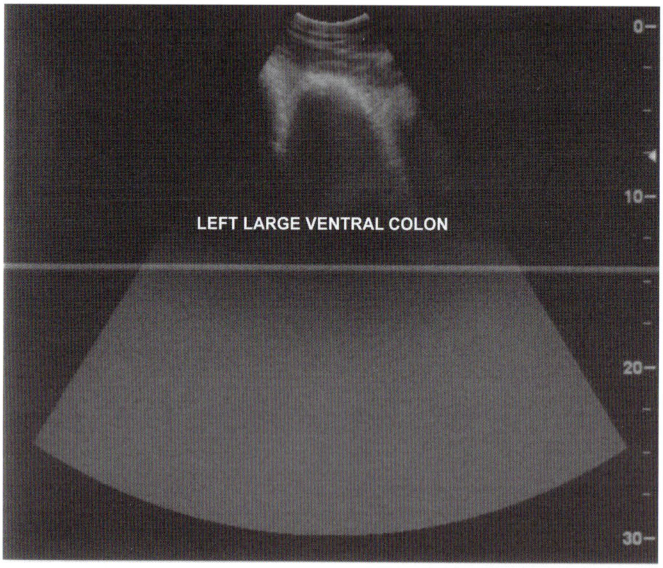

a

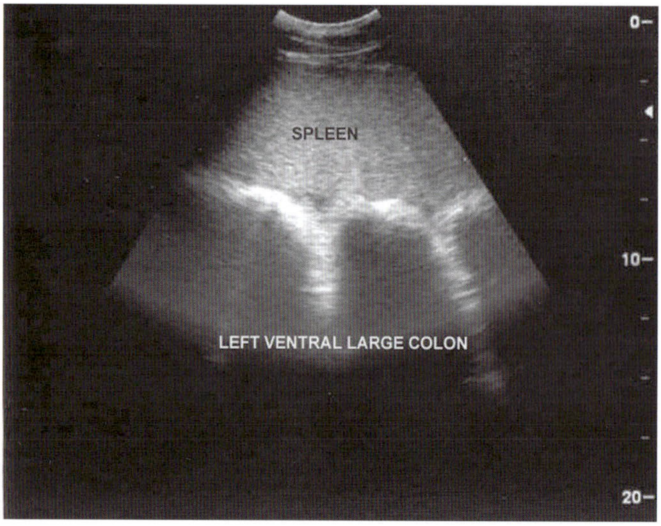

b

Figures 1.129a,b Ultrasonographic images of the abdomen in a normal horse as outlined in fig. 1.128. The large ventral colon is sacculated, while the dorsal is not. In normal horses, ultrasonography of the left ventral abdomen reveals the presence of the sacculated left large ventral colon next to the body wall (a) and sometimes close to the spleen (b). (Images used with permission from Abutarbush SM, Use of ultrasonography to diagnose large colon volvulus in horses, Journal of the American Veterinary Medical Association, 2006; 228[3] 409–13)

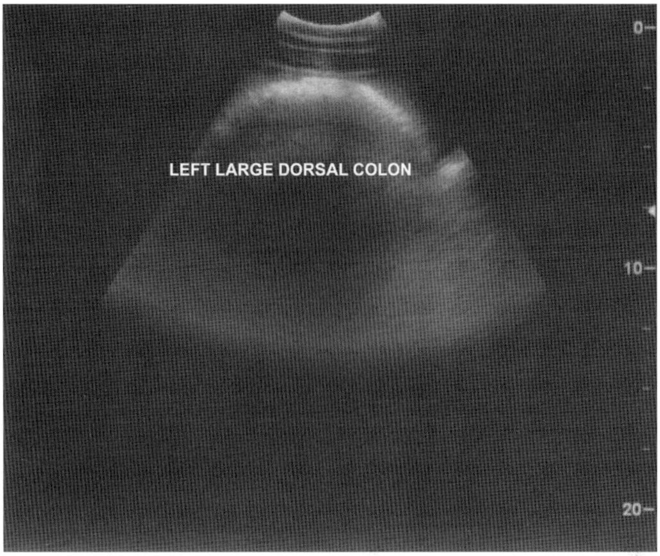

a

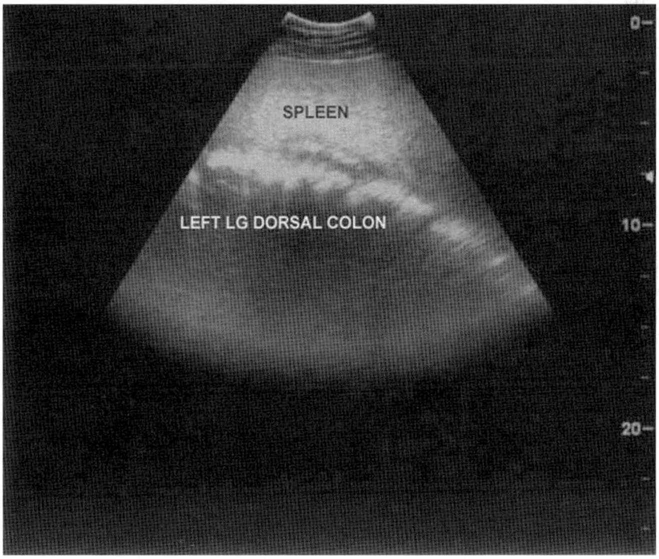

b

Figures 1.130a,b Ultrasonographic images of the left ventral abdomen in a horse with a 540° large colon volvulus as outlined in fig. 1.127. Note the abnormal ventral location of the left dorsal large colon (no sacculation) next to the body wall (a) or the spleen and body wall (b). The principle of using ultrasonography to diagnose LCV is to identify the left dorsal colon in a ventral position. The presence of the nonsacculated large colon, when ultrasounding the left ventral abdomen, is indicative of a LCV, which means that the dorsal left colon is in a ventral position. LCV with a rotation of 360° or 720° will not be diagnosed using this method because the ventral colon will be in a ventral location (fig. 1.127). (Images used with permission from Abutarbush SM, Use of ultrasonography to diagnose large colon volvulus in horses, Journal of the American Veterinary Medical Association, 2006; 228[3] 409–13)

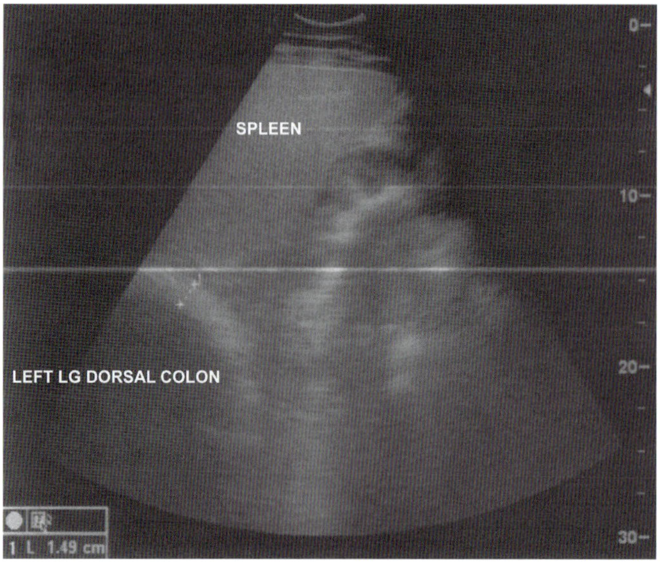

Figure 1.131 Ultrasonographic image of the left ventral abdomen in a horse with large colon volvulus. Note the thickened large colon that can be seen in cases of LCV.

Large Colon Displacement (LCD)

Not an uncommon cause of abdominal pain in horses. There are two main classifications for LCD: left LCD and right LCD.

Right Displacement of the (Left) Large Colon (RDLC)

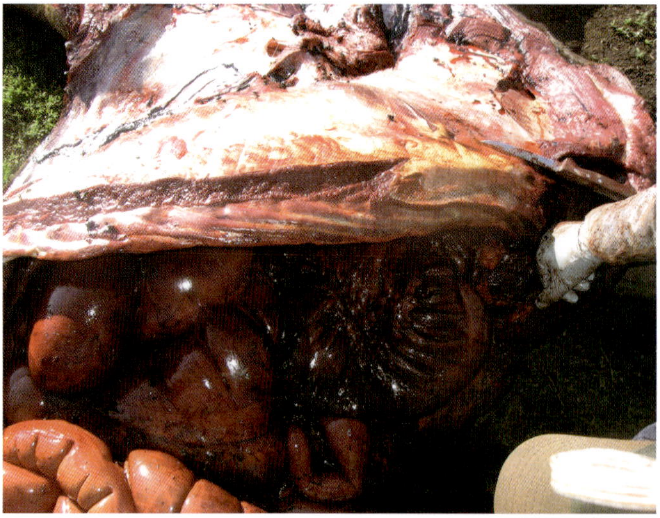

1.132

Figures 1.132–1.133 Postmortem photograph of a horse with right displacement of the large colon. The horse is on lateral position with the left side down and the right side up. Note the presence of the pelvic flexure (the connection between the left dorsal and ventral large colon) in the right side of the abdomen lateral to the cecum fig. 1.133. With RDLC, the colon displaces to the right of the cecum (lateral).

Figures 1.132–1.133 *Continued*

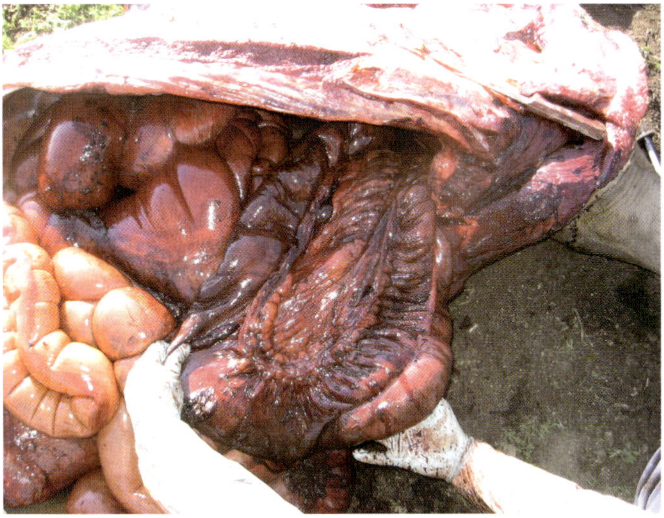

1.133

Left Dorsal Displacement of the Large Colon (LDLC)

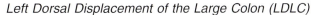

Figures 1.134a,b Cross-section diagrams of the abdomen of a horse with early (a) and advanced (b) left dorsal displacement of the large colon (nephrosplenic entrapment). The left large colon can be entrapped between the left kidney and spleen (nephrosplenic entrapment) or between the spleen and the left body wall; both are referred to as left dorsal displacement of the large colon. Nephrosplenic entrapment occurs over a wide age range, 8 months to 16 years, and is more frequently observed in middle-aged horses. Geldings are more frequently affected, but displacement can occur in any gender. Large-framed or large horses are at higher risk of developing NSELC. The cause is unknown. Diagnosis of LCD can be made by transrectal palpation, percutaneous ultrasonography of the upper left flank (nephrosplenic entrapment), or exploratory laparotomy. (Drawings by Dr. Juliane Deubner, WCVM, University of Saskatchewan)

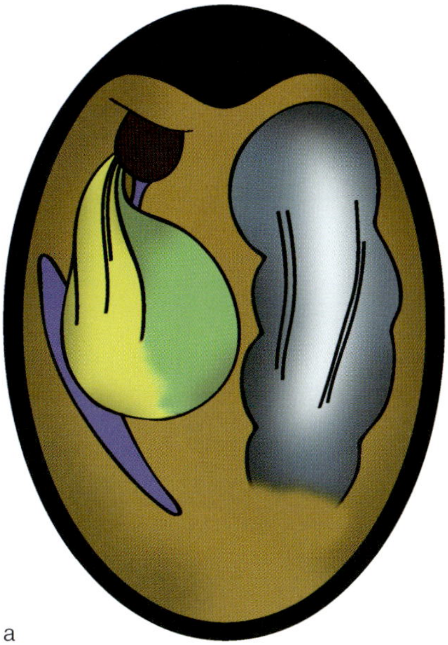

a

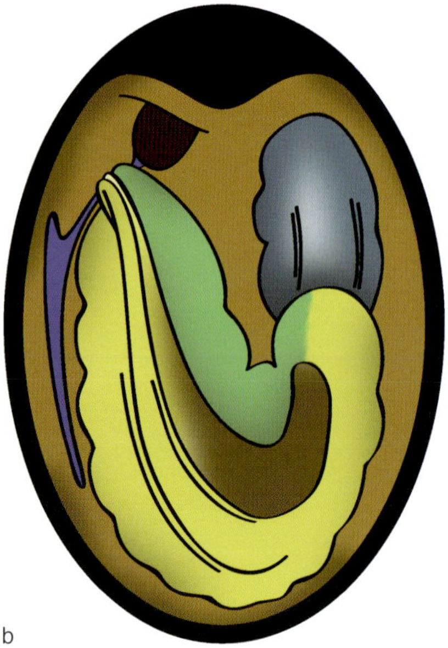

b

Figures 1.134a,b *Continued*

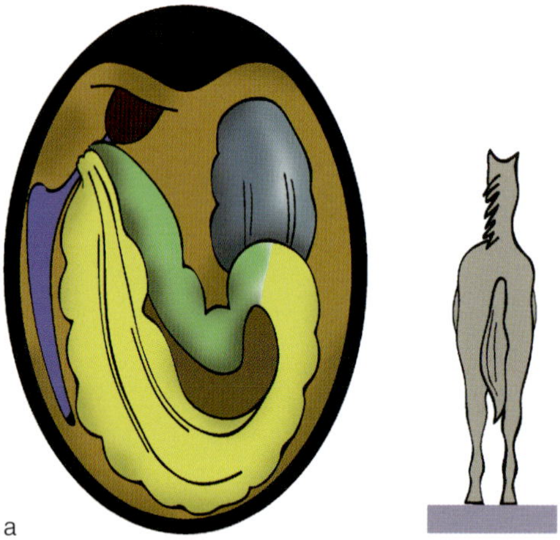

a

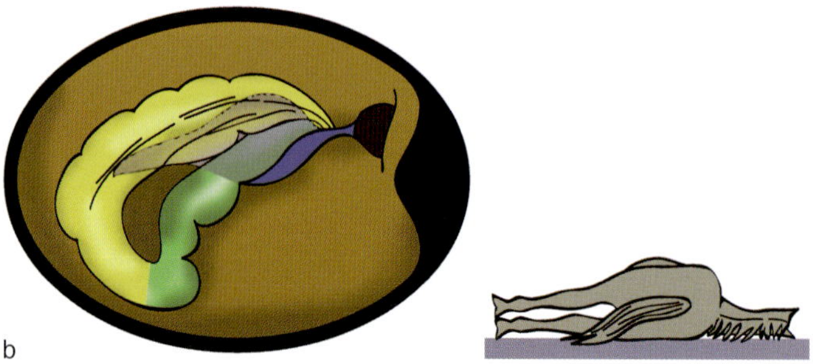

b

Figures 1.135a–e Cross-section diagrams of the abdomen of a horse with left dorsal displacement of the large colon (nephrosplenic entrapment) and its treatment by rolling. Treatment by rolling should be performed under general anesthesia. The horse is anesthetized and placed in right lateral recumbency (b), then rotated up to dorsal recumbency. The abdomen is rocked back and forth for a few minutes. Then the hind limbs are hooked to a chain hoist and the hind quarters are elevated off the ground (c). The horse is then rolled to the left lateral side and evaluated (d) or rolling is continued to the right lateral side and then evaluated (e). Correction is evaluated by both rectal examination and per cutaneous ultrasound of the left flank. (Drawings by Dr. Juliane Deubner, WCVM, University of Saskatchewan)

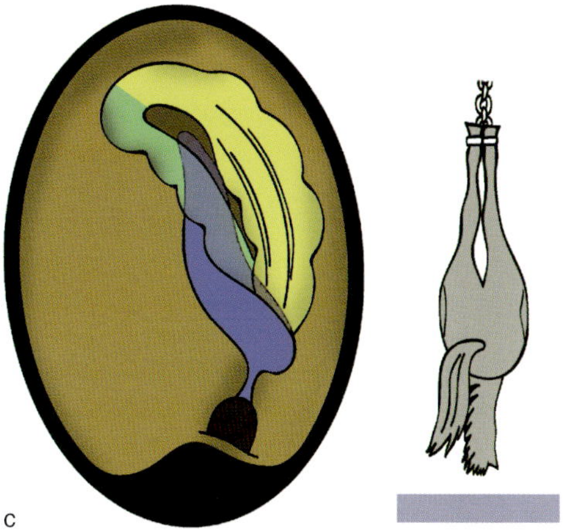

c

d

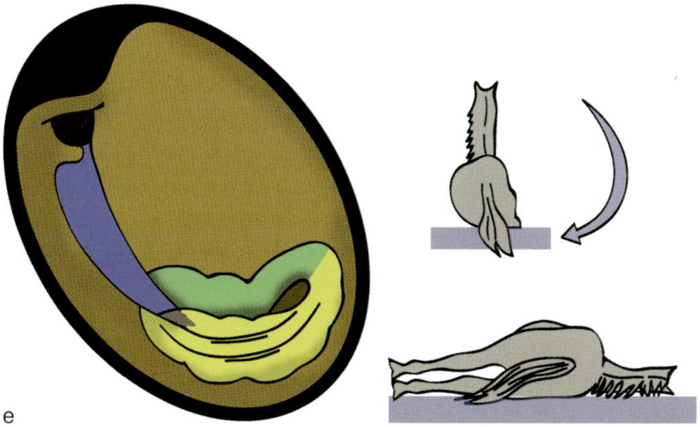

e

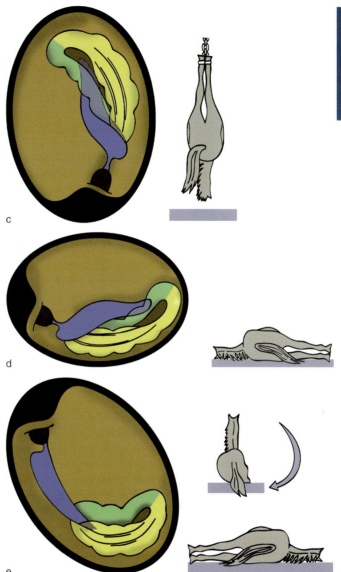

Figures 1.135a–e *Continued*

1

Large Colon Impaction (LCI)

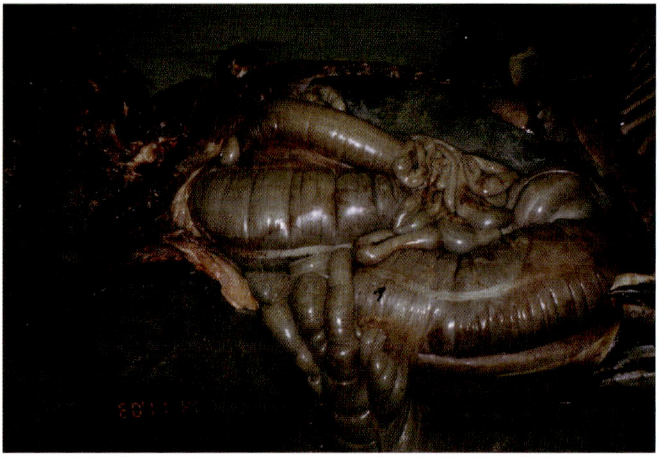

Figure 1.136a Postmortem photograph of a horse with large colon impaction (a). LCI could occur at any location in the large colon, but occurs commonly at areas of natural narrowing of the diameter of the lumen of the large colon, pelvic flexure, transverse colon. Risk factors include exercise restriction, large concentrate meals, and restricted access to water in cold climates (frozen water sources). Clinically it is manifested by an onset of mild pain and sometimes diarrhea. The production of watery fecal fluids followed by boluses of fibrous ingesta can be seen. If not treated, severe cases may result in colitis or rupture of the colon (figs. 1.136b,c). Doughy, ingesta-filled viscus may be felt rectally, however, it depends on the location of the impaction, whether it is reachable by hand or not. Large colon impaction should be treated with IV fluid therapy, analgesics, and oral laxatives.

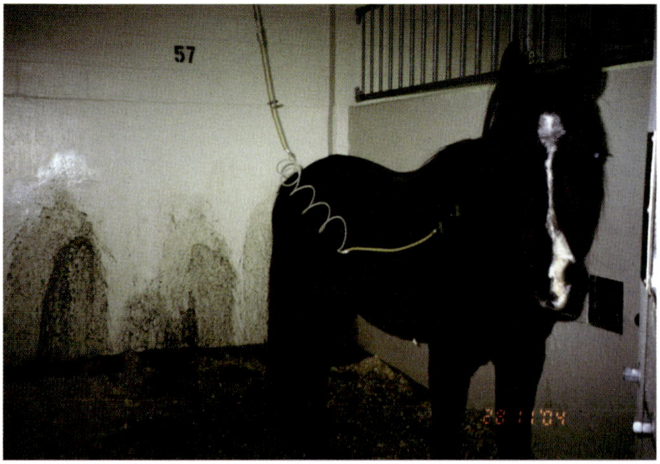

Figure 1.136b An adult horse with long-standing large colon impaction that has developed colitis and diarrhea.

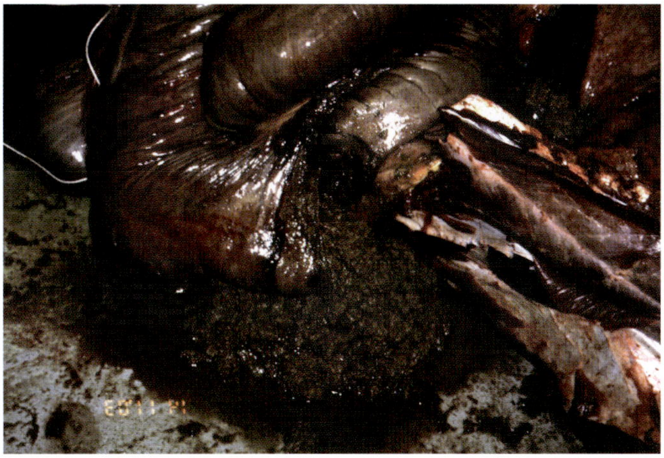

Figure 1.136c Postmortem photograph of a horse with long-standing large colon impaction. Note the ruptured colon.

Large Intestinal Intussusception

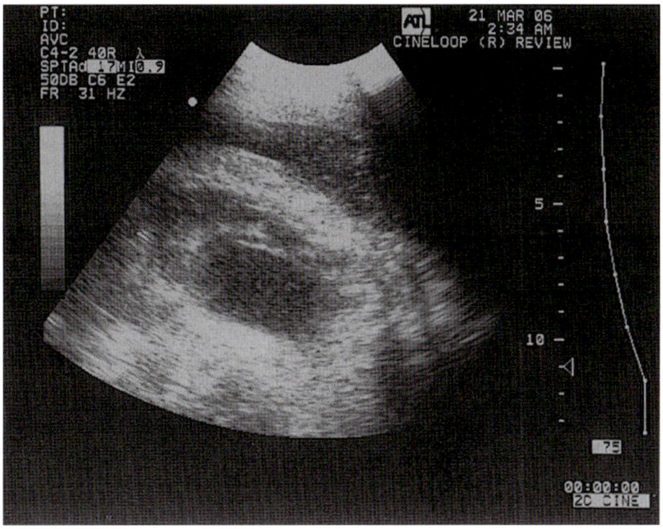

Figure 1.137 Ultrasonographic image of the right paralumbar fossa showing a classic target lesion (bull's-eye) of intussusception of the large intestine. It is an uncommon cause of colic that is usually seen in young horses (2–3 years old). It can occur at different locations in the large intestine and the most common one is the cecocolic intussusception. Clinical signs are usually associated with acute onset of abdominal pain that differs in the severity according to the severity of the intussusception. Intussuscept may be felt transrectally.

Salmonellosis

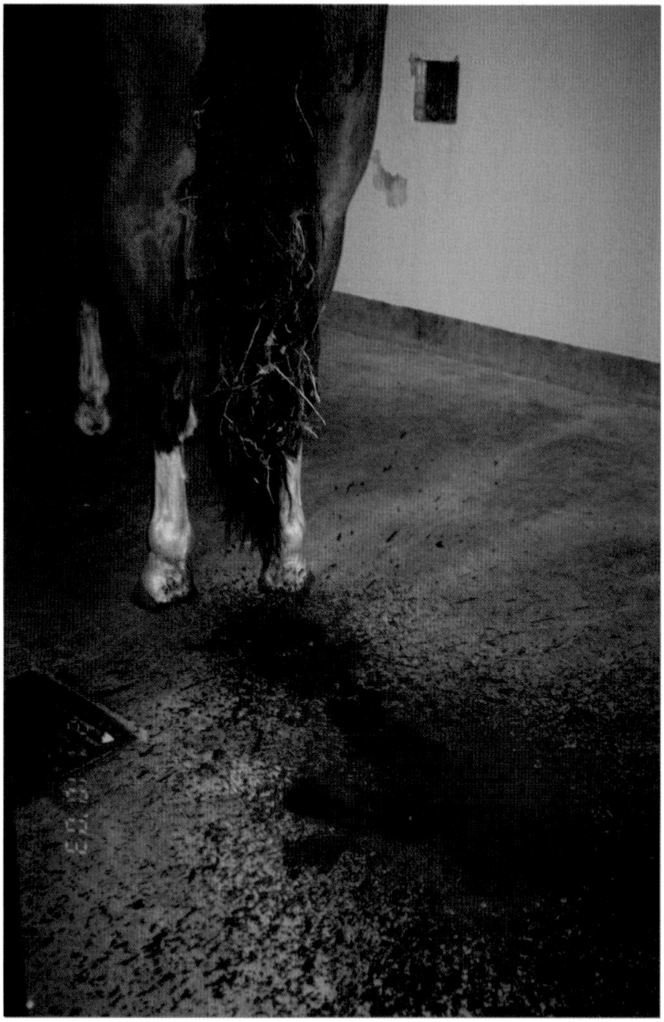

Figure 1.138 Horse affected with salmonellosis. Note the watery diarrhea. Salmonellosis is a serious disease and can be fatal. It is zoonotic and can cause serious sickness in humans. *S. typhimurium* and *agona* are common isolates, but other serotypes can cause the disease. *Salmonella* infection can be latent and horses may become carriers.

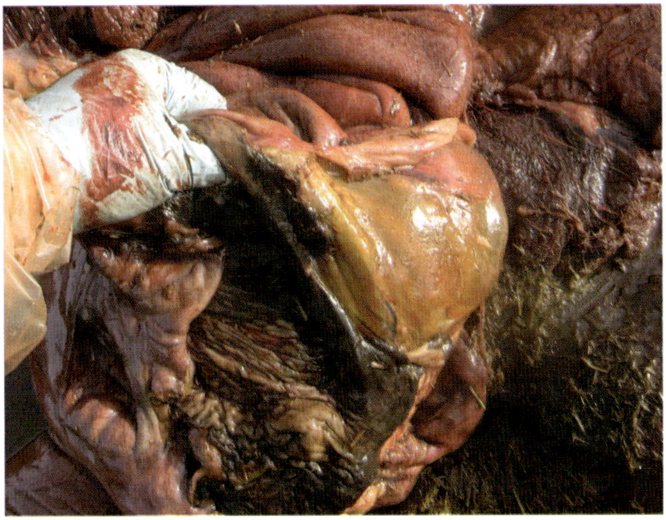

a

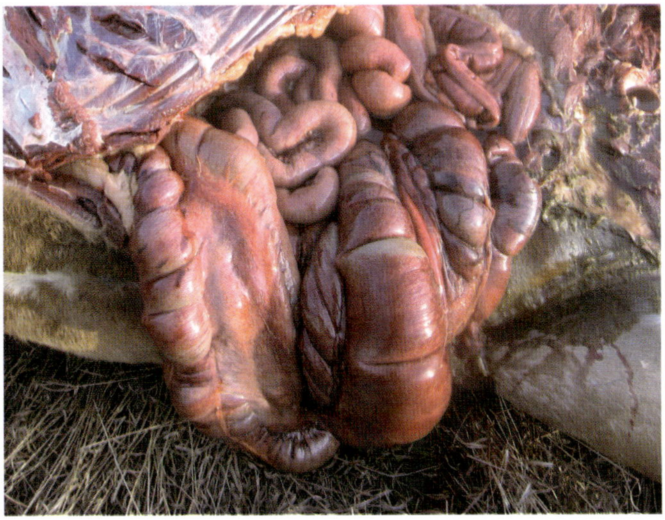

b

Figures 1.139a–d Postmortem photograph of a horse affected with acute salmonellosis. Note the severe enterocolitis. The large colon is edematous (a), thickened, and very inflamed (b, c). Small intestines can be affected also (d).

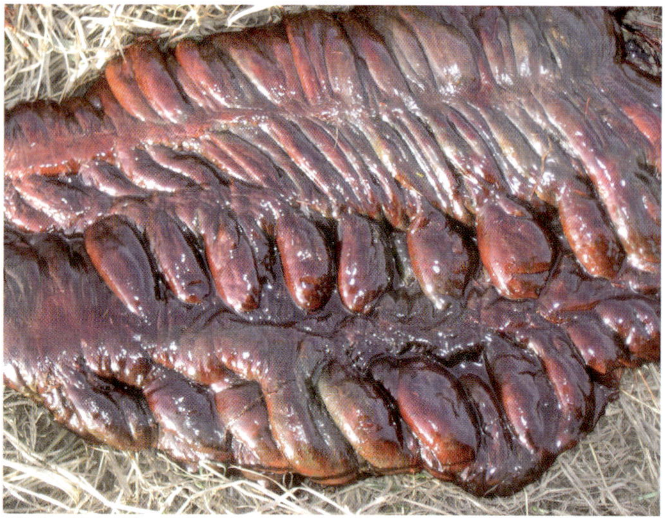

c

Figures 1.139a–d *Continued*

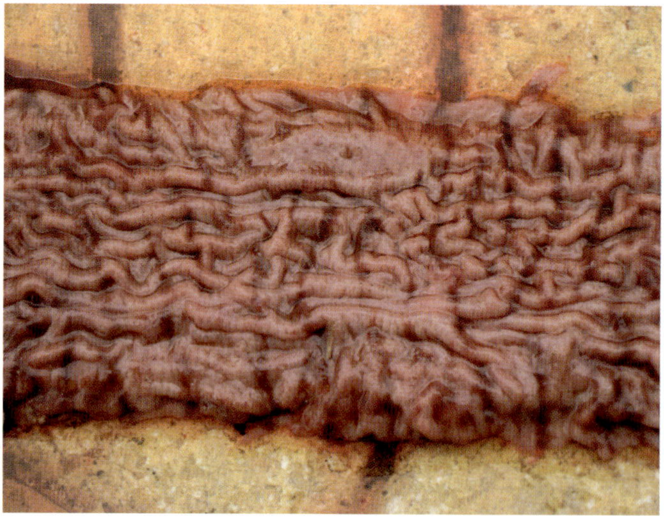

d

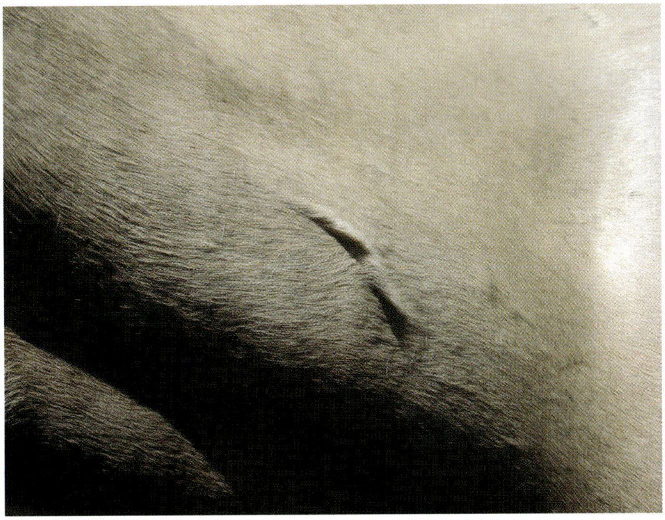

Figure 1.140 Horse affected with salmonellosis. Note the severe dehydration and skin tenting.

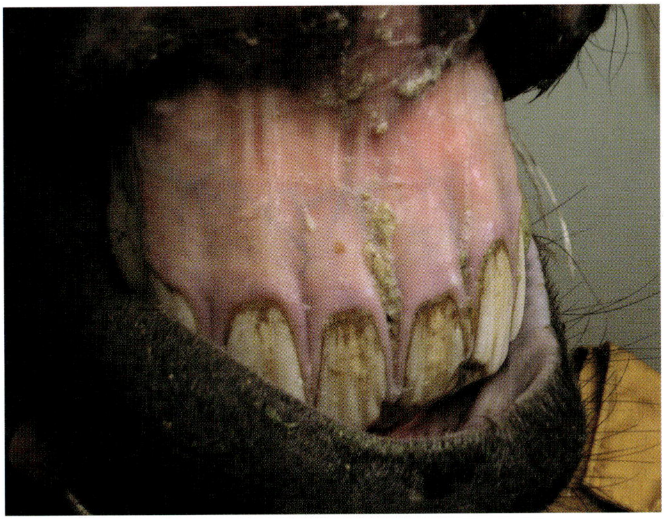

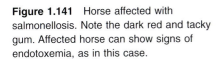

Figure 1.141 Horse affected with salmonellosis. Note the dark red and tacky gum. Affected horse can show signs of endotoxemia, as in this case.

Strongylosis

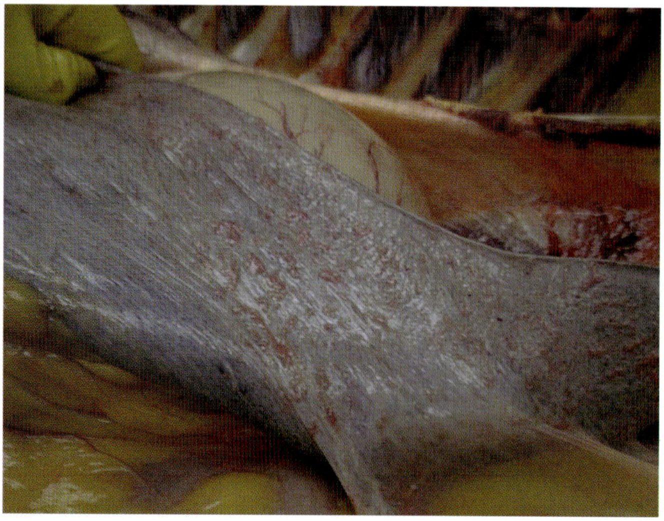

Figure 1.142 Postmortem photograph of a horse. Note the presence of fibrous tags on the spleen, which is indicative of parasitic migration, mainly due to *Strongylus* spp. Strongylosis is caused by *Strongylus vulgaris, Strongylus edentatus, Strongylus equinuus. S. vulgaris* by far is the most important. Diarrhea is caused by larval migration through the intestinal wall causing inflammation and abnormal intestinal motility and function. Fibrous tags, as in this figure, on the abdominal organs and heamomalasma ilii (fig. 1.143) are found in necropsy as evidence of larval migration. It is more commonly seen in young and naive horses. Clinical signs include fever, depression, poor weight gain, intermittent mild colic and diarrhea. Diagnosis is based on clinical signs, elevated alpha- and beta-globulin, and IgG(T). Fecal analysis might be unrewarding.

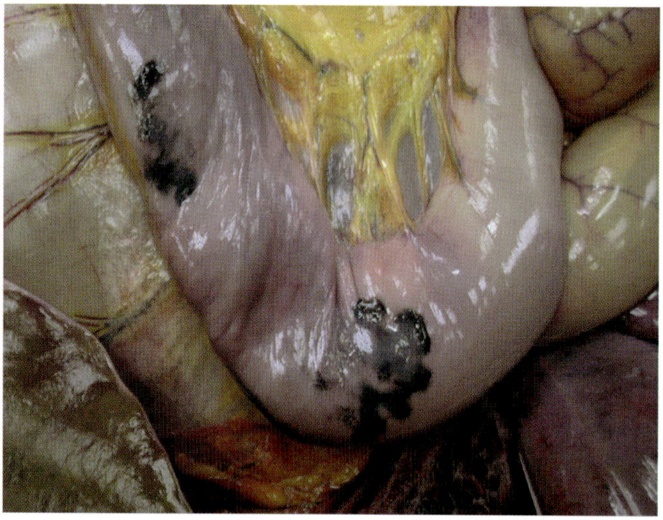

Figure 1.143 Postmortem photograph of the small intestine of a horse. Note the heamomalasma ilii. It can be found in necropsy and is an evidence of larval migration.

Figure 1.144 Postmortem photograph of the cecum of a horse. Note the presence of black dots on the mucosa, which are encysted small strongyles larvae (cyathostomes). This can be found incidentally on postmortem examination, as in this case. Cyathostomiasis is caused by small strongyles (cyathostomes) and typhlocolitis is usually precipitated by intramural larval stages, and sudden emergence of the encysted larvae triggers severe mucosal inflammation (figs. 1.145 and 1.146). In the northern temperate zones, it is usually seen in the late winter or early spring; in the southern temperate zones, it occurs in the fall or winter. Cyathostomiasis is usually associated with chronic diarrhea, but can cause severe acute diarrhea that becomes chronic. In addition to diarrhea, affected horses exhibit ill thrift and have a fever, weight loss, ventral edema, and intermittent mild episodes of abdominal pain. Appetite is usually normal. Diagnosis is based on clinical signs, the presence of hypoalbuminemia, and histopathological examination of cecal and ascending colon biopsies. Fecal analysis might be unrewarding.

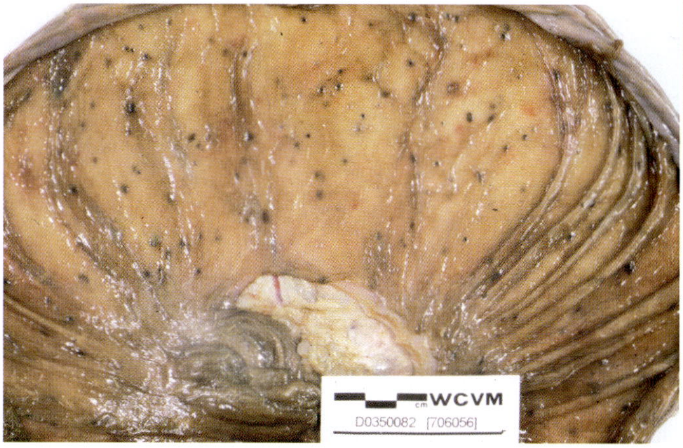

Figures 1.145–1.146 Postmortem photograph of the large colon of a horse affected with typhlocolitis caused by cyathostomes. Note the thickened, edematous colon with the encysted larvae (black dots) embedded in the intestinal wall.

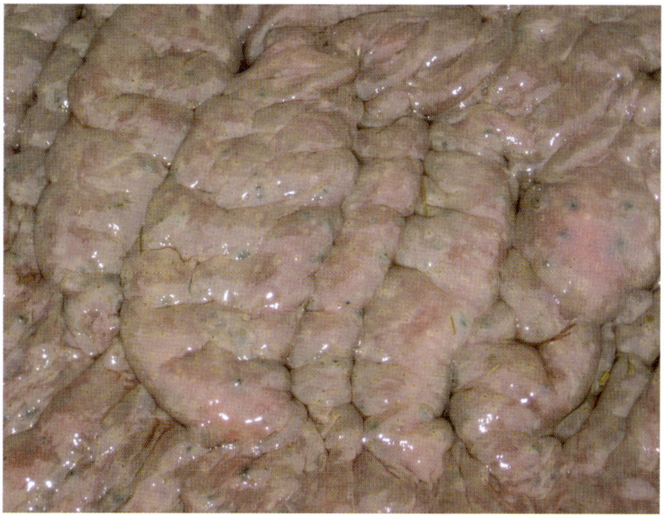

1.145

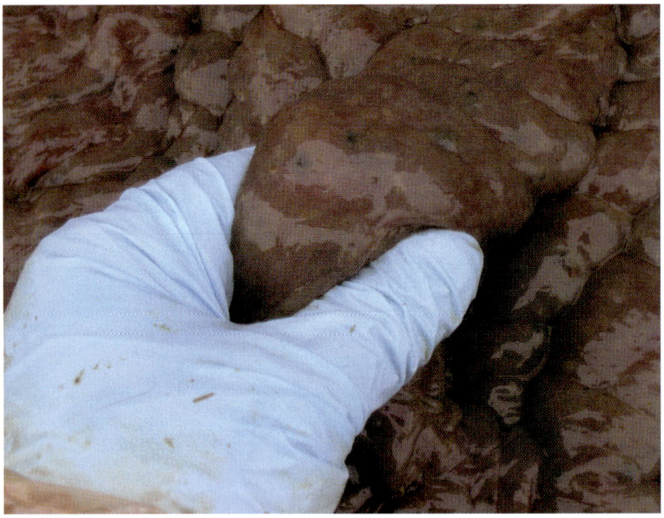

1.146

Figures 1.145–1.146 *Continued*

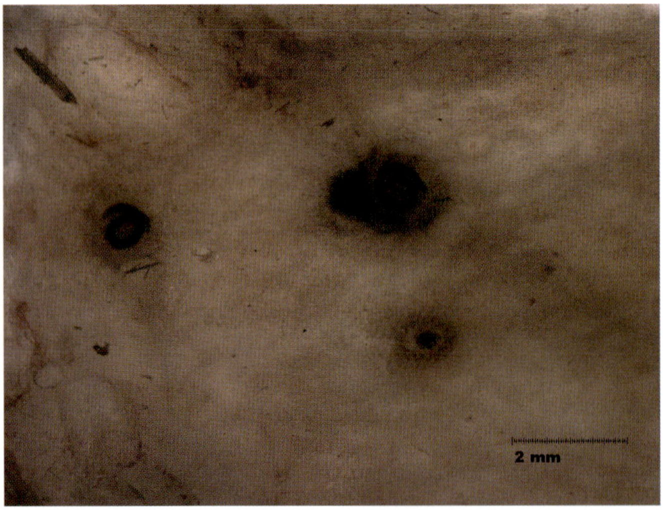

1.147

Figures 1.147–1.148 Microscopic examination of the encysted larvae (black mucosal dots) in the intestinal mucosa seen in fig. 1.144.

Figures 1.147–1.148 *Continued*

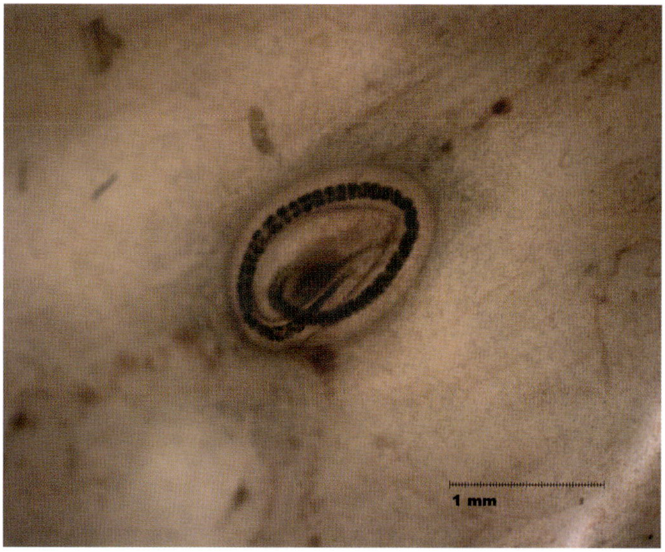

1.148

Nonsteroidal Anti-inflammatory Drugs (NSAIDs) Toxicity

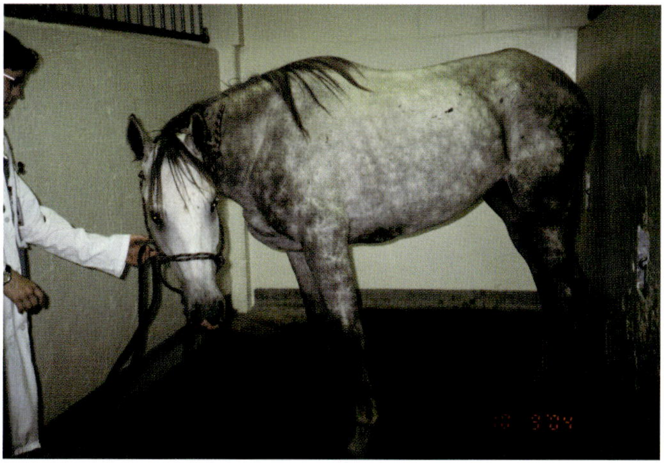

Figure 1.149 An adult horse affected with NSAIDs toxicity. Note the weight loss and ventral edema. Toxicity with NSAIDs can cause GI and renal disease. All NSAIDs can invariably cause toxicity, but phenylbutazone is the drug that is commonly reported to cause toxicity in horses. Overdose or dosage error are the common scenario, however, toxicity has been reported in horses that have been administered the correct dose. Clinical signs include generalized ulceration of the GI tract, starting from the mouth (fig. 1.150), colitis (right dorsal colitis) (fig. 1.151), anorexia, colic, depression, fever, diarrhea, weight loss (protein losing enteropathy), endotoxemia, hypoproteinemia, and ventral and peripheral edema (figs. 1.152 and 1.153). Horses might be presented with chronic clinical signs of mild recurrent colic and protein losing enteropathy. Diagnosis is based on history, clinical signs, ultrasonographic finding of thickened right dorsal colon (>0.5 cm) (fig. 1.154).

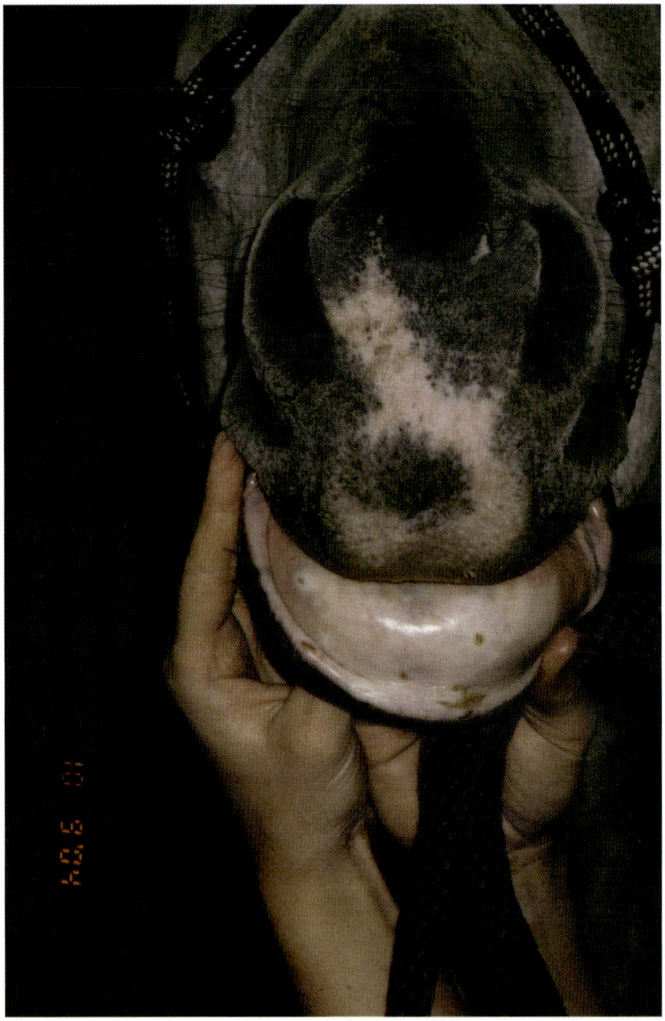

Figure 1.150 An adult horse affected with NSAIDs toxicity. Note the oral ulcers.

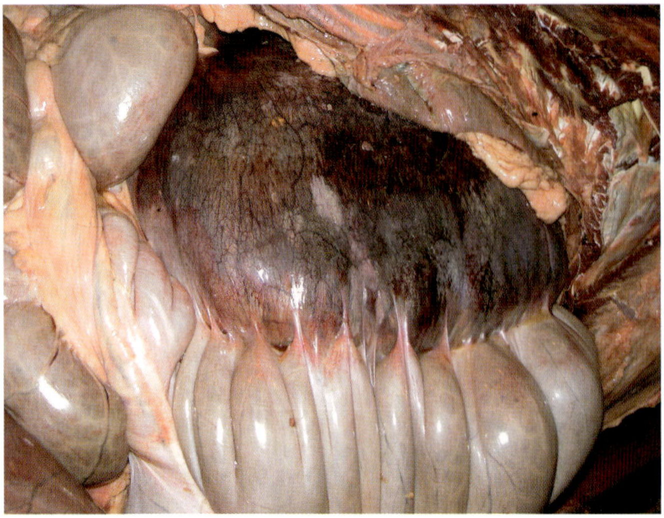

Figure 1.151 Postmortem examination of an adult horse affected with NSAIDs toxicity. Note the severe necrotic right dorsal colon.

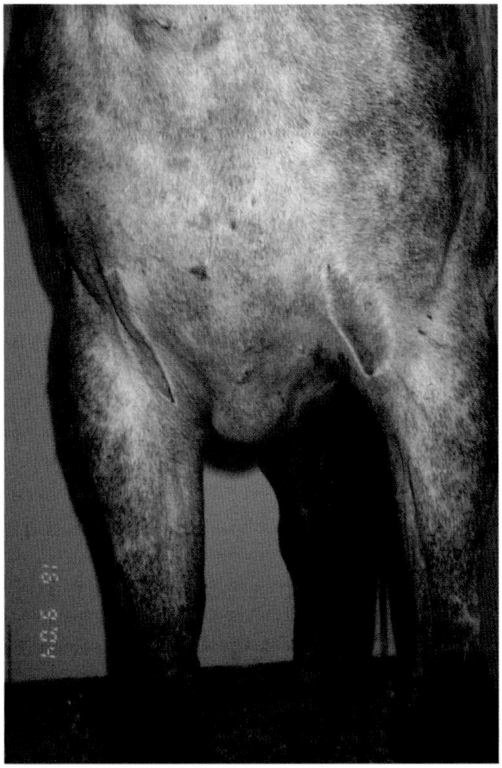

Figure 1.152 Brisket edema in an adult horse affected with NSAIDs toxicity.

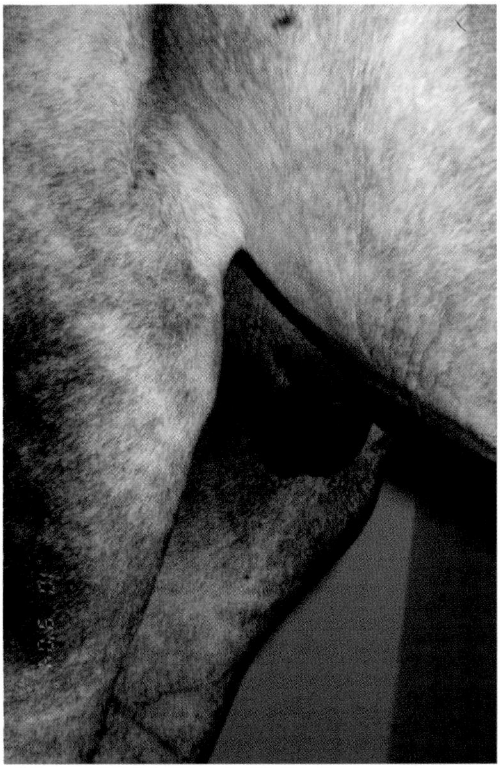

Figure 1.153 Preputial edema in an adult horse affected with NSAIDs toxicity.

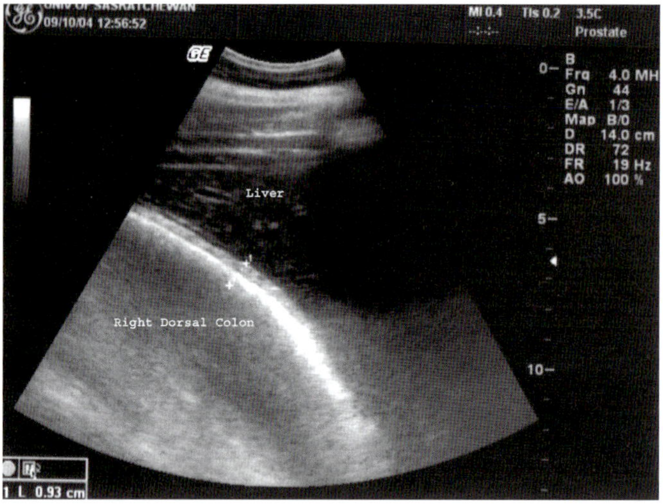

Figure 1.154 An ultrasonographic image of the right dorsal colon in an adult horse affected with NSAIDs toxicity. Note the thickened wall of the right dorsal colon. This figure was captured during ultrasonographic imaging of the right 11th to 14th intercostal spaces.

Grain (Carbohydrate) Overload

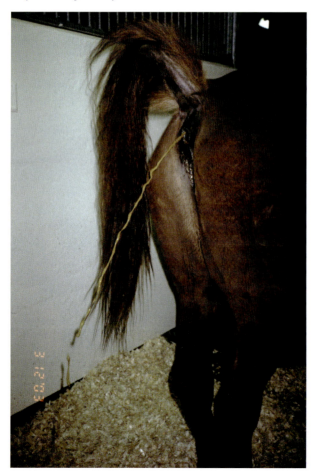

Figure 1.155 An adult horse with severe diarrhea due to grain overload. Grain overload results from feeding horses unusual amounts of grain (corn, barley, wheat). It can cause osmotic diarrhea and colitis. Clinical signs depend on the amount of grain ingested. Clinical signs are identical to those of enterocolitis and range from mild diarrhea to fatal enterocolitis and death. Other clinical signs include the presence of large amounts of undigested grain in the feces, colic, abdominal distention, depression, dehydration, and signs of endotoxemia and laminitis (fig. 1.156). Diagnosis is based on history, clinical signs, the presence of hypocalcemia and metabolic acidosis.

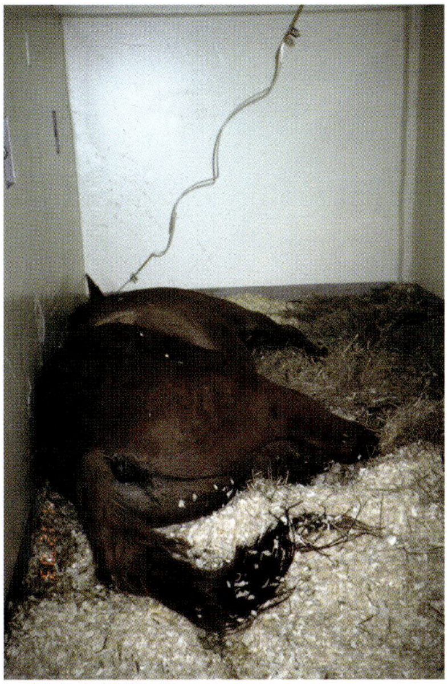

Figure 1.156 The same horse seen in fig. 1.155 after he developed laminitis. The horse had severe and painful laminitis due to which he spent a lot of time laying down.

Small Colon Impaction

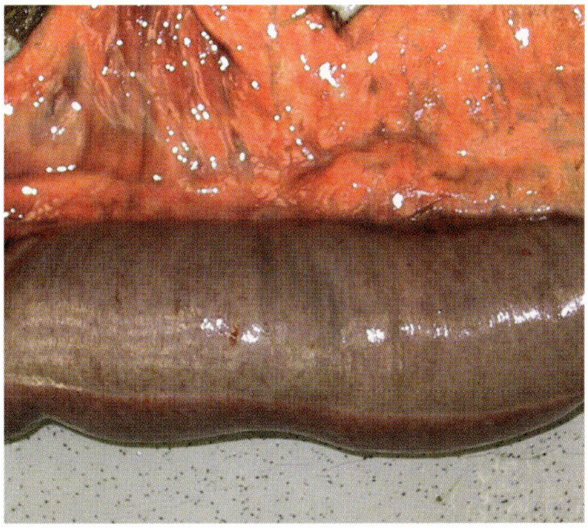

a

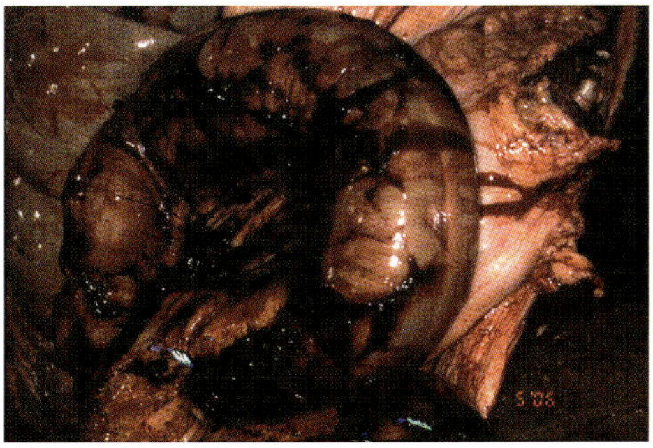

b

Figures 1.157a,b Postmortem photographs of a horse with small colon impaction. It is the most common abnormal condition of the small colon. The small colon gets impacted with firm ingesta. It occurs usually in the fall and winter. Salmonella is implicated as the cause of small colon impaction. Medical treatment includes aggressive IV fluid therapy and judicious use of analgesics and oral laxatives. Severe surgical intervention is indicated if no improvement is noticed, or if the affected horse becomes progressively painful and develops severe abdominal distension.

Intraluminal Obstruction of the Small Colon with Enteroliths, Fecaliths, or Foreign Bodies

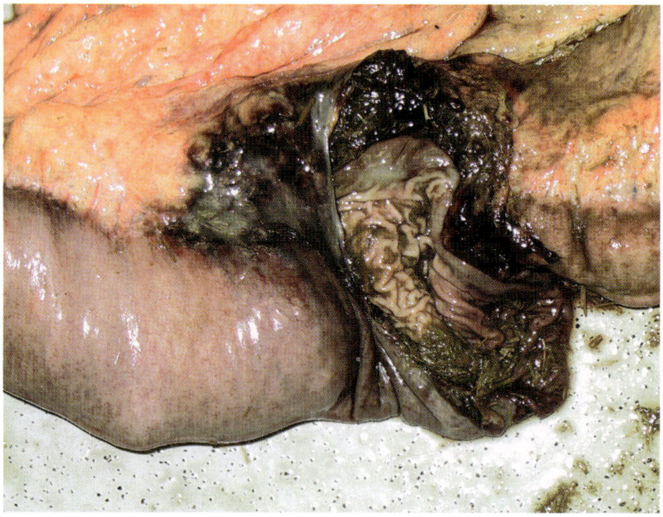

Figure 1.158 Postmortem photographs of a horse with small colon rupture as a result of a foreign body; this is a known complication. Fecaliths (inspissated feces), enteroliths (fig. 1.159), and foreign bodies can lodge in the small colon and cause secondary backup of ingesta and small colon impaction. Fecaliths causing small colon impaction are more common in miniature horses and are thought to be caused by feeding coarse forage.

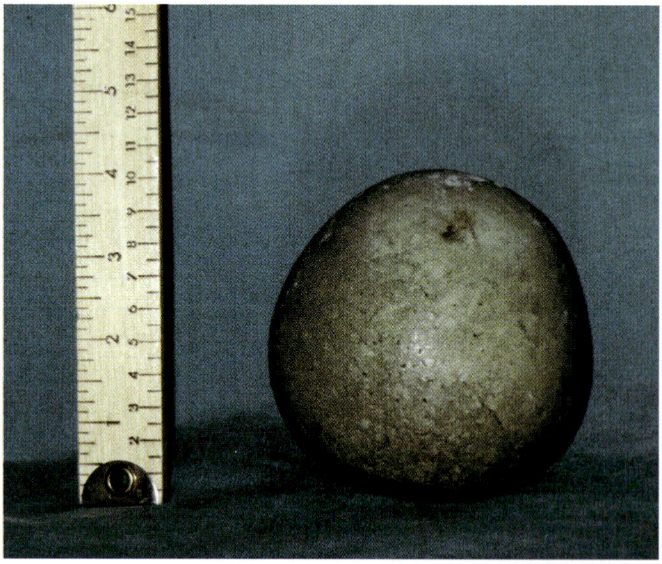

Figure 1.159 A photograph of an enterolith. Enteroliths are more common in the Arabian breed. It is usually seen in the southwestern United States and California. Abdominal radiography may aid in the diagnosis of obstructive enterolith.

Idiopathic Inflammatory Bowel Disease (Granulomatous Enteritis, Basophilic Enterocolitis, Lymphocytic-Plasmocytic Enterocolitis, Multisystemic Eosinophilic Epitheliotropic Disease, and Idiopathic Eosinophilic Enterocolitis)

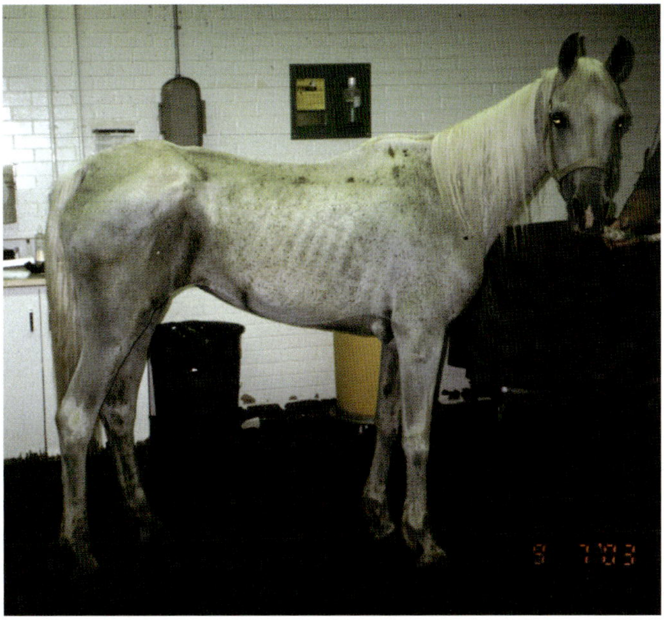

Figure 1.160 A horse affected with idiopathic inflammatory bowel disease (basophilic enterocolitis). Note the severe weight loss. Affected horses are usually presented with weight loss, ill thrift, diarrhea (fig. 1.161) and hypoproteinemia.

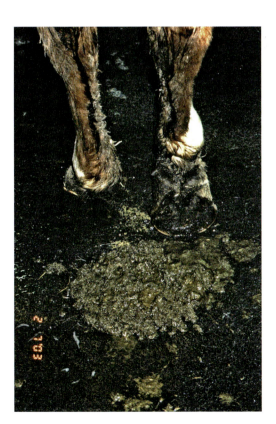

Figure 1.161 A horse affected with idiopathic inflammatory bowel disease. Note the loose feces (cow-pie-like diarrhea).

Antibiotic Induced Colitis

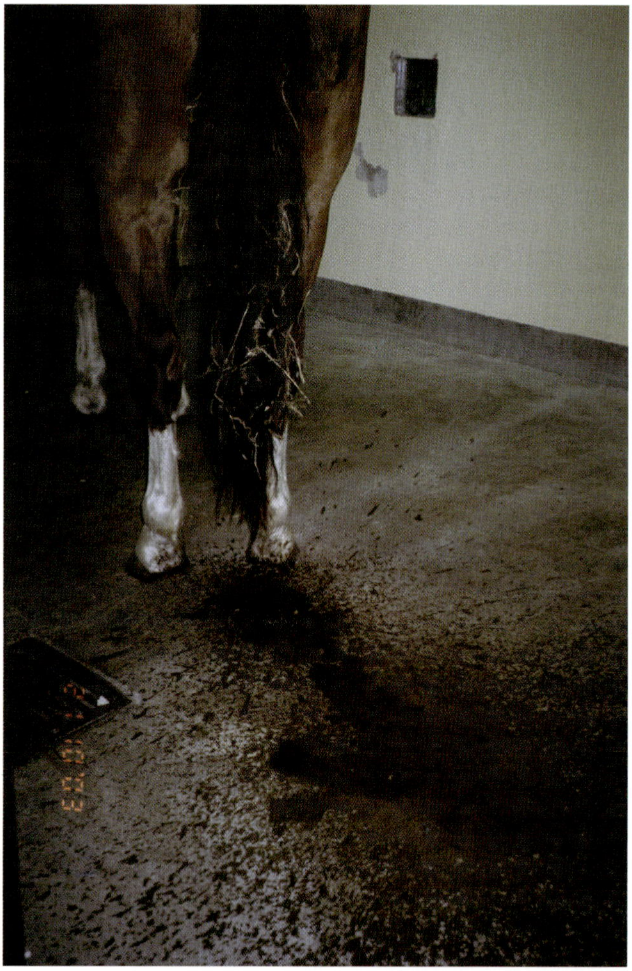

Figure 1.162 A horse affected with antibiotic induced colitis. Note the watery diarrhea. Clinical signs are similar to those seen in colitis caused by different reasons. Clinical signs include diarrhea, fever, and endotoxemia. Antibiotic induced colitis can be caused by treatment with most antibiotics and is suspected to be bacterial in origin.

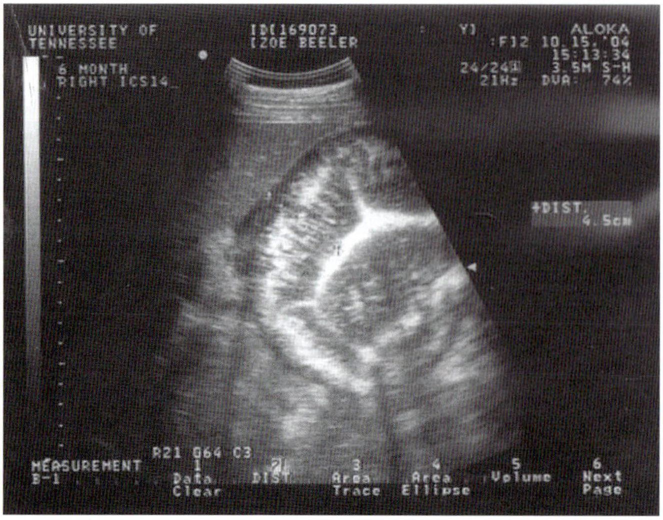

Figure 1.163 Ultrasonographic image of the right dorsal colon of a 6-month-old foal with antibiotic induced colitis. Dorsal is to the left. A small piece of the liver is visible on the left side of the image. The right dorsal colon with tremendous edema is visible on the right. Thickened large colon is usually seen on ultrasonography in cases of colitis.

Abdominal Abscessation

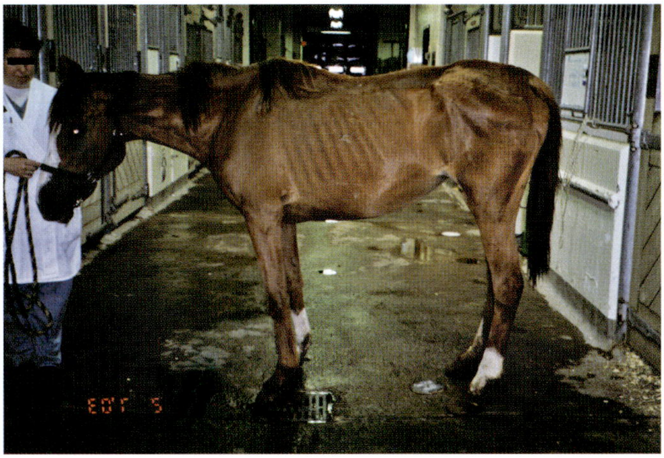

Figure 1.164 An adult horse affected with abdominal abscessation. Note the severe weight loss. Abdominal abscessation occurs as a sequel to respiratory infection, peritonitis, foaling accidents, foreign body penetration of the small intestine, verminous arteritis, umbilical infections, and septicemia. Clinical signs include anorexia, depression, weight loss, and intermittent colic.

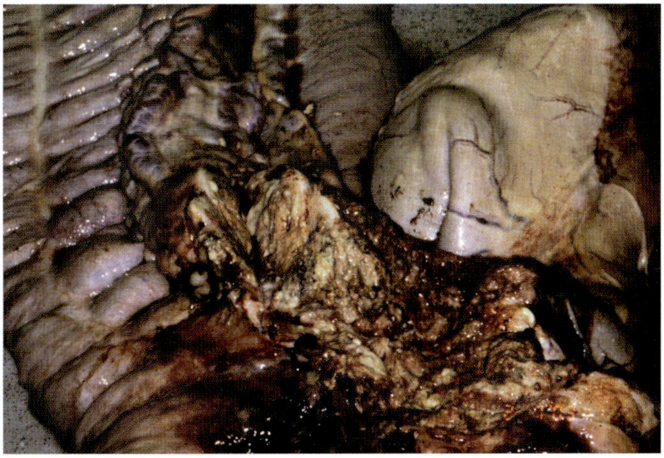

Figure 1.165 Postmortem examination of an adult horse affected with abdominal abscessation. Most abdominal abscesses occur in or around the mesentery.

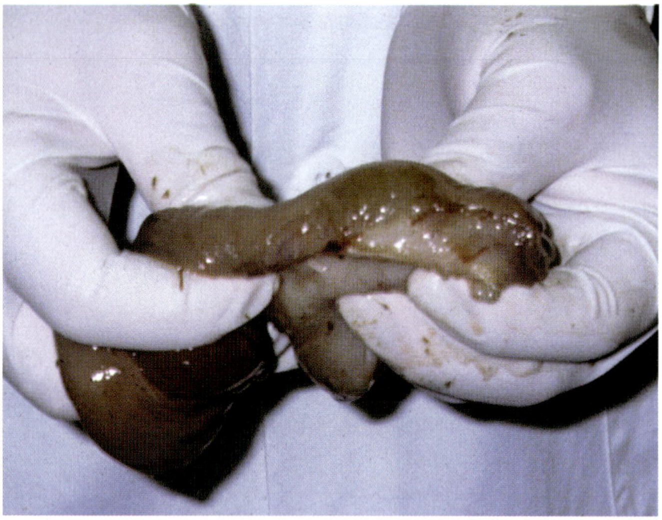

Figure 1.166 Thickened large colon in a horse affected by abdominal abscessations that were pinging on the lymphatic vessels; this resulted in edematous and thickened intestines.

Abdominal Adhesions

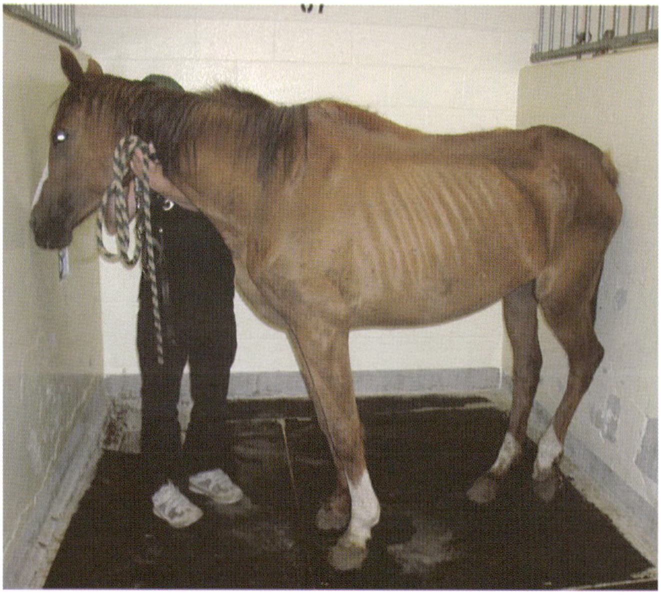

Figure 1.167 An adult horse with severe weight loss caused by abdominal adhesions. Abdominal adhesions usually occur secondary to inflammatory and traumatic injuries to the intestine. It is also seen in horses that have had exploratory laparotomy and reproductive surgeries. Clinical signs include colic due to intestinal obstruction, chronic weight loss, and sometimes soft feces (diarrhea) as in fig. 1.168.

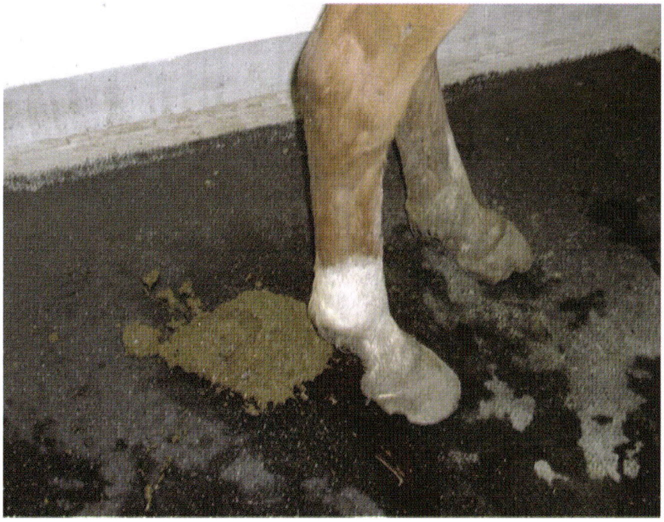

Figure 1.168 An adult horse with abdominal adhesions. Note the diarrhea and "cow pie feces."

Peritonitis

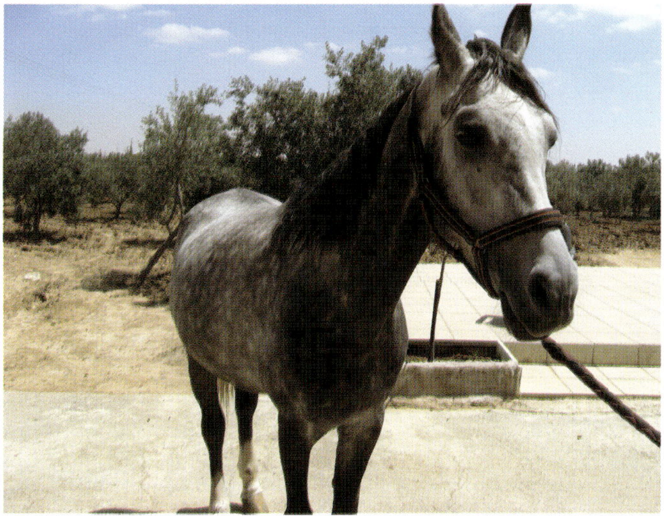

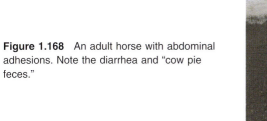

Figure 1.169 An adult horse affected with peritonitis. Although the abdomen seems full, the horse has lost weight. Depending on the cause, peritonitis can be localized or diffuse, septic or nonseptic, primary or secondary. Primary causes include intestinal or gastric rupture, abdominal abscess rupture, and leakage of bacteria to the abdomen from an infected uterus in postpartum mares. Usually it is diffuse and caused by contamination with intestinal bacteria. Clinical signs are variable depending on the primary cause and disease duration. They include depression, anorexia, fever, reluctance to move, splinting of the abdomen, and sensitivity to external pressure, colic, weight loss, signs of intestinal ileus, and endotoxemia. Cases with peracute peritonitis may die in hours. The disease is confirmed by abdominocentesis (figs. 1.170 and 1.171). Abdominal ultrasonography is also helpful in the diagnosis (figs. 1.172 and 1.173).

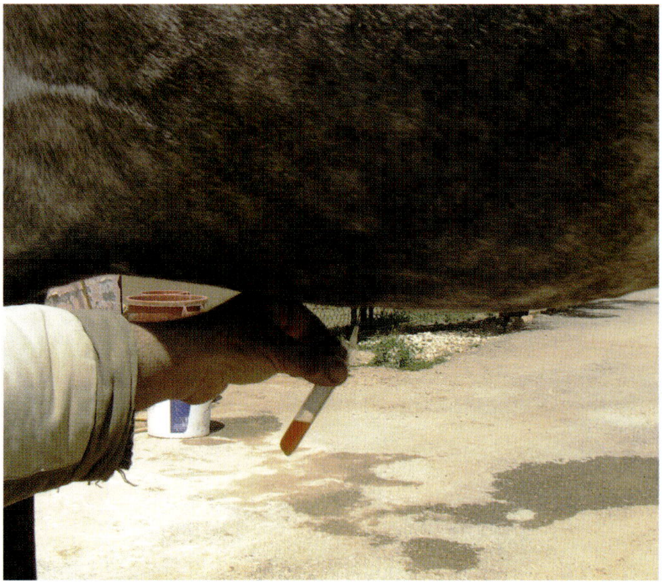

Figure 1.170 Abdominocentesis in a horse affected with peritonitis. Note the serosanguinous abdominal fluid. Normal peritoneal fluid is clear and straw-colored and has low protein content. In case of peritonitis, the fluid is usually cloudy and blood tinged (serosanguinous). Peritonitis cannot be diagnosed based on the gross appearance of the peritoneal fluid, and microscopic (cytological) examination of the fluid should be done.

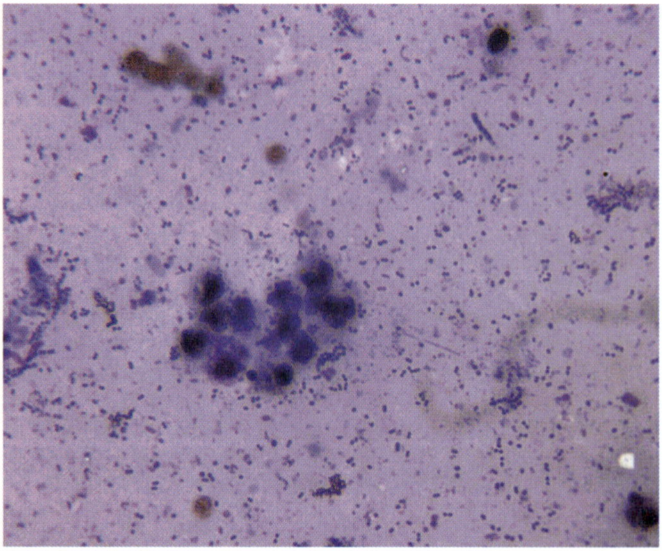

Figure 1.171 Microscopic (cytological) examination of a smear made from peritoneal fluid of a horse with diffuse peritonitis secondary to intestinal rupture. Note the presence of bacteria in the cytoplasm of the neutrophils.

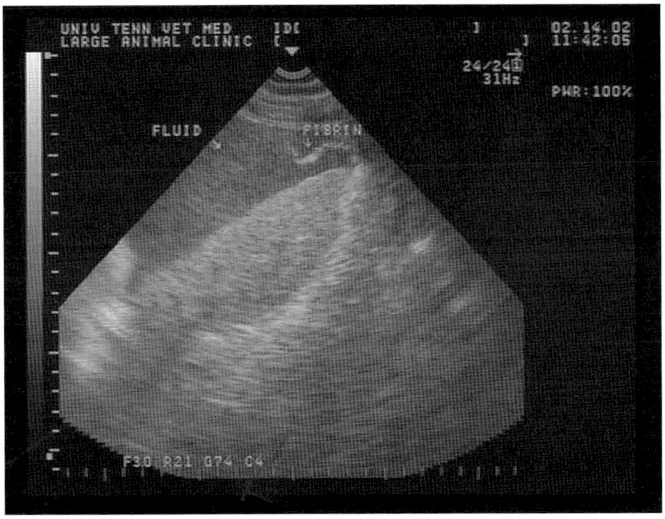

Figure 1.172 Ultrasonographic image of the abdomen in a horse affected with peritonitis (dorsal is to the left). Note the cellular fluid and fibrin tag.

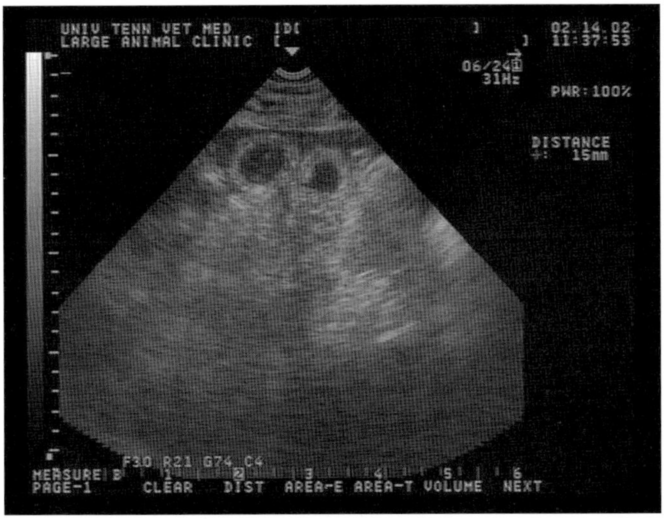

Figure 1.173 Ultrasonographic image of the abdomen in a horse affected with peritonitis (dorsal is to the left). Note the thickened small intestine shown on the top of the picture, surrounded by cellular fluid.

Enterocutaneous Fistula and Parietal (Richter's) Hernia

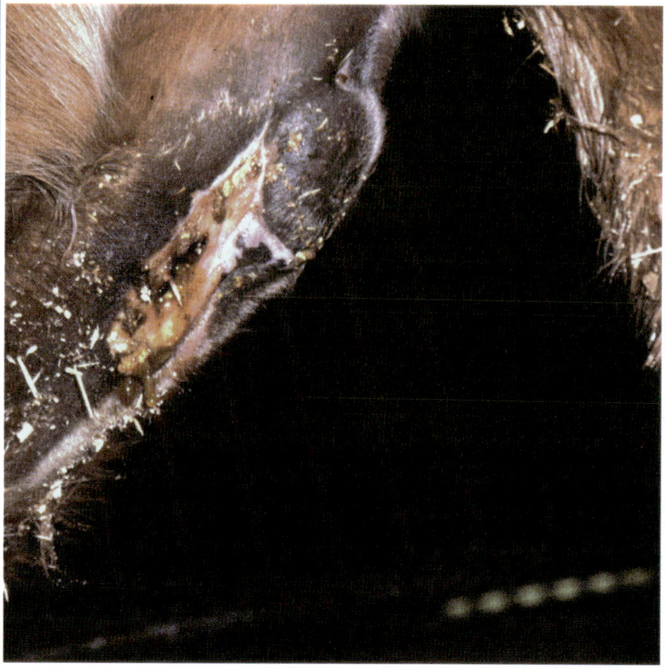

Figure 1.174a Enterocutaneous fistula in a horse as a sequela to parietal (Richter's) hernia. Note the drainage of digesta from the fistula. Parietal or Richter's hernia occurs when the small intestinal (ileum) incarceration, in case of umbilical hernia (fig. 1.174b), involves only a portion of the antimesenteric wall.

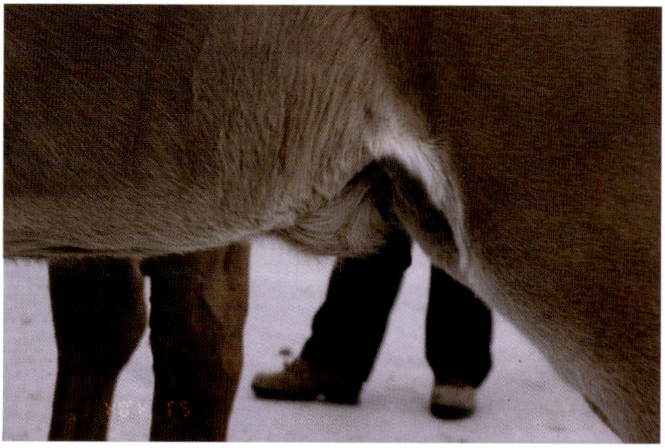

Figure 1.174b Umbilical hernia in a foal.

Omental Hernia

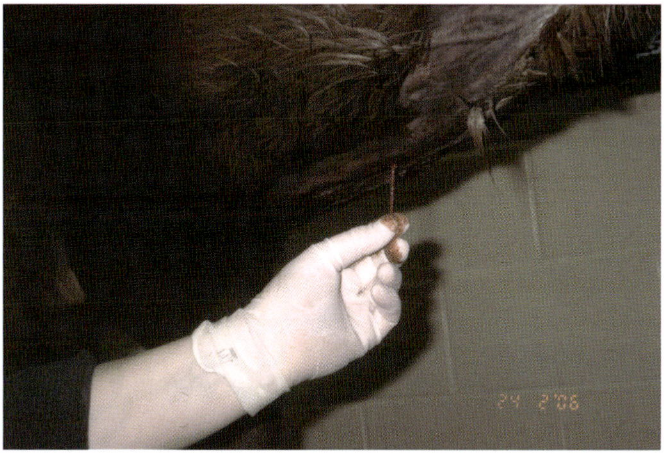

Figure 1.175 Omental hernia in a foal. It usually occurs subsequent to abdominocentesis using a teat cannula in a small percentage of foals. This is usually a benign complication. The prolapsed part of the omentum should be cut close to the skin.

Grass Sickness (Equine Dysautonomia)

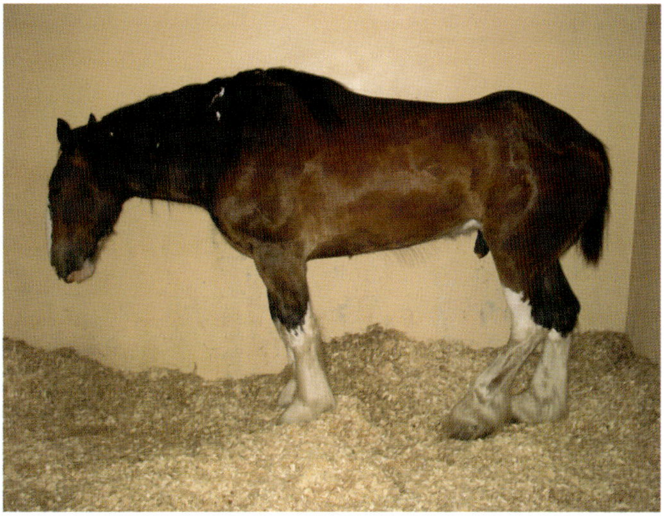

Figure 1.176 An adult horse affected with grass sickness. Note the dullness and weight loss. Grass sickness is a disease of unknown etiology. It is reported in Europe and Australia. A similar disease, *mal seco*, has been reported in Argentina and southern Chile. The disease is sporadic and often fatal. Grass sickness is an acquired degenerative neuropathy that mainly affects the autonomic and enteric nervous system. It has three clinical forms: acute, subacute, and chronic forms. Clinical signs of the three forms overlap from one form to the other. Clinical signs include depression, dullness, fever, "tucked up" appearance (fig. 1.177), weight loss, dysphagia (fig. 1.178), signs of intestinal ileus and large colon impaction (fig. 1.179), nasogastric reflux, abdominal pain (fig. 1.180), piloerection (fig. 1.181), patchy sweating (fig. 1.182), muscle fasciculation, rhinitis sicca (figs. 1.183 and 1.184), gait abnormalities, narrow base stance, leaning against the walls (fig. 1.185), ptosis (fig. 1.186), pica, and penile prolapse and paralysis (fig. 1.187). Antemortem diagnosis of grass sickness can be confirmed only by histological examination of ileal biopsy obtained via laparotomy. There is no curative treatment for grass sickness. (Image courtesy of Dr. R. Scott Pirie, University of Edinburgh, Scotland)

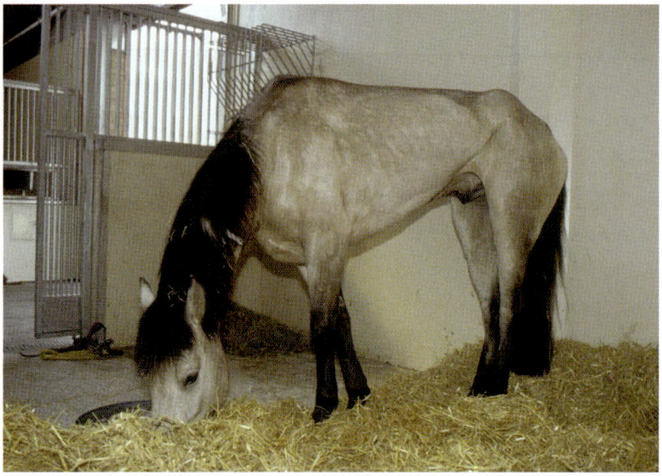

Figure 1.177 A "tucked up" appearance and weight loss in a horse affected with grass sickness. (Image courtesy of Dr. R. Scott Pirie, University of Edinburgh, Scotland)

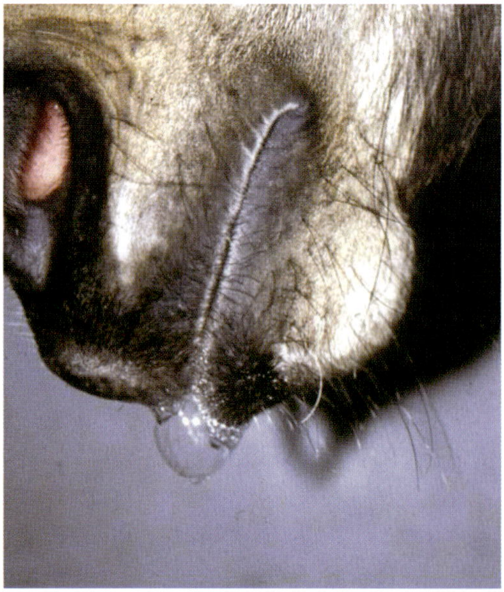

Figure 1.178 Drooling of saliva and dysphagia in a horse affected with grass sickness. (Image courtesy of Dr. R. Scott Pirie, University of Edinburgh, Scotland)

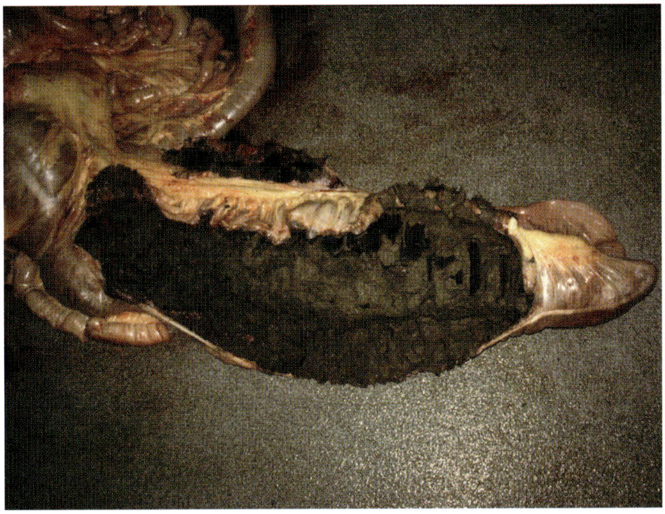

Figure 1.179 Large colon impaction found during postmortem examination of a horse affected with grass sickness. (Image courtesy of Dr. R. Scott Pirie, University of Edinburgh, Scotland)

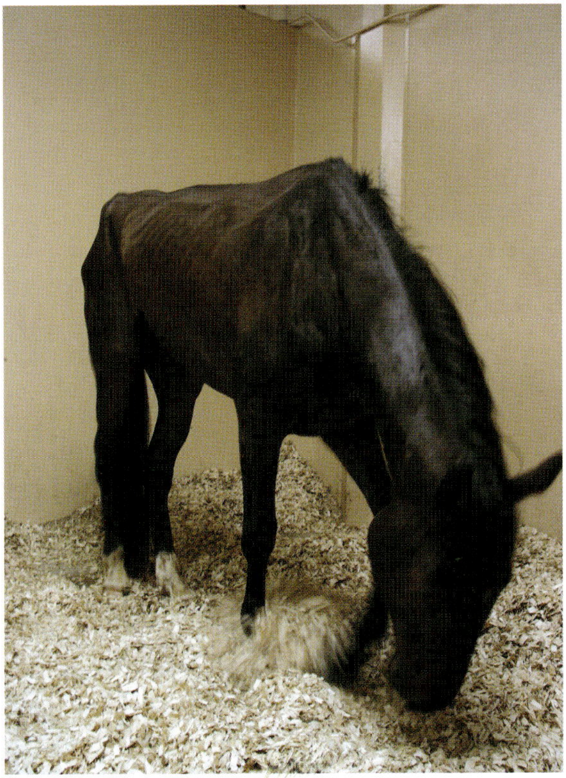

Figure 1.180 Abdominal pain (colic) in a horse affected with grass sickness. (Image courtesy of Dr. R. Scott Pirie, University of Edinburgh, Scotland)

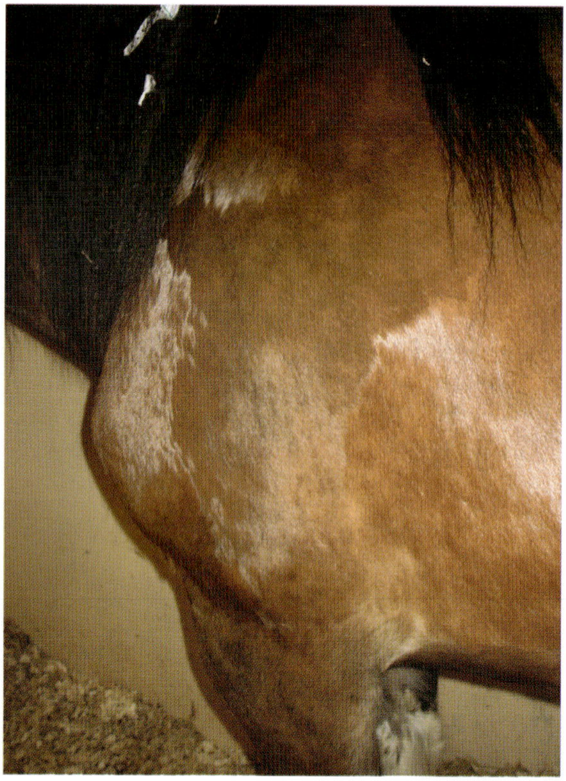

Figure 1.181 Piloerection (erection of hair) in a horse affected with grass sickness. (Image courtesy of Dr. R. Scott Pirie, University of Edinburgh, Scotland)

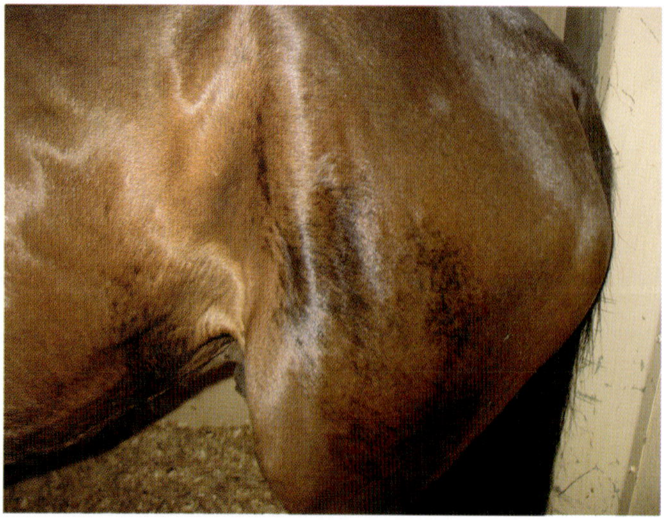

Figure 1.182 Patchy sweating in a horse affected with grass sickness. (Image courtesy of Dr. R. Scott Pirie, University of Edinburgh, Scotland)

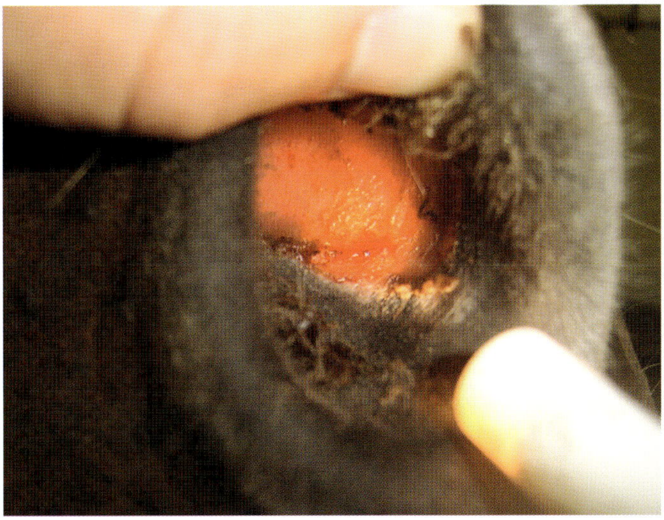

Figure 1.183 Rhinitis sicca in a horse affected with grass sickness. (Image courtesy of Dr. R. Scott Pirie, University of Edinburgh, Scotland)

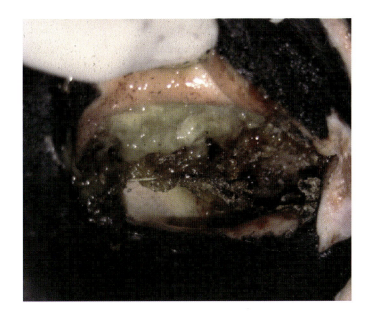

Figure 1.184 Rhinitis sicca in a horse affected with grass sickness. Note the accumulation of mucopurulent material in the nasal passages. (Image courtesy of Dr. R. Scott Pirie, University of Edinburgh, Scotland)

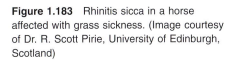

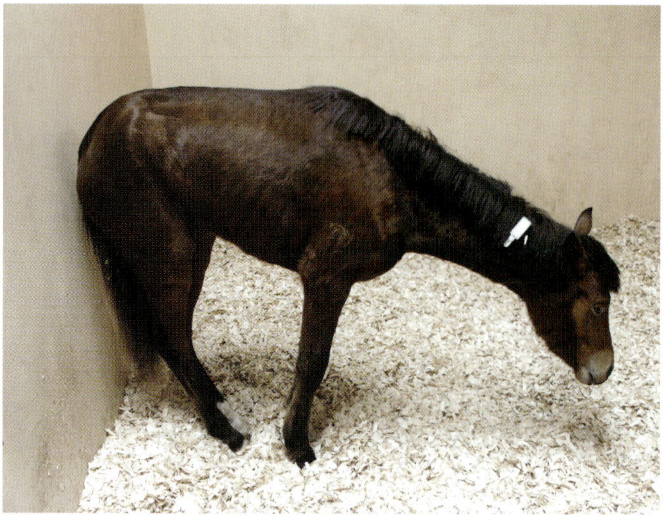

Figure 1.185 Narrow base stance and leaning against the walls in a horse affected with grass sickness. (Image courtesy of Dr. R. Scott Pirie, University of Edinburgh, Scotland)

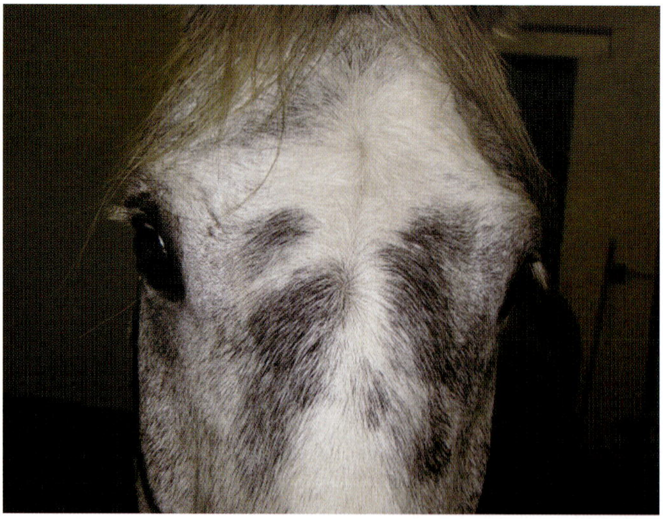

Figure 1.186 Ptosis (droopy upper eyelid), in a horse affected with grass sickness. (Image courtesy of Dr. R. Scott Pirie, University of Edinburgh, Scotland)

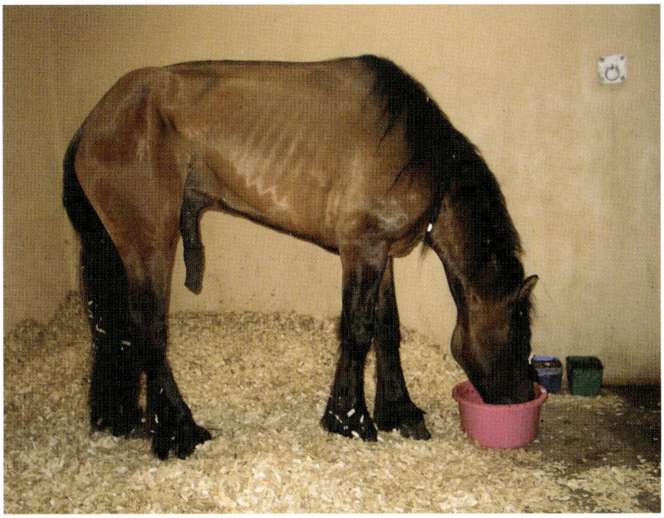

Figure 1.187 Penile prolapse and paralysis in a horse affected with grass sickness. (Image courtesy of Dr. R. Scott Pirie, University of Edinburgh, Scotland)

HYPERLIPEMIA AND HYPERLIPIDEMIA

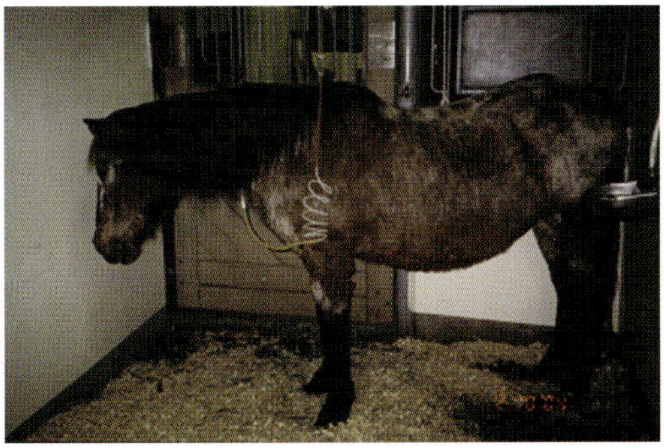

Figure 1.188 Hyperlipemia in a pony. Note the depression. Hyperlipemia/hyperlipidemia is caused by negative energy balance. The disease is mainly seen in ponies. It is characterized by serum triglyceride elevation. In hyperlipidemia, serum triglyceride elevation is up to 500 mg/dL, while it is much over that in cases of hyperlipemia. In cases of hyperlipemia, which is much more severe than hyperlipidemia, the plasma is milky and hepatic lipidosis is present (fig. 1.189). Clinical signs of hyperlipemia include anorexia, depression, weakness, icterus (fig. 1.190), and incoordination. Fatty and swollen liver is usually seen on postmortem examination (fig. 1.191).

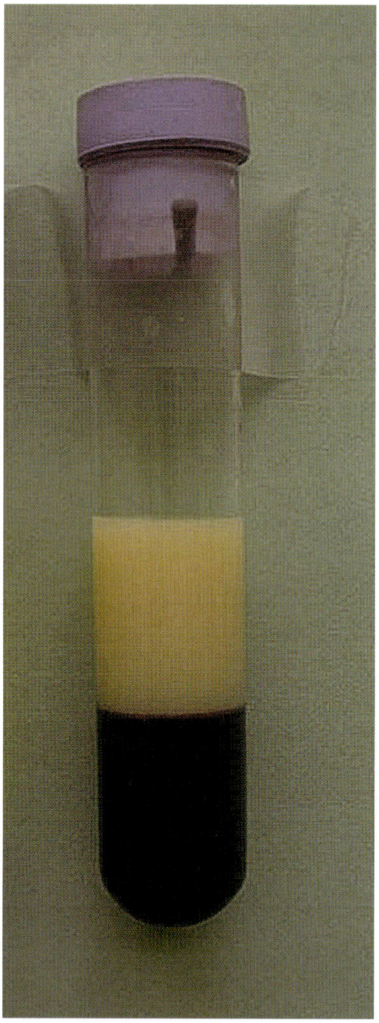

Figure 1.189 Milky plasma in a pony affected with hyperlipemia.

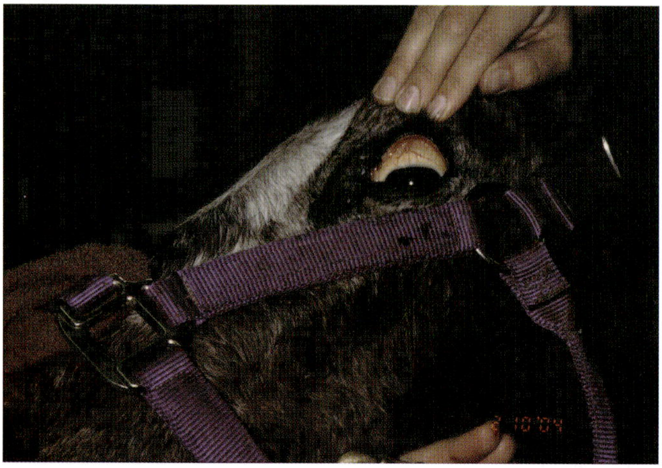

Figure 1.190 Icteric mucous membranes of a pony affected with hyperlipemia.

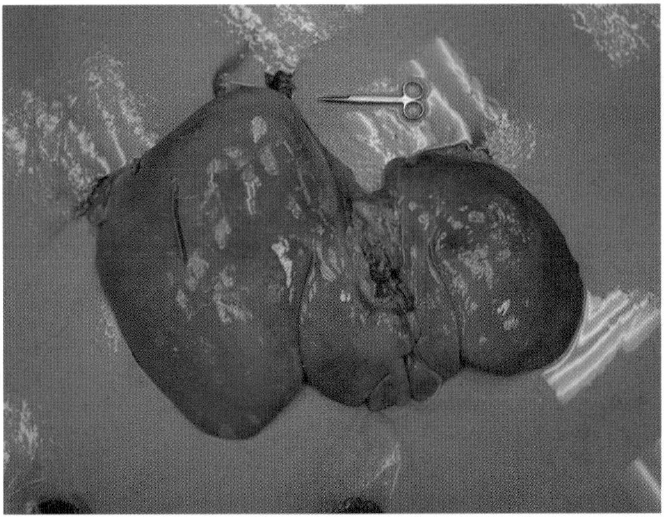

Figure 1.191 Fatty and swollen liver obtained during postmortem examination from a pony affected with hyperlipemia.

RECOMMENDED READINGS

Abutarbush SM. Dysphagia in horses. Large Animal Veterinary Rounds 4(2), 2004.

Abutarbush SM. Use of ultrasonography to diagnose large colon volvulus in horses. J Am Vet Med Assoc. 228(3):409–13, 2006.

Abutarbush SM, Carmalt JL. Endoscopy and arthroscopy for the equine practitioner. Made Easy Series. Jackson, WY: Teton NewMedia, 2008.

Abutarbush SM, et al. Clinical West Nile virus infection in 2 horses in western Canada. Can Vet J. 45(4):315–17, 2004.

Abutarbush SM, Carmalt JL, Shoemaker RW. Causes of gastrointestinal colic in horses in western Canada: 604 cases (1992–2002). Can Vet J. 46:800–805, 2005.

Abutarbush SM, Naylor JM. Comparison of surgical versus medical treatment of nephrosplenic entrapment of the large colon in horses: 19 cases (1992–2002). J Am Vet Med Assoc. 227:603–5, 2005.

Abutarbush SM, Shoemaker RW, Bailey JV. Strangulation of small intestines by a mesodiverticular band in 3 adult horses. Can Vet J. 44(12):1005–6, 2003.

Alder HA, Arey LB, Barr ML, et al. Dorland's illustrated medical dictionary, 24th ed. Philadelphia: WB Saunders Co, 1965.

Baum KH, Halpern NE, Banish LD, Modransky PD. Dysphagia in horses: the differential diagnosis—part II. Compendium Contin Educ Pract Vet. 10(12):1405–10, 1988.

Baum KH, Modransky PD, Halpern NE, Banish LD. Dysphagia in horses: the differential diagnosis-part I. Compendium Contin Educ Pract Vet. 10(11):1301–7, 1988.

Brown CM. Problems in equine medicine. Philadelphia: Lea & Febiger, 67–80, 1989.

Burba DJ, Moor RM. Renosplenic entrapment: a review of clinical presentation and treatment. Equine Vet Educ. 9:180–84, 1997.

Cohen ND. Neurologic evaluation of the equine head and neurogenic dysphagia. Vet Clin North Am Eq Pract. 9(1):231–40, 1993.

Craig DR, Shivy DR, Pankowski, Erb HN. Esophageal disorders in 61 horses results of nonsurgical and surgical management. Vet Surg. 18(6):432–43, 1989.

Dart AJ, Snyder JR, Pasco JR, Farver TB, Galuppo LD. Abnormal conditions of the equine descending (small) colon: 102 cases (1979–1989). J Am Vet Med Assoc. 200:971–78, 1992.

Edwards GB. Duodenitis-proximal jejunitis (anterior enteritis) as a surgical problem. Eq Vet Edu. 12:411–14, 2000.

Greet T. Dysphagia in the horse. In Practice 11(6):256–62, 1989.

Hance SR, Noble J, Holcomb S, Rush-Moore B, Beeard W. Treating choke with oxytocin. Am Assoc Eq Pract Proceedings 43:338–39, 1997.

Heath SE, Artsob H, Bell RJ, Harland RJ. Equine encephalitis caused by snowshoe hare (California serogroup) virus. CVJ 30:669–71, 1989.

Hillyer M. Management of oesophageal obstruction ("choke") in horses. Practice 17(10):450–56, 1995.

Howarth S, Lane JG. Multiple cranial nerve deficits associated with auditory tube (guttural pouch) diverticulitis: three cases. Eq Vet Edu. 2(4):206–7, 1990.

Jones SL, Zimmel D, Tate LP, Campbell N, Redding WR, Carlson GP. Dysphagia caused by squamous cell carcinoma in two horses. Compendium Contin Educ Pract Vet. 23(11):1020–24, 2001.

Klohnen A, Vachon AM, Fischer AT, Jr. Use of diagnostic ultrasonography in horses with signs of acute abdominal pain. J Am Vet Med Assoc. 209(9):1597–601, 1996.

MacKay RJ. On the true definition of dysphagia. Compendium Contin Educ Pract Vet. 1988(11):1024–28, 2001.

Mair T, Divers T, Ducharme N. Manual of equine gastroenterology. London: WB Saunders, 63–67, 2002.

Modransky PD, Reed SM, Barbee DD. Dysphagia associated with guttural pouch empyema and dorsal displacement of the soft palate. Equine Practice 4(8):3–38, 1982.

Murray MJ, Smith BP. Diseases of the alimentary tract. In Smith BP, ed. Large animal internal medicine. 3rd ed. St Louis: Mosby, 593–789, 2002.

Pascoe R. Differential diagnosis of diseases of horses. University of Sydney Post Graduate Foundation in Veterinary Sciences, 190–95, 1994.

Radostits OM, Gay CC, Blood DC, et al. Diseases of the alimentary tract—1 Veterinary medicine: a textbook of the diseases of cattle, sheep, pigs, goats, and horses. 9th ed. London: WB Saunders, 169–258, 2000.

Swerczek TW. Toxicoinfectious botulism in foals and adult horses. JAVMA 176(3):217–20, 1980.

Wagner PC, Rantanen NW, Grant BD. Differential diagnosis of dysphagia in the horse. Modern Vet Pract. 60(12): 1029–33, 1979.

2 Diseases of the Cardiovascular System

Congenital Cardiac Defects
- Ventricular Septal Defect (VSD)
- Truncus Arteriosus
- Tetralogy of Fallot

Pericardial Diseases
- Pericarditis
- Neoplasia

Myocardial Diseases
- Cardiomyopathy
- Myocarditis
- Cor Pulmonale

Endocardial and Valvular Diseases
- Mitral Valve Insufficiency
- Aortic Valve Insufficiency
- Tricuspid Valve Insufficiency
- Endocarditis

Cardiac Arrhythmias
- Sinus Rhythm
- Atrioventricular Block
- Supraventricular Arrhythmias
- Atrial Fibrillation
- Ventricular Arrhythmias

Vascular Diseases
- Thrombosis and Thrombophlebitis
- Aortic Root Disease
- Purpura Hemorrhagica

Ventricular Septal Defect (VSD)

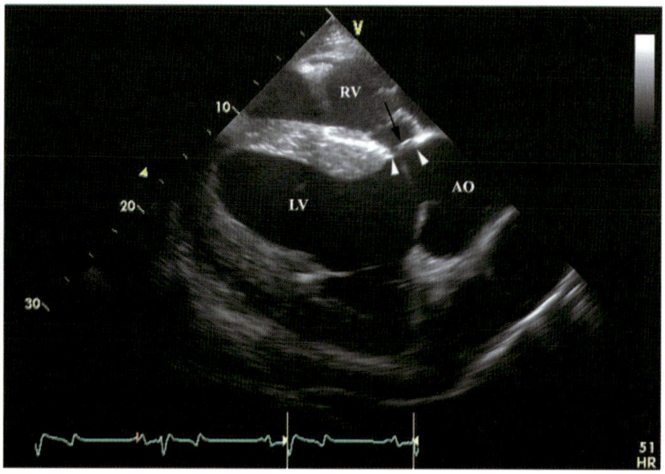

Figure 2.1 Membranous ventricular septal defect (VSD). Two-dimensional echocardiographic image of a 2-year-old Thoroughbred gelding with a history of poor racing performance. Note the defect in the interventricular septum just below the aortic valve (between arrowheads). An aortic valve cusp (arrow) prolapsed into the defect and occluded it partially. The membranous VSD is the most common congenital cardiac defect in the horse. There are two murmurs associated with a VSD: a grade 4-6/6 pansystolic coarse band shaped murmur (fig. 2.2) over the tricuspid valve. This is caused by flow through the defect. The second one is a grade 4-6/6 holosystolic crescendo decrescendo murmur over the pulmonic valve secondary to relative pulmonic stenosis. Outflow and muscular VSDs occur less commonly (figs. 2.3 and 2.4). A VSD should be measured in both the long and short axis views (figs. 2.5 and 2.6). Color flow Doppler can be used to confirm flow through the defect (fig. 2.7). The velocity of the jet should be obtained using continuous wave Doppler (fig. 2.8). LV, left ventricle; RV, right ventricle; AO, aorta.

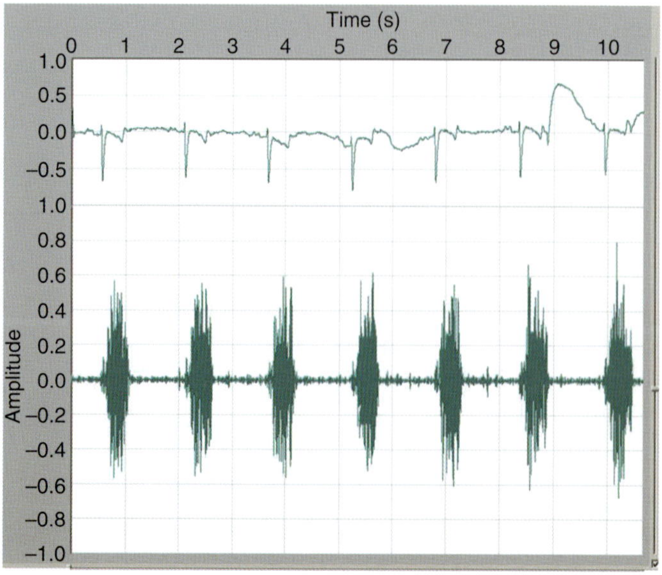

Figure 2.2 Phonocardiogram from horse in fig. 2.1 showing pansystolic band shaped murmur recorded over tricuspid valve.

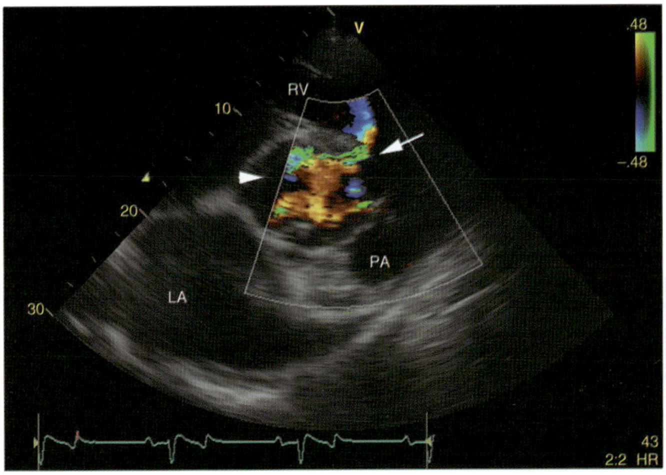

Figure 2.3 Outflow (supracristal) ventricular septal defect (VSD). Color flow Doppler image of an outflow VSD (between arrows), right parasternal short axis view of aorta. PA, pulmonary artery; RV, right ventricle; LA, left atrium.

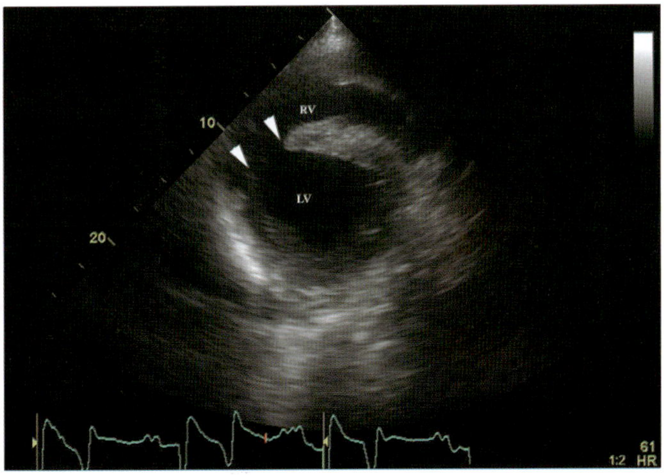

Figure 2.4 Muscular ventricular septal defect (VSD). Two-dimensional echocardiographic image of an apical muscular VSD (between arrows) obtained from right parasternal short axis view of left ventricle (LV). Muscular VSDs can occur as single or multiple defects ("Swiss cheese septum") or in combination with complex cardiac defects. Small muscular VSDs may spontaneously close. RV, right ventricle; LV, left ventricle.

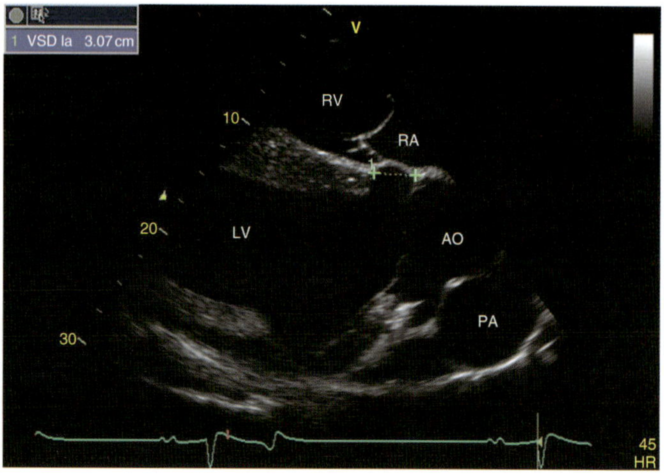

Figure 2.5 Echocardiographic image of a membranous ventricular septal defect (VSD) measured in the right parasternal long axis view of the left ventricular outflow tract. Small VSDs measure <2.5 cm and have velocities >4 m/sec (fig. 2.8). Horses with small defects have an excellent prognosis for a normal life expectancy and a good prognosis for athletic activity such as racing. Medium defects measure 2.5–3.5 cm and large defects are >3.5 cm. Horses with large defects rarely live beyond 5 years of age. LV, left ventricle; AO, aorta; PA, pulmonary artery; RV, right ventricle; RA, right atrium.

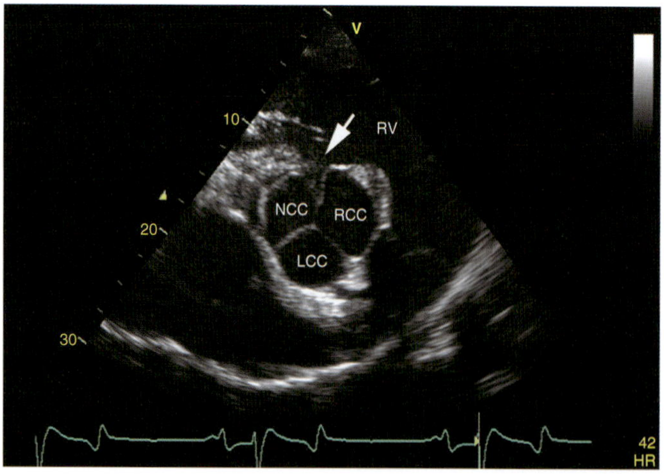

Figure 2.6 Echocardiographic image of ventricular septal defect (VSD) from the right parasternal short axis view of the aorta. Note the defect in the septum seen between the right coronary cusp (RCC) and noncoronary cusp (NCC) of the aortic valve. RV, right ventricle; LCC, left coronary cusp of aortic valve; RCC, right coronary cusp of aortic valve; NCC, noncoronary cusp (NCC).

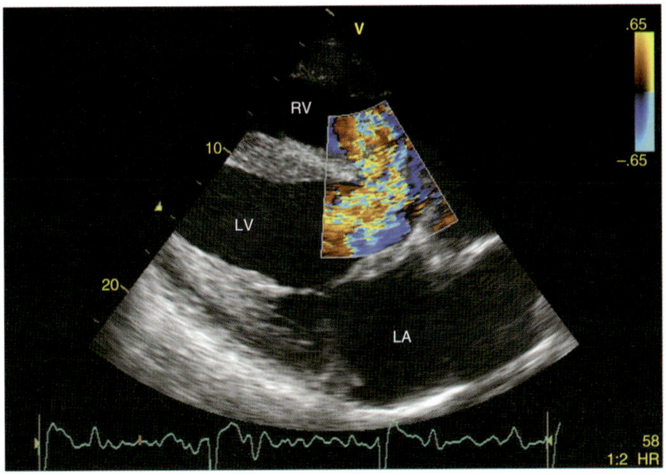

Figure 2.7 Color flow Doppler image of ventricular septal defect (VSD). Notice the turbulent flow through the septal defect. LA, left atrium; LV, left ventricle; RV, right ventricle.

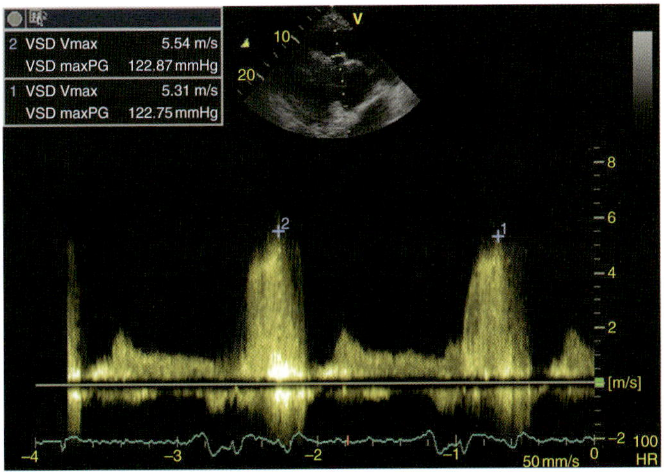

Figure 2.8 Continuous wave Doppler image of flow through VSD. Velocities greater than 4 m/sec are consistent with a small, restrictive VSD.

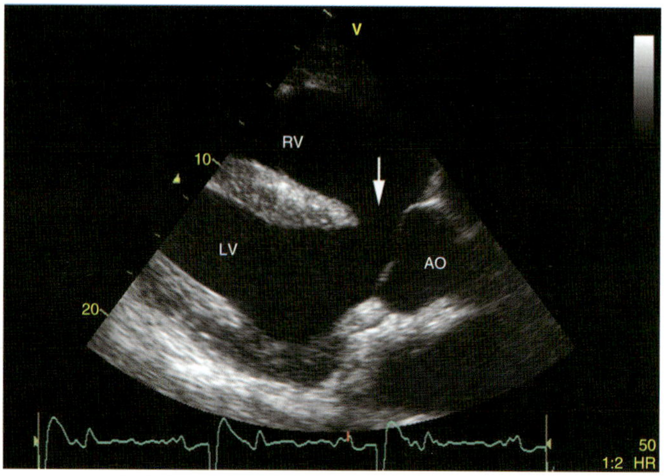

Figure 2.9 Echocardiographic image of Welsh pony with large membranous ventricular septal defect (VSD) (arrow) and pulmonic stenosis (fig. 2.10). VSDs are particularly common in Welsh ponies and often occur in association with abnormalities of the pulmonic valve or main pulmonary artery. The left-sided volume overload associated with a large VSD eventually leads to left heart failure and pulmonary edema (fig. 2.11). LV, left ventricle; RV, right ventricle; AO, aorta.

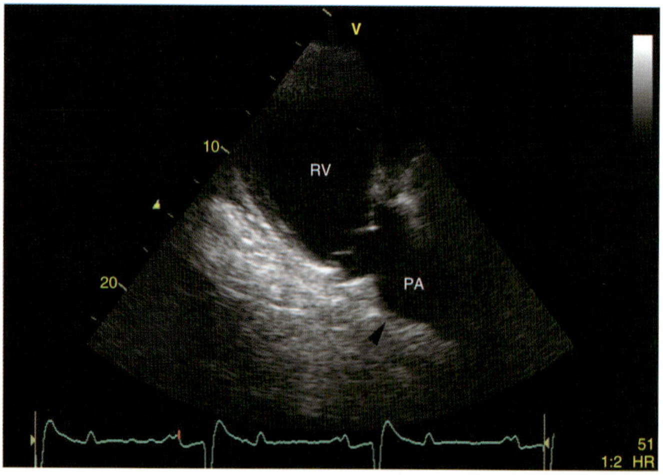

Figure 2.10 Poststenotic dilatation (arrowhead) of the pulmonary artery (PA) is evident in this right parasternal long axis view of the right ventricular outflow tract. RV, right ventricle; PA, pulmonary artery.

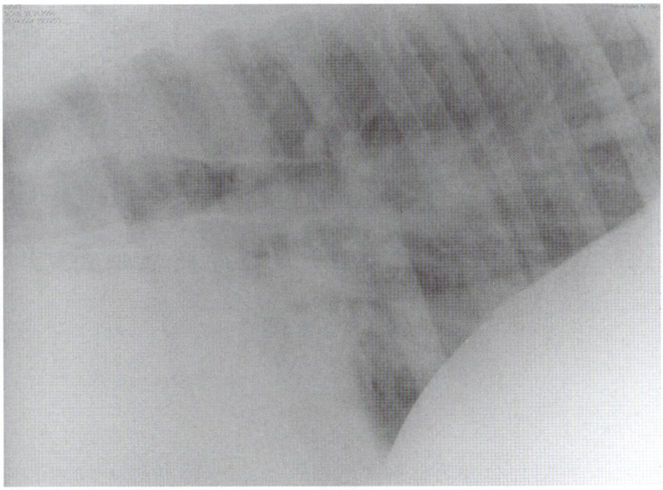

Figure 2.11 Radiographic image of pulmonary edema in pony with heart failure due to large VSD.

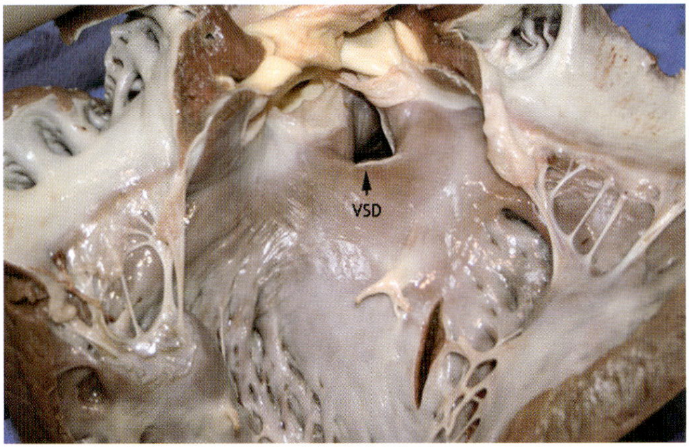

Figure 2.12 Postmortem image of a large membranous VSD.

Truncus Arteriosus

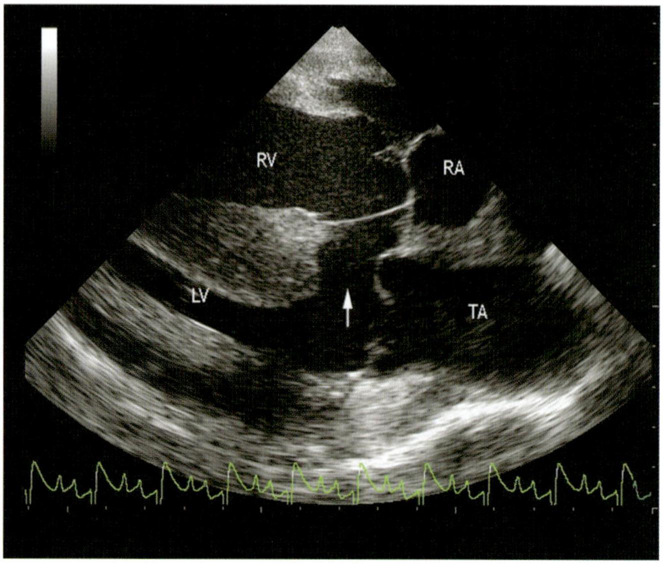

Figure 2.13 Truncus arteriosus in a neonatal foal; right parasternal left ventricular outflow tract view. Truncus arteriosus results from failure of the aorticopulmonary septum to develop and separate the truncus arteriosus into the aorta and the pulmonary artery. Truncus arteriosus is characterized by a large ventricular septal defect (arrow) over which a single great vessel arises (TA). This single vessel carries mixed venous and arterial blood to both the lungs and body resulting in cyanosis (fig. 2.15). Prognosis for life is grave. RA, right atrium; RV, right ventricle; LV, left ventricle; TA, truncus arteriosus.

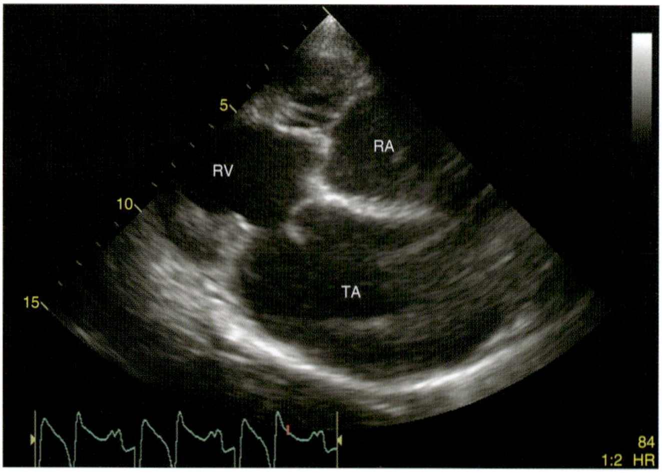

Figure 2.14 Truncus arteriosus; right parasternal right ventricular outflow tract view. Normally, both the aorta and pulmonary artery can be seen in this view. Instead a single great vessel (TA) is visualized. This view is important for distinguishing truncus arteriosus from pseudotruncus arteriosus (severe atresia of the pulmonary artery). RA, right atrium. RV, right ventricle; TA, truncus arteriosus.

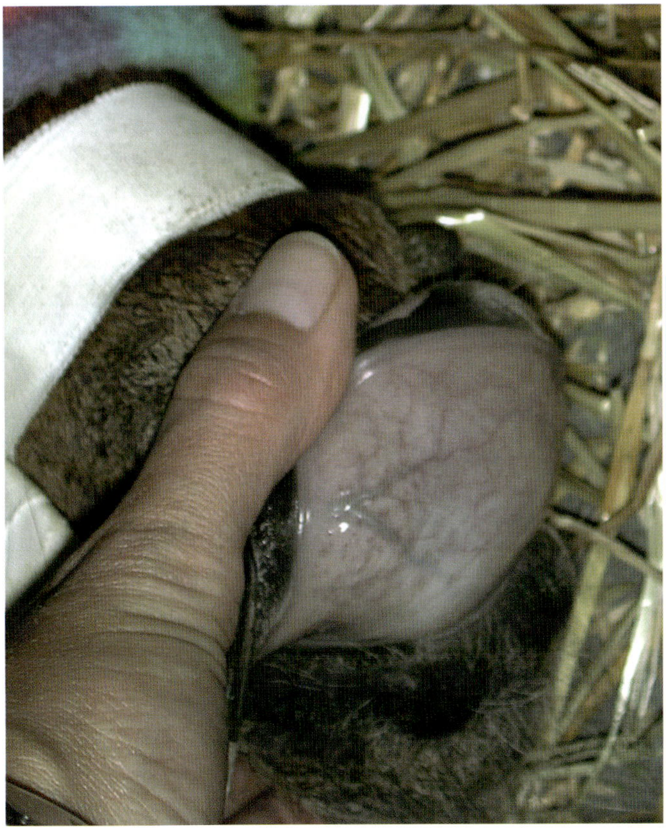

Figure 2.15 Cyanotic mucous membranes in a foal with truncus arteriosus.

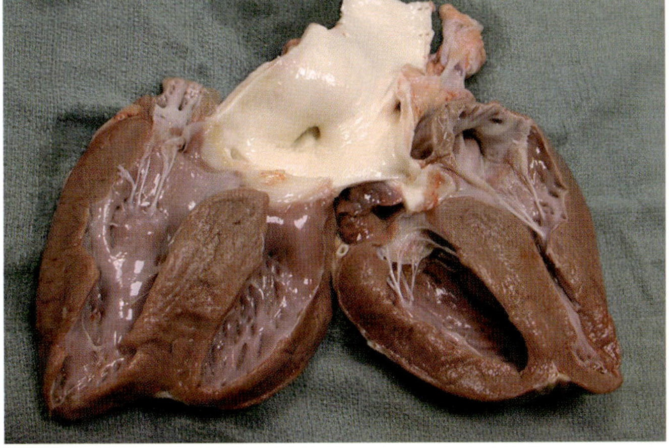

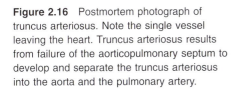

Figure 2.16 Postmortem photograph of truncus arteriosus. Note the single vessel leaving the heart. Truncus arteriosus results from failure of the aorticopulmonary septum to develop and separate the truncus arteriosus into the aorta and the pulmonary artery.

Tetralogy of Fallot

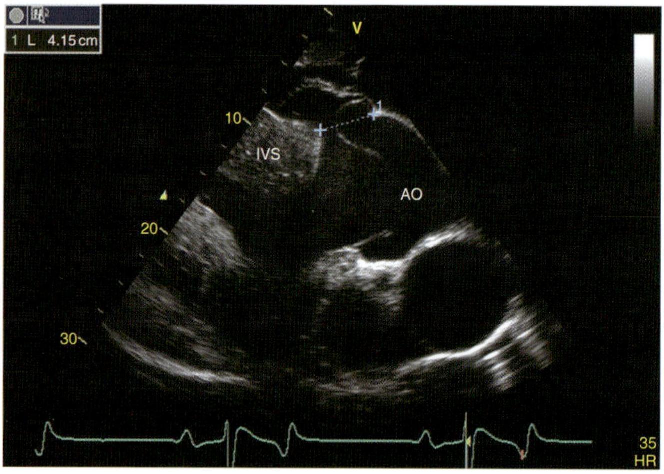

Figure 2.17 Tetralogy of Fallot in a 3-year-old Thoroughbred gelding. Tetralogy of Fallot is characterized by ventricular septal defect, pulmonary artery stenosis, right ventricular hypertrophy and biventricular origin (overriding) aorta. Note large VSD measuring 4.15 cm, overriding aorta (AO) and small pulmonary artery (fig. 2.18). Tetralogy of Fallot is a common complex congenital defect in the horse. The size of the VSD and the severity of the right ventricular outflow obstruction determine the hemodynamic significance and degree of cyanosis. IVS, interventricular septum; AO, aorta.

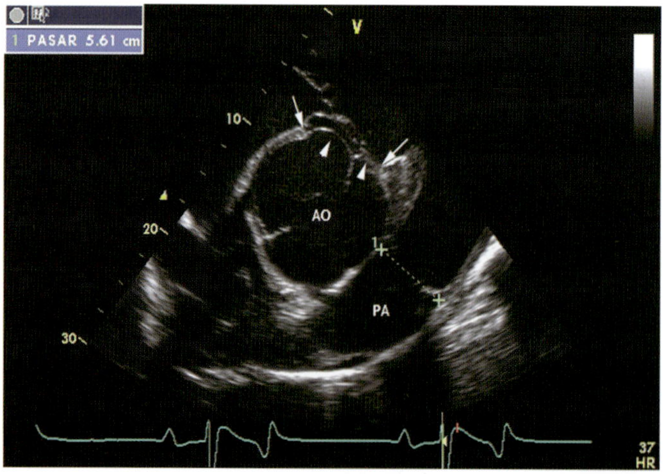

Figure 2.18 Right parasternal short axis image of the horse shown in fig. 2.17. Note the large ventricular septal defect (VSD) (between arrows) and hypoplastic pulmonary artery (PA) measuring 5.61 cm. The noncoronary and right coronary cusps of the aortic valve (arrowheads) prolapsed into the VSD, partially patching the defect. AO, aorta; PA, pulmonary artery.

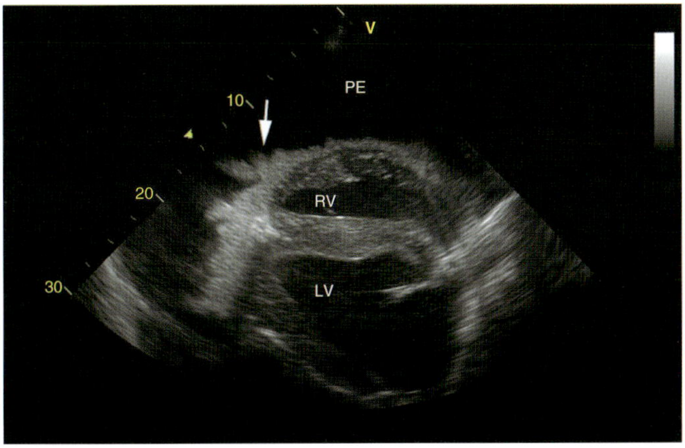

Figure 2.19 Fibrinoeffusive pericarditis. Two-dimensional echocardiographic image from horse with large pericardial effusion (PE) and fibrin (arrow) on epicardial surface. Horses with pericarditis present with lethargy and fever. Physical examination findings include tachycardia, muffled heart sounds, and/or pericardial friction rubs sound. Cardiac tamponade (fig. 2.20) and dampening of the ECG complexes (fig. 2.21) may be present with large effusions. Arrhythmias can be present if there is concurrent myocarditis and may only be detected with a 24-hour ECG recording. Diagnosis is confirmed by echocardiography (figs. 2.19 and 2.22). Pericardial drainage and lavage are critical with large effusions (fig. 2.23). Fluid should be submitted for cytology and culture. The definitive cause is often not identified although causes can be bacterial or viral. The prognosis is good when the condition is recognized early and treated aggressively. Left untreated, constrictive pericarditis may result (fig. 2.24). LV, left ventricle; RV, right ventricle; PE, pericardial effusion.

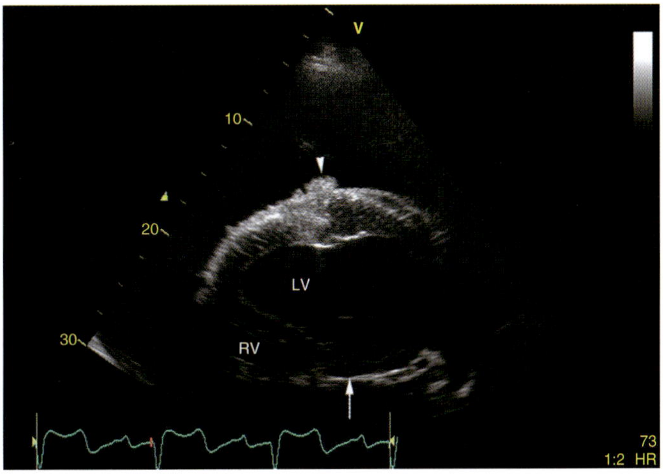

Figure 2.20 Pericardial effusion can result in cardiac tamponade. Echocardiographic image obtained from a pony with large pericardial effusion causing right atrial (arrow) and ventricular (RV) collapse. Fibrin (arrowhead) can be seen on the epicardium of the left ventricle (LV). The pony had generalized venous distension, jugular pulsations, ventral edema, ascites (fig. 2.25), pleural effusion, and altered mentation most likely secondary to poor cerebral perfusion. Signs resolved once 22 liters of fluid were removed via pericardiocentesis. The pony recovered completely. RV, right ventricle; LV, left ventricle.

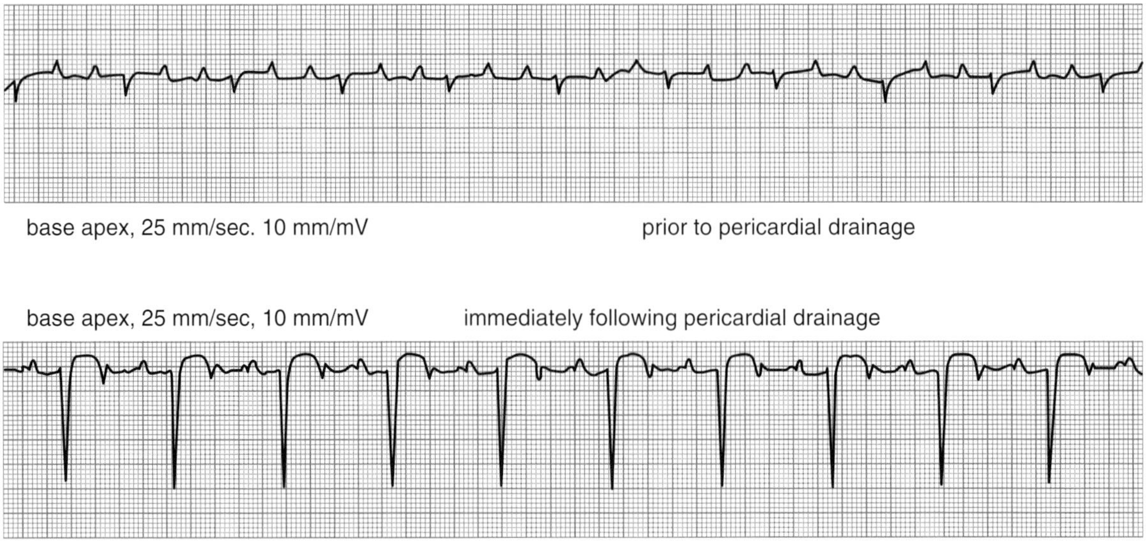

Figure 2.21 Electrocardiograms obtained prior to and immediately after drainage of a large amount of pericardial effusion. Note that both ECG strips were obtained with a sensitivity of 10 mm/mV. There is marked dampening of the complexes prior to drainage. Sinus tachycardia is present in both recordings.

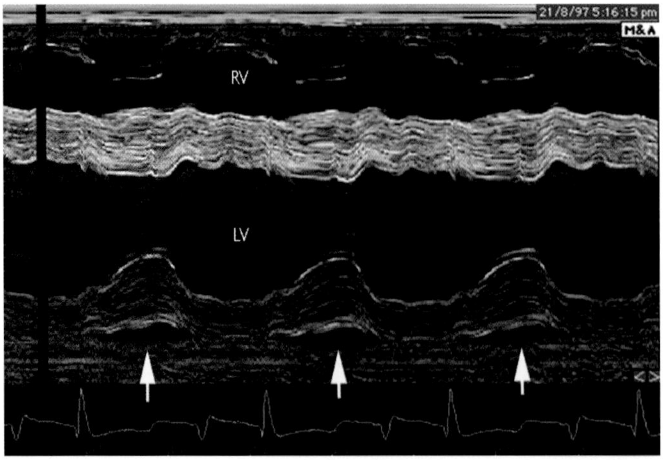

Figure 2.22 M-mode echocardiographic image demonstrating small pericardial effusion. Note the anechoic fluid visible within the pericardium only during systole (arrows). RV, right ventricle; LV, left ventricle.

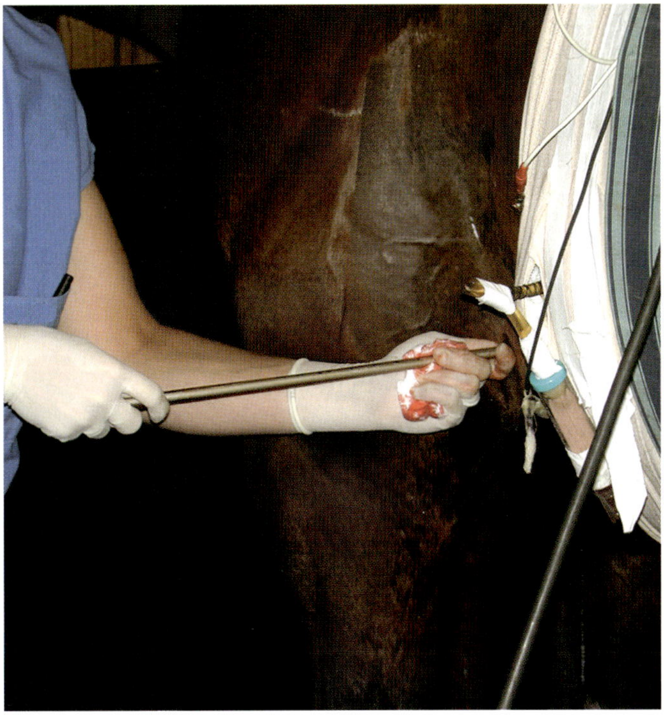

Figure 2.23 Placement of pericardial catheter. Pericardiocentesis can be performed in the standing horse. The optimal site can be determined echocardiographically. Placement of a large indwelling tube allows for pericardial drainage, lavage, and antibiotics instillation. Placement of the drain should be performed under continuous ECG monitoring as potentially fatal arrhythmias may develop if the myocardium is irritated during the procedure.

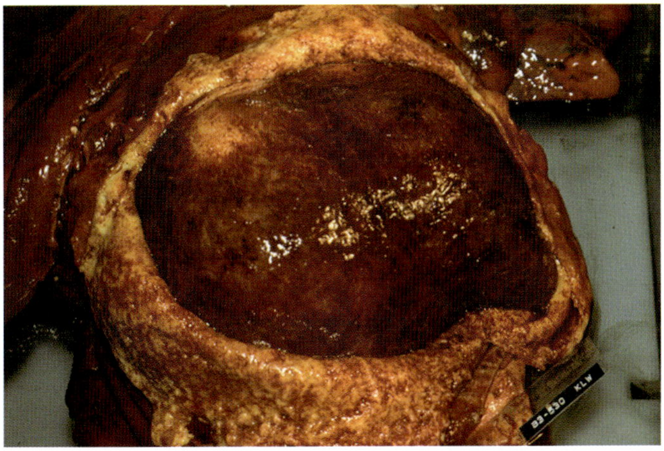

Figure 2.24 Postmortem photograph from a 3-year-old colt with constrictive pericarditis. Note the markedly thickened pericardium peeled back off the epicardium. Constrictive pericarditis is uncommon in horses but can occur in chronic cases.

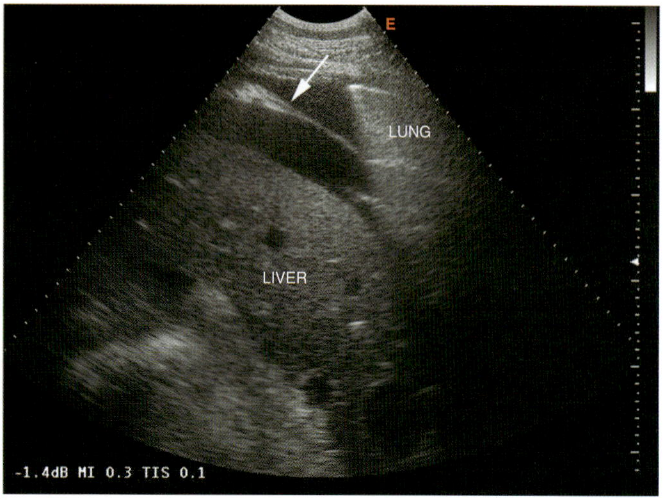

Figure 2.25 Ultrasonographic image of ascites and pleural effusion in a pony with large pericardial effusion that have caused cardiac tamponade and decreased venous return. Note the fluid on either side of the diaphragm (arrow). Both the ascites and pleural effusion resolved within 48 hours of draining the pericardium.

Neoplasia

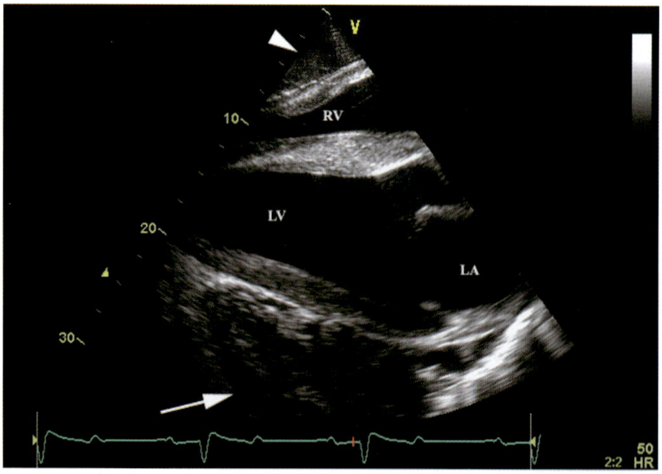

Figure 2.26 Pericardial mesothelioma, echocardiographic image, right parasternal long axis, four chamber view. Notice the large mass within the pericardium (arrows) on both the long axis and short axis (fig. 2.27) views. Clinical signs included weight loss, tachycardia, jugular vein distension, and muffled heart sounds. LV, left ventricle; LA, left atrium; RV, right ventricle.

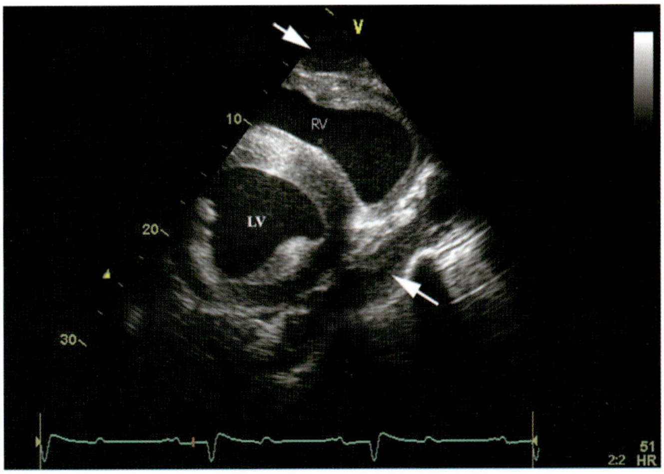

Figure 2.27 Echocardiographic image of pericardial mesothelioma, right parasternal short axis view of ventricles. Note hypoechoic tissue within the pericardium (arrows) compressing the right ventricle (RV). There is no pericardial effusion noted. LV, left ventricle; RV, right ventricle

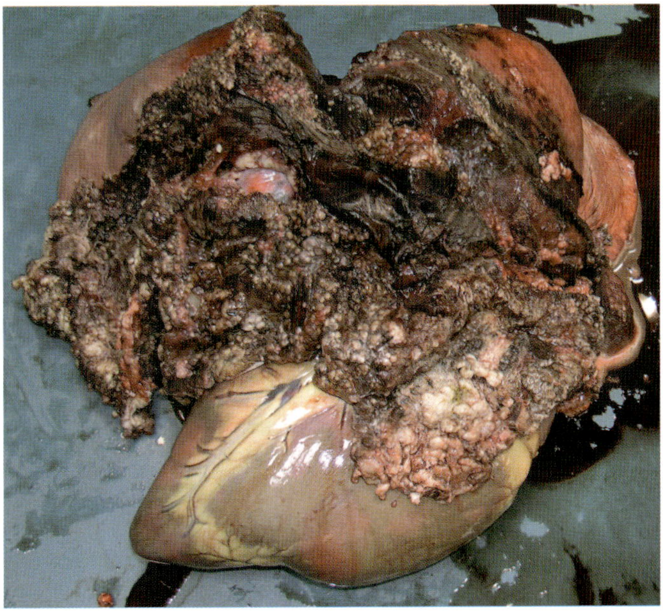

Figure 2.28 Postmortem examination of the horse in figs. 2.26 and 2.27. The parietal pleura, parietal pericardium, and mediastinum are diffusely covered with coalescing cobblestone nodules. Histopathology confirmed the diagnosis of mesothelioma.

Cardiomyopathy

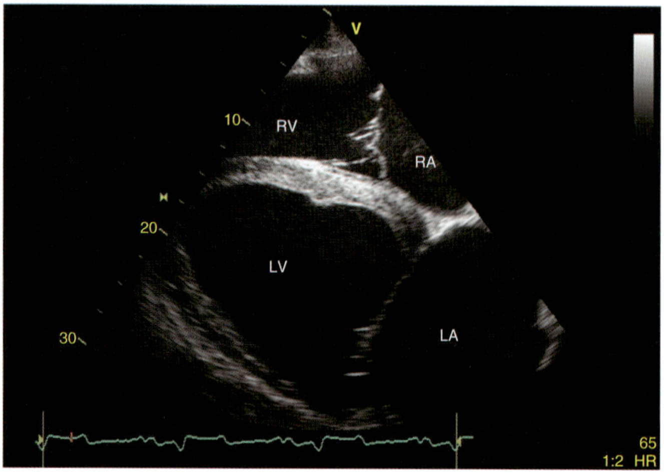

Figure 2.29 Dilated cardiomyopathy (DCM). Two-dimensional echocardiographic image from a broodmare in late gestation with dilated cardiomyopathy and congestive heart failure. Note the marked dilation of both the right and left heart with marked left ventricular dysfunction. Color flow evaluation showed mitral and tricuspid regurgitation (fig. 2.31). Mare was presented in late gestation with anorexia and marked peripheral edema (fig. 2.32). DCM is an uncommon condition in the horse and when diagnosed should prompt investigation into possible ionophore exposure. Treatment is limited to management of heart failure with positive inotropes, diuretics, and afterload reducers. Prognosis is grave. LA, left atrium; LV, left ventricle; RA, right atrium; RV, right ventricle.

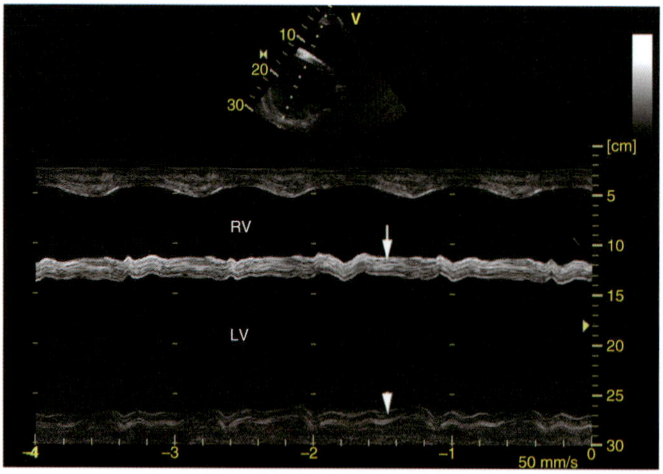

Figure 2.30 M-mode echocardiographic image from a horse with dilated cardiomyopathy (DCM). Note the markedly reduced contractility with a fractional shortening between 1% and 6% (normal 30%–40%), thinning of the interventricular septum (arrow) and left ventricular free wall (arrowhead). LV, left ventricle; RV, right ventricle.

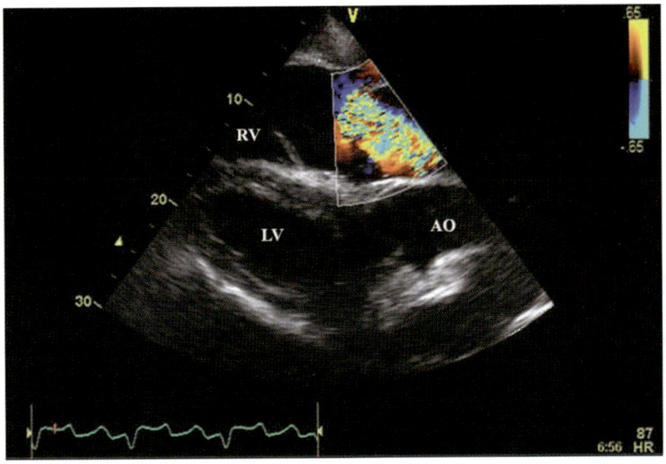

Figure 2.31 Color flow Doppler evaluation of tricuspid valve from the horse in fig. 2.29. RV, right ventricle; LV, left ventricle; AO, aorta.

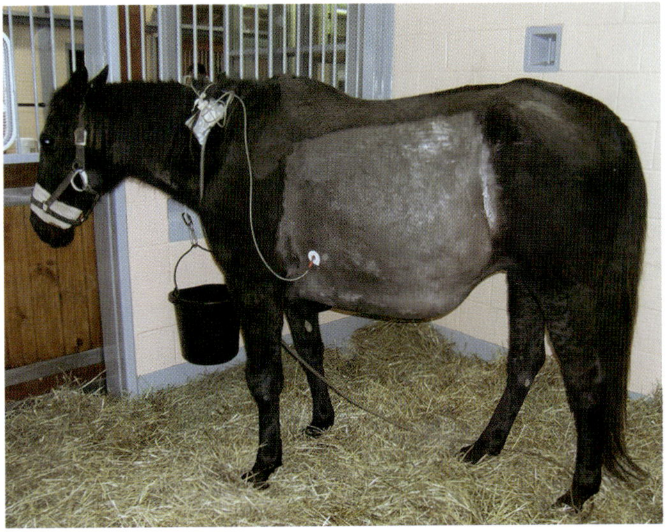

Figure 2.32 A mare with congestive heart failure and cardiac cachexia. Note the muscle wasting and large plaque of ventral edema. Mare received intranasal oxygen therapy and was under constant telemetric monitoring.

2

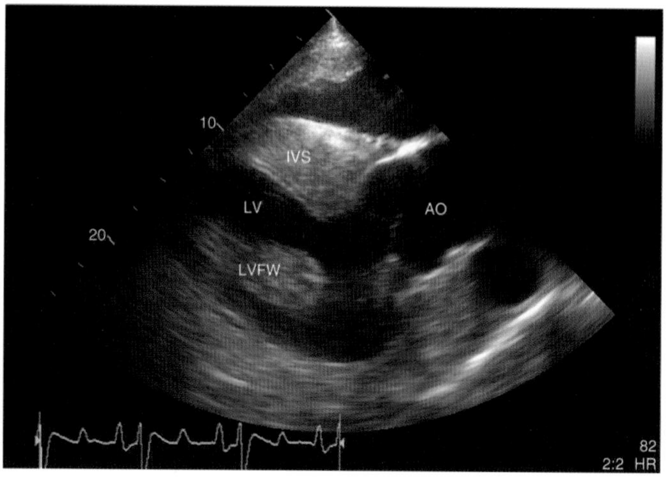

Figure 2.33 Hypertrophic cardiomyopathy (HCM). Two-dimensional echocardiographic image showing markedly thickened left ventricular free wall (LVFW) and interventricular septum (IVS). HCM is rarely reported in the horse. When identified it is almost exclusively due to systemic hypertension secondary to renal failure or chronic pain, as in chronic laminitis. AO, aorta; LV, left ventricle; IVS, interventricular septum; LVFW, left ventricular free wall.

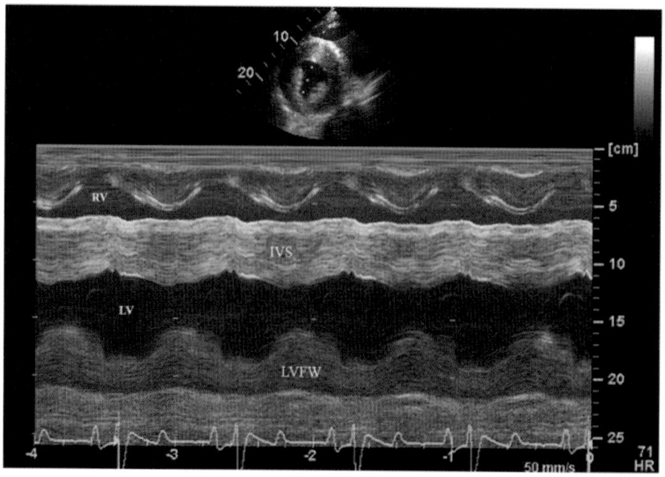

Figure 2.34 M-mode echocardiographic image of left ventricle from a horse with hypertrophic cardiomyopathy. Note the marked thickening of the interventricular septum (IVS) and left ventricular free wall (LVFW). This horse had end-stage renal failure and a systemic blood pressure of 254/183 mmHg. LV, left ventricle; RV, right ventricle; IVS, interventricular septum; LVFW, left ventricular free wall.

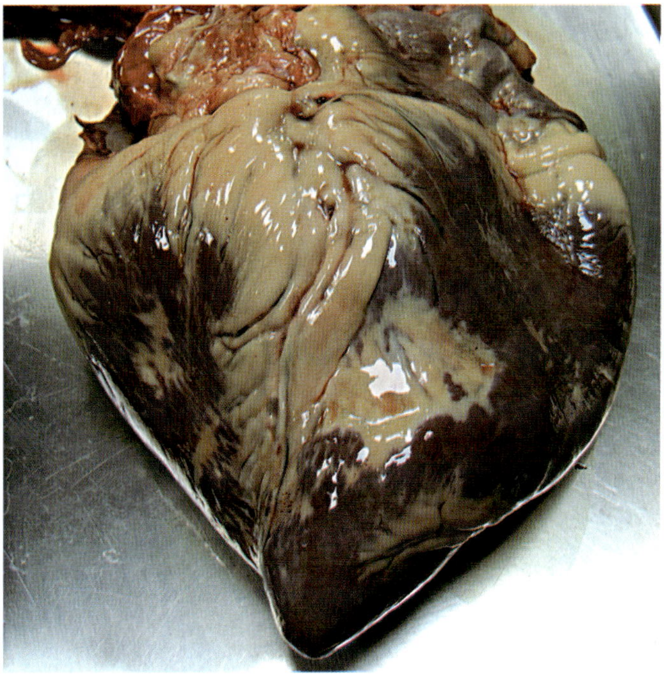

Figure 2.35 Myocarditis in an adult horse. Postmortem photograph of heart from a horse that died from a ventricular dysrhythmia. Note the numerous yellow-tan, depressed regions along the myocardium. Histopathology revealed fibrofatty metaplasia. This horse had chronic arteriosclerotic changes of the aorta and right coronary artery (fig. 2.98) with thromboemboli secondary to verminous arteritis. Arrhythmogenic right ventricular dysplasia is the primary differential for arrhythmogenic death and fibrofatty metaplasia without arteritis.

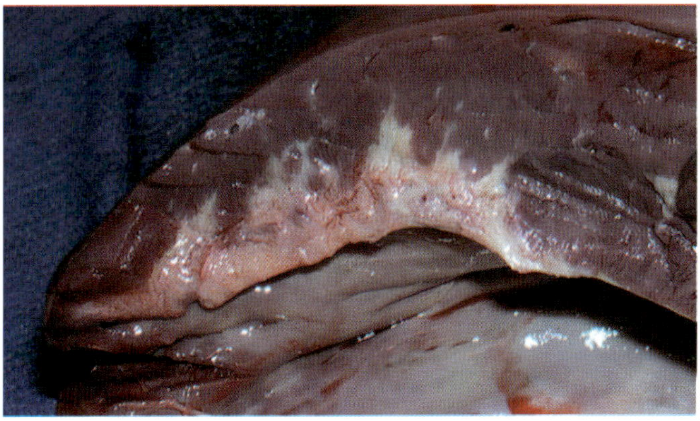

Figure 2.36 Cut section of fibrofatty metaplasia from horse in fig. 2.35.

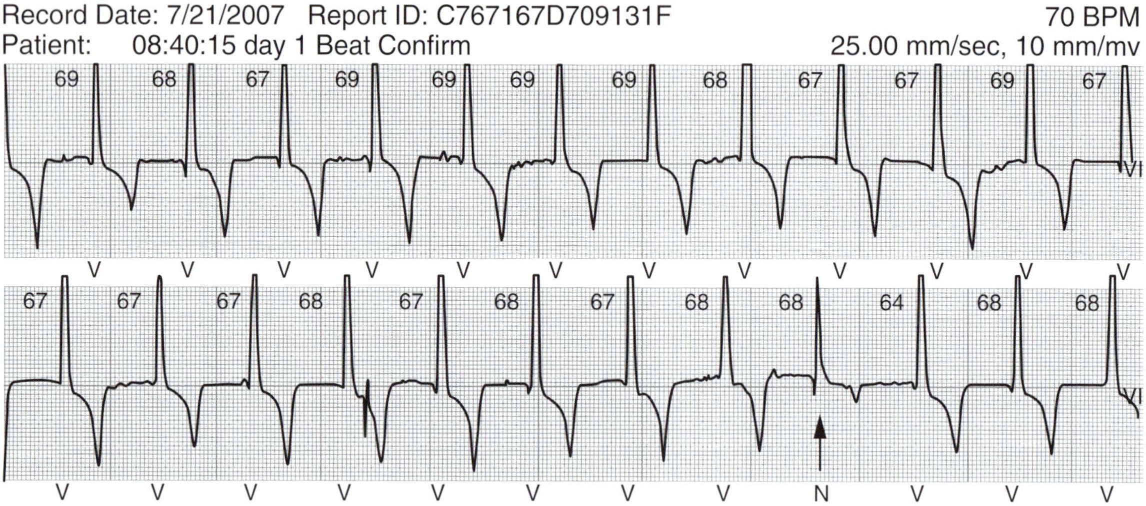

Figure 2.37 Holter recording from horse with myocarditis. Note the widened QRS complexes and slightly elevated rate consistent with an idioventricular rhythm. A single capture beat is present (arrow). Myocarditis is a poorly characterized disease in the horse. Signs may be vague and include lethargy and poor performance. Recent respiratory disease may be part of the history. Auscultation may or may not reveal cardiac arrhythmias and a 24 ECG recording (Holter monitor) is often necessary to document arrhythmias. Cardiac troponin I level may be elevated. Echocardiographic examination may reveal myocardial dysfunction. Treatment includes rest (paddock turnout with no forced exercise) and anti-inflammatory medication, usually corticosteroids.

Cor Pulmonale

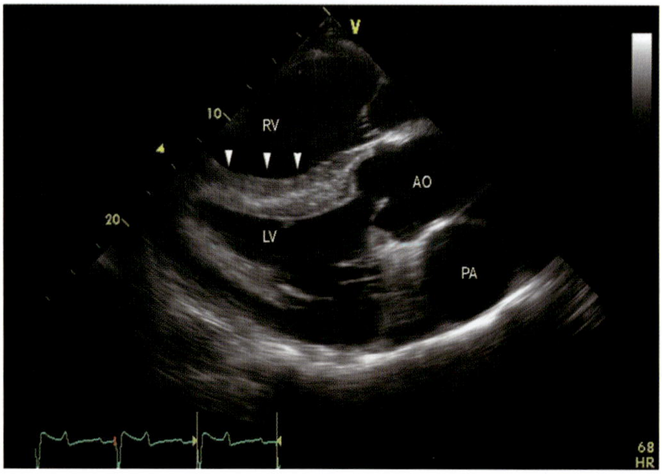

Figure 2.38 Cor pulmonale. Two-dimensional echocardiographic image from a horse with cor pulmonale secondary to recurrent airway obstruction. Image is of the left ventricular outflow tract during diastole. Note how the interventricular septum (arrows) bulges toward the left ventricle (LV) indicating that right ventricular pressure exceeds that of the left ventricle. The pulmonary artery (PA) is markedly dilated when compared to the aorta (AO). Cor pulmonale is a term used to describe right ventricular failure secondary to pulmonary arterial hypertension caused by primary pulmonary disease. It can be acute or chronic. Acute cor pulmonale is usually secondary to pulmonary thromboembolism or acute respiratory distress syndrome. Cardiac output can be severely compromised. LV, left ventricle; RV, right ventricle; PA, pulmonary artery; AO, aorta.

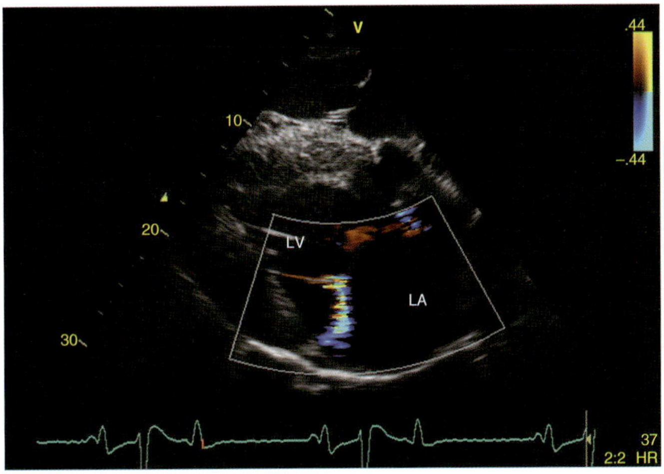

Figure 2.39 Mitral valve insufficiency. Color flow Doppler image from the right parasternal long axis view showing small eccentric jet of mitral regurgitation (MR). MR can occur secondary to degenerative valvular disease, mitral valve prolapse, mitral valve dysplasia, ruptured chordae tendineae (figs. 2.41), noninfective valvulitis, and bacterial endocarditis (fig. 2.44). Valvular insufficiency is likely to lead to poor performance and heart failure. Enlargement of the left atrium can lead to atrial fibrillation (fig. 2.45). LA, left atrium; LV, left ventricle.

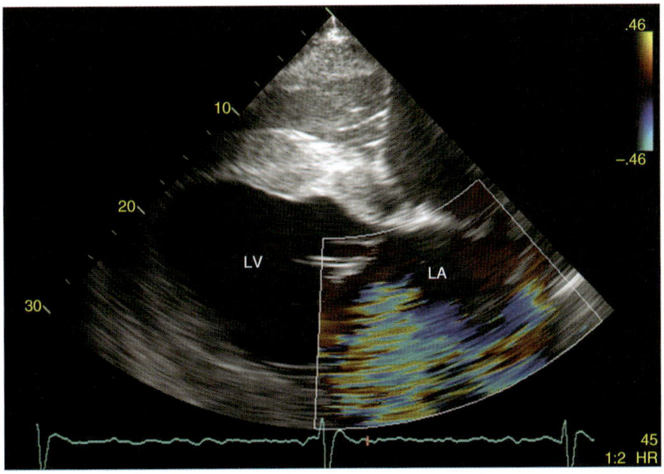

Figure 2.40 Severe mitral valve insufficiency. Color flow Doppler image from the right parasternal long axis view showing large jet of mitral regurgitation occupying almost the entire left atrium (LA). LV, left ventricle; LA; left atrium.

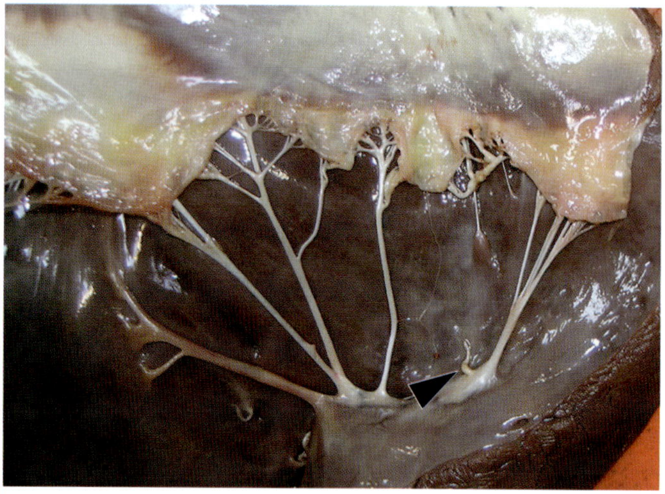

Figure 2.41 Postmortem photograph of a ruptured chorda tendinea (RCT) (arrowhead). RCT results in acute severe mitral valve regurgitation and heart failure. The ruptured chorda may be seen echocardiographically as a linear echo everting into the left atrium during systole. The left atrium is usually only mildly enlarged as it has not had time to dilate in response to the increased left atrial pressure. Pulmonary edema is usually present (fig. 2.43). Atrial splitting (fig. 2.42) and jet lesions (fig. 2.46) may be seen at postmortem examination.

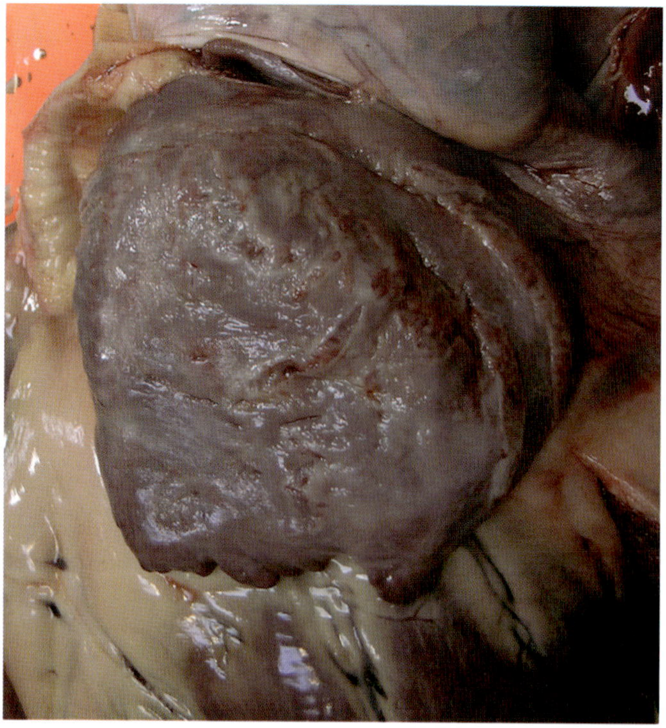

Figure 2.42 Postmortem photograph shows splitting of the atrial epicardium secondary to rupture of a chorda tendinea and acute mitral valve regurgitation.

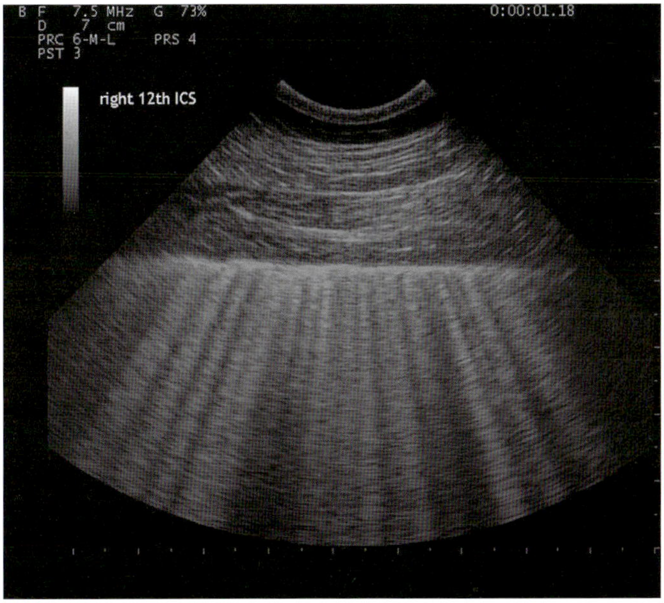

Figure 2.43 Sonographic image of pulmonary edema in horse with a ruptured chorda tendinea and congestive heart failure. Note the numerous coalescing comet tail artifacts consistent with interruption of the normal aeration at the visceral pleural surface.

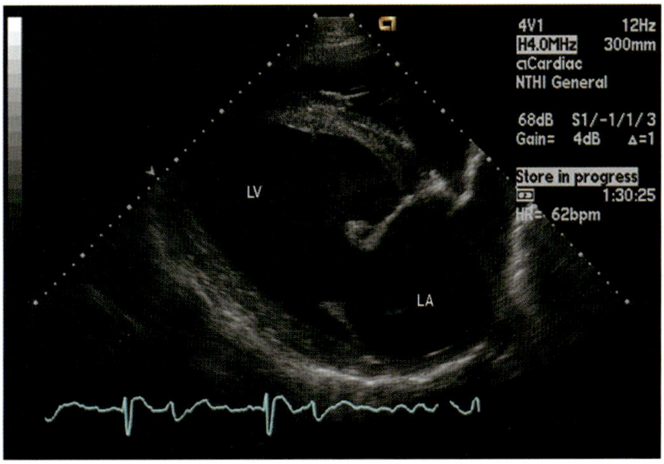

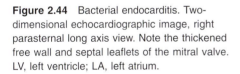

Figure 2.44 Bacterial endocarditis. Two-dimensional echocardiographic image, right parasternal long axis view. Note the thickened free wall and septal leaflets of the mitral valve. LV, left ventricle; LA, left atrium.

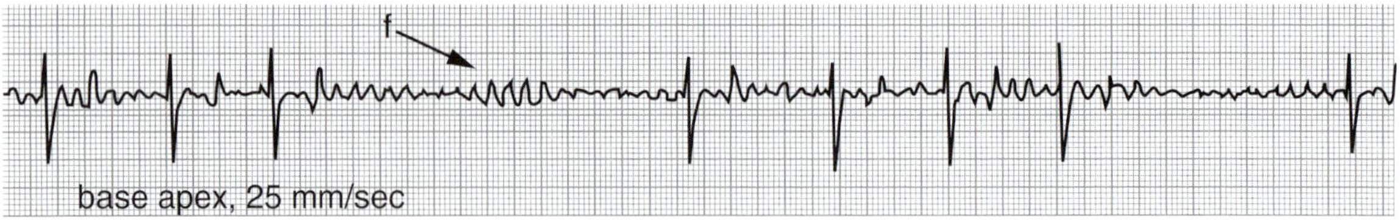

Figure 2.45 Atrial fibrillation secondary to mitral regurgitation and left atrial enlargement. Note the irregularly irregular rhythm, normal QRS complexes, and fibrillation waves (f).

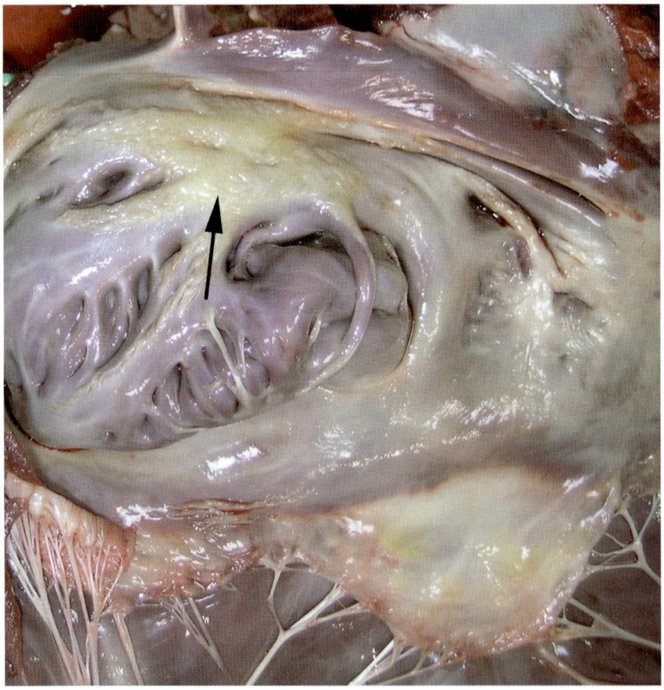

Figure 2.46 Jet lesion. Postmortem image of localized areas of subendocardial fibrosis in the left atrium (arrow) secondary to the jet of mitral valve regurgitation.

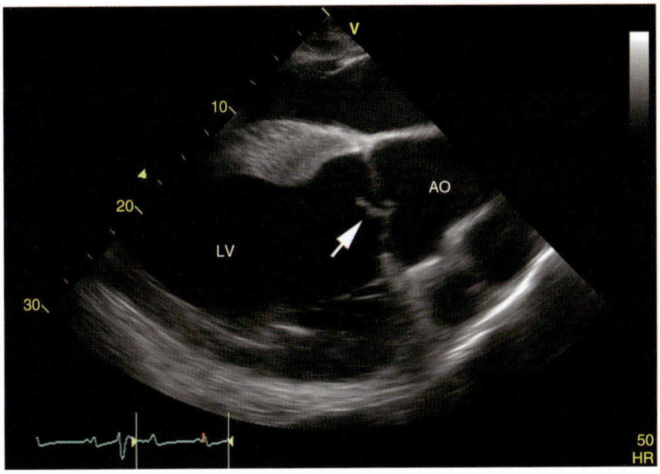

Figure 2.47 Aortic valve insufficiency (AI). Echocardiographic image; right parasternal long axis left ventricular outflow view. Note the tear in the aortic valve (arrow). Aortic insufficiency is usually a disease of older horses and occurs most commonly secondary to degenerative valve changes. Fenestrations or tears in the valve leaflets occur less commonly. Congenital malformations of the aortic valve are rare and bacterial endocarditis occurs uncommonly (fig. 2.52). Horses with AI have a characteristic murmur (fig. 2.51). Progression of the disease is usually slow if due to degenerative valve disease. Tears of the valve progress more quickly. Diagnosis is confirmed by echocardiography (figs. 2.48 and 2.49). LV, left ventricle; AO, aorta.

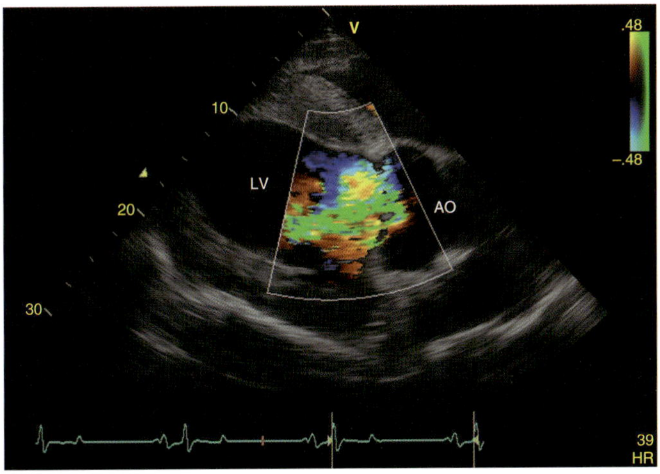

Figure 2.48 Color flow Doppler image of aortic insufficiency, right parasternal long axis view. LV, left ventricle; AO, aorta.

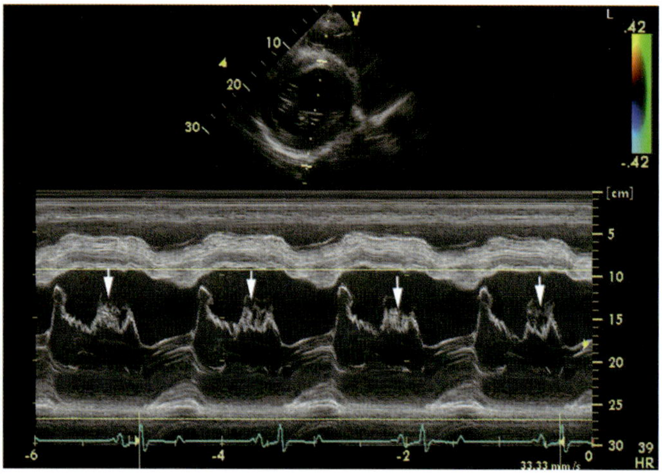

Figure 2.49 M-mode image of the mitral valve from a horse with aortic insufficiency. High frequency vibrations (arrows) are present on the septal leaflet of the mitral valve secondary to the jet of aortic regurgitation striking the mitral valve. This finding is diagnostic of aortic regurgitation without color flow Doppler interrogation.

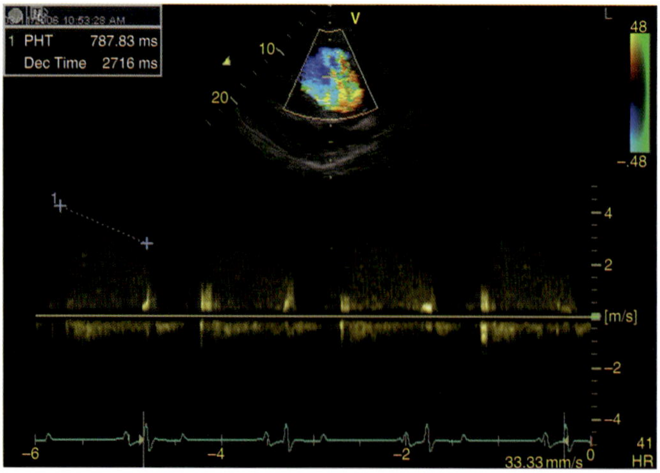

Figure 2.50 Continuous wave Doppler evaluation of aortic regurgitation. Pressure half time is used to assess the severity of aortic regurgitation. As left ventricular pressure rises, the velocity of the regurgitant jet drops off quickly, producing a steep slope to the velocity profile. Pressure half time <250 ms is consistent with severe aortic regurgitation. PHT, pressure half time.

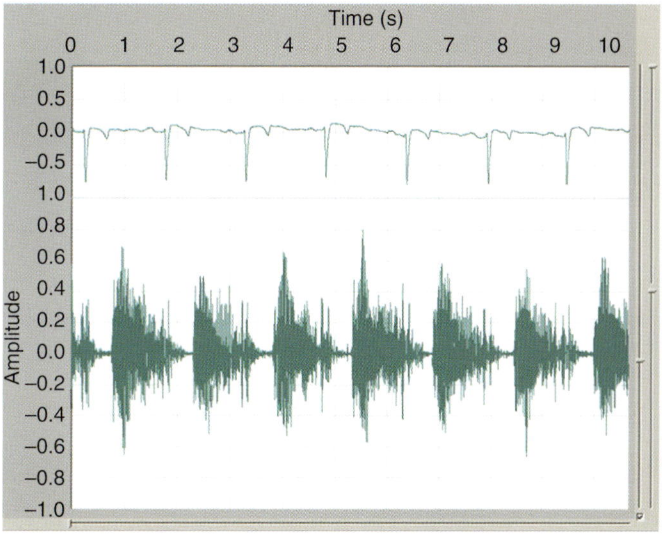

Figure 2.51 Phonocardiogram of aortic valve insufficiency. Diastolic decrescendo murmurs over the aortic to mitral valve region are almost always due to aortic insufficiency as valvular stenosis is rare in the horse. Murmurs may be blowing, coarse, or musical in quality.

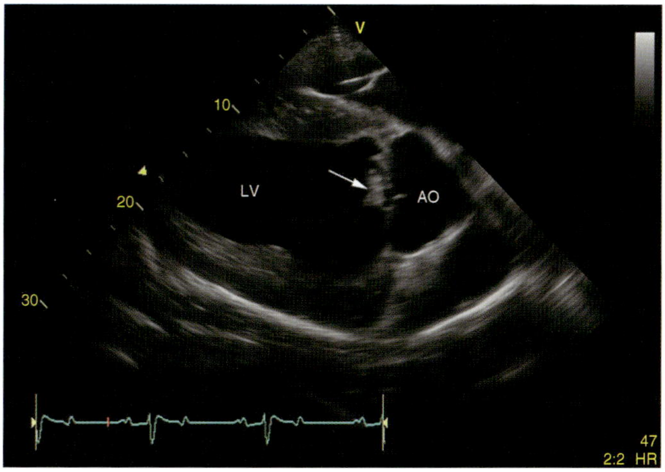

Figure 2.52 Bacterial endocarditis of the aortic valve. Note the thickened aortic valve leaflets (arrow). AO, aorta; LV, left ventricle.

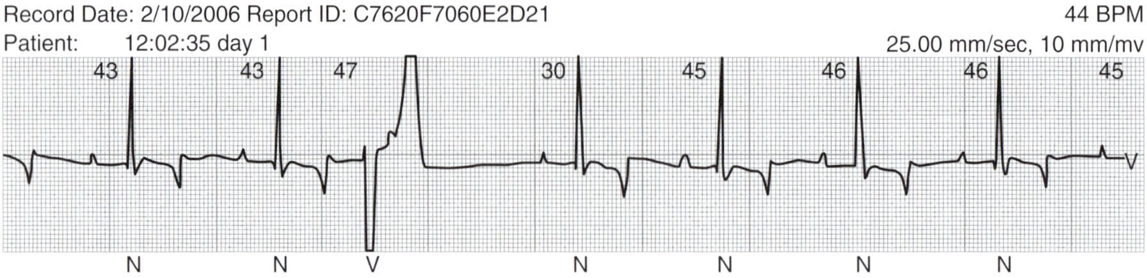

Figure 2.53 Electrocardiogram from a horse with chronic degenerative valve disease, aortic insufficiency, ventricular premature contraction, and aortic valve insufficiency. Note the early, wide and bizarre QRS complex (V) that is not associated with a P wave. Horses with moderate to severe aortic insufficiency should be evaluated for the presence of ventricular dysrhythmias. Horses with aortic insufficiency may be predisposed to ventricular arrhythmias because of diastolic runoff and poor myocardial perfusion.

Tricuspid Valve Insufficiency

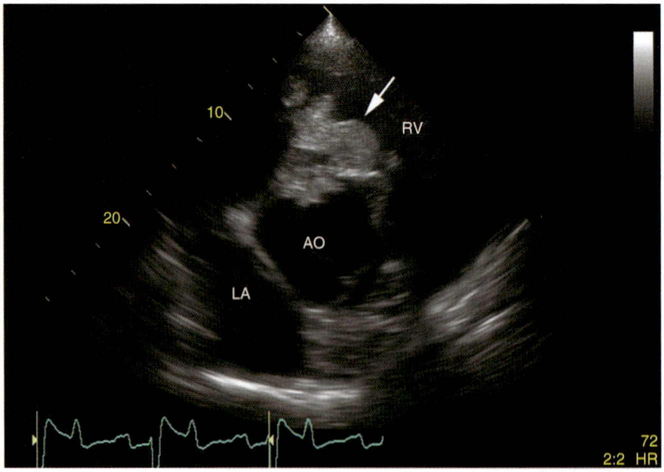

Figure 2.54 Tricuspid insufficiency and bacterial endocarditis. Two-dimensional echocardiographic short axis view of vegetative endocarditis. Note the marked thickening of the tricuspid valve leaflets (arrow). Endocarditis of the tricuspid valve occurs less frequently than mitral valve endocarditis. Septic jugular vein thrombophlebitis is a predisposing cause. AO, aorta; RV, right ventricle; LA, left atrium.

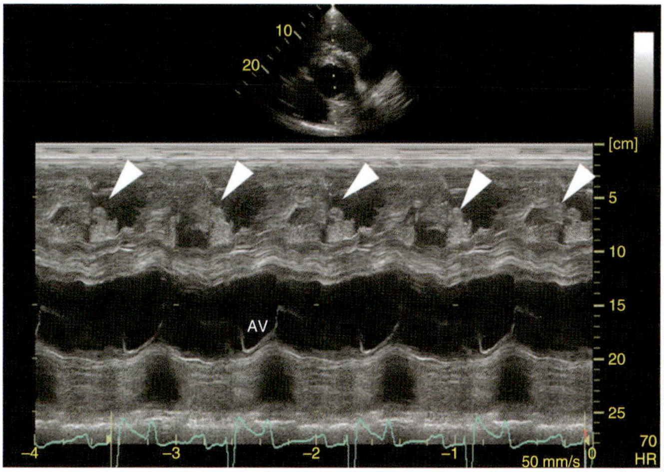

Figure 2.55 M-mode echocardiographic image from the horse shown in fig. 2.54. Note the marked thickening of the tricuspid valve leaflets (arrowheads). AV, aortic valve.

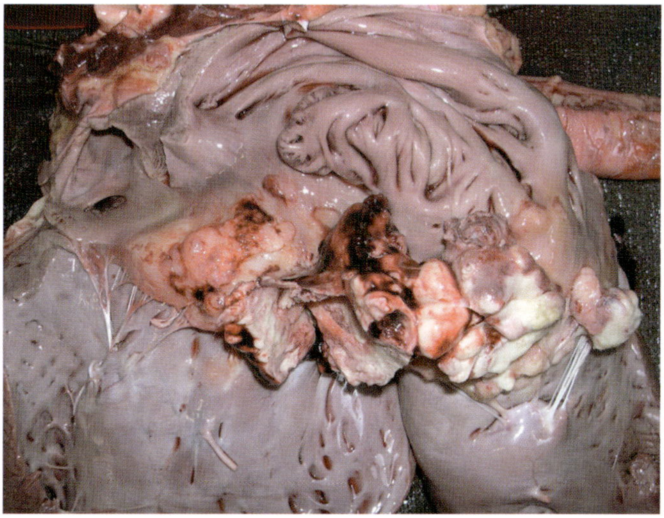

Figure 2.56 Postmortem photograph of the horse shown in fig. 2.54. Note the massive proliferative lesions on all three cusps of tricuspid valve.

Endocarditis

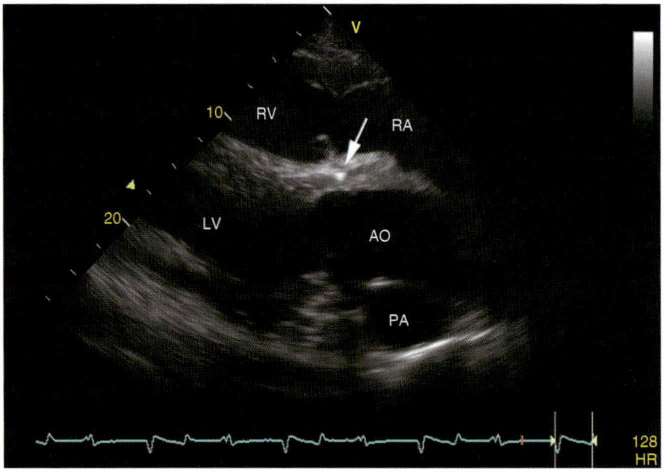

Figure 2.57 Atrial endocarditis. Echocardiographic image from a horse with a history of weakness and near collapse during exercise. Note the thickening along the right atrial septum and echogenic foci consistent with calcification (arrow) within this thickened tissue. ECG showed third degree heart block (fig. 2.60). Atrial endocarditis involving the AV node was diagnosed on postmortem examination (fig. 2.59). RV, right ventricle; LV, left ventricle; AO, aorta; RA, right atrium; PA, pulmonary artery.

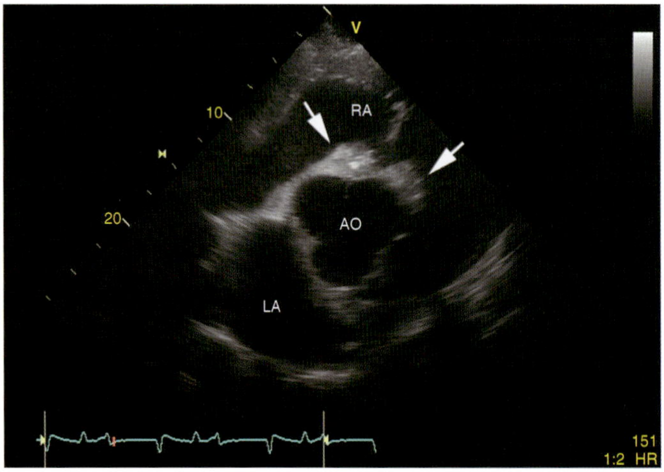

Figure 2.58 Short axis echocardiographic image from the same horse shown in fig. 2.57. RA, right atrium; AO, aorta; LA, left atrium.

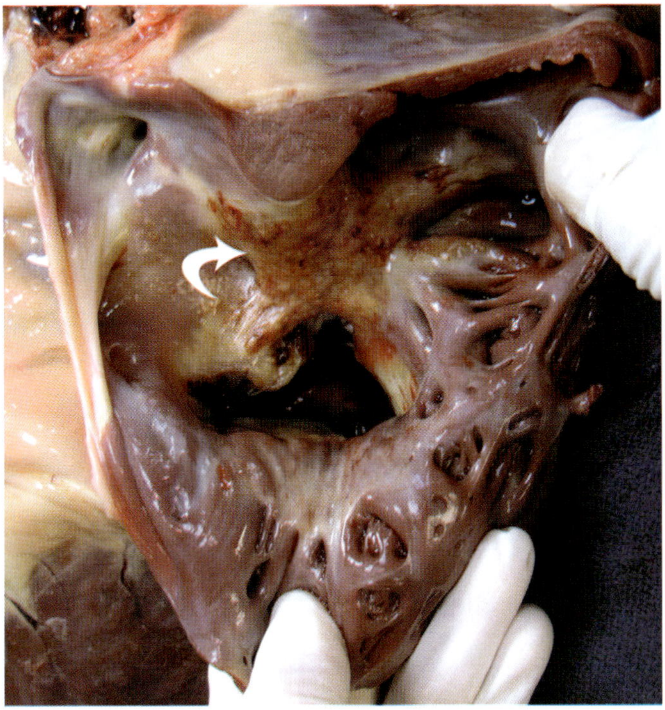

Figure 2.59 Postmortem examination of the horse shown in figs. 2.57 and 2.58 showed raised irregular tan areas along right atrial septum (arrow). The connective tissue between the atrium and aortic root was thickened with gritty foci of mineralization. Dense fibrous tissue and granulomas were identified histologically. No organisms were seen.

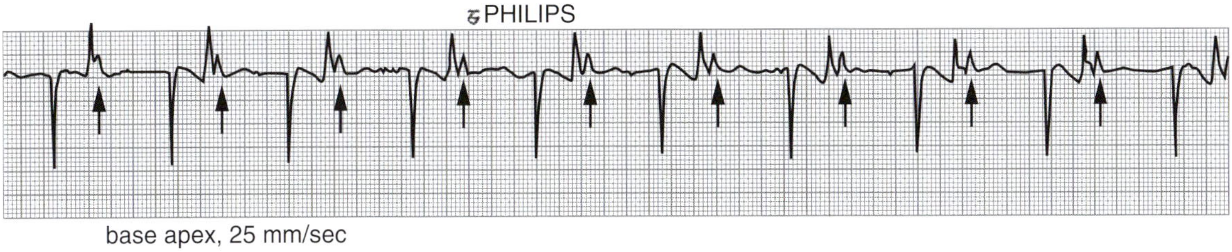

Figure 2.60 ECG from a horse with atrial endocarditis involving the AV node region. Note the P waves (arrows) not associated with QRS complexes. P-R interval exceeds 500 milliseconds. Atrial rate is slightly higher than ventricular rate. QRS complexes are narrow and appear at regular intervals consistent with a junctional escape rhythm. Diagnosis was third degree (complete) AV block.

Sinus Rhythm

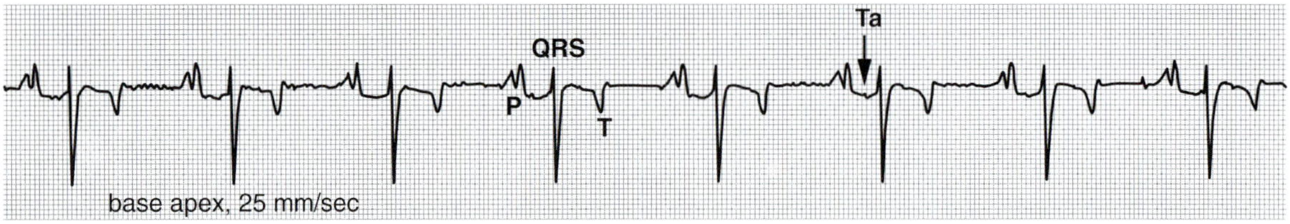

Figure 2.61 Normal resting sinus rhythm; base apex lead. Note the upright, notched P waves, negative QRS complexes, and biphasic T waves. P wave notching occurs because the slow resting heart rate and large atrial mass permit visualization of the right atrial and then left atrial depolarization. This is a normal finding and not an evidence of atrial enlargement. The slight dip below baseline following P wave is called a T_a wave and represents an atrial repolarization. T waves can be very variable in their appearance, being positive, negative, or biphasic.

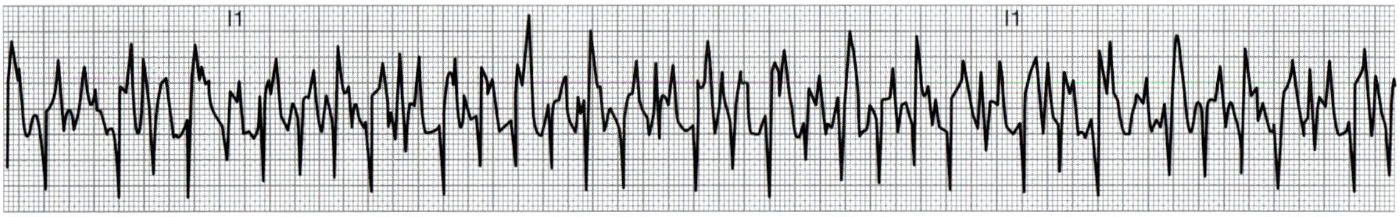

Figure 2.62 Sinus tachycardia during exercise. P waves become difficult, if not impossible, to identify and T waves become very large. Footfall and respiratory effort cause significant artifactual changes in the ECG recording. Care must be taken not to overinterpret artifact as dysrhythmia. Remembering that a QRS complex must always have an associated T wave will help avoid misinterpretation. Calipers should always be used to determine if the rhythm is regular or not.

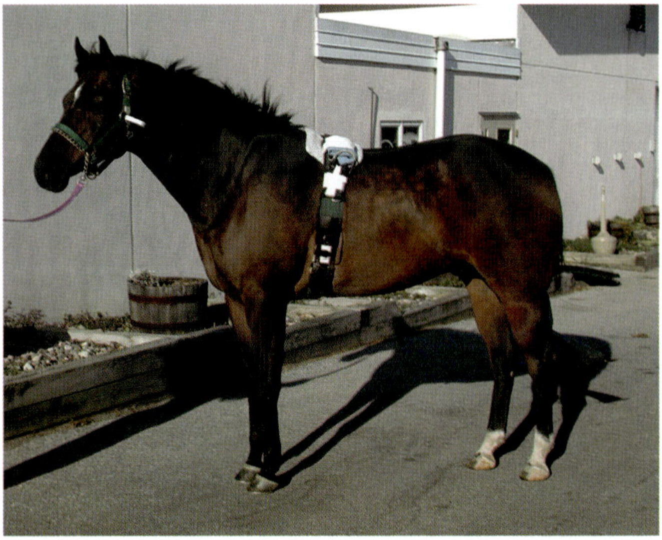

Figure 2.63 Photograph of horse fitted with Holter monitor and telemetry. Holter monitor recordings are necessary for identifying intermittent arrhythmias at rest. They are easily placed and their recordings are of excellent quality when the horse is stall restricted. Exercising ECGs and emergency monitoring of the cardiac rhythm is best performed using telemetric equipment.

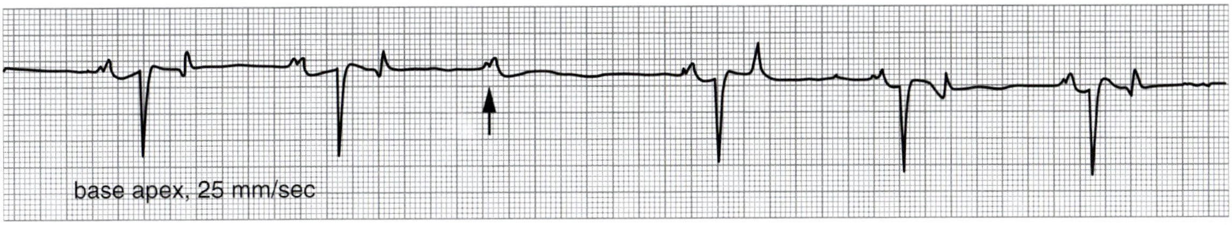

Figure 2.64 Type I second degree atrioventricular (AV) block. High vagal tone in the fit resting horse results in conduction block at the AV node level. This physiologic form of AV block is characterized by variable PR intervals and "on-time" P waves (arrow) not followed by QRS complexes. Auscultation findings include a regularly irregular rhythm with isolated fourth heart sounds (S4-atrial contraction sound). The rhythm will disappear with reduction in vagal tone such as occurs with exercise or vagolytic drug administration.

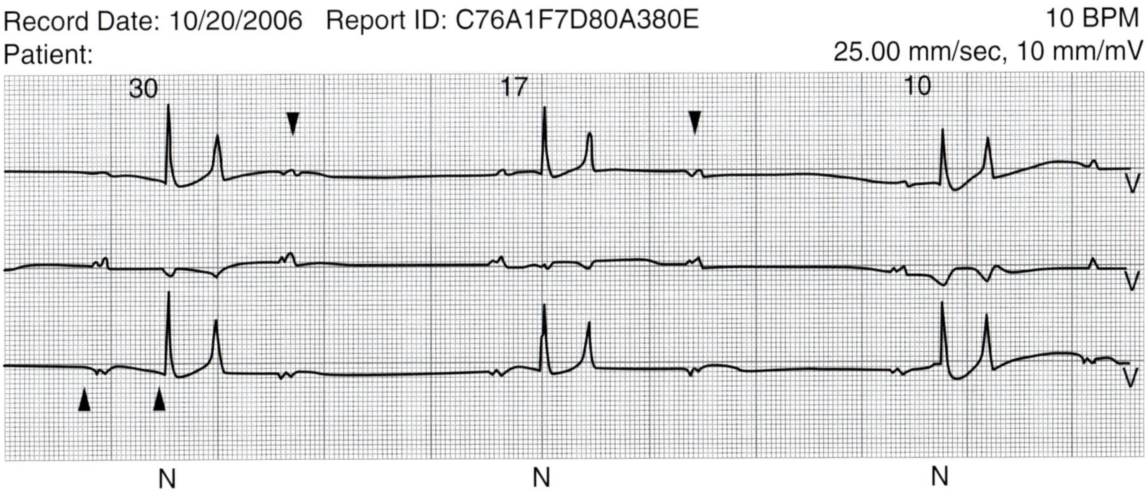

Figure 2.65 First and second degree AV block; Holter monitor recording of a horse receiving reserpine. Note P-R interval prolongation, which was greater than 0.5 seconds (between blue arrowheads). The second and fourth P waves are blocked (black arrowheads). The horse is bradycardic with a heart rate of 18–20 bpm. Reserpine is an adrenergic blocking agent that acts by depleting catecholamine stores. Cardiovascular side effects are rare but may include a decrease in atrioventricular conduction, potentiation of digitalis toxicity, and precipitation of ventricular arrhythmias.

base apex, 25 mm/sec

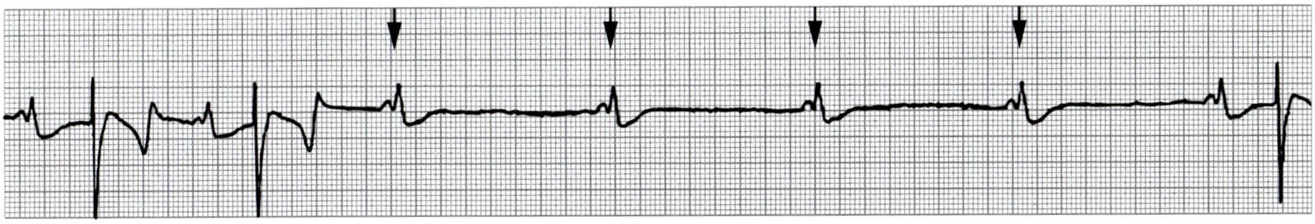

Figure 2.66 Advanced second degree AV block. Base apex recording from a horse with severe exercise intolerance. Note the sequential P waves (arrows) not followed by QRS complexes. Neither exercise nor glycopyrrolate administration resulted in improved conduction, which is consistent with a diagnosis of AV node disease.

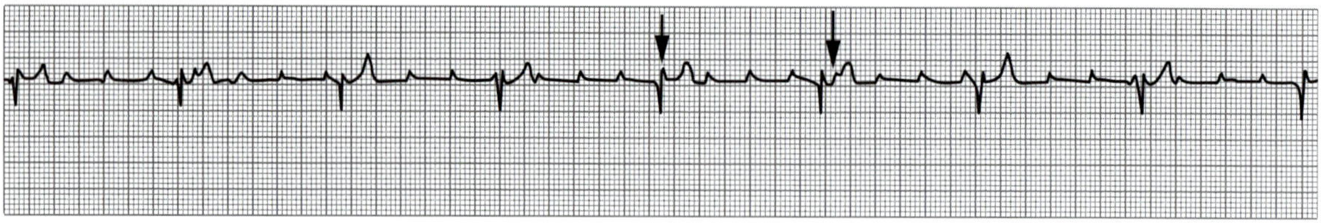

Figure 2.67 Third degree (complete) AV block. Base apex recording from a neonatal foal with septic myocarditis. Note the complete lack of association of the P waves with the QRS complexes with some of the P waves being buried in QRS complexes or T waves (arrows). The P-P intervals and R-R intervals are regular. The atrial rate is elevated at 150 bpm and the ventricular rate is slow at 40 bpm (healthy age matched foal should have HR of about 100 bpm). The slow ventricular rate is the result of an escape rhythm and should not be suppressed. The elevated atrial rate is most likely secondary to the underlying disease (sepsis). Temporary pacemaker insertion should be considered for treatment of complete heart block secondary to sepsis since the risk of sudden death is high. On postmortem examination there was myocellular necrosis and interstitial edema of the right atrial septum and AV node.

Supraventricular Arrhythmias

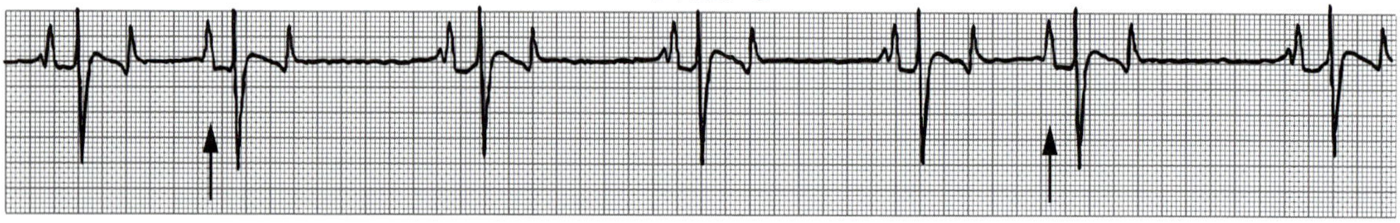

Figure 2.68 Atrial premature contraction (APC) with a normal ventricular conduction. Note the early P' wave (arrows) followed by a normal QRS complex. Because P' waves (premature P waves) originate from a focus outside the sinus node, they are different in appearance from the normal sinus-generated P waves.

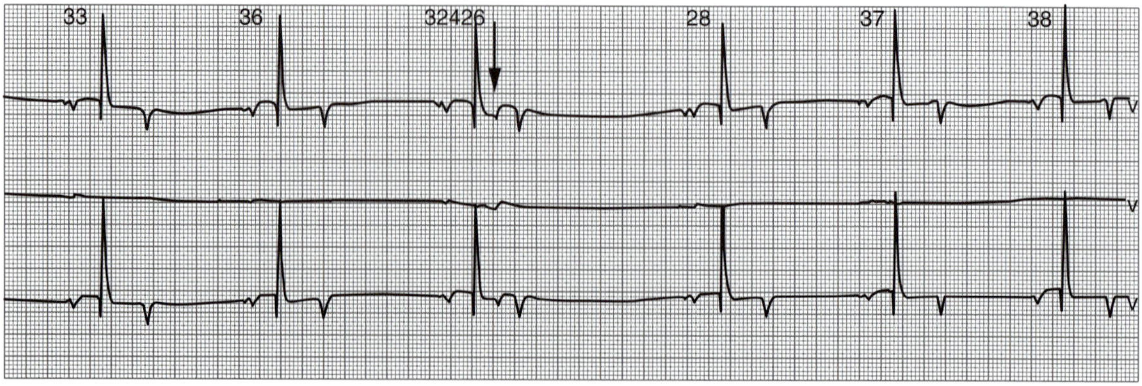

Figure 2.69 Nonconducted atrial premature contraction (APC). Holter monitor recording (*not* a standard base apex lead). Note the premature P' wave present between the QRS and T wave of the previous beat (arrow). APC is not conducted to the ventricles because the AV node is still in its refractory period. The electrical activity does reach the sinus node causing it to reset, creating the appearance of a pause following the blocked APC.

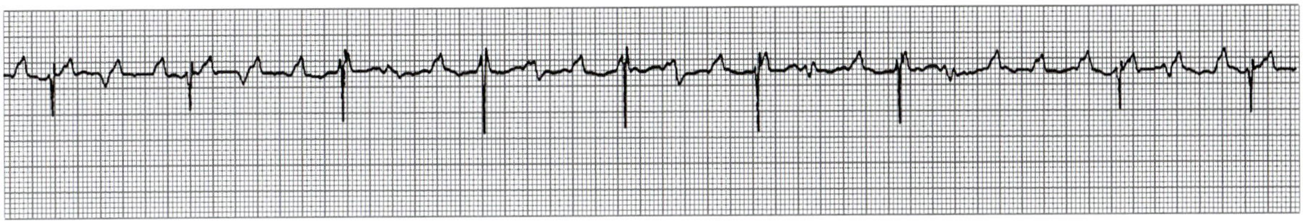
base apex, 25 mm/sec

Figure 2.70 Atrial tachycardia with second degree AV block at rest. Base apex lead from horse experiencing exercise intolerance. Note the rapid atrial rate of 170 bpm and the normal ventricular rate of 50 bpm. The QRS complexes are normal in appearance but irregular in timing. Horses with atrial tachycardia usually block most of the premature atrial depolarizations at the AV node. This results in a normal resting heart rate but irregular rhythm due to variable conduction through the AV node (similar to atrial fibrillation). This is in contrast to what can happen during exercise when vagal tone is reduced (fig. 2.71).

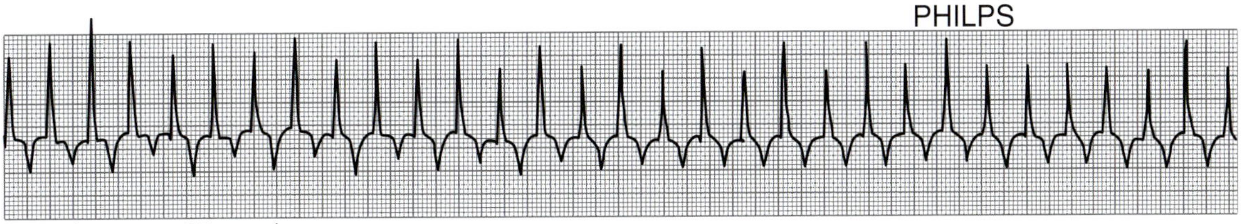

telemetry, 25 mm/sec

Figure 2.71 Atrial tachycardia during trotting exercise (same horse as in fig. 2.70). Telemetric recording from horse with atrial tachycardia and second degree AV block at rest. Note how during exercise the atrial premature depolarizations are no longer blocked at the AV node and conduction is 1:1 resulting in a heart rate of 170 bpm. A normal horse at the trot would have a heart rate of 80–120 bpm. QRS complexes are upright because of placement of telemetry (not base apex configuration). Horses with atrial tachycardia may be extremely weak or collapse if forced to exercise.

Atrial Fibrillation

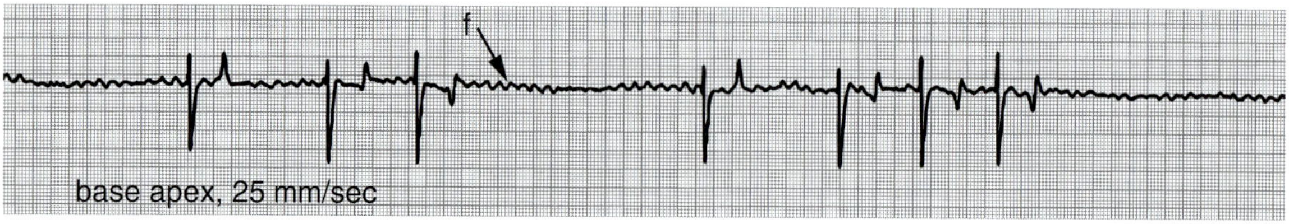

Figure 2.72 ECG from a horse with atrial fibrillation secondary to mitral regurgitation and left atrial enlargement. Note the irregularly irregular rhythm, normal QRS complexes, absence of P waves, and presence of fibrillation or "f" waves. Atrial fibrillation can occur as an idiopathic condition or secondary to atrial enlargement or electrolyte abnormalities. Horses with atrial fibrillation have normal resting heart rate, unless in heart failure or systemically ill (fig. 2.73). Exercising heart rates are elevated (fig. 2.74). Auscultation reveals an irregularly irregular rhythm with variable intensity heart sounds and absence of the fourth heart sound. Echocardiographic examination is indicated to rule out underlying heart disease. Horses without underlying heart disease may spontaneously convert to normal sinus rhythm once systemic illness or electrolyte abnormalities are corrected (fig. 2.75). Treatment is indicated in horses unable to perform their intended job. Treatment options include quinidine sulfate or quinidine gluconate (fig. 2.76), electrical cardioversion (figs. 2.77–2.80), or other antiarrhythmics such as flecainide or amiodarone.

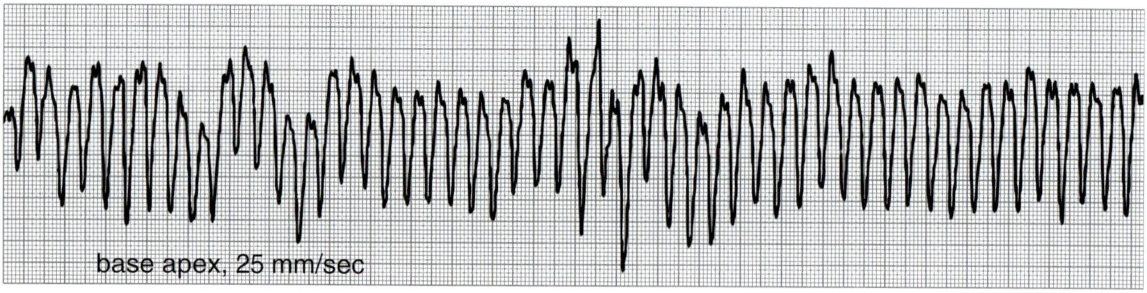

Figure 2.73 Rapid atrial fibrillation in a horse with a history of weakness during exercise. Careful examination of the R-R intervals using calipers is necessary to differentiate this rhythm from ventricular tachycardia. Note that the rhythm is irregularly irregular in contrast to unifocal ventricular tachycardia, which is a regular rhythm.

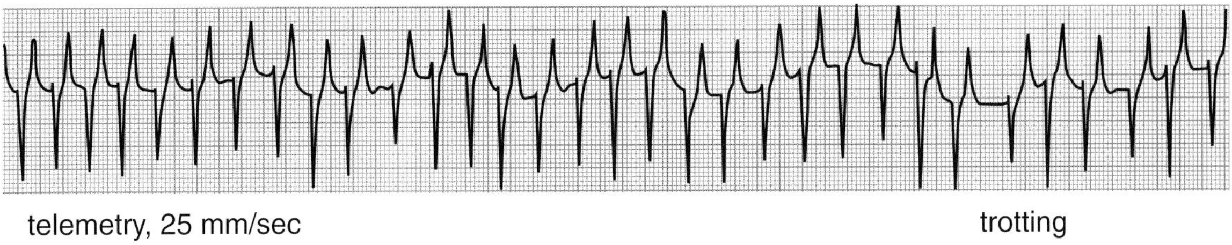

Figure 2.74 Exercising ECG from a horse with lone atrial fibrillation. Horses with atrial fibrillation have exercising heart rates that are 40–70 beats higher for each level of exercise than a horse with normal sinus rhythm. This horse has a heart rate of 150 bpm at the trot. A horse in sinus rhythm would have a heart rate of 80–120 bpm at the trot. The increase in heart rate is necessary to maintain cardiac output in the face of reduced atrial contribution to ventricular filling and stroke volume. It is the limiting factor in a horse's ability to perform at speed while in atrial fibrillation. Racehorses, upper-level event horses, and approximately 50% of Grand Prix–level jumpers are unable to perform successfully while in atrial fibrillation.

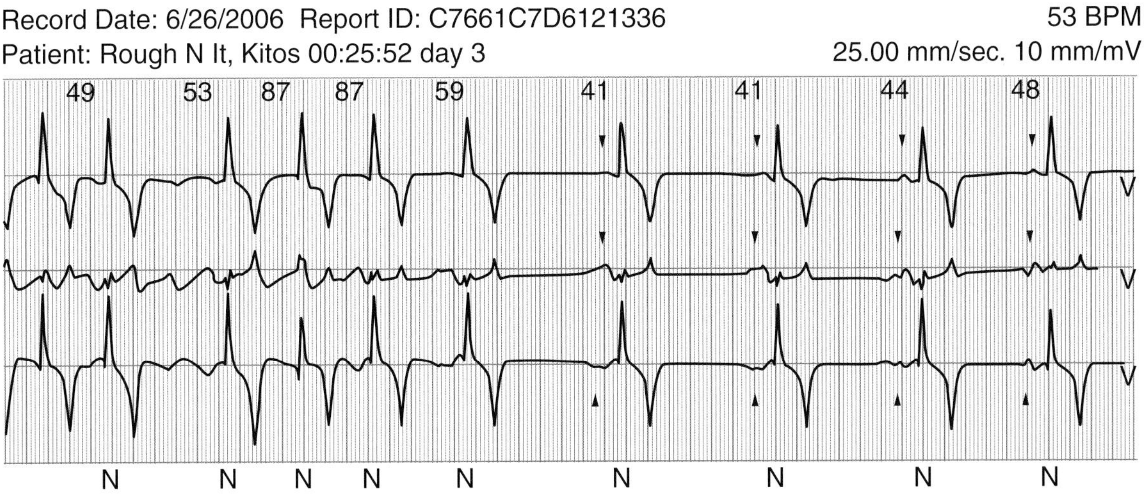

Figure 2.75 Holter monitor recording of horse converting from atrial fibrillation to normal sinus rhythm. Note the leads are not the standard base apex arrangement. P waves (arrowheads) following conversion are best seen in the middle lead.

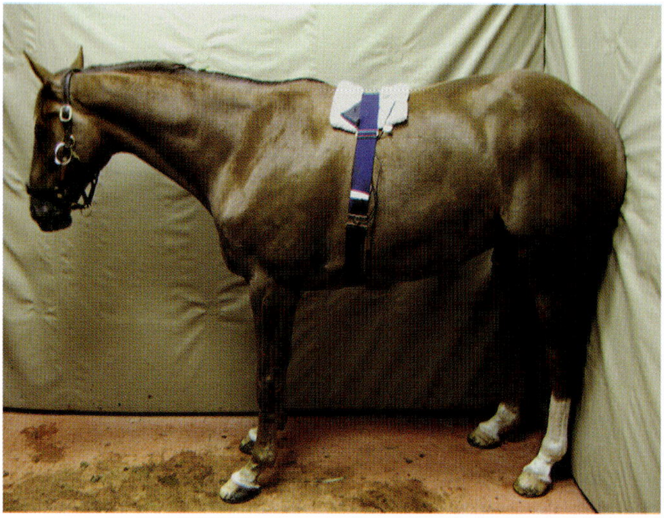

Figure 2.76 A horse fitted with telemetry during quinidine sulfate treatment. Idiosyncratic and toxic reactions can occur quickly with quinidine administration. Horses undergoing treatment should be monitored closely for development of various arrhythmias and other side effects. This horse demonstrated subtle neurologic signs manifested by positioning himself in the corner of the stall and leaning against the wall for support. Hypotensive horses may show this behavior as well. It is important that these signs be recognized and the horse not be moved as collapse may occur.

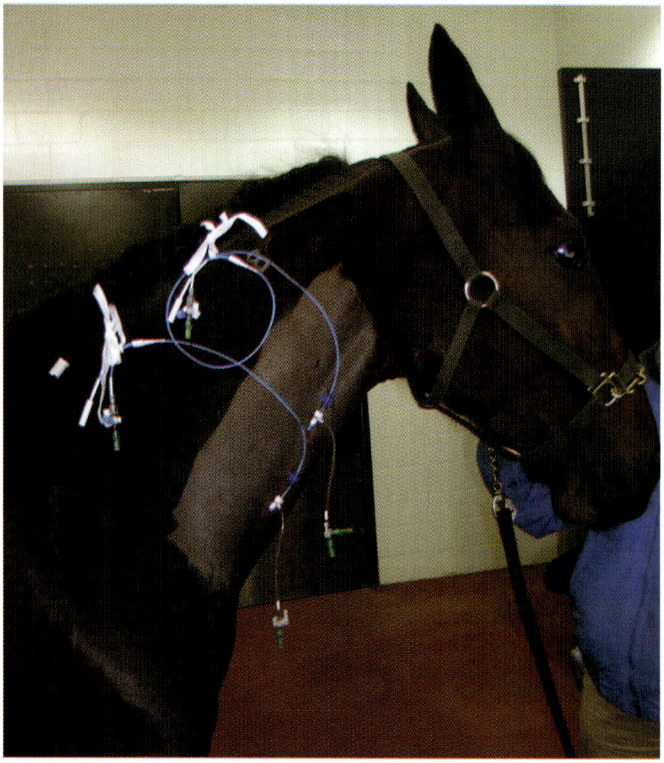

Figure 2.77 Photograph of horse fitted with electrical cardioversion catheters. Catheters are placed into the right atrium and left pulmonary artery via the jugular vein under ultrasound and pressure transducer guidance. Positioning of the pulmonary arterial catheter is confirmed radiographically (fig. 2.78). Defibrillation is performed under general anesthesia.

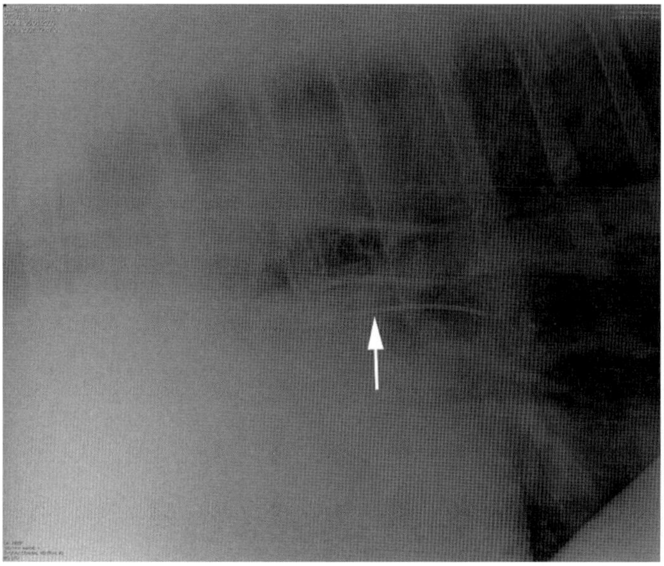

Figure 2.78 Radiographic image of radiopaque electrical cardioversion catheter in the pulmonary artery (arrow).

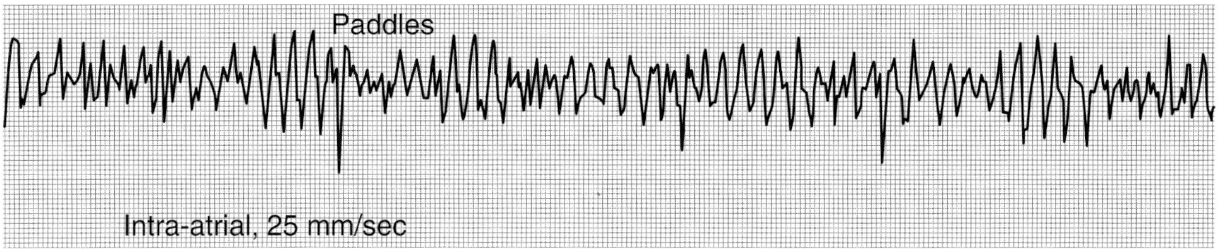

Figure 2.79 Intra-atrial ECG obtained from horse undergoing electrical cardioversion. Note rapid and chaotic atrial depolarization consistent with atrial fibrillation.

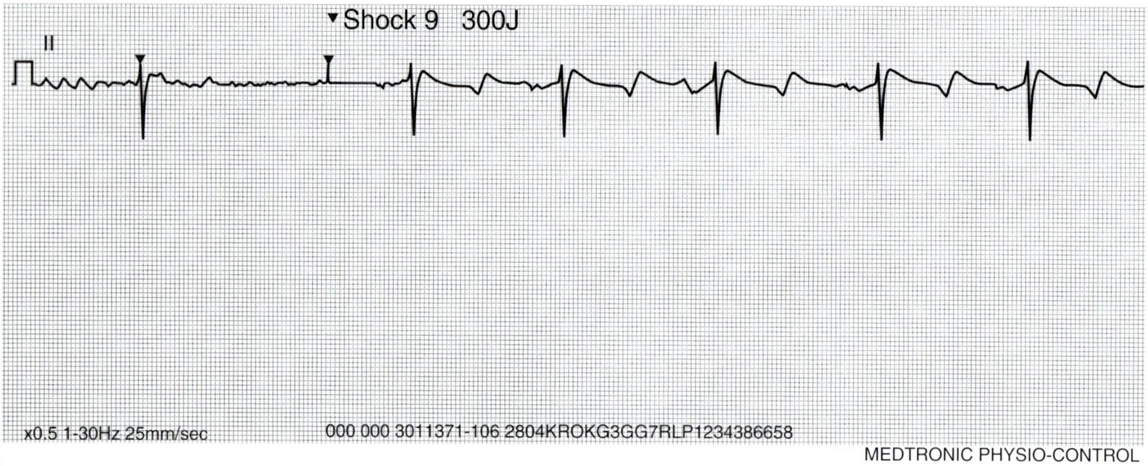

Figure 2.80 Base apex surface ECG showing atrial fibrillation, delivery of electrical shock, and conversion to normal sinus rhythm.

Ventricular Arrhythmias

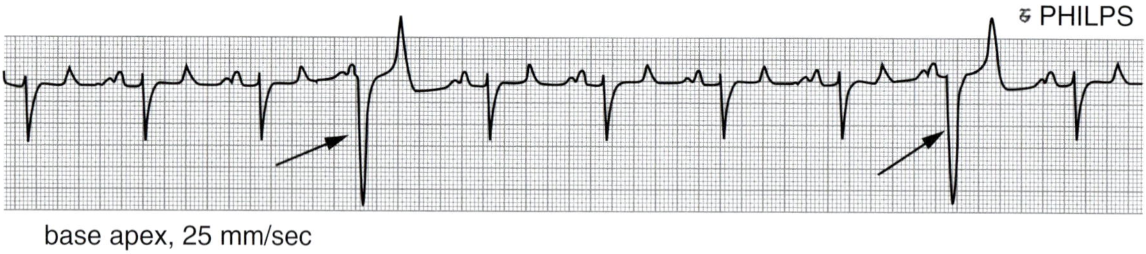

Figure 2.81 Ventricular premature depolarization (VPC, VPD, PVC). Note the premature, wide, and bizarre QRS complexes (arrows) and extremely short P-R interval. VPCs can occur secondary to a number of conditions including myocardial disease, electrolyte abnormalities, various drugs, ischemia, and high sympathetic tone. Normal horses may have up to 1 VPC per hour on a 24-hour Holter recording.

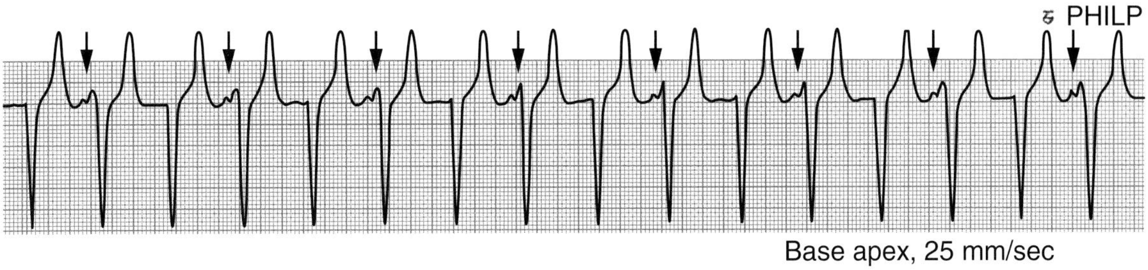

Figure 2.82 Sustained unifocal ventricular tachycardia. Note the rapid regular rhythm. QRS complexes are wide and not associated with P waves although P waves can be seen at regular intervals throughout the strip (arrows). The QRS complexes are all similar in appearance indicating a single irritable focus in the ventricle. The regularity of the rhythm is an important feature to note as this distinguishes rapid ventricular tachycardia (where the P waves are often not visible due to rate) from rapid atrial fibrillation, an irregularly irregular rhythm lacking in P waves.

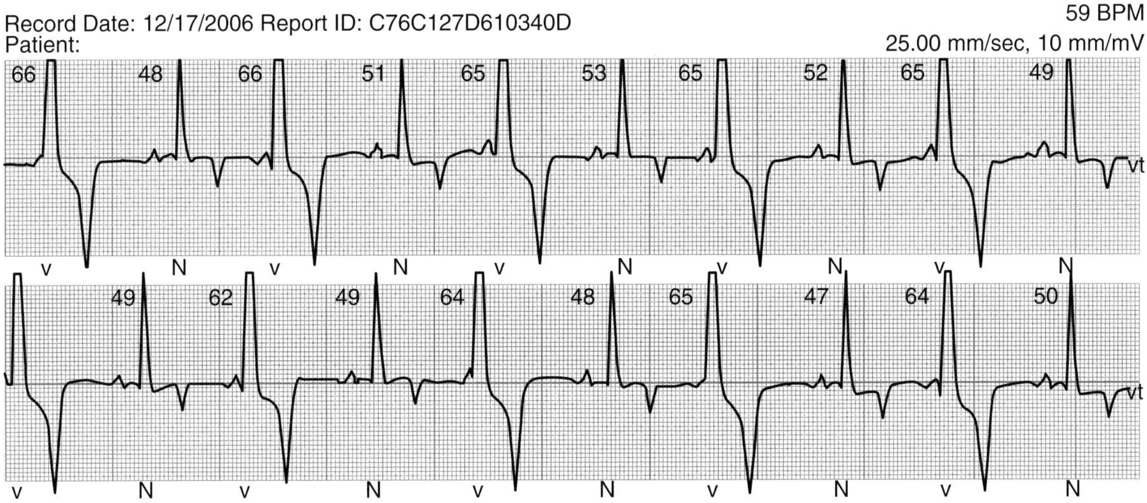

Figure 2.83 Ventricular bigeminy; Holter recording. Occasionally an irritable ventricular focus will repeatedly couple to the end of a normal cycle. The pattern is referred to as ventricular bigeminy. N, normal sinus beat; V, ventricular premature beat.

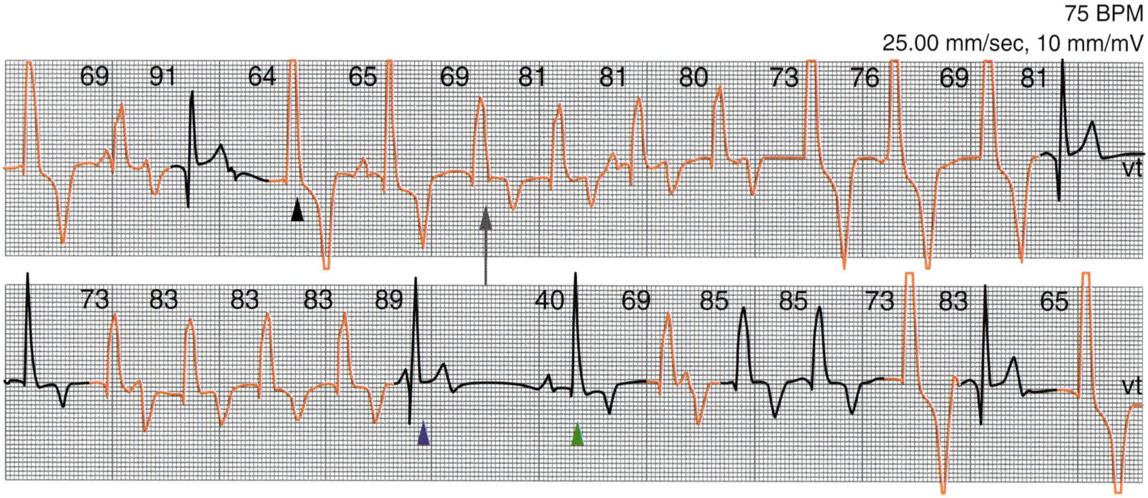

Figure 2.84 Multiform ventricular tachycardia. Holter recording. When several irritable foci are present within the ventricles, wide and bizarre QRS complexes that differ in appearance to each other will be present. Note the two forms of VPCs (black and gray arrows). Capture beats (blue arrow) and fusion beats (green arrow) are also present.

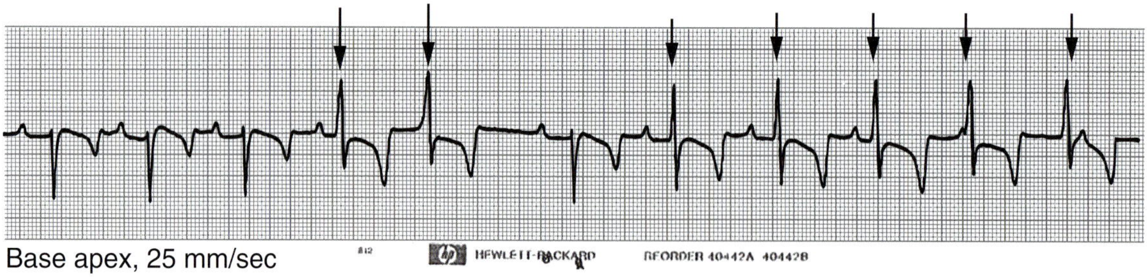

Figure 2.85 Paroxysmal ventricular tachycardia. Note the intermittent runs of unifocal ventricular premature beats (arrows).

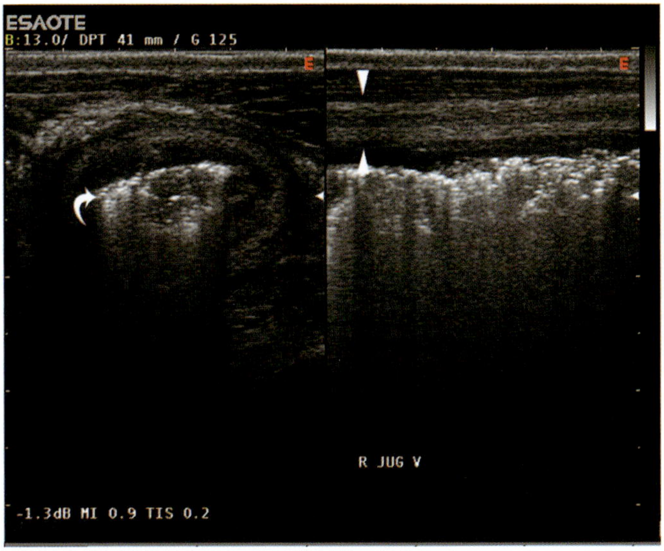

Figure 2.86 Sonogram of septic thrombophlebitis of the jugular vein. Note the hyperechoic luminal gas echoes (arrow) consistent with anaerobic infection. The vein is thick walled (between arrowheads) and the surrounding tissue is thick and echogenic consistent with a perivasculitis. Jugular vein thrombophlebitis almost always occurs secondary to venipuncture or use of indwelling catheters particularly in animals predisposed by a hypercoagulable state. The thrombus may or may not be septic (fig. 2.87). Complications may include profound edema of the head (mostly in bilateral jugular vein thrombosis–fig. 2.89b), endocarditis and pulmonary thromboembolism. Ultrasound-guided aspirate will aid in selecting appropriate antibiotics. Treatment may include systemic anti-inflammatory drugs, antibiotics, surgical drainage, or removal of the vein (fig. 2.90)

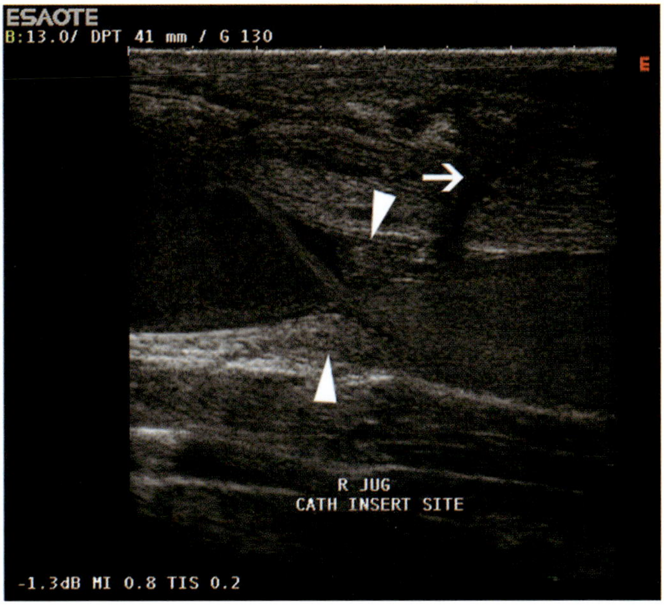

Figure 2.87 Thrombus (arrowheads) at previous catheter site (arrow) with no sign of infection. Note the echogenic swirling blood as it slows just proximal to the thrombus (to the right of the image). Palpation of the vein did not identify heat or elicit a painful response.

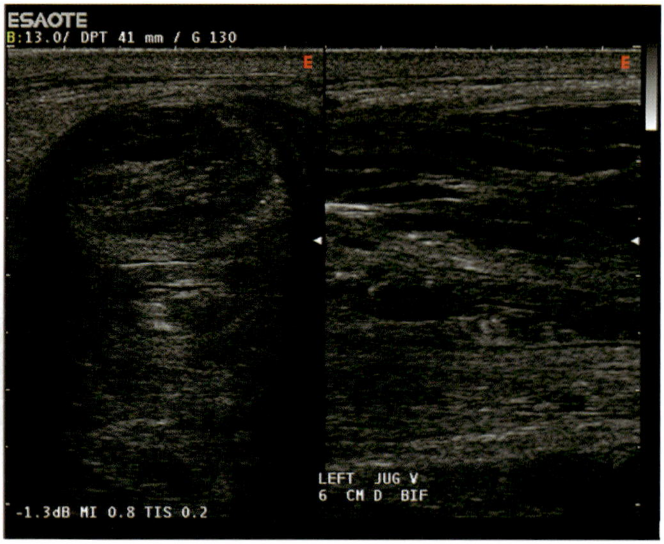

Figure 2.88 Multiloculated, cavitated thrombus in jugular vein consistent with septic thrombophlebitis.

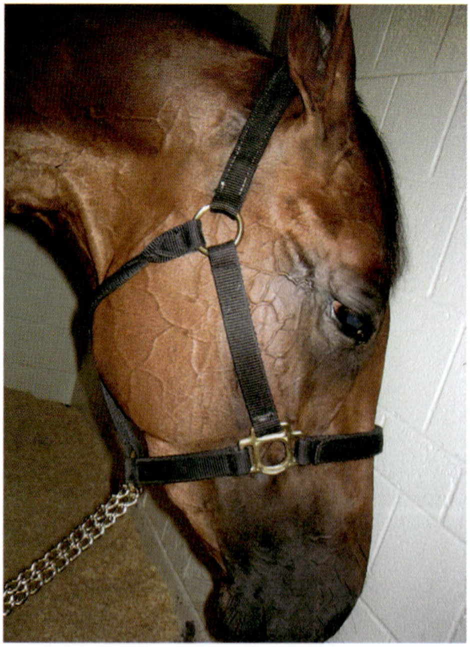

Figure 2.89a Photograph of a horse with venous distension of the head and neck secondary to acute thrombophlebitis.

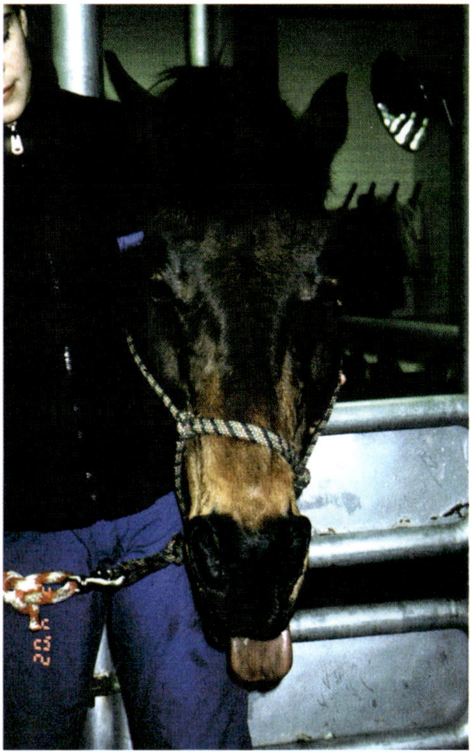

Figure 2.89b Edema of the head and tongue in a horse affected with bilateral jugular thrombosis.

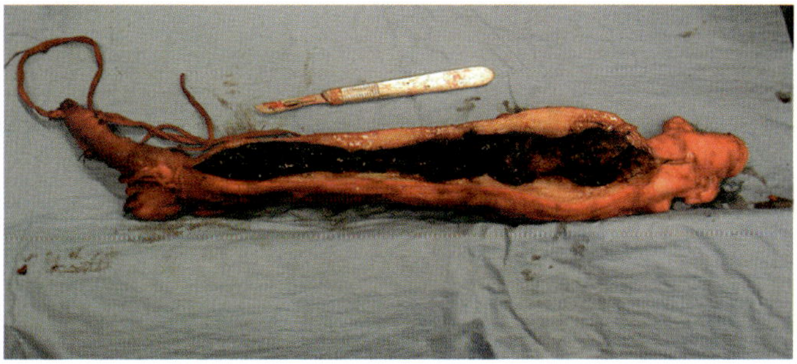

Figure 2.90 Jugular vein; postsurgical removal. Surgical removal should be considered for treatment of jugular vein thrombophlebitis when the infection is nonresponsive to medical therapy and the thrombus does not extend beyond the thoracic inlet.

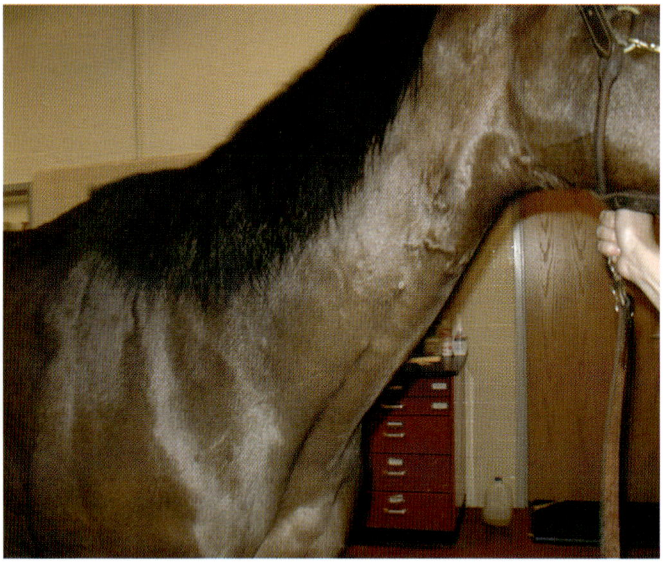

Figure 2.91 Postoperative appearance of the horse from which images in figs. 2.86 and 2.90 were obtained.

Aortic Root Disease

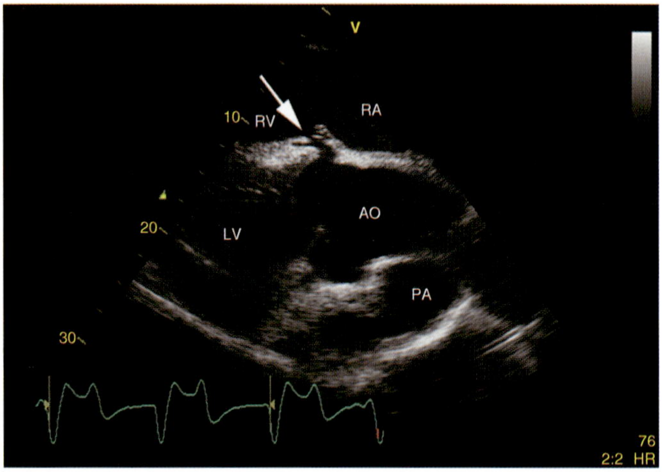

Figure 2.92 Echocardiographic image of an aortocardiac fistula. Note the defect in the wall of the aorta (arrow) just distal to the sinus of Valsalva. Flow through the defect can be confirmed with color flow Doppler (fig. 2.94). Horses with aortocardiac fistulas will usually present in acute distress with ventricular tachycardia (fig. 2.95) and a continuous right-sided murmur. The ventricular arrhythmia may self correct or respond to antiarrhythmic therapy. An aortic aneurysm (fig. 2.96) may be present prior to rupture. Rupture can occur into the right atrium (fig. 2.97) or right ventricle or dissect along the interventricular septum. Older male horses are overrepresented. Affected horses live up to 4 years with an aortocardiac fistula. These horses are unsound and should never be ridden. AO, aorta; LV, left ventricle; RA, right atrium; RV, right ventricle; PA, pulmonary artery.

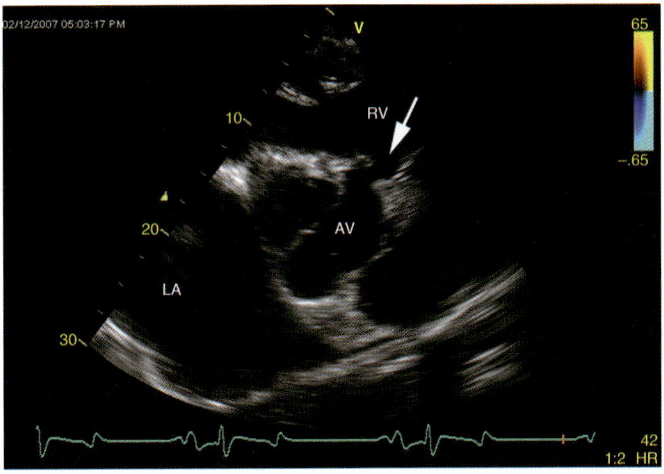

Figure 2.93 Echocardiographic image of aortocardiac fistula (arrow) in right parasternal short axis view of the aortic valve (AV). LA, left atrium; RV, right ventricle.

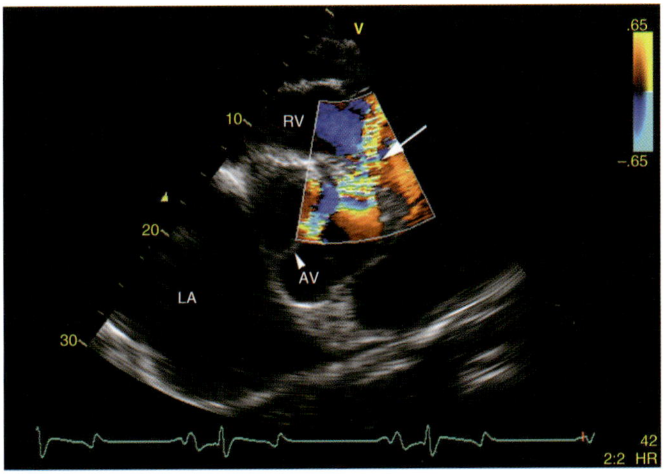

Figure 2.94 Color flow Doppler image of an aortocardiac fistula. Note the flow (arrow) from the aorta into the right ventricle (RV). This left to right shunt eventually causes left-sided volume overload and congestive heart failure similar to congenital left to right shunts. RV, right ventricle; LA, left atrium; AV, aortic valve.

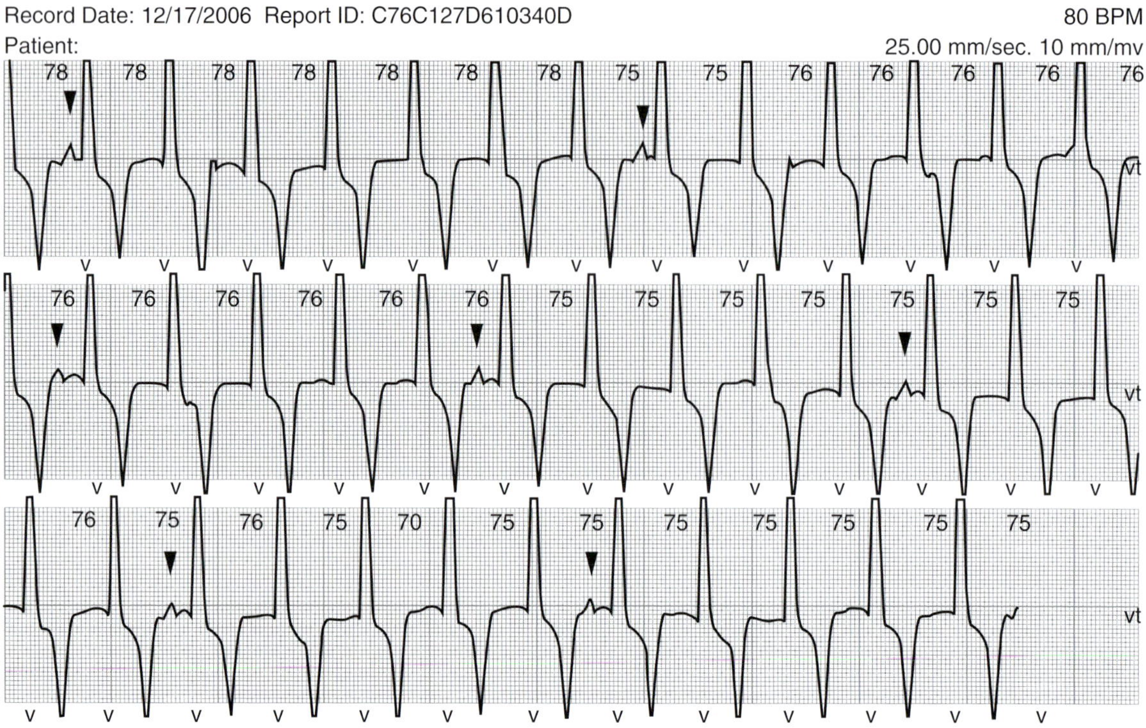

Figure 2.95 Uniform ventricular tachycardia secondary to rupture of the aorta into the right ventricle; Holter monitor recording. The rhythm may spontaneously resolve in some horses. Anti-arrhythmic therapy should be employed in any horse that is hemodynamically unstable, has a heart rate greater than 120 bpm, the rhythm is multiform, or the R on T phenomenon is detected. Arrowheads point out P waves. V, ventricular premature beat.

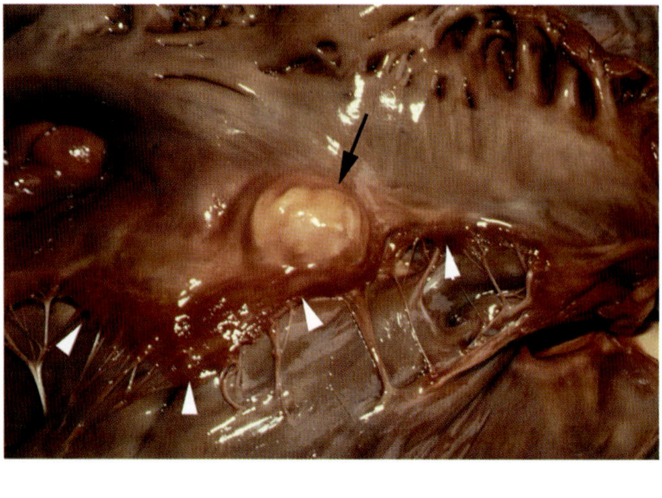

Figure 2.96 Postmortem photograph of aortic aneurysm viewed from the right side of the heart at the level of tricuspid valve. Note bulging of sinus of Valsalva (arrow) just proximal to tricuspid valve (arrowheads).

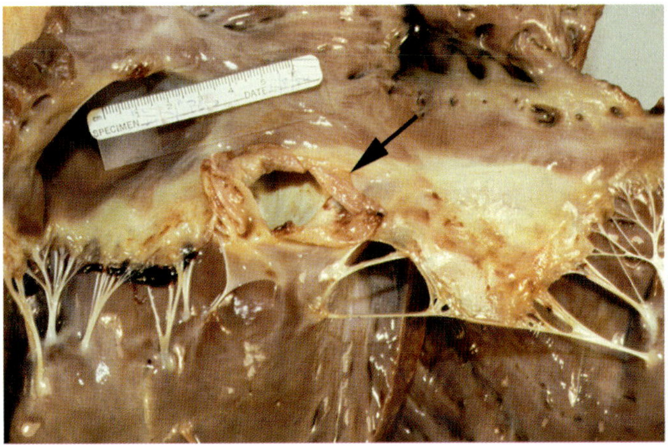

Figure 2.97 Postmortem photograph of aortocardiac fistula rupture (arrow) into right atrium.

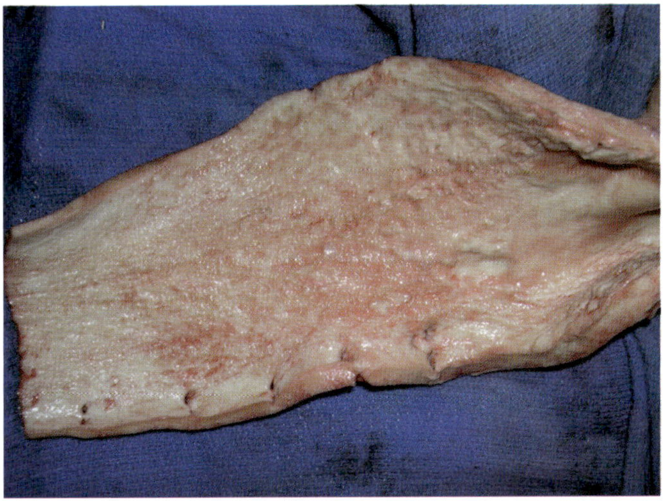

Figure 2.98 Postmortem photograph of verminous arteritis (aorta). Note the corrugated appearance of the intimal lining of the aorta. Fibrinous thrombi and several raised firm areas consistent with mineralization were present. The lesion extended 30 cm out the ascending aorta and into the right coronary artery. Coronary artery thromboemboli caused numerous myocardial infarcts (figs. 2.35 and 2.36). The horse died from a ventricular dysrhythmia.

2

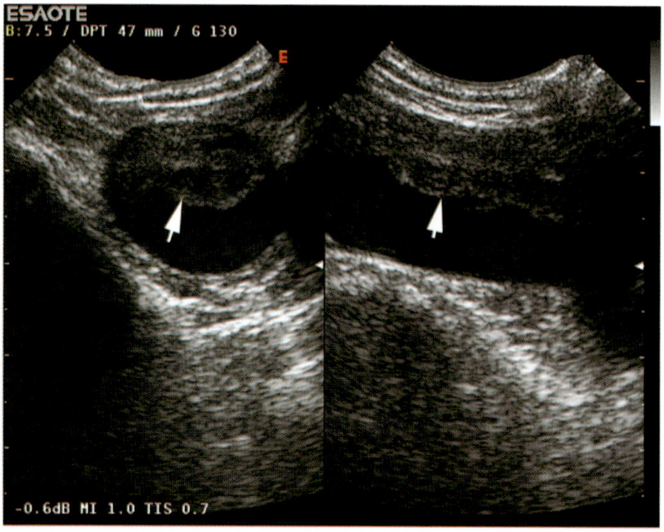

Figure 2.99 Sonogram of an aortoiliac thrombus (arrows). Etiology of this disease process is not fully understood. Horses are usually young intact males with a history of poor performance and hind limb lameness or stiffness. In severe cases the horse may have rigid hind limbs and an arched back, and may walk on its toes or go down. The limbs are cool to the touch and saphenous vein refill time is prolonged. Treatment is limited to aspirin therapy and continued exercise in horses that can tolerate it. Prognosis is poor to grave if the thrombus is large and occludes the terminal aorta.

Purpura Hemorrhagica

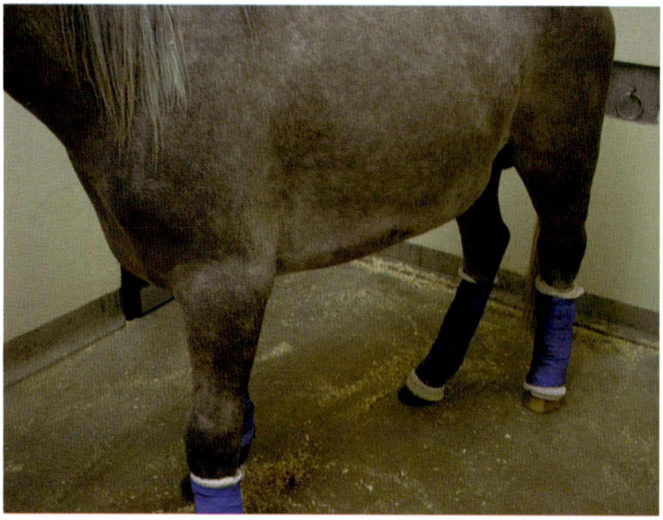

Figure 2.100 An adult horse affected with purpura hemorrhagica. Note the ventral and limb edema. Purpura hemorrhagica appears to be immune-complex-mediated vasculitis that is caused by type III hypersensitivity reaction. The disease is usually a sequela to *Streptococcus equi* infection. However, it can also follow other infection such as equine influenza. Clinical signs include ventral, head, and limb edema (figs. 2.101 and 2.102), and mucosal petechiae and ecchymoses (figs. 2.103–2.106). Fever and anorexia are uncommon. Edema may progress to serum exudation, crusting, sloughing, and ulceration (figs. 2.107–2.109). Treatment is usually achieved by the administration of antibiotics and corticosteroids as well as supportive therapy.

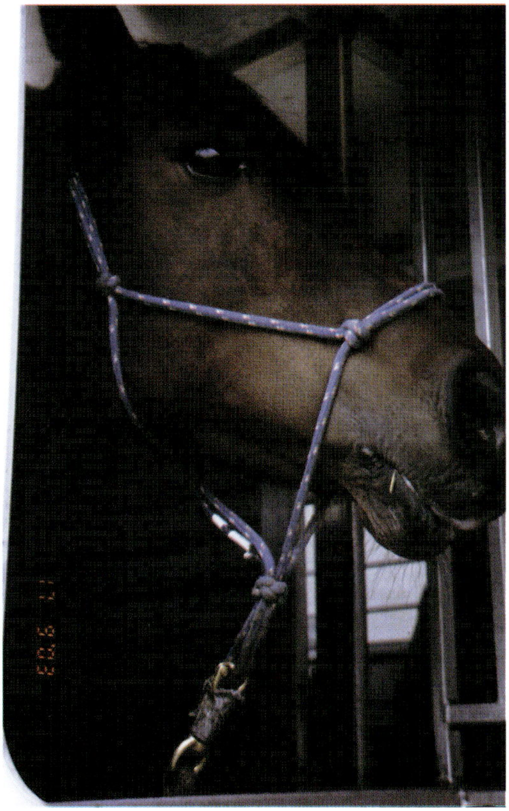

Figure 2.101 Edema of the head (cheek) in a horse affected with purpura hemorrhagica.

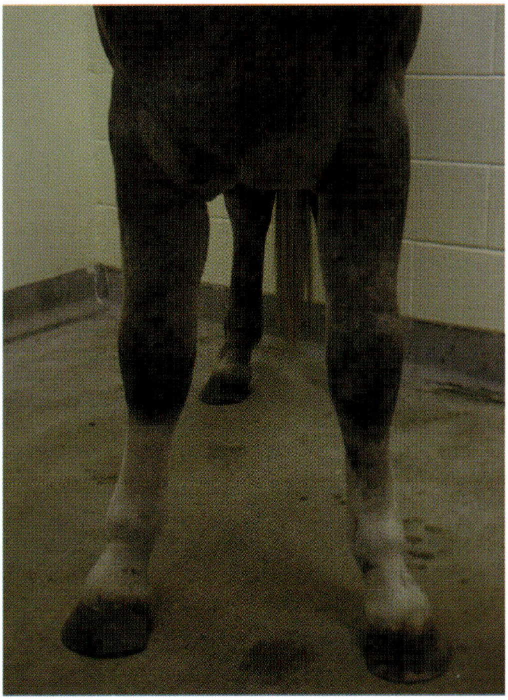

Figure 2.102 Limb edema in a horse affected with purpura hemorrhagica.

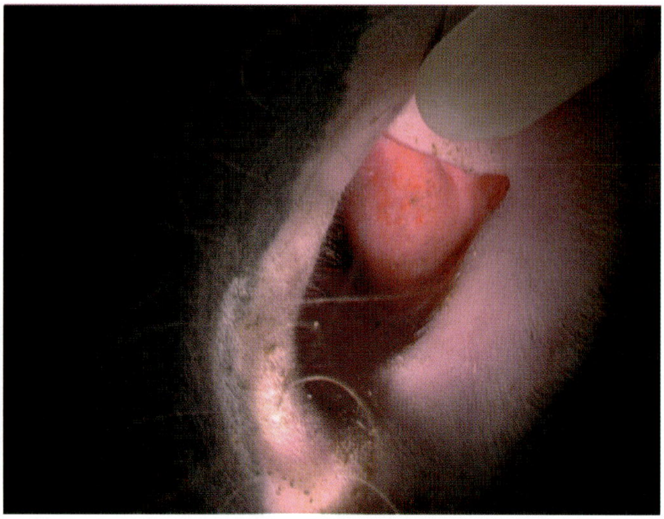

Figure 2.103 Petechiae in the nasal mucosa in a horse affected with purpura hemorrhagica.

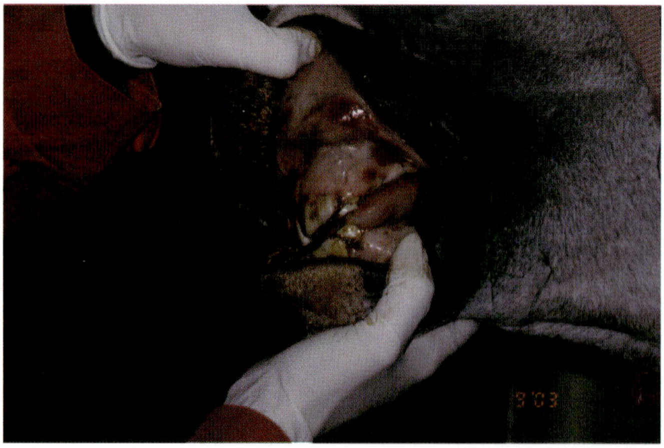

Figure 2.104 Ecchymoses in the oral mucosa in a horse affected with purpura hemorrhagica.

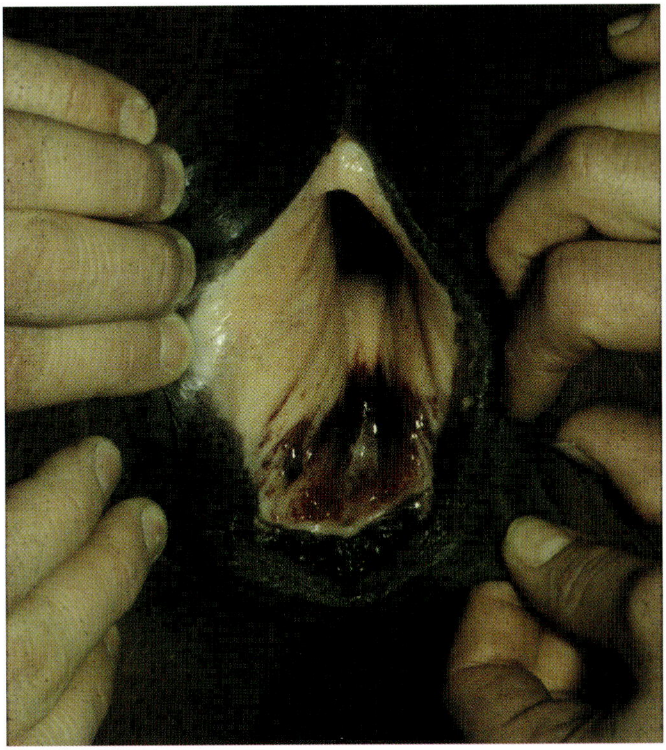

Figure 2.105 Ecchymoses in the vulvar mucosa in a mare affected with purpura hemorrhagica.

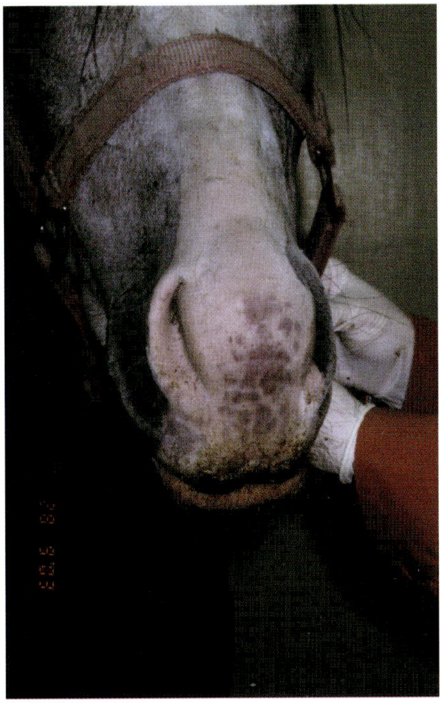

Figure 2.106 Ecchymotic hemorrhage on the muzzle of a horse affected with purpura hemorrhagica.

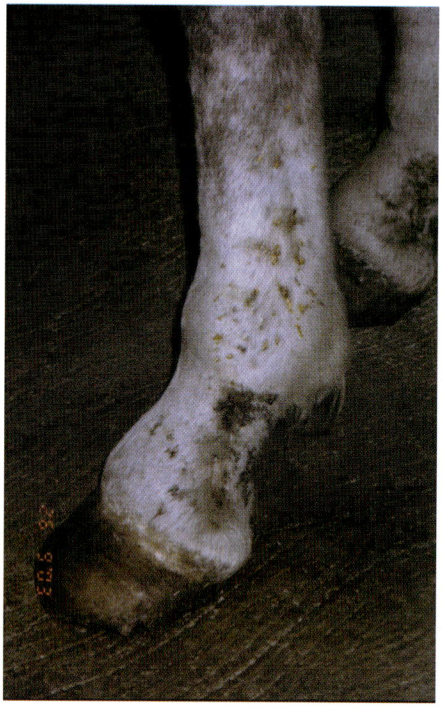

Figure 2.107 Serum exudation and limb edema in a horse affected with purpura hemorrhagica.

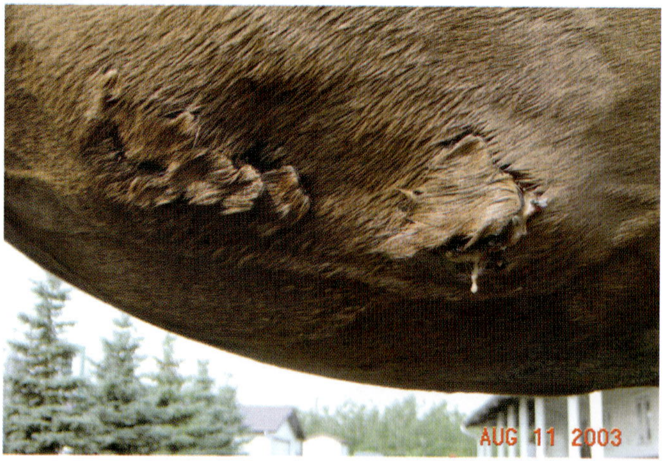

Figure 2.108 Skin crusting in a horse affected with purpura hemorrhagica.

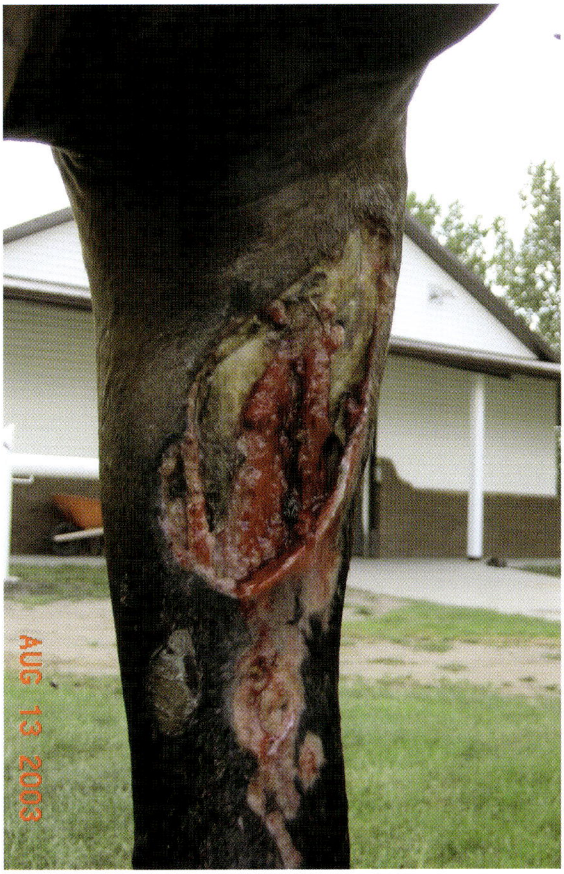

Figure 2.109 Skin sloughing in a horse affected with purpura hemorrhagica.

Recommended Reading

Bonagura, JD, Reef, VB. Disorders of the cardiovascular system. In Reed SM, Bayly WM, Sellon DC, eds. Equine internal medicine. 2nd ed. Philadelphia: WB Saunders, 355–459, 2004.

Marr, CM, Reef, VB, Brazil, TJ, et al. Aorto-cardiac fistulas in seven horses. Veterinary Radiology & Ultrasound 39(1):22–31, 1998.

Reef, VB. Cardiovascular ultrasonography. In Reef VB, ed., Equine diagnostic ultrasound. Philadelphia: WB Saunders, 215–72, 1998.

Sage, AM, Worth, L. Fever: Endocarditis and pericarditis. In Marr CM, ed., Cardiology of the horse. Philadelphia: WB Saunders, 256–67, 1999.

3 Diseases of the Respiratory System

Diseases of the Extrathoracic Airways
- Nasal Passages
  - Wry Nose
  - Progressive Ethmoid Hematoma
- Sinus Diseases
  - Sinusitis
  - Sinus Cyst
  - Sinonasal Neoplasia and Polyps
- Guttural Pouch Diseases
  - Guttural Pouch Empyema
  - Guttural Pouch Tympany
  - Guttural Pouch Mycosis
- Pharyngeal Diseases
  - Dorsal Displacement of the Soft Palate (DDSP)
  - Pharyngitis
- Laryngeal Diseases
  - Subepiglottic Cyst
  - Epiglottic Entrapment
  - Arytenoid Chondropathy
  - Laryngeal Hemiplegia
- Tracheal Collapse

Diseases of the Intrathoracic Airways
- Noninfectious Pulmonary Diseases
  - Recurrent Airway Obstruction (RAO, Heaves)
  - Inflammatory Airway Disease (IAD)
  - Exercise-induced Pulmonary Hemorrhage (EIPH)
- Infectious Pulmonary Diseases
  - Bacterial Pneumonia in Adult Horses
  - Aspiration Pneumonia
  - Pleuropneumonia
  - Interstitial Pneumonia in Adult Horses

Diseases of the Thoracic Wall and Pleura
- Pneumothorax

Strangles

African Horse Sickness

Nasal Passages

Wry Nose

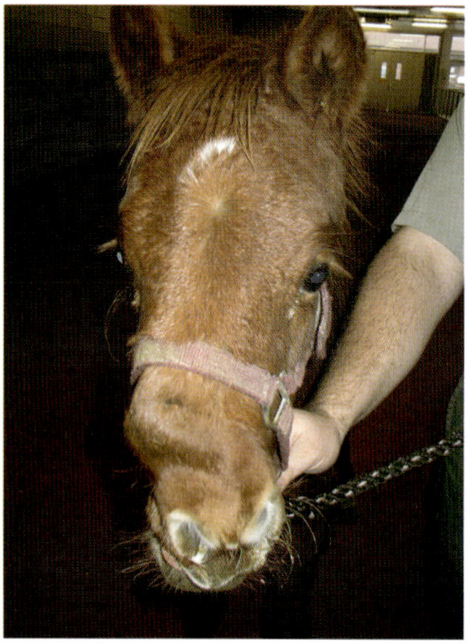

Figure 3.1a Foal born with a wry nose. Congenital shortening and deviation of the maxillae, premaxillae, nasal bones, and vomer bone. It is also called campylorrhinus lateralis. Wry nose is a rare deformity encountered in newborn foals. The condition is thought to be secondary to abnormal fetal position. Mildly affected cases may not need immediate treatment. Severely affected cases can be corrected surgically.

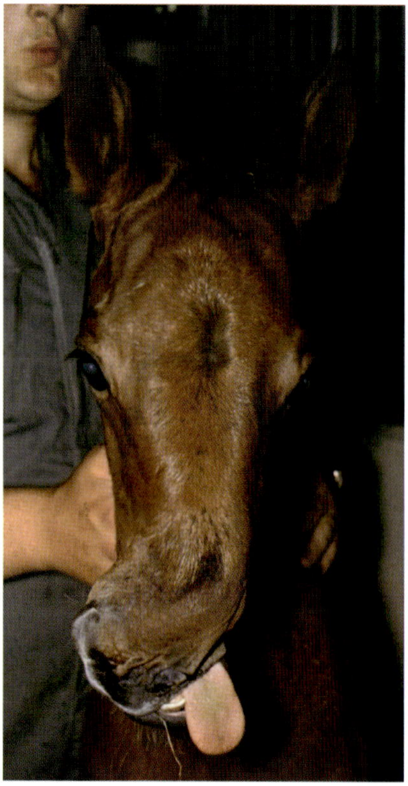

Figure 3.1b Another foal affected with wry nose. (Photograph is courtesy of Dr. Peter Fretz, WCVM, University of Saskatchewan.)

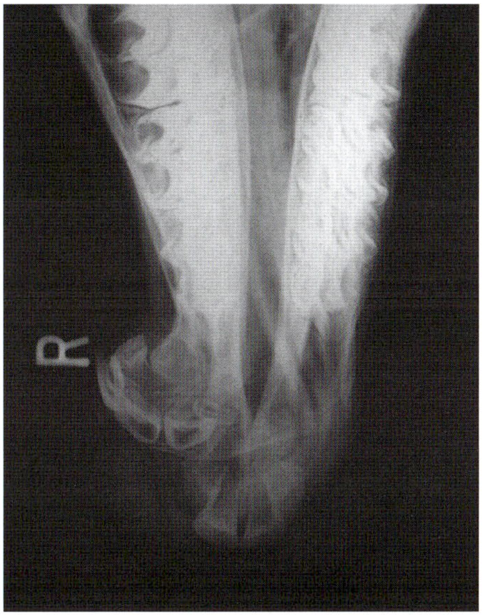

Figure 3.1c Radiograph of the maxilla of the foal seen in fig. 3.1b. (Photograph is courtesy of Dr. Peter Fretz, WCVM, University of Saskatchewan.)

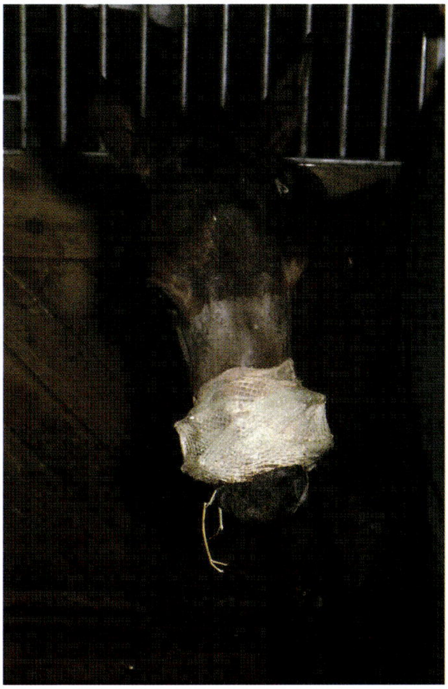

Figure 3.1d The same foal seen in fig. 3.1b after surgical correction. (Photograph is courtesy of Dr. Peter Fretz, WCVM, University of Saskatchewan.)

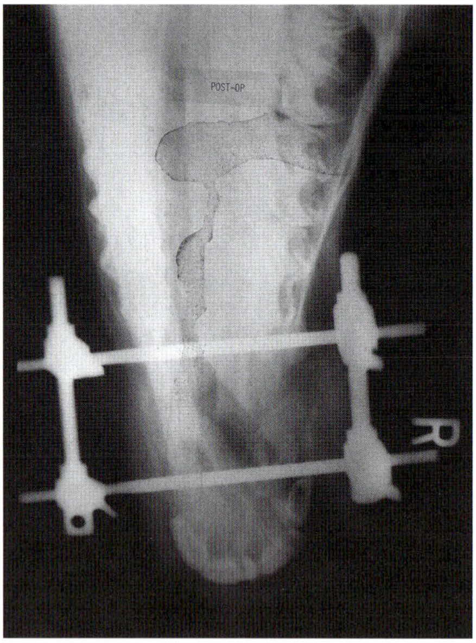

Figure 3.1e Radiograph of the maxilla of the foal seen in fig. 3.1b after surgical correction. (Photograph is courtesy of Dr. Peter Fretz, WCVM, University of Saskatchewan.)

Progressive Ethmoid Hematoma

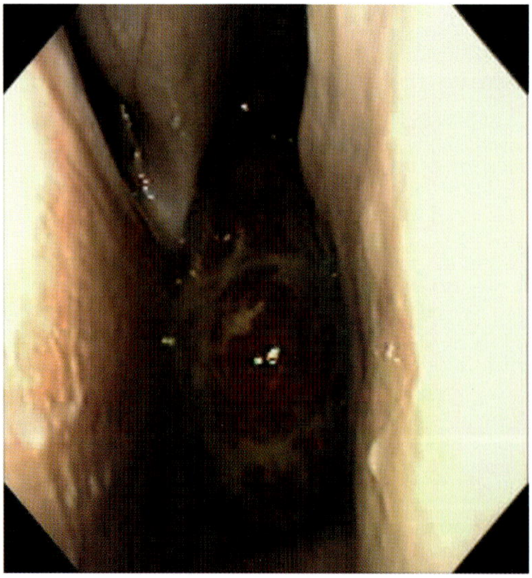

Figure 3.2 Endoscopy of the caudal nasal passage revealing a red, smooth, glistening ethmoid hematoma protruding from the ethmoid region. The brown-green discoloration on the surface of the ethmoid hematoma is caused by hemosiderin deposition. Repeated submucosal hemorrhages originating from the ethmoid turbinate region or paranasal sinuses result in a progressively growing mass that may obstruct airflow. Epistaxis or blood-tinged nasal discharge are typically associated with the lesion. Treatment of ethmoid hematoma includes surgical or cryogenic ablation, laser photoablation, and intralesional injection of formalin.

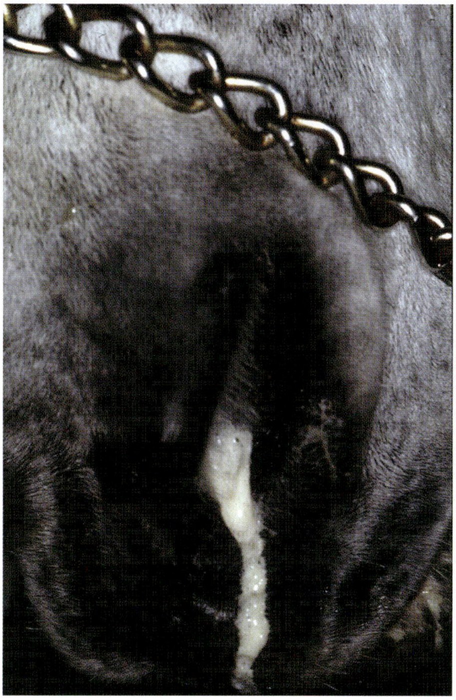

Figure 3.3 Unilateral purulent nasal discharge in a horse with chronic sinusitis. Sinusitis may result from primary infection (viral, bacterial, or fungal) or be secondary to dental disorders or neoplasia. Sinusitis secondary to dental disease is often associated with purulent, foul-smelling, unilateral nasal discharge.

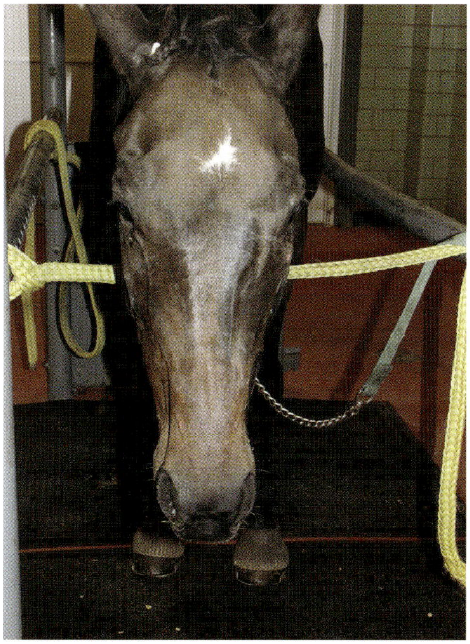

Figure 3.4 Deformation of the face over the left maxillary region in a horse with chronic sinusitis. Percussion of the sinuses while maintaining the mouth open may reveal dullness on the affected side but the technique is poorly sensitive.

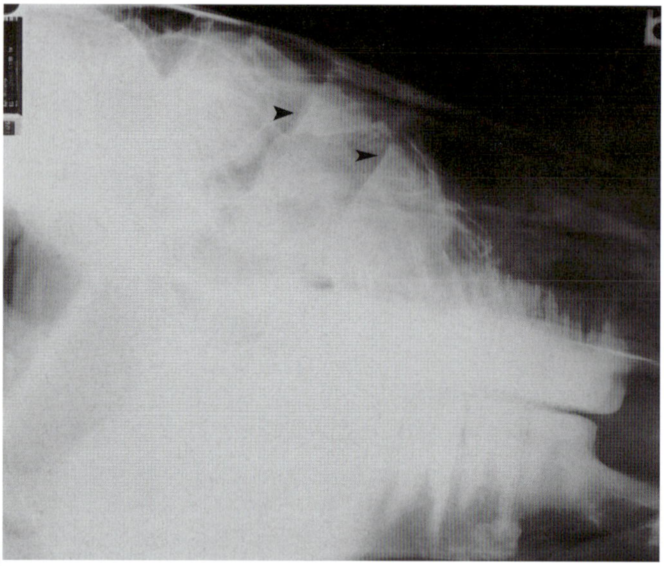

Figure 3.5 Lateral skull radiograph showing parallel fluid-air interfaces in the frontal and maxillary (rostral and caudal) sinuses in a horse with sinusitis (arrowheads). Particular attention should be paid to the cheek teeth (second to fourth) for evidence of periodontal or dental disease such as broken tooth, lytic changes, or increased opacity.

Sinus Cyst

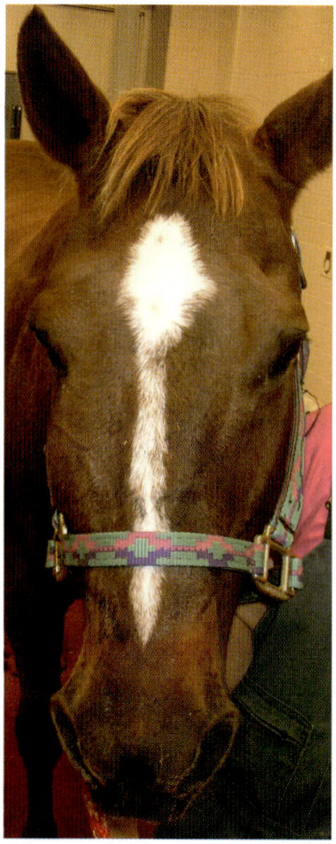

Figure 3.6a Deformation of the face over the right maxillary region in a horse with sinus cyst. The space-occupying cyst may result in nasal airway obstruction or deformation of the face. Fluid-filled cystic lesions arise from the maxillary or ventral conchal sinus. Serous to serohemorrhagic nasal discharge may be observed.

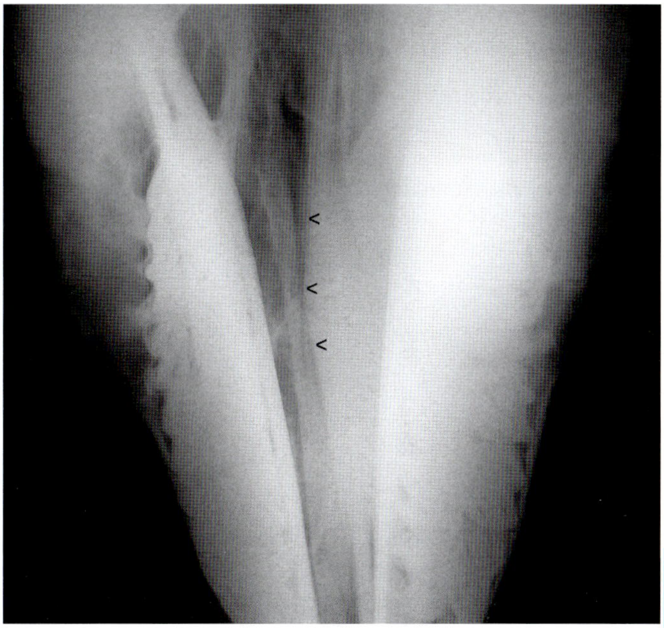

Figure 3.6b Skull radiograph typically reveals rounded, well-demarcated opacity. If the cyst is large, it can deviate the nasal septum as seen in this radiograph (arrowheads). Fluid lines may be detected if the cyst impairs sinus drainage. Needle aspiration of amber-colored cyst fluid provides confirmation of the presumptive diagnosis. Surgical resection of the cyst is curative.

Sinonasal Neoplasia and Polyps

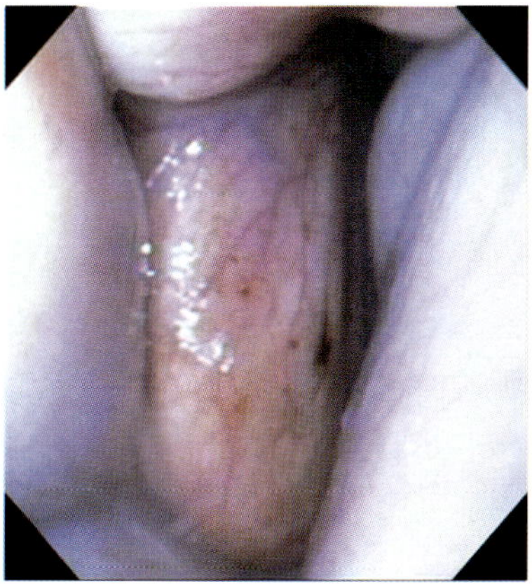

Figure 3.7 Tumors and polyps are rare tissue growths that may arise from sinuses or nasal passages. Osteoma, fibroma, chondroma, adenocarcinoma, squamous cell carcinoma, and other nasal tumors have been reported in horses. Clinical signs include unilateral purulent nasal discharge, epistaxis, facial swelling, and nasal obstruction. A combination of endoscopy, radiography, and tissue biopsy are required to differentiate neoplasia from polyps. The histopathological diagnosis may be complicated by the fact that neoplasia and polyps often contain large necrotic, cystic, and fibrotic areas. This is an endoscopic view of an osteoma of the nasal passages.

Guttural Pouch Diseases

Horses are the only domestic species that have large auditory tube diverticulae, also called guttural pouches. The stylohyoid bone protrudes through the ventral aspect of each pouch dividing it into a medial and a lateral compartment. Branches of several cranial nerves (VII, IX, X, XI, and XII), sympathetic trunk, and major arteries (internal carotid, external carotid, and maxillary) run in the wall of the guttural pouches. As a result, guttural pouch diseases may be accompanied by neurological deficits or hemorrhage. Each pouch opens into the nasopharynx via a fibrocartilaginous ostium (opening) that is kept closed during normal breathing.

Guttural Pouch Empyema

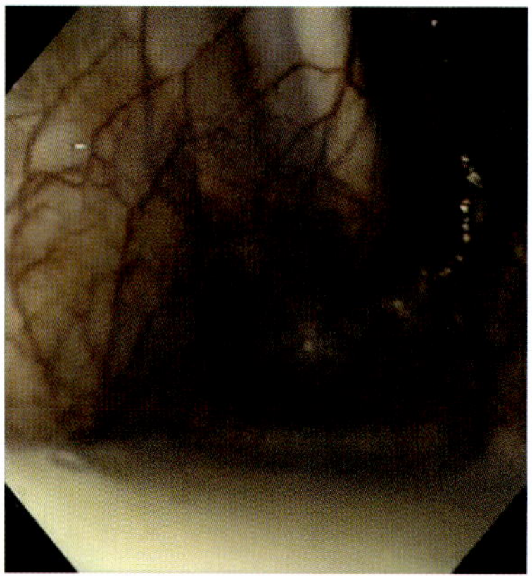

Figure 3.8 Endoscopic view of guttural pouch empyema secondary to streptococcal infection. Accumulation of purulent exudate in the guttural pouches may result from upper respiratory infection or rupture of abscessed retropharyngeal lymph node inside the ventral aspect of the medial compartment. The most common cause of guttural pouch empyema is *Streptococcus equi* subsp. *equi* infection "strangles" but other beta-hemolytic streptococci such as *S. equi* subsp *zooepidemicus* may also cause empyema.

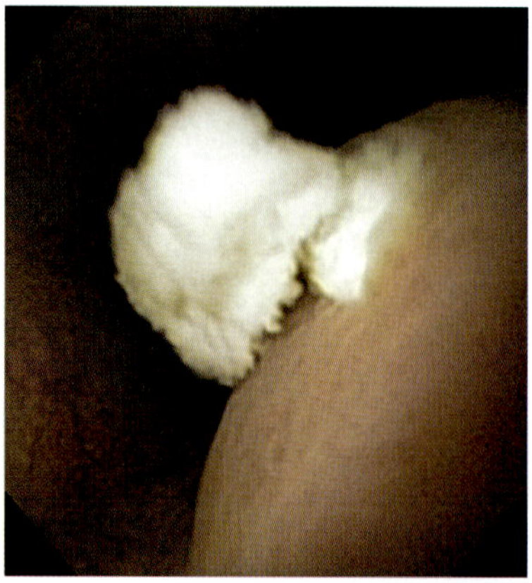

Figure 3.9 Endoscopic examination revealing purulent exudate draining from a swollen retropharyngeal lymph node inside the medial compartment of the guttural pouch.

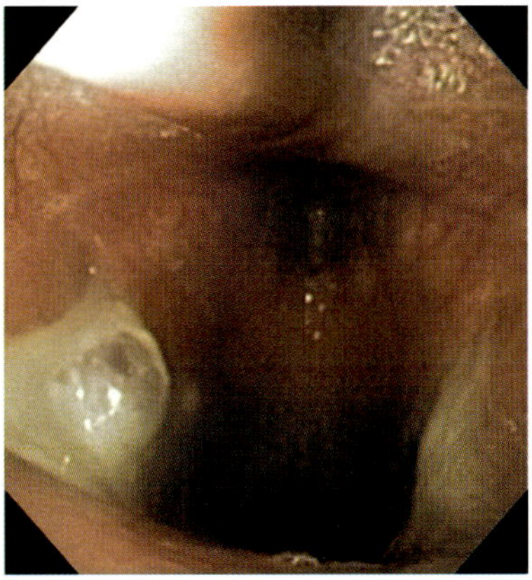

Figure 3.10 Endoscopy of the nasopharynx of a horse with strangles showing purulent discharge draining from both guttural pouch openings. Endoscopy of each guttural pouch is essential in any horse with a history of purulent nasal discharge or retropharyngeal swelling because empyema is not always accompanied by visible purulent discharge.

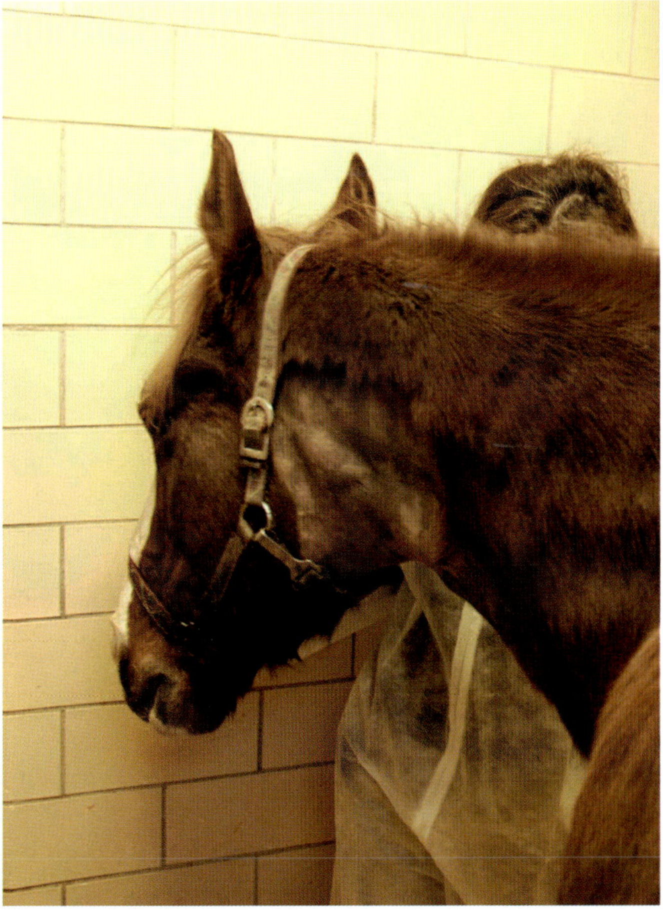

Figure 3.11 Enlarged retropharyngeal lymph nodes in a horse with strangles.

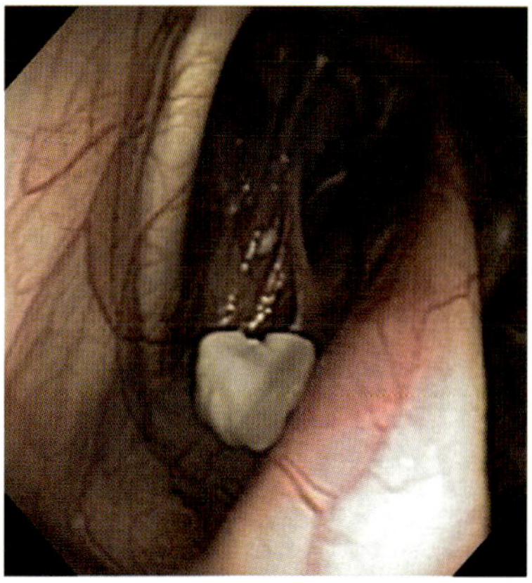

Figure 3.12 A chondroid located in the lateral compartment of the guttural pouch. Chronic empyema may result in formation of inspissated concretions called chondroids, as in this case.

Guttural Pouch Tympany

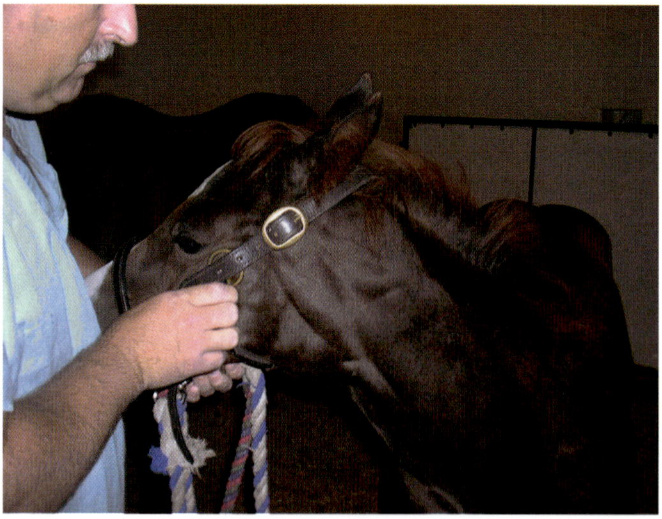

Figure 3.13 Marked distension of the throat latch region in a foal with guttural pouch tympany. Tympany is a rare disease of foals resulting from the accumulation of air within one or both guttural pouches secondary to abnormal function of the ostium. Marked swelling of guttural pouches may cause breathing difficulties, dysphagia, and secondary aspiration pneumonia.

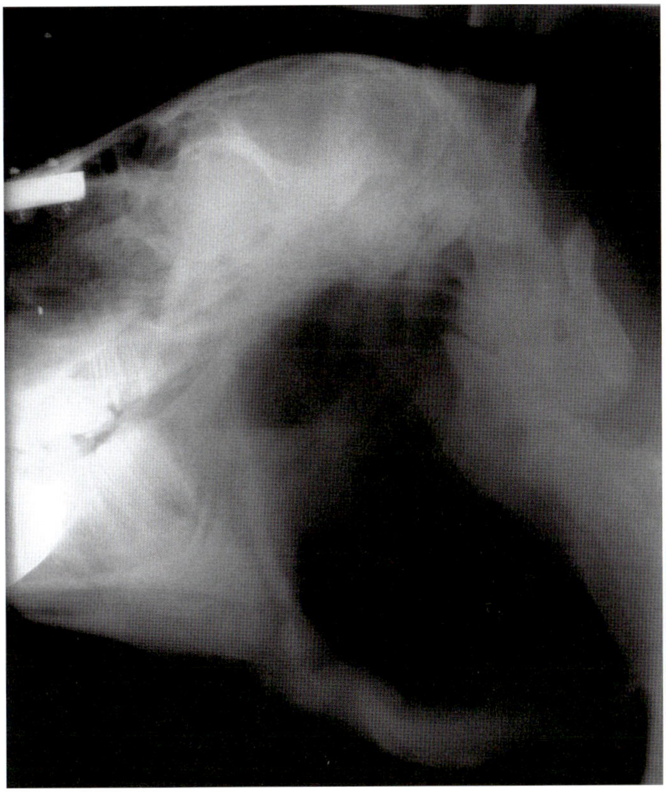

Figure 3.14 Lateral radiograph of a foal with guttural pouch tympany.

Guttural Pouch Mycosis

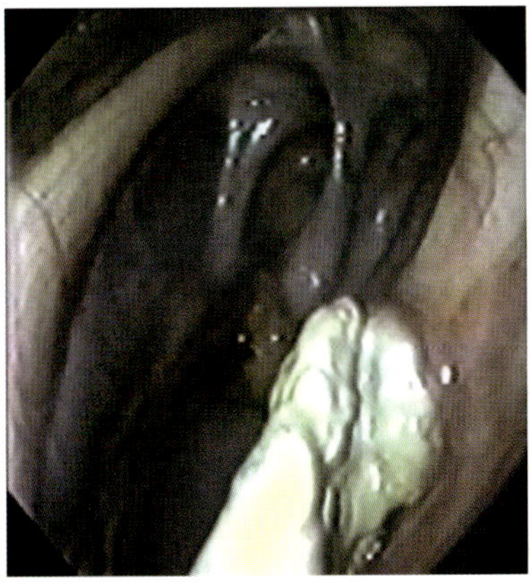

Figure 3.15 Fungal plaque on the wall of the right guttural pouch in a case of guttural pouch mycosis (GPM). GPM is a fungal infection of the guttural pouch. It could be unilateral or bilateral. Clinical signs of GPM include bloody nasal discharge and signs of cranial nerve deficits, such as dysphagia. Bloody nasal discharge is seen when fungal plaques are located on and erode guttural pouches blood vessels, such as the internal and external carotid arteries. Diagnosis is confirmed by endoscopic examination of the guttural pouches.

Pharyngeal Diseases

Dorsal Displacement of the Soft Palate (DDSP)

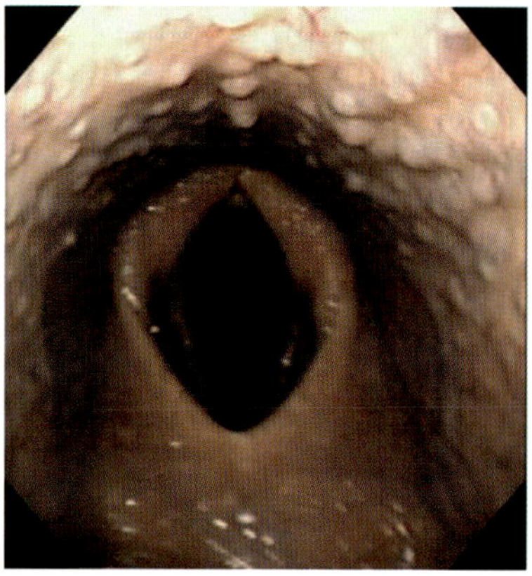

Figure 3.16 Dorsal displacement of the soft palate (DDSP) visualized by endoscopy at rest in a horse with dysphagia. DDSP can be intermittent or persistent. Intermittent DDSP can have many causes including pharyngeal inflammation, excitement, fatigue, and placing the tongue over the bit. Persistent DDSP can be caused by guttural pouch mycosis, epiglottic hypoplasia, flaccidity, and entrapment, or other epiglottic abnormalities. Clinical signs include respiratory noises and immediate exercise intolerance. Persistent DDSP can cause signs of dysphagia. Diagnosis is confirmed by endoscopy. Several conservative and surgical treatments have been suggested for DDSP.

Pharyngitis

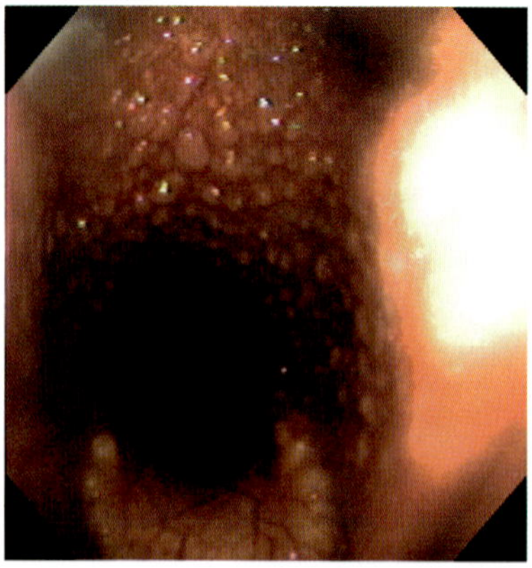

Figure 3.17 Grade 4/4 pharyngeal lymphoid hyperplasia in a 2-year-old racehorse. Lymphoid hyperplasia is a response to antigenic exposure such as bacteria and viruses. Pharyngitis is commonly observed in young horses and resolves on its own as they age. Lymphoid follicle hyperplasia is usually not observed in horses above 5 years of age.

Subepiglottic Cyst

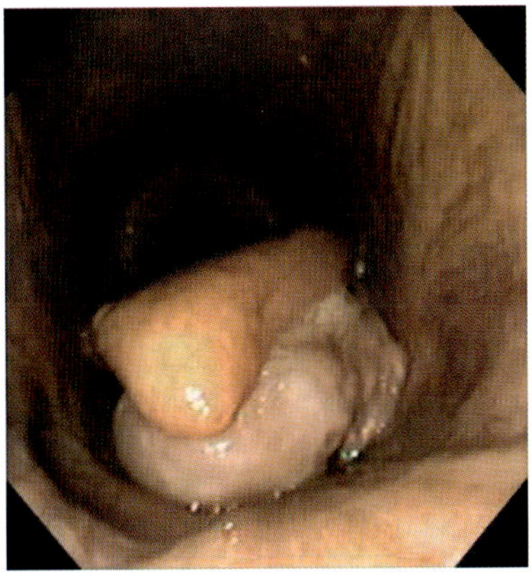

Figure 3.18 Subepiglottic cyst in a 4-year-old racehorse presented for poor performance and abnormal respiratory noise associated with exercise. Subepiglottic cyst can cause epiglottic entrapment and is usually treated surgically.

Epiglottic Entrapment

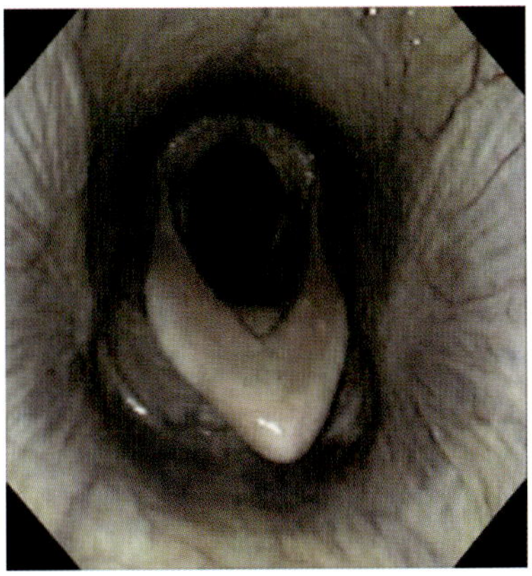

Figure 3.19 Epiglottis entrapped by aryepiglottic membrane in a racehorse presented for poor performance and abnormal respiratory noise associated with exercise. Treatment is usually surgical.

Arytenoid Chondropathy

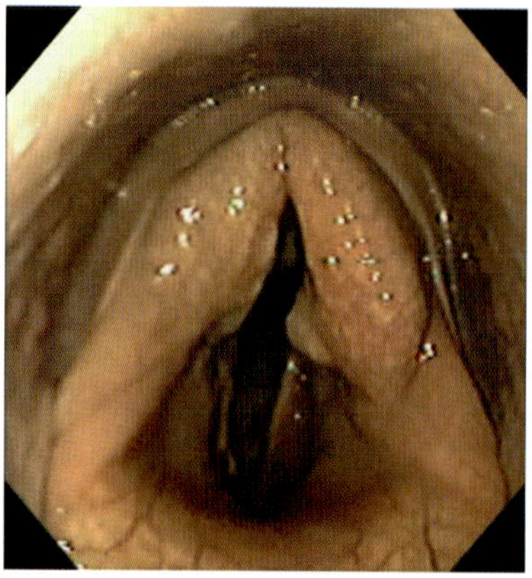

Figure 3.20 Chondropathy of the left arytenoid cartilage with "kissing" lesion on the right arytenoid. Arytenoid chondropathy can be caused by trauma or inflammation of the arytenoid cartilages secondary to mucosal damage. It most often is unilateral. Signs include exercise intolerance and upper respiratory noise or distress. Treatment varies depending on the severity of the lesion and degree of upper respiratory tract obstruction.

Laryngeal Hemiplegia

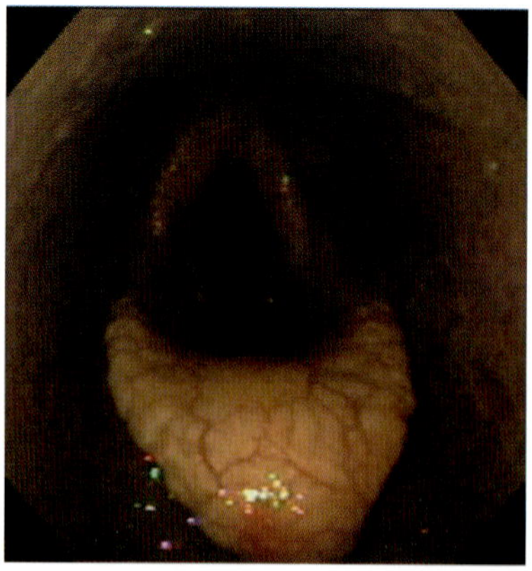

Figure 3.21 Left laryngeal hemiplegia in a horse with a complaint of exercise intolerance and inspiratory stridor. Laryngeal hemiplegia is caused by damage or degeneration of the laryngeal nerve(s), most commonly the left recurrent laryngeal nerve. It can be treated surgically.

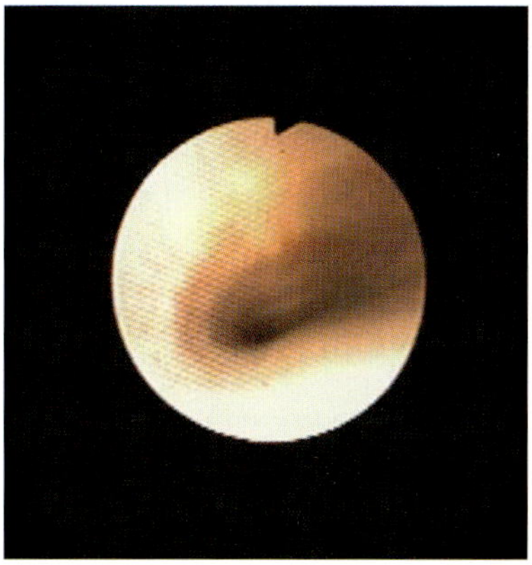

Figure 3.22 Endoscopic view of a collapsed trachea in a miniature foal with a complaint of respiratory stridor and exercise intolerance. It can be congenital, as in Shetland ponies and miniature horses, or caused by trauma. Surgical treatment may be attempted.

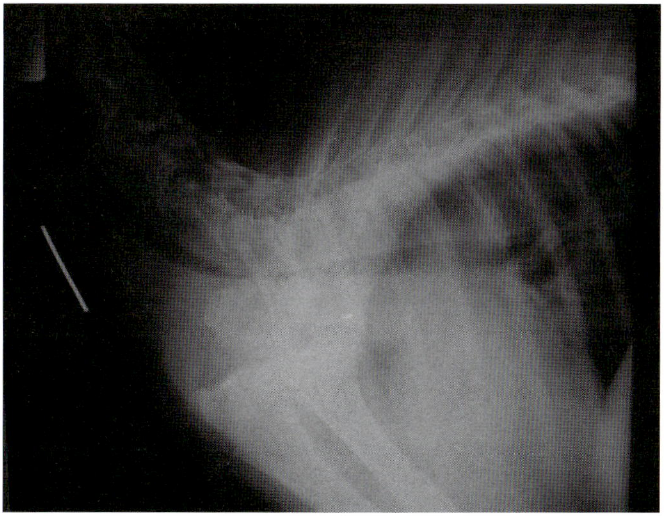

Figure 3.23 Lateral cervical and thoracic radiograph of a miniature foal with tracheal collapse at the level of the thoracic inlet.

Noninfectious Pulmonary Diseases

Recurrent Airway Obstruction (RAO, Heaves)

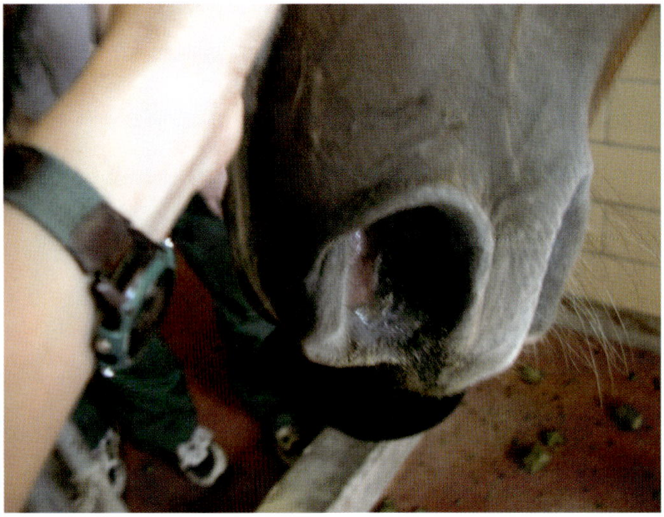

Figure 3.24 Horse flaring its nostrils during an attack of heaves. Heaves or RAO is an allergic response to airborne dust from hay and straw. Some horses are allergic to inhaled mold or pollen present on pasture during the summer. Exposure to allergens results in severe airway inflammation, increased respiratory secretions, coughing, bronchoconstriction, and increased respiratory efforts at rest (nostril flaring, increased abdominal contraction).

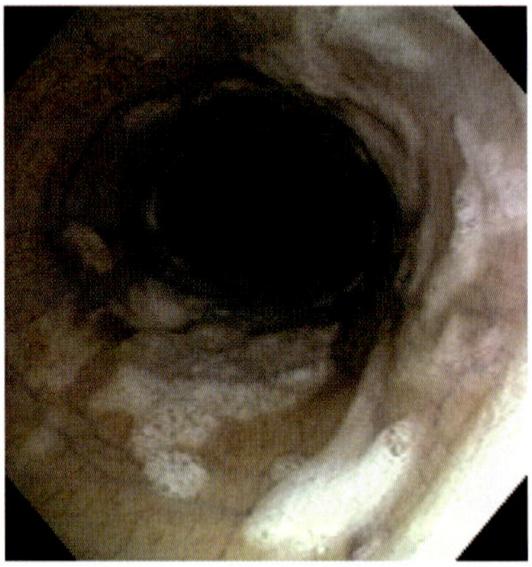

Figure 3.25 Accumulation of mucopurulent respiratory secretions in the trachea of a horse with heaves. Cytological examination typically reveals marked neutrophilic inflammation without evidence of sepsis.

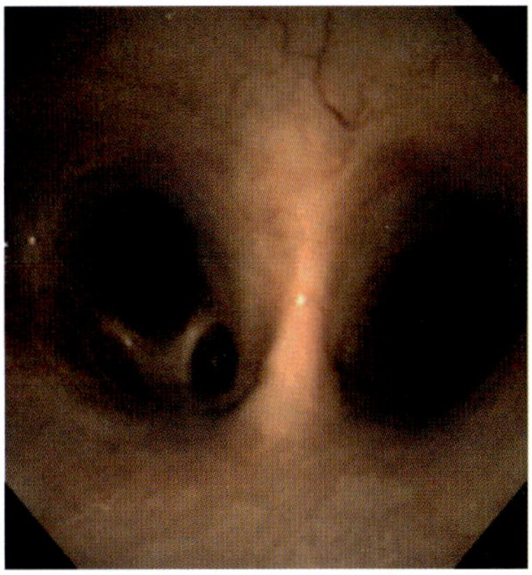

Figure 3.26 Endoscopy of the carina revealing rounded airway bifurcation and hyperemia consistent with bronchial edema. Some horses with heaves may exhibit marked airway obstruction without gross evidence of bronchial edema. Treatment focuses on environmental management, use of anti-inflammatory medications, and bronchodilators.

Inflammatory Airway Disease (IAD)

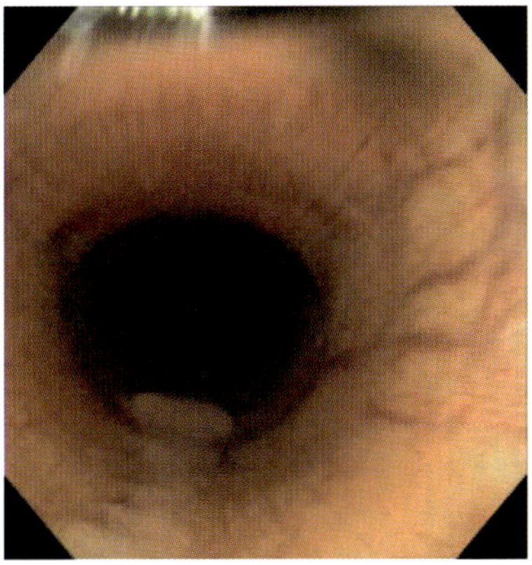

Figure 3.27 Mucopurulent exudates is visible by endoscopic examination of the trachea of a racehorse with inflammatory airway disease. Horses commonly present with a history of decreased performance and coughing. The degree of airway inflammation is much less than that of RAO (heaves) and horses with IAD do not show increased respiratory efforts at rest. Cytological examination or respiratory secretion may reveal mild neutrophilic, eosinophilic, or mastocytic inflammation.

Exercise-induced Pulmonary Hemorrhage (EIPH)

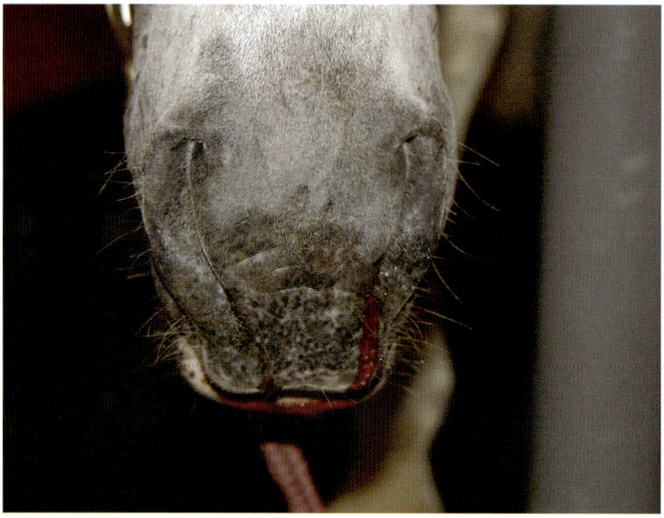

a

Figures 3.28a,b (a) Epistaxis postexercise in a horse with exercise-induced pulmonary hemorrhage (EIPH). Only 1% of horses with EIPH develop epistaxis. Endoscopy of the trachea is much more sensitive for detection of lung hemorrhage. (b) A Thoroughbred racehorse with EIPH and epistaxis. EIPH occurs frequently in horses that are strenuously exercised. There are no definitive clinical signs that can be used to diagnose EIPH, however, depending on the volume of blood in the trachea, horses may cough, swallow repeatedly, have epistaxis, and reduced performance. The etiology of EIPH is unclear; however, it is suspected that increased transmural capillary pressures cause stress failure of the pulmonary capillaries and accumulation of blood in the interstitial and alveolar spaces. Diagnosis is based upon clinical signs, postexercise tracheobronchoscopy, or cytological analysis of bronchoalveolar lavage fluid (figs. 3.29a–e). No specific therapy for horses with EIPH exists; however, rest is recommended and enforced by racing jurisdictions.

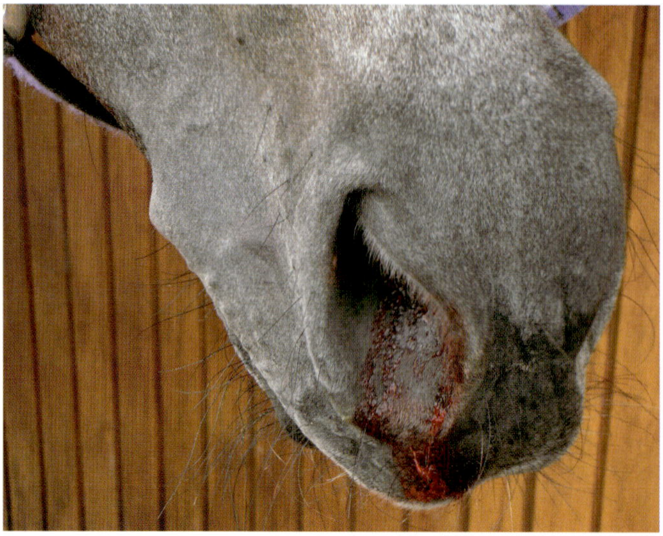

b

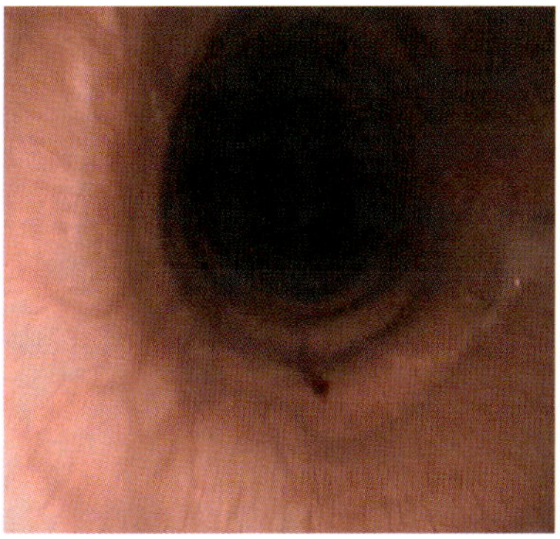

Figure 3.29a A racehorse with grade 1 EIPH as detected by tracheobronchoscopy. EIPH Score 1: Presence of one or more flecks of blood or two or fewer short (<1/4 length of the trachea), narrow (<10% of the tracheal surface area) streams of blood in the trachea or main stem bronchi visible from the tracheal bifurcation.

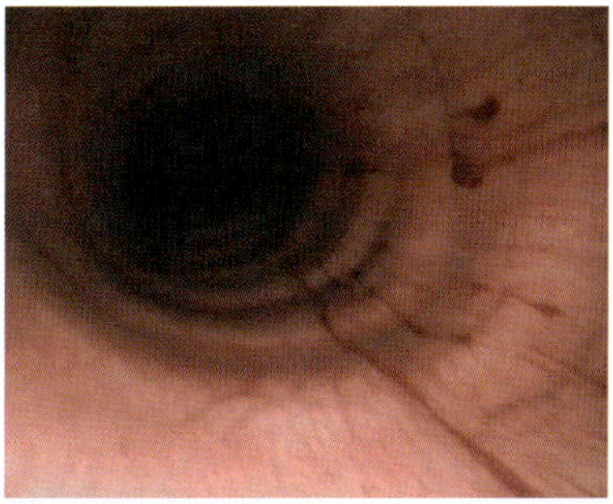

Figure 3.29b A racehorse with grade 2 EIPH as detected by tracheobronchoscopy. EIPH Score 2: one long stream of blood (greater than half the length of the trachea) or more than two short streams of blood are occupying less than a third of the tracheal circumference.

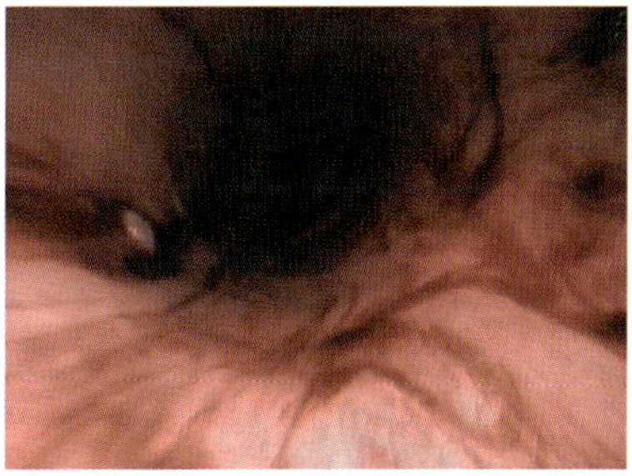

Figure 3.29c A racehorse with grade 3 EIPH as detected by tracheobronchoscopy. Multiple, distinct streams of blood covering more than one-third of the tracheal circumference, with no blood pooling at the level of the thoracic inlet.

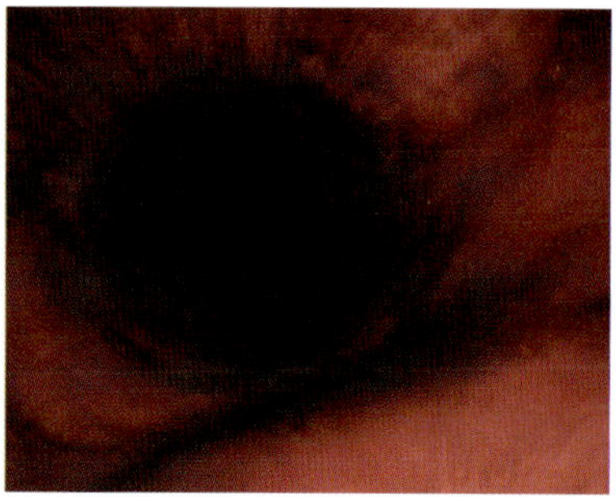

Figure 3.29d A racehorse with grade 4 EIPH as detected by tracheobronchoscopy. EIPH Score 4: Multiple, coalescing streams of blood covering >90% of the tracheal surface, with blood pooling at the thoracic inlet.

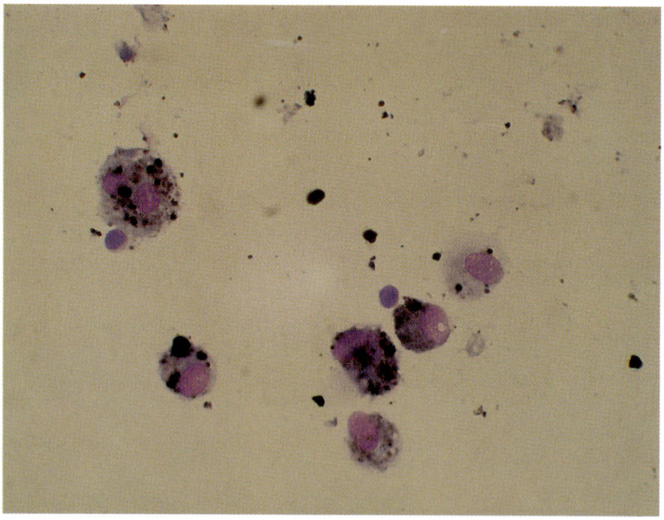

Figure 3.29e Photomicrograph of bronchoalveolar lavage fluid showing hemosiderophages in a racehorse with EIPH (Diff-Quick stain).

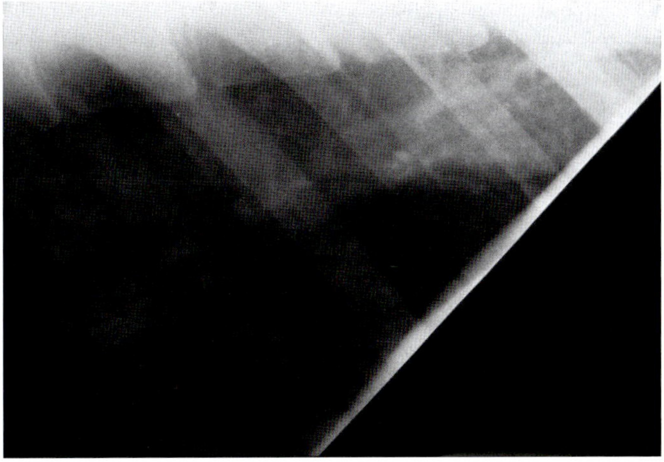

Figure 3.30 Lateral thoracic radiograph of a racehorse with chronic EIPH. An area of marked increased opacity is visible in the caudodorsal lung region consistent with pulmonary fibrosis and remodeling secondary to chronic lung bleeding. Most, if not all strenuously exercising horses (e.g., racehorses) experience some degree of EIPH. Repeated bleeding episodes result in lung fibrosis, which over time predisposes horses to more severe bleeding that may negatively affect performance.

Infectious Pulmonary Diseases

Bacterial Pneumonia in Adult Horses

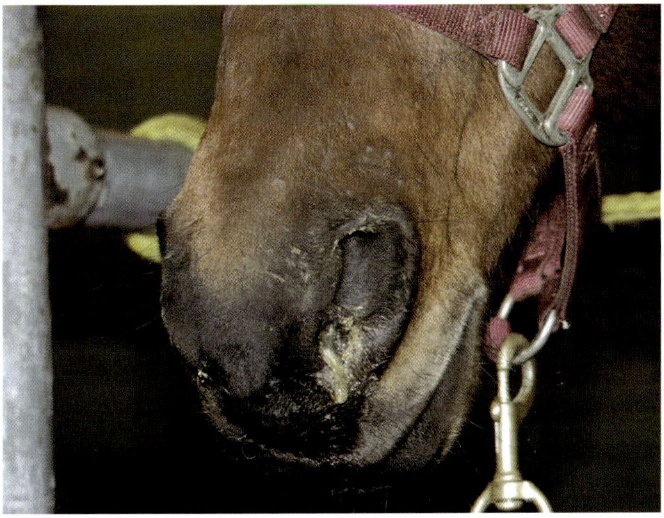

Figure 3.31 Mucopurulent nasal discharge in an adult horse with pneumonia. The color and aspect of the nasal discharge is not sufficient to differentiate infectious from noninfectious respiratory diseases. One should use other clinical and diagnostic findings to differentiate. Bacterial pneumonia in the adult horse can be caused by opportunistic, environmental, or commensal bacterial pathogens. However, the infection with the previous pathogens is usually preceded by events that suppress the pulmonary immunity. Clinical signs include fever, depression, lethargy, and inappetence.

Aspiration Pneumonia

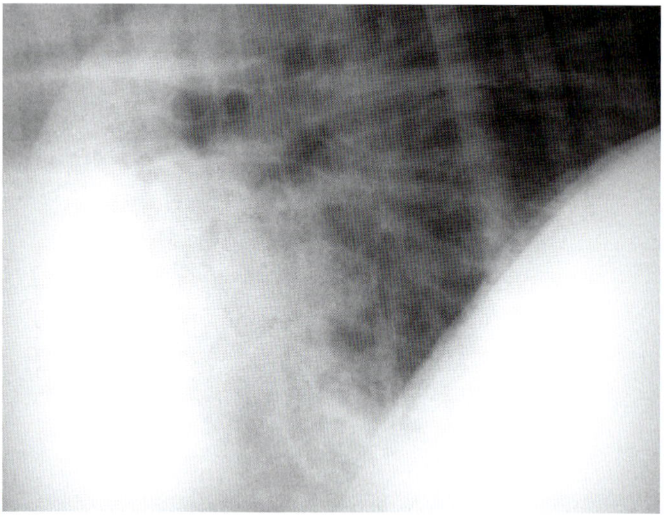

Figure 3.32 Lateral thoracic radiograph (caudoventral view) in a horse with aspiration pneumonia secondary to esophageal obstruction. The cardiac silhouette is obscured by marked alveolar infiltrate consistent with pneumonia. Aspiration pneumonia can result from any condition that causes dysphagia and subsequently feed aspiration. Inadvertent deposition of mineral oil in the lungs during nasogastric intubation is another cause of aspiration pneumonia.

Pleuropneumonia

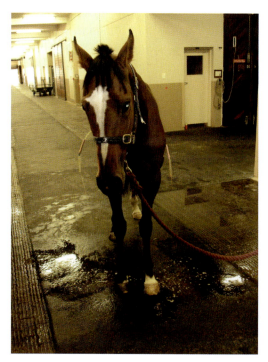

Figure 3.33a A racehorse with acute pleuropneumonia after long-distance transportation. Risk factors may include transportation, dysphagia, respiratory viral infections, anesthesia, and strenuous exercise. Affected horses are depressed, febrile, and dyspnoic, cough, and may have nasal discharge. Thoracic ultrasonography and radiography provide a definitive diagnosis (figs. 3.33b–d). Cytological examination of pleural fluid (fig. 3.34a) and a transtracheal aspirate may show suppurative inflammation with intracellular and extracellular bacteria. Treatment may include placement of indwelling chest tubes and drainage (figs. 3.34b and c), pleural lavage, and the use of anti-inflammatories and broad spectrum antibiotics. Extensive pleural disease (figs. 3.34d and e) may require a thoracotomy.

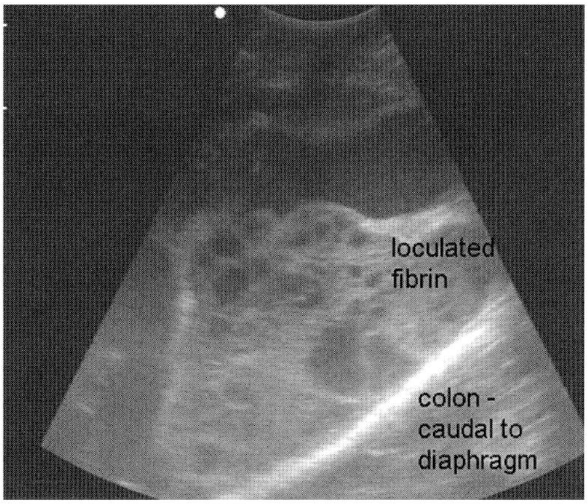

Figure 3.33b Intercostal transverse ultrasonographic image of ventral midthorax of a racehorse with acute pleuropneumonia. Pleural effusion seen contained in multiple hyperechoic loculated fibrin strands. Dorsal is to the left. (Image is courtesy of Professor Ann Carstens, Faculty of Veterinary Science, University of Pretoria.)

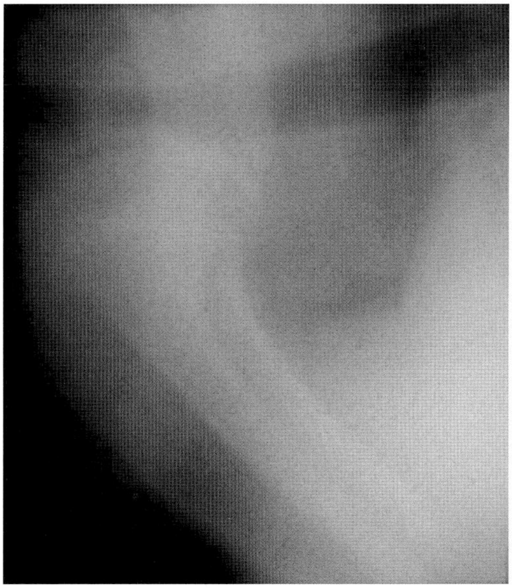

Figure 3.33c Lateral radiograph of the cranioventral thorax of a racehorse with acute pleuropneumonia. The pleural effusion is seen with soft tissue radio-opacity border that is effacing the cranial border of the cardiac silhouette and the cranioventral aspect of the diaphragm. (Image is courtesy of Professor Ann Carstens, Faculty of Veterinary Science, University of Pretoria.)

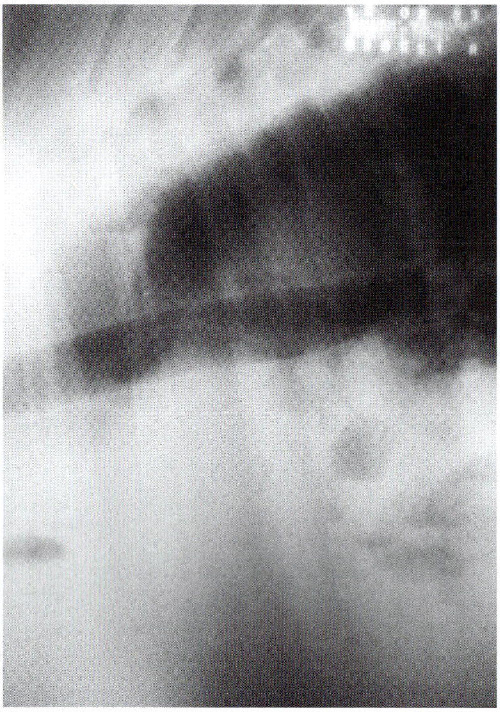

Figure 3.33d Lateral thoracic radiograph of a horse with pleuropneumonia showing marked increased opacity (ground-glass appearance) obscuring most of the ventral thorax below the trachea.

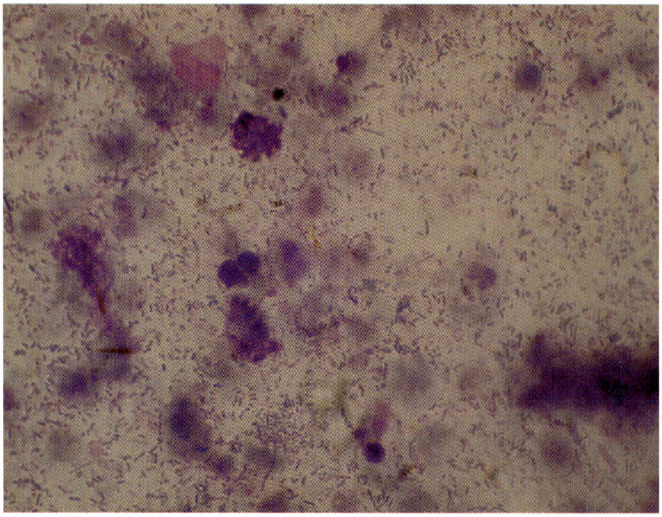

Figure 3.34a Photomicrograph of pleural fluid showing degenerate white blood cells and mixed bacteria in a racehorse with pleuropneumonia (Diff-Quick stain).

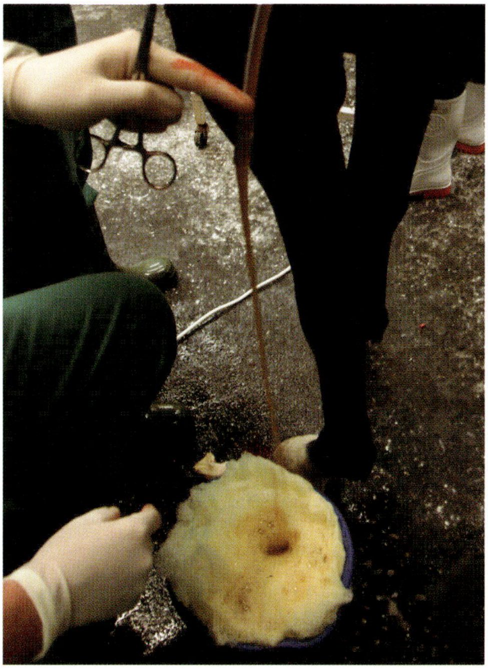

Figure 3.34b Pleural fluid draining from an indwelling chest tube.

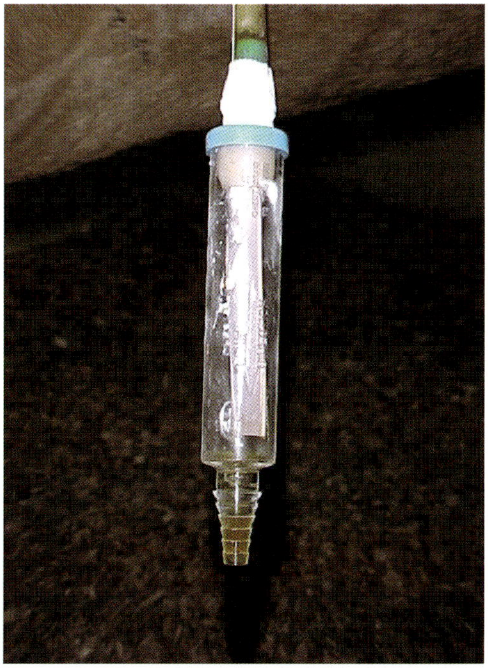

Figure 3.34c A Heimlich valve attached to the indwelling chest tube to allow drainage of pleural fluid while preventing development of a pneumothorax.

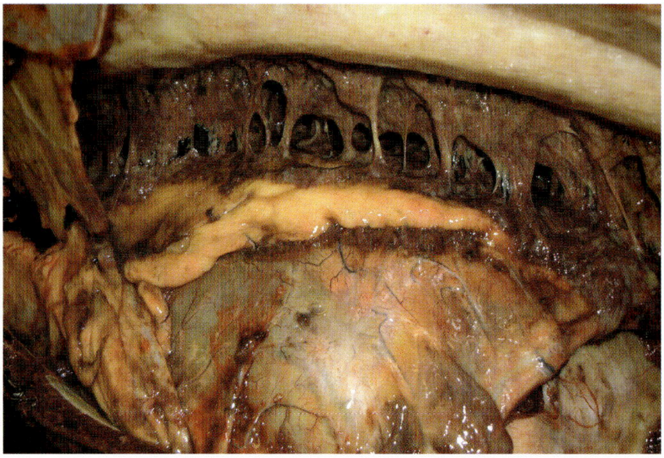

Figure 3.34d Severe pyogranulomatous pericarditis in a horse with pleuropneumonia.

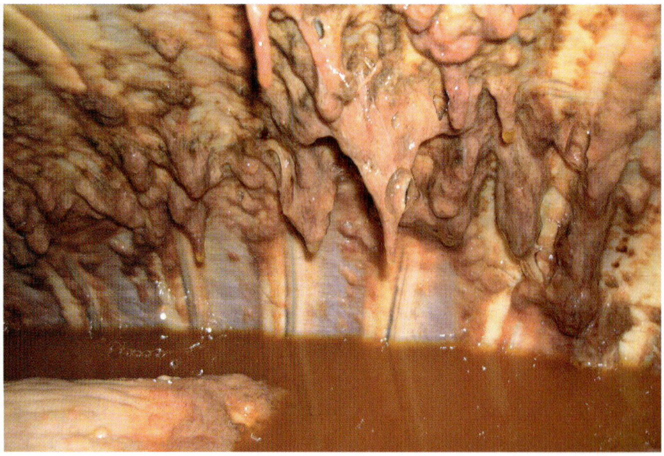

Figure 3.34e Severe pyogranulomatous pleuritis and pyothorax in a horse with pleuropneumonia.

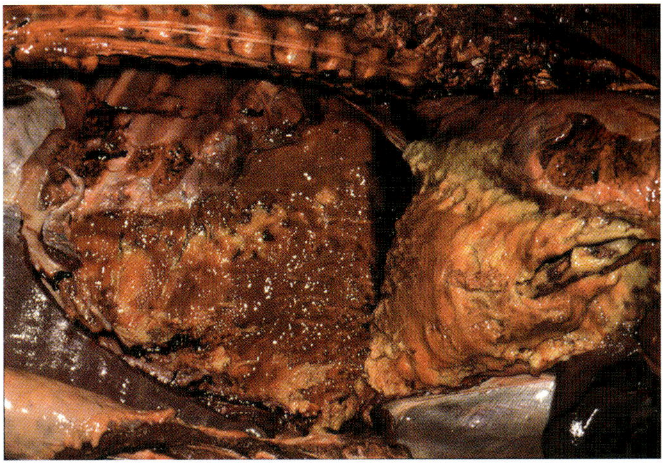

Figure 3.35 Gross examination of the chest cavity in a horse with pleuropneumonia. The lung has been lifted off the chest wall revealing a thick layer of fibrin adhesions and purulent exudate covering both pleural and parietal pleura.

Interstitial Pneumonia in Adult Horses

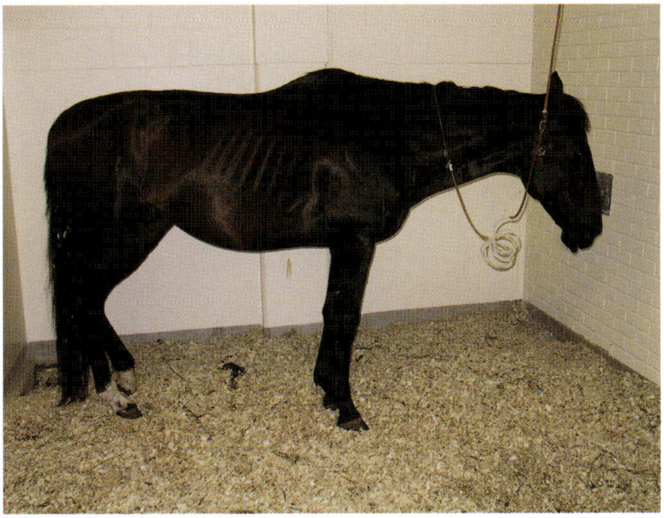

Figure 3.36a An adult horse with acute interstitial pneumonia. Interstitial pneumonia in adult horses is poorly defined. Several viruses have been implicated as the cause. Other suggested causes include drug reaction, hypersensitivity, plant toxicity, smoke inhalation, and inhaled chemicals. Clinical signs include fever, weight loss, and, as in this horse, exercise intolerance and progressive respiratory distress. Cytological examination of transtracheal and bronchoalveolar aspirates usually reveals variable results. Bacterial culture of transtracheal and bronchoalveolar aspirates reveals no significant growth. Radiography and lung biopsy are valuable tools of diagnosis.

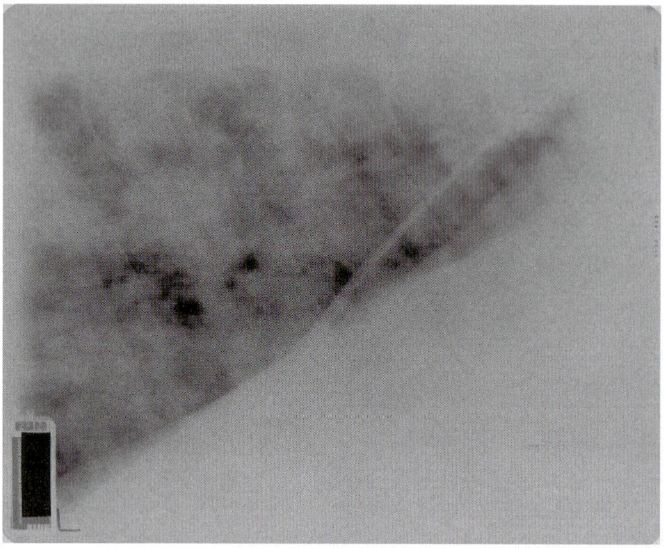

Figure 3.36b Lateral thoracic radiograph (caudodorsal view) of a horse with interstitial pneumonia. Patchy opacities are due to marked widespread interstitial infiltration.

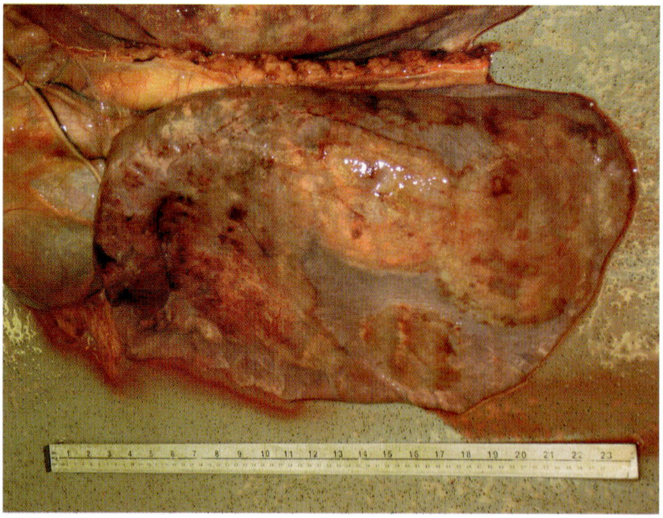

Figure 3.36c Postmortem photograph of a lung with interstitial pneumonia.

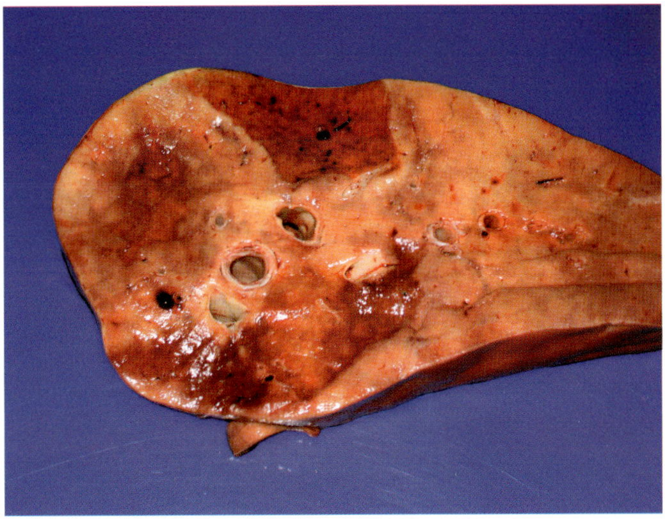

Figure 3.36d Postmortem photograph of a lung with interstitial pneumonia (cross section).

Diseases of the Thoracic Wall and Pleura

Pneumothorax

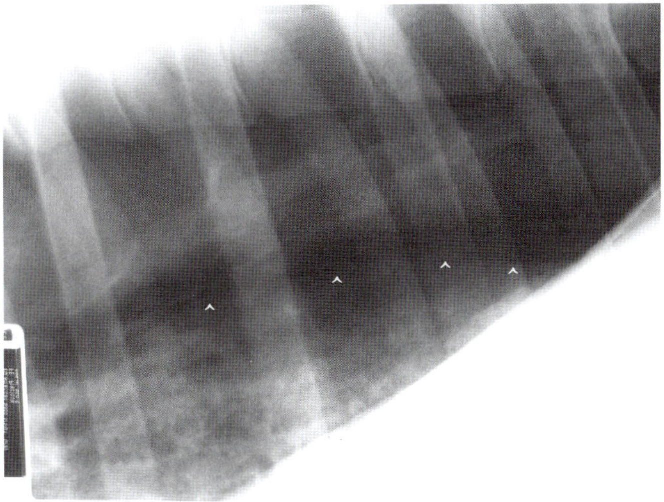

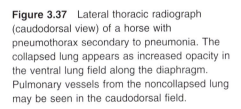

Figure 3.37 Lateral thoracic radiograph (caudodorsal view) of a horse with pneumothorax secondary to pneumonia. The collapsed lung appears as increased opacity in the ventral lung field along the diaphragm. Pulmonary vessels from the noncollapsed lung may be seen in the caudodorsal field.

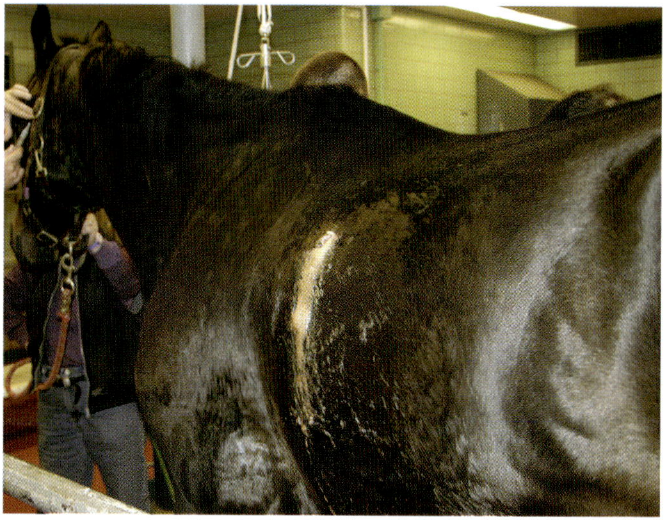

Figure 3.38 Pleural exudate is draining from the chest of a horse that was injured in a trailer accident resulting in pneumothorax and pleuritis. Trauma and penetration of the thorax is another cause of pneumothorax.

STRANGLES

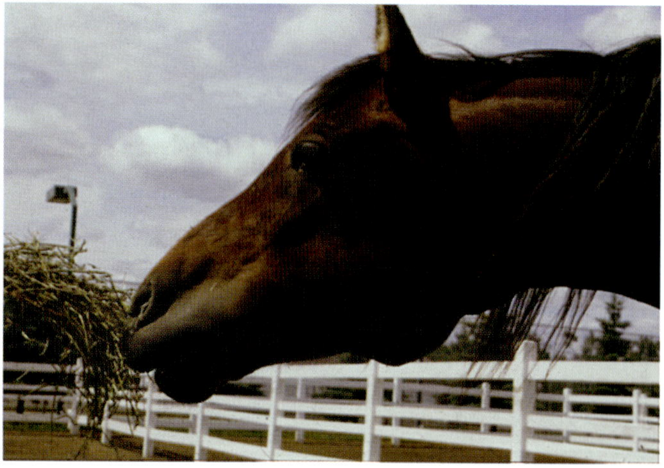

Figure 3.39 Enlarged submandibular lymph node in a horse with strangles. Strangles is a highly contagious disease especially in young horses. It is caused by *Streptococcus equi* subsp. *equi.* Clinical signs include fever, depression, anorexia, and serous to mucopurulent nasal discharge. Enlargement and abscessation of the submandibular, submaxillary, retropharyngeal, and cervical lymph nodes are characteristic. Purpura hemorrhagica (see Chapter 2) and 'bastard strangles' (see brain abscess in Chapter 4) are serious complications of strangles.

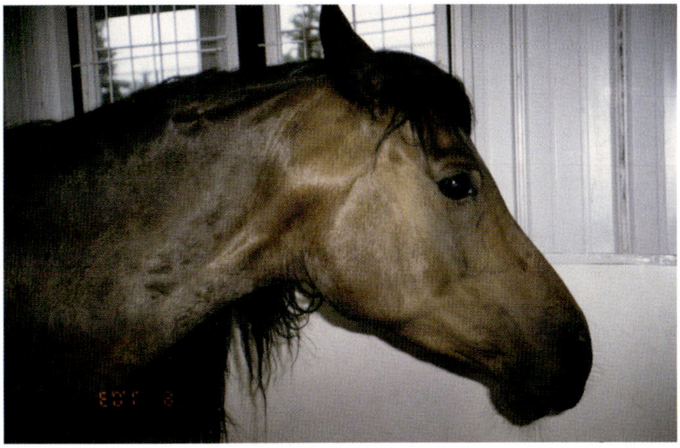

Figure 3.40 Enlarged retropharyngeal lymph nodes in an adult horse affected with strangles.

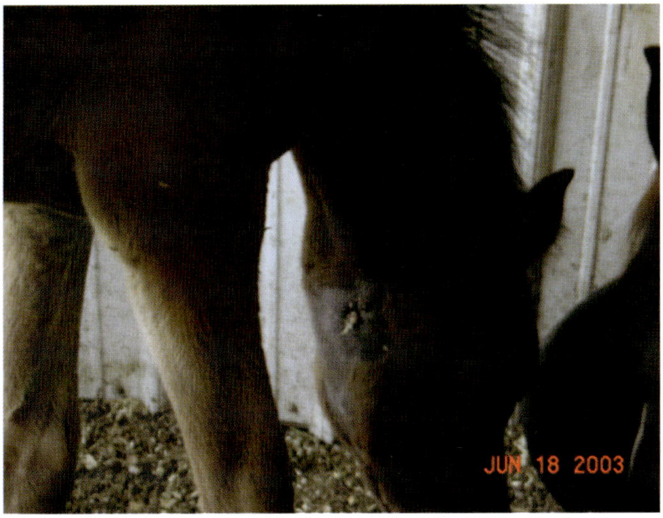

Figure 3.41 Enlarged submandibular lymph nodes in a foal. The abscess has ruptured, which is usually the case.

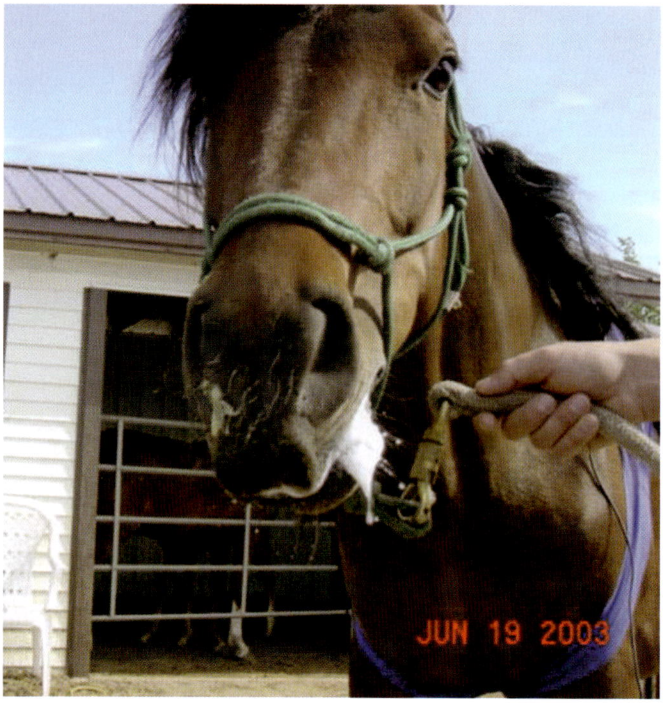

Figure 3.42 Enlarged lymph node can compress the esophagus and cause choke as in this adult horse. This horse had signs of dysphagia including the presence of froth at the mouth.

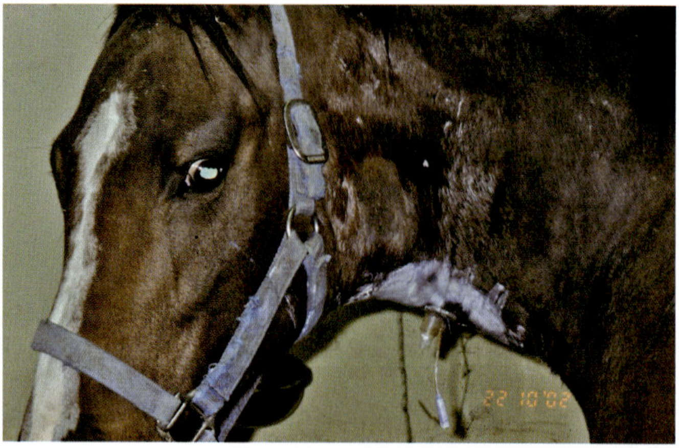

a

Figures 3.43a,b Enlarged lymph node can compress the pharynx and impede respiration. Affected horses are presented with respiratory noises and distress and may need emergency temporary tracheostomy. Once respiratory distress has resolved, tracheostomy tube is removed and tracheostomy site usually heals nicely as shown in fig. 3.43b, which is the same horse as in fig. 3.43a.

Figures 3.43a,b *Continued*

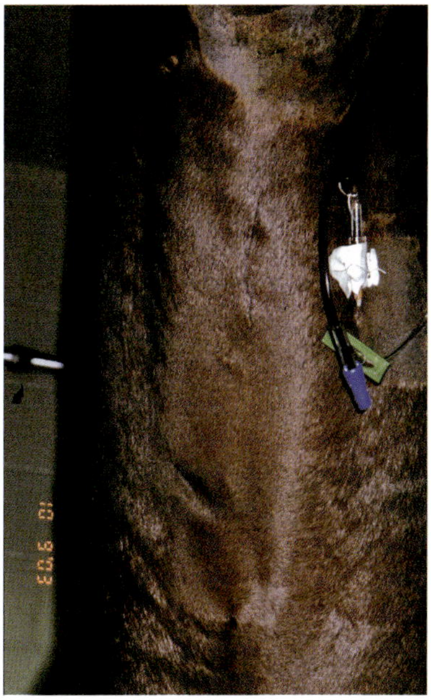

b

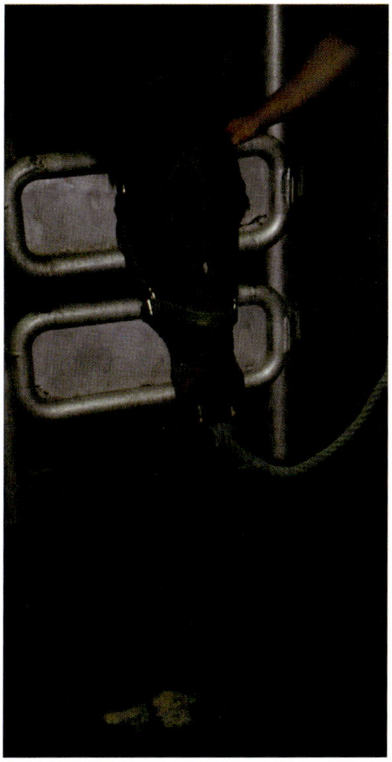

Figure 3.44 The mucopurulent nasal discharge seen in horses with strangles can originate from the ruptured abscessed retropharyngeal lymph nodes in the medial compartment of the guttural pouches (see guttural pouch empyema above) as shown in this horse.

African Horse Sickness

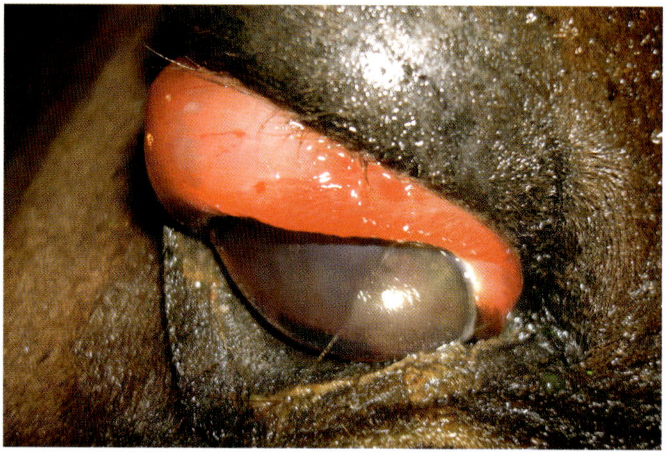

Figure 3.45 A Thoroughbred racehorse with severe conjunctival edema due to African horse sickness. This is an infectious disease of horses caused by an orbivirus and transmitted by Culicoides midges. Clinical signs include inappetence, pyrexia, and diffuse edema of subcutaneous (fig. 3.46), intermuscular (fig. 3.47) and pulmonary tissues, effusions into body cavities, and serosal (fig. 3.48) and visceral hemorrhage. Diagnosis is based on clinical signs and viral isolation from blood, lung, spleen, and lymph nodes. Differential diagnoses include equine encephalosis, equine viral arteritis, and purpura hemorrhagica. There is no specific therapy for African horse sickness; however, prophylactic immunization should be performed yearly in endemic regions.

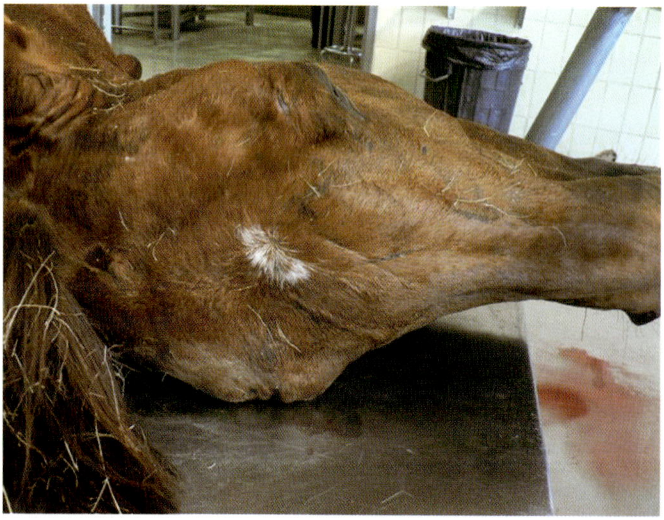

Figure 3.46 Subcutaneous edema of the supraorbital fossae. (Image is courtesy of Section of Pathology, Faculty of Veterinary Science, University of Pretoria.)

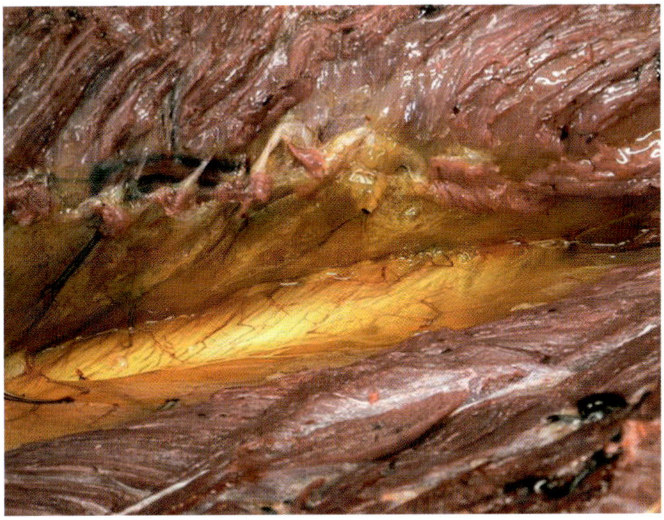

Figure 3.47 Severe intermuscular edema. (Image is courtesy of Section of Pathology, Faculty of Veterinary Science, University of Pretoria.)

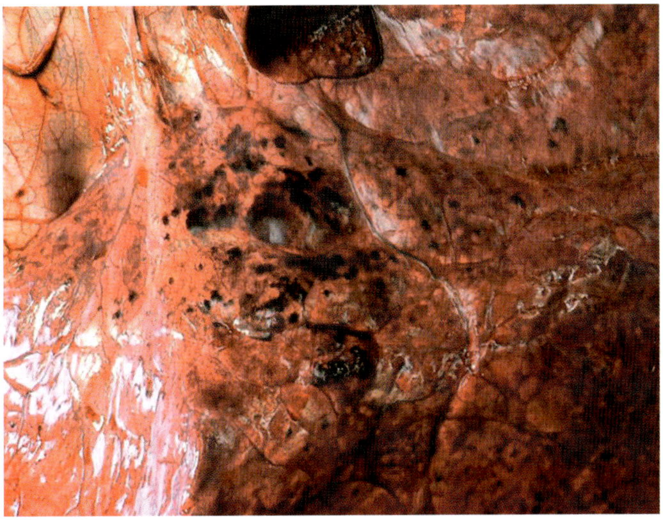

Figure 3.48 Pulmonary subserosal petechiae and ecchymoses. (Image is courtesy of Section of Pathology, Faculty of Veterinary Science, University of Pretoria.)

Recommended Reading

Couetil LL, Hinchcliff KW. Non-infectious respiratory diseases. In Hinchcliff KW, Kaneps A, and Geor RJ, eds. Equine sports medicine and surgery. Philadelphia: Saunders Elsevier, 2004.

Couetil LL, Hoffman AM, Hodgson J, Buechner-Maxwell V, Viel L, Wood JL, Lavoie JP. Inflammatory airway disease of horses. J Vet Intern Med. 21:356–61, 2007.

Dixon P, Schumacker J. Disorders of the upper respiratory tract. In McGorum B, Dixon P, Robinson N, et al., eds. Equine respiratory medicine and surgery. Philadelphia: Saunders Elsevier, 369–562, 2007.

Hinchcliff KW, Jackson MA, Brown JA, Dredge AF, O'Callaghan PA, McCaffrey JP, Morley PS, Slocombe RE, Clarke AF. Tracheobronchoscopic assessment of exercise-induced pulmonary hemorrhage in horses. Am J Vet Res. 66:596–98, 2005.

Lakritz J, Wilson D, Berry C, Schrenzel M, Carlson G, Madigan J. Bronchointerstitial pneumonia and respiratory distress in young horses: clinical, clinicopathologic, radiographic, and pathologic findings in 23 cases (1984–1989). J Vet Intern Med. 7:277–88, 1993.

Mair TS, Lane JG. Pneumonia, lung abscesses and pleuritis in adult horses: a review of 51 cases. Equine Vet J. 21:175–80, 1989.

Seltzer KL, Byars TD. Prognosis for return to racing after recovery from infectious pleuropneumonia in Thoroughbred racehorses: 70 cases (1984–1989). J Am Vet Med Assoc. 208:1300–1301, 1996.

4 Diseases of the Nervous System

Diseases of the Nervous System

- Brain Abscess
- Head Trauma
- Hepatoencephalopathy
- Leukoencephalomalacia (Moldy Corn Disease)
- West Nile Virus (WNV)
- Verminous Meningoencephalomyelitis
- Equine Herpes Virus I (EHV-1) Myeloencephalitis
- Equine Protozoal Myeloencephalitis (EPM)
- Equine Wobbler Syndrome (Cervical Vertebral Stenosis/ Instability, Cervical Vertebral Malformation, Cervical Spinal Cord Compression)
- Equine Motor Neuron Disease (EMND)
- Rabies
- Stringhalt
- Tetanus (Lockjaw)
- Lead Poisoning
- Cholesterol Granuloma (Cholesteatomas)
- Horner's Syndrome
- Otitis Media-Interna (Temporohyoid Osteoarthropathy)
- Radial Nerve Paralysis
- Facial Nerve Trauma
- Meningitis

Brain Abscess

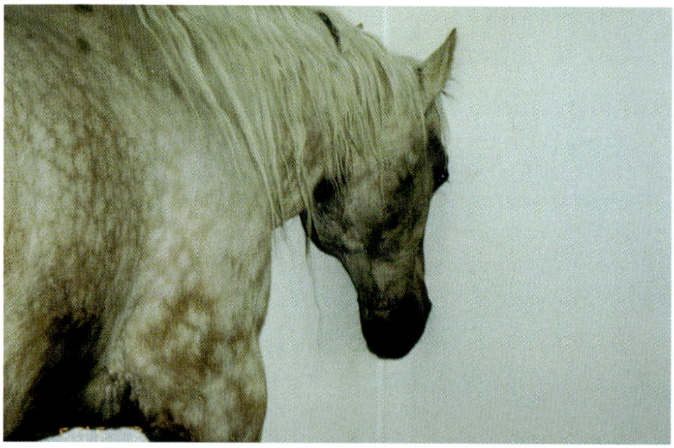

Figure 4.1 A mature horse affected with brain abscess. Note the depressed mentation. Brain abscess occurs sporadically in horses. It is mainly caused by *Streptococcus equi*, as in this horse, and *Streptococcus zooepidemicus*. Clinical signs include depression, blindness, head-pressing (fig. 4.2), propulsive walking, circling, mania, asymmetrical cranial nerve deficits (fig. 4.3). Response to antimicrobial therapy is poor.

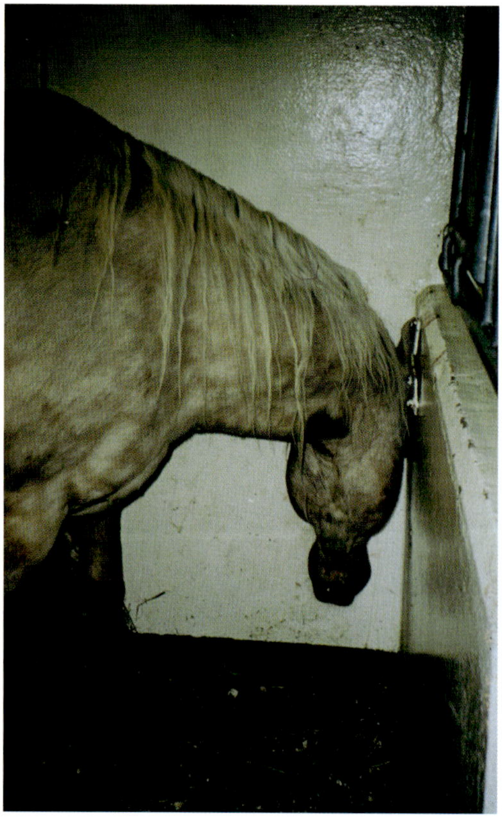

Figure 4.2 Head-pressing in a horse affected with brain abscessation.

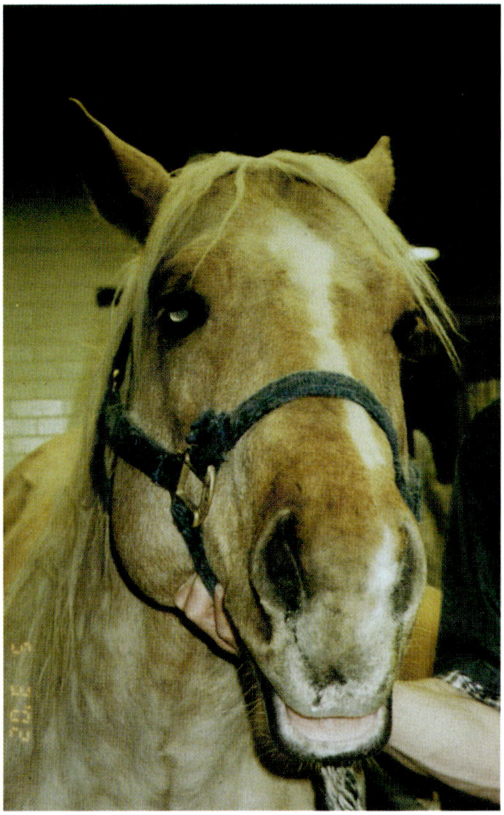

Figure 4.3 A horse affected with brain abscessation showing droopy lip due to cranial nerve VII deficit.

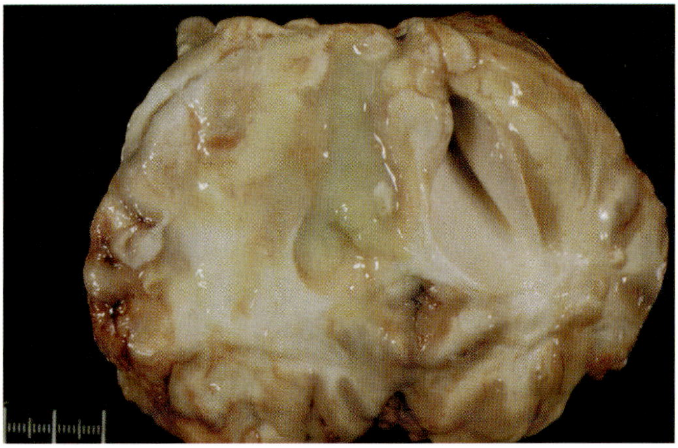

Figure 4.4 Postmortem photograph of a brain of a horse with brain abscess.

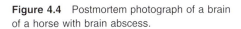

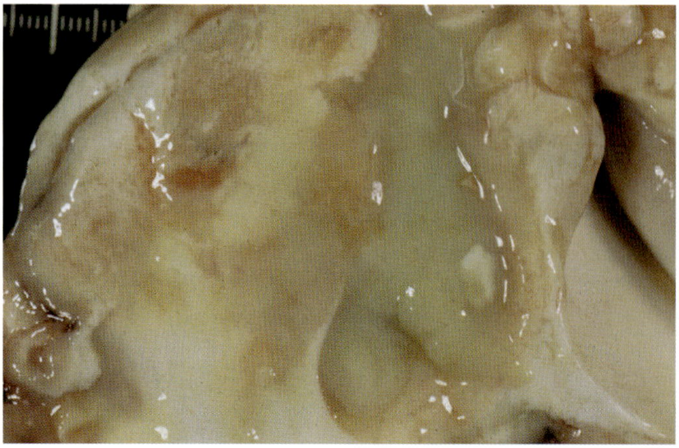

Figure 4.5 A close-up view of fig. 4.4.

Head Trauma

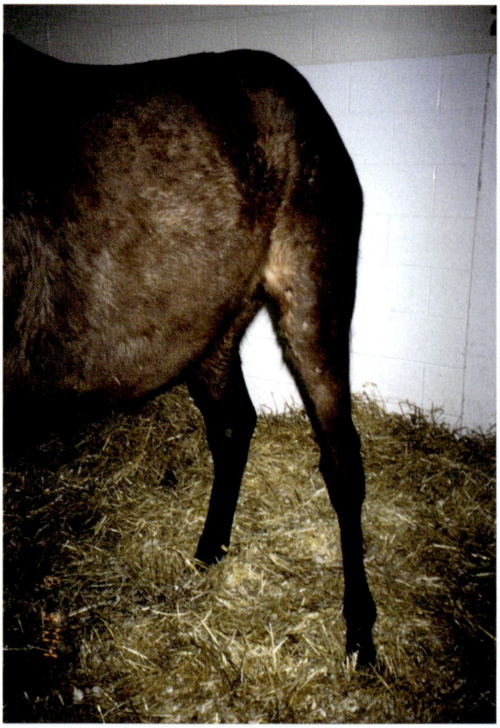

Figure 4.6 An adult horse affected with head trauma. Note the abnormal stance (wide-base stance). Horses are susceptible for head trauma due to their nature and reaction. It results from kicks, sharp blows, or falling over backward (especially foals). Head trauma leads to membrane disruption, cerebral edema, and increased intracranial pressure. A hematoma is usually formed. There are two main scenarios: poll impact, as in this horse, and frontal/parietal impact.

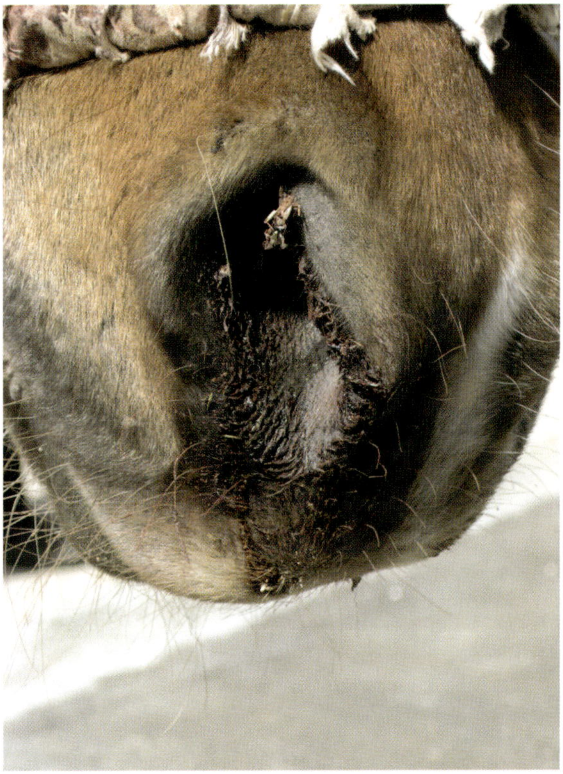

Figure 4.7 An adult horse with head trauma due to poll impact. Note the bloody nasal discharge. The horse flipped over backward and stroked its poll. When the downward motion is arrested by striking the ground, the head flips into extension. The longus and rectus capitis muscles are convulsively stretched by the sudden extension. These muscles course ventrally between the guttural pouches from their attachment to the basisphenoid and basioccipital bones. This may result in fracture of the basilar bones at or close to the suture (figs. 4.8 and 4.9). Hematomas form at fracture site and extend into membranous labyrinths and basilar areas of brain, which leads to vestibular (fig. 4.10) and occipital cortex dysfunction. A boney tubercle is ripped from the basilar bones and adjacent large vessels are lacerated. This results in bleeding into the guttural pouches, into the meninges, or around the brainstem and stretching and tearing of the cranial nerves V, IX, and/or X. Affected horses are presented with neurological signs (figs. 4.6, 4.10, and 4.11) and bloody nasal discharge as in this horse.

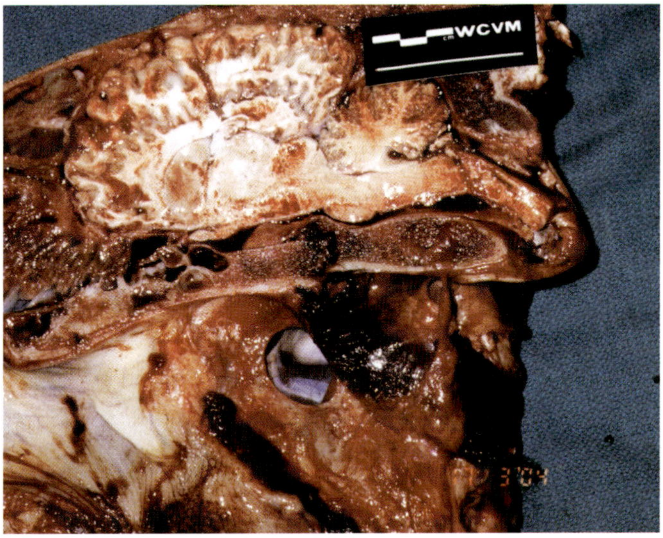

Figure 4.8 Postmortem photograph of a horse (skull) with basilar fracture.

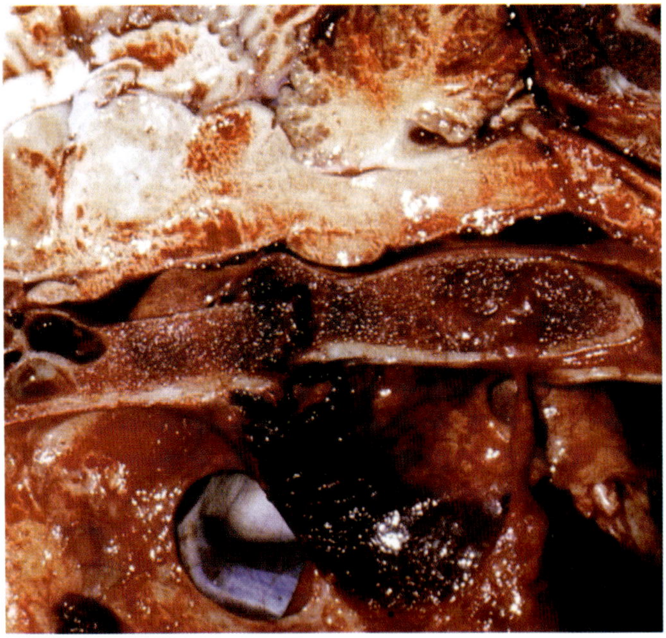

Figure 4.9 A close-up view of fig. 4.8. Fracture is at the center of the photograph.

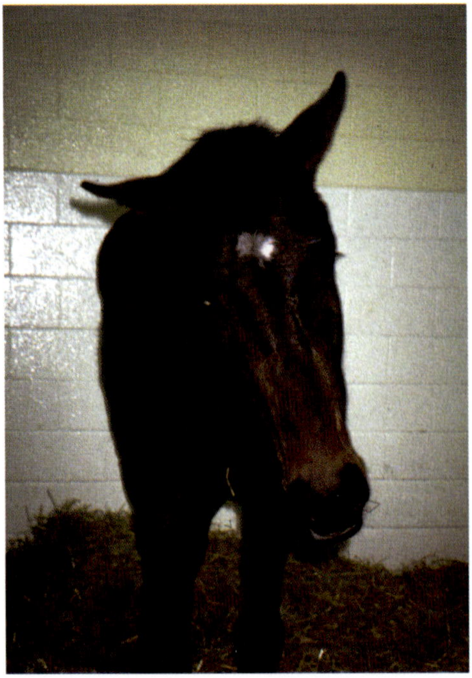

Figure 4.10 An adult horse with head trauma due to poll impact. Note the head tilt and facial asymmetry due to the damage to the facial nerve and vestibular apparatus.

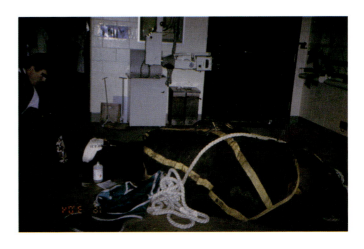

Figure 4.11 An adult horse with recumbency caused by head trauma due to poll impact. The horse flipped over backward and stroked its poll.

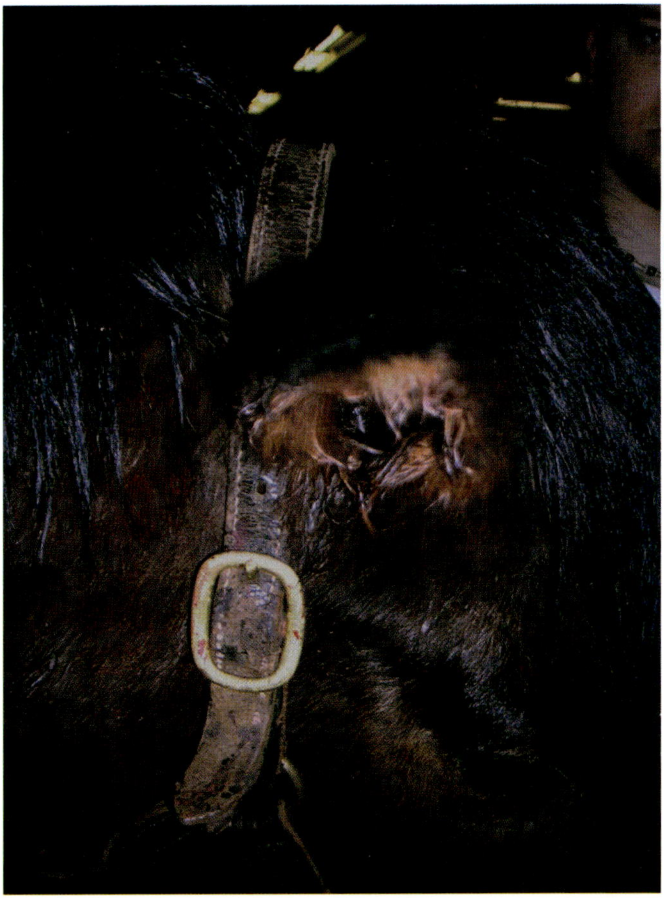

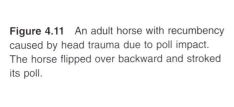

Figure 4.12 An adult horse with head trauma due to poll impact. Note the bloody discharge from the ear. Hemorrhage into the inner/middle ear may result from fracture of the petrous temporal bone.

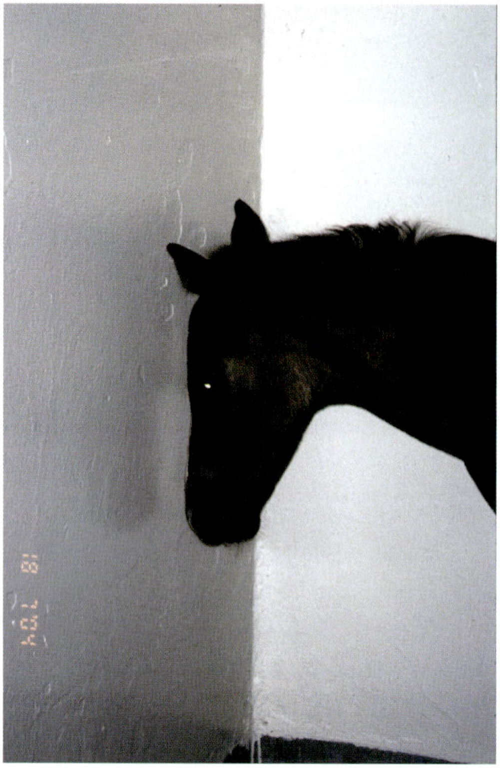

Figure 4.13 Blindness and optic nerve dysfunction due to a head trauma in a foal. The pupils were permanently dilated. Optic nerve dysfunction is caused by caudal displacement of the brain and stretching and avulsion of the optic nerve (fig. 4.14).

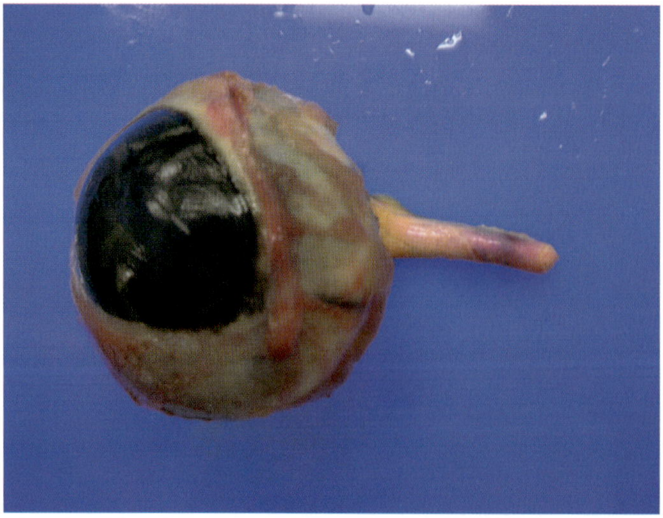

Figure 4.14 A postmortem photograph of the eyeball and optic nerve from the foal in fig. 4.13. Note the stretched and damaged optic nerve.

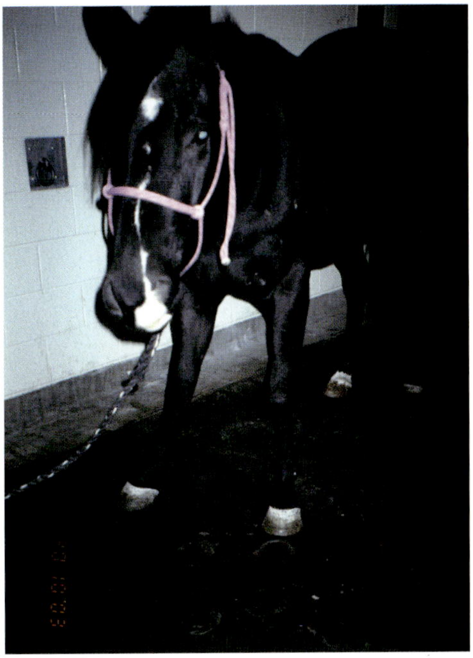

Figure 4.15 An adult horse affected with head trauma (poll impact). Note the wide-base stance. Occasionally poll impact may result in fracture of the paramastoid processes (jugular) or occipital condyles (fig. 4.16), as in this case.

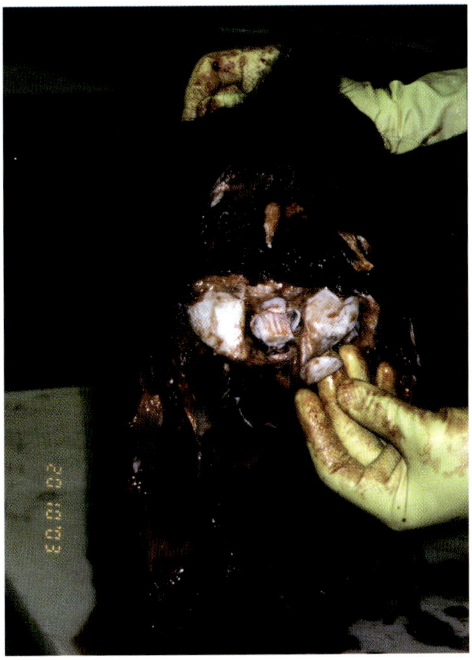

Figure 4.16 A postmortem photograph of the skull from a horse affected by a head trauma and fracture of the occipital condyles.

4

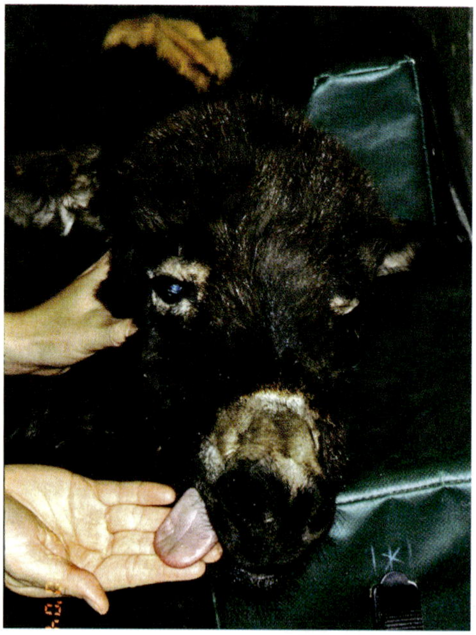

Figure 4.17 A donkey foal affected with head trauma (frontal impact). The foal was paralyzed and blind. Forehead trauma or frontal/parietal impact may result in depression fractures of dome of calvarium and brain swelling. A blow anywhere to the dorsal surface of the head as in case of a kick or collision with a narrow post. This may lead to brain contusions or lacerations. Additional injuries can result if the brain is tossed around in the calvarium.

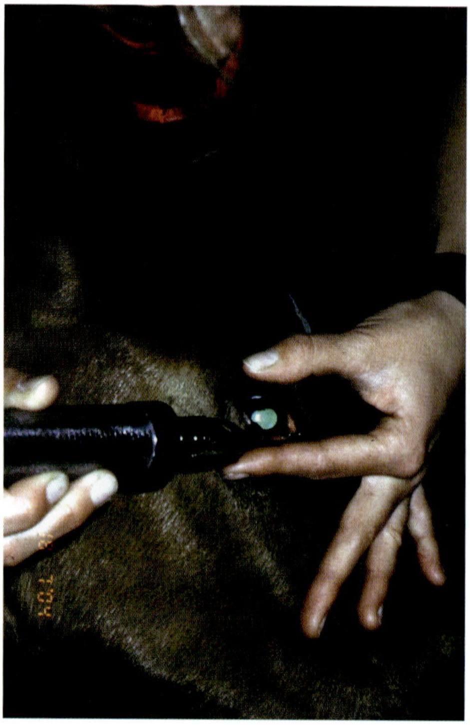

Figure 4.18 Permanent dilatation of the pupils in a foal. The foal had optic nerve dysfunction, which resulted from frontal/parietal impact.

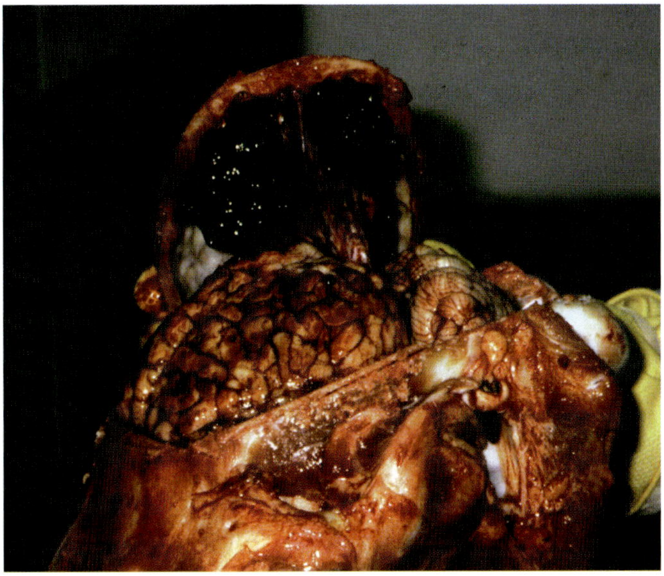

Figure 4.19 Postmortem photograph of a foal with head trauma. Note the severe intracranial hemorrhage.

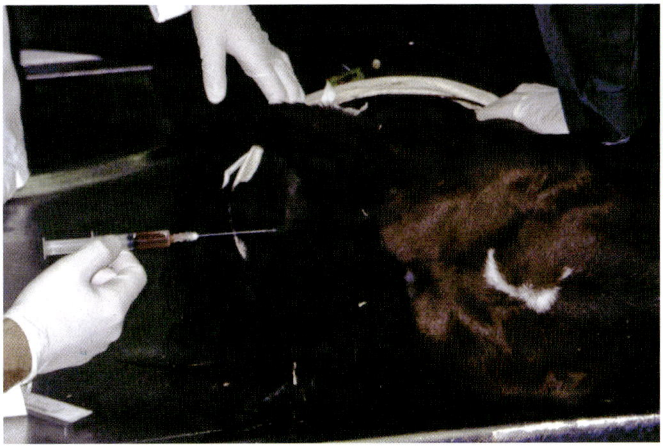

Figure 4.20 Cerebrospinal fluid sample from a horse affected with head trauma. Note the presence of frank blood due to the acute hemorrhage.

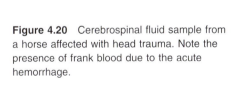

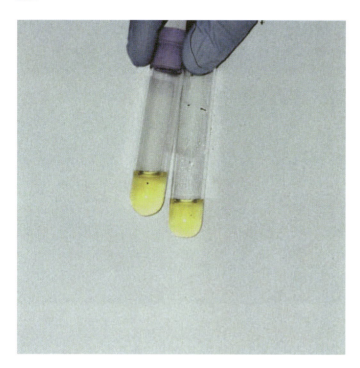

Figure 4.21 Cerebrospinal fluid sample from a horse affected with head trauma. Note the yellowish color, xanthochromia, which is seen in longer standing cases of head trauma.

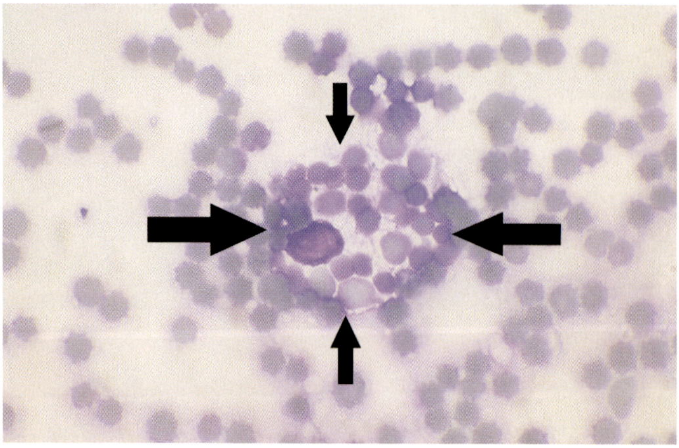

Figure 4.22 Cytological examination of the cerebrospinal fluid sample from a horse affected with head trauma. Note the presence of a hemosiderophage (arrows) and many erythrocytes.

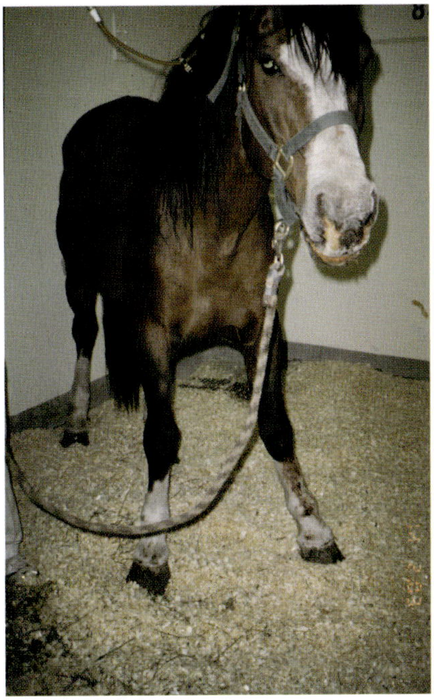

Figure 4.23 An adult horse affected with hepatoencephalopathy as a result of diffuse hepatitis. Note the wide-base stance. This horse had photodermatitis and episodes of incoordination, aimless walking, and yawning. Other clinical signs of hepatoencephalopathy include depression, stupor, and head-pressing. Hepatoencephalopathy occurs in animals with acute or chronic liver failure, which causes impairment of cerebral function. Any age can be affected, but most are adults.

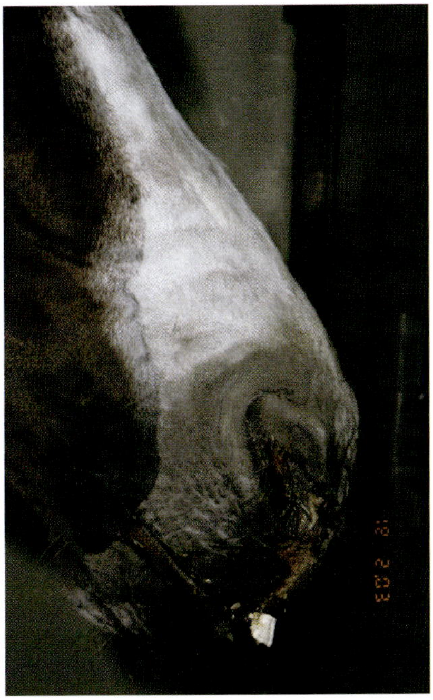

Figure 4.24 An adult horse affected with hepatoencephalopathy as a result of diffuse hepatitis. Note the signs of photodermatitis where the white skin is affected and the sharp demarcation between the affected and nonaffected areas.

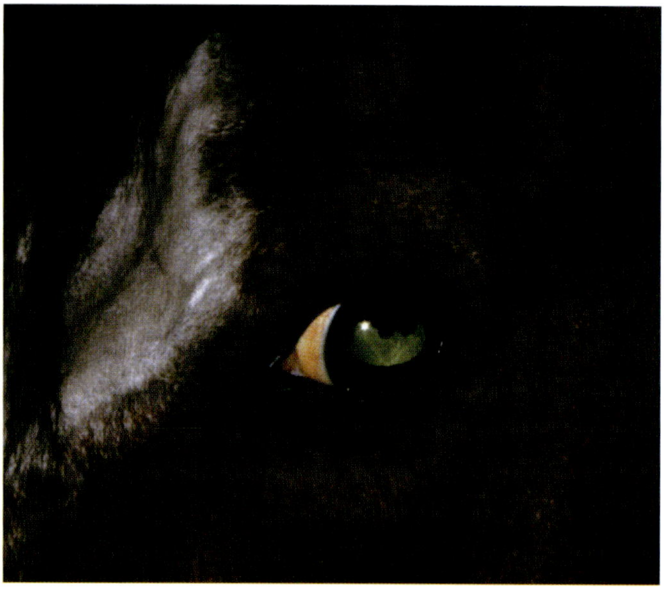

Figure 4.25 An adult horse affected with hepatoencephalopathy, note the icteric sclera.

Leukoencephalomalacia (Moldy Corn Disease)

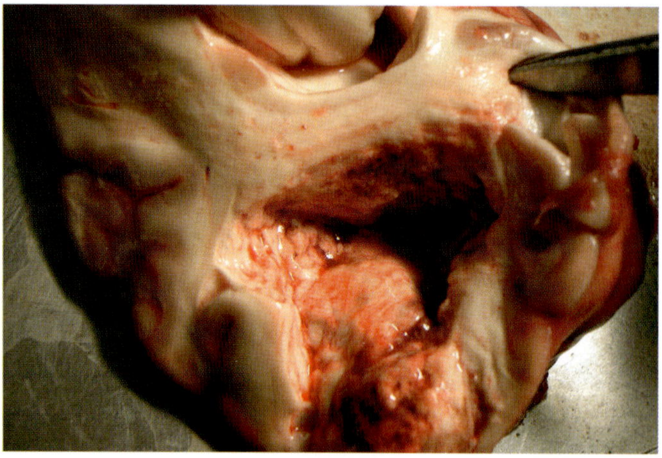

Figure 4.26 Postmortem examination of the brain in a horse affected with leukoencephalomalacia. Note the liquefactive necrosis and degeneration of the white matter of the right cerebral hemisphere due to *Fusarium moniliforme*. Leukoencephalomalacia is caused by ingestion of corn infected with the fungus *Fusarium moniliforme,* which produces fumonisin B1 toxin. Clinical signs of this are those of neurotoxicosis due to fumonisin B1 intoxication. Those include ataxia, depression, blindness, head-pressing, and manic behavior. There may be signs of hepatotoxicosis, however, this occurs less commonly. Definitive diagnosis is based on feed analysis and identification of fumonisin B1 toxin. Therapy is mainly supportive as there is no specific antidote for exposure to this toxic metabolite.

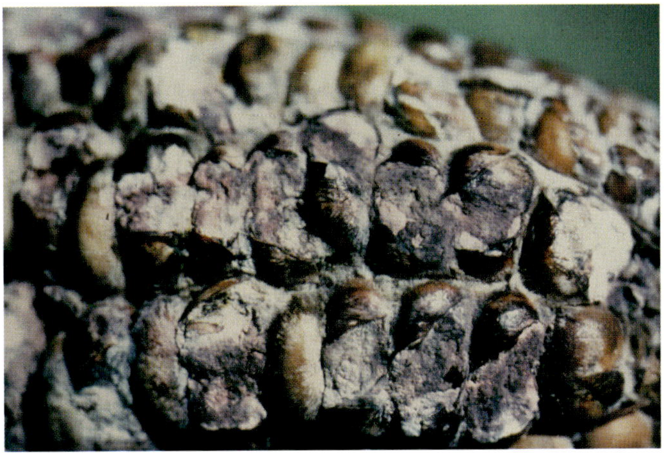

Figure 4.27 Moldy corn infected with *Fusarium moniliforme*. (Image courtesy of the Section of Pathology, Faculty of Veterinary Science, University of Pretoria.)

West Nile Virus (WNV)

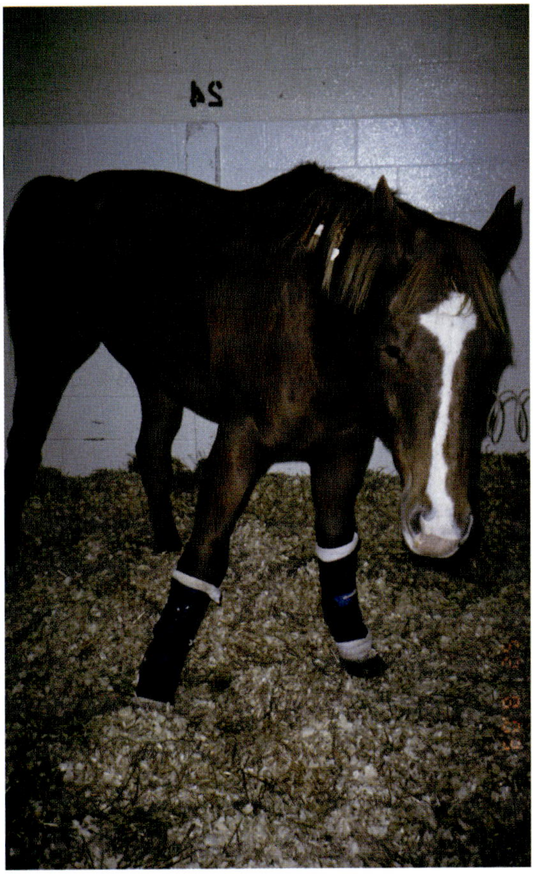

Figure 4.28 An adult horse affected with West Nile Virus (WNV). Note the wide-base stance. The horse was ataxic in all four legs. WNV causes encephalomyelitis in horses. The disease is seasonal and its transmission is via mosquito bites from viremic birds to dead-end hosts (horses). All ages are affected and the course of disease ranges from 5 to 15 days. Clinical signs include fever, acute onset of ataxia in all four limbs (figs. 4.28 and 4.29). Seizures, depression (fig. 4.30), somnolence, blindness, circling, head tremors, lip twitching (fig. 4.31), hypersensitivity to touch and sound, hyperexcitability, recumbency, coma, or death can be seen. Cranial nerve deficit signs may also be seen (fig. 4.32). Treatment is mainly supportive.

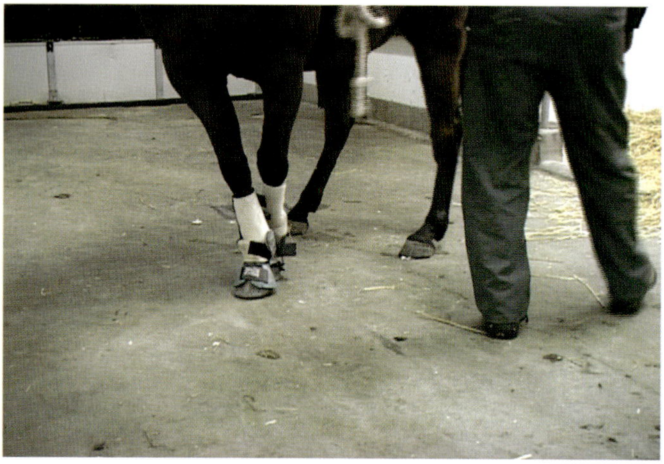

Figure 4.29 An adult horse affected with WNV. The horse was stepping on its feet when turned in a circle.

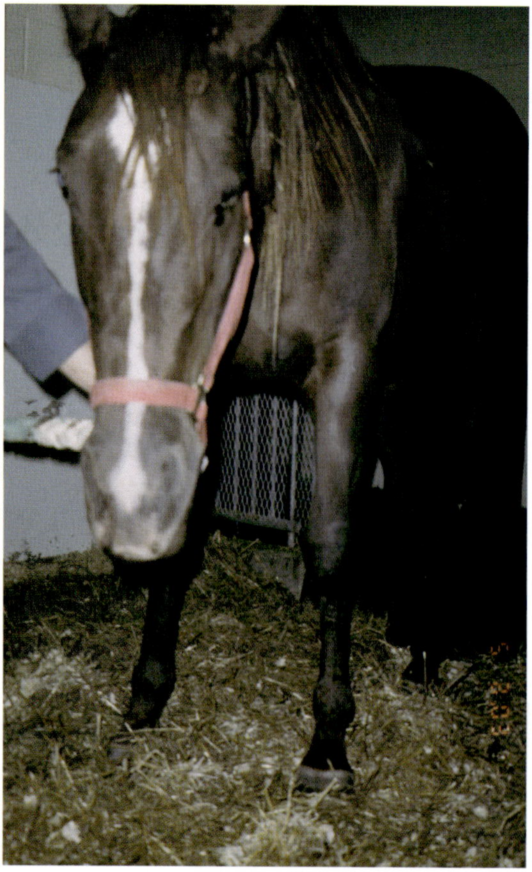

Figure 4.30 An adult horse affected with WNV. Note the depression.

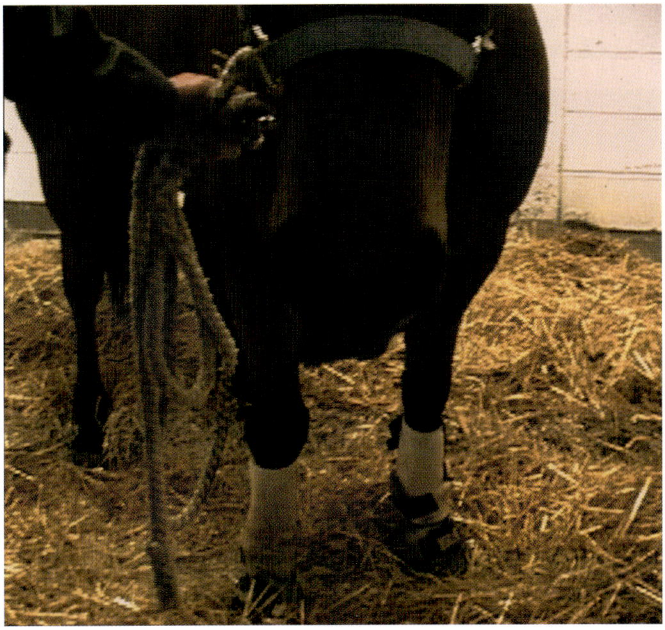

Figure 4.31 An adult horse affected with WNV. Note lip twitching.

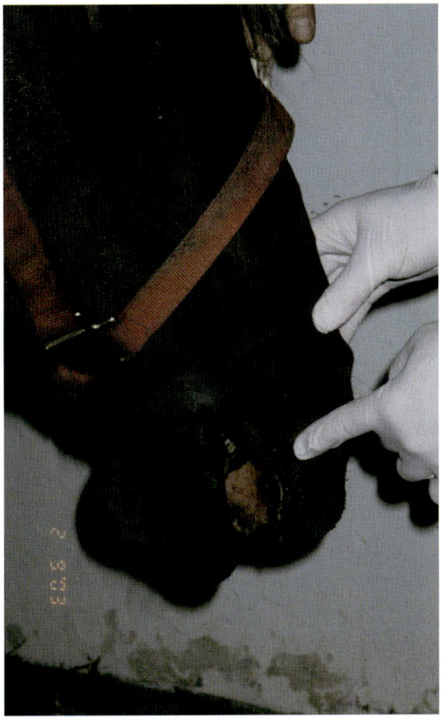

Figure 4.32 An adult horse affected with WNV. Note the droopy lips due to cranial nerve VII deficit.

Verminous Meningoencephalomyelitis

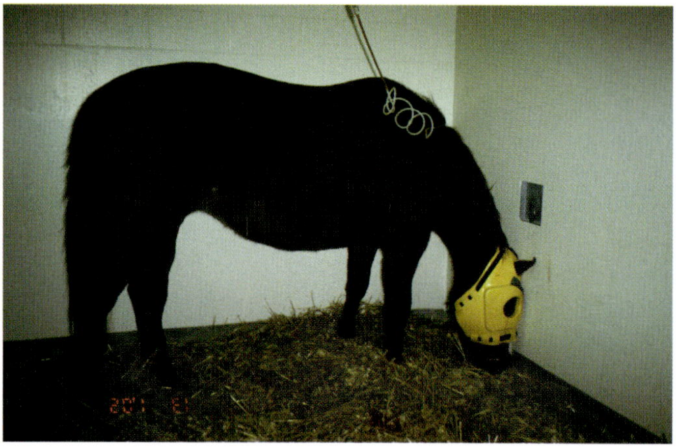

Figure 4.33 An adult horse affected by verminous meningoencephalomyelitis. The horse had stupor (fig. 4.33), head-pressing (fig. 4.34), seizures, ataxia, and weakness in all four limbs (fig. 4.35). The disease is caused by migration of nematodes and insect larvae through the central nervous system. Parasitic agents that have been reported to cause the disease include, *Hypoderma* spp., *Strongylus vulgaris*, and *Setaria* spp.

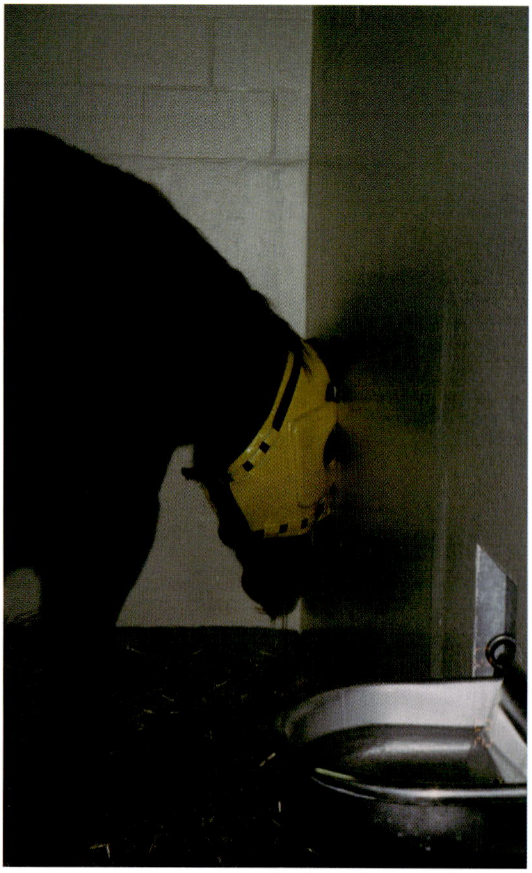

Figure 4.34 Head-pressing in a horse affected with verminous meningoencephalomyelitis.

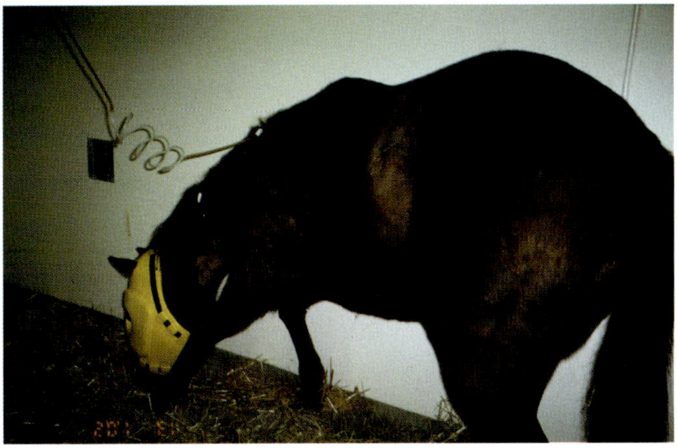

Figure 4.35 Ataxia and weakness in all four limbs in a horse affected with verminous meningoencephalomyelitis.

Equine Herpes Virus I (EHV-1) Myeloencephalitis

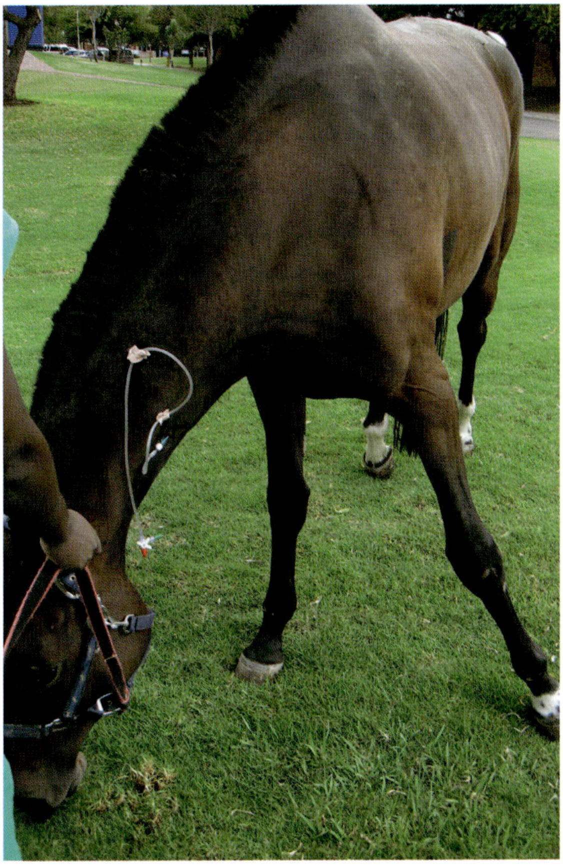

Figure 4.36 A mare affected with equine herpes myeloencephalitis due to equine herpes virus (EHV)-1. Note the wide-based forelimb stance and knuckling of the hind limb. The disease is characterized by an acute onset of ataxia (more severe in the hind limbs) and a mixture of brain stem and cerebral cortex dysfunction. There might be a recent history of upper respiratory tract infection or abortion on the premises. Clinical signs include acute onset of fever, ataxia, tetraplegia (fig. 4.37), tetraparesis, urinary incontinence (fig. 4.38), dilation of the bladder, flaccid anus and tail (fig. 4.39), and variable areas of perineal desensitization. The hind legs are usually more affected than the front legs (fig. 4.40). Some horses may show signs of cranial nerve deficits and patchy sweating (fig. 4.41). Other clinical signs include colic, dysuria, urine scalding of the perineum, and cystitis. Differential diagnosis includes cervical vertebral instability, equine protozoal myeloencephalitis, abscess or trauma affecting the central nervous system, cervical fractures, viral encephalitis, and degenerative myelopathy. Diagnosis is based on the collection (fig. 4.42) and analysis of cerebrospinal fluid (CSF), isolation of EHV-1 from the respiratory tract, buffy coat or CSF and serology. CSF may be xanthrochromic (fig. 4.43) and have a normal or mild mononuclear pleocytosis (fig. 4.44). Treatment includes anti-inflammatory medication, antibiotics, and antiviral agents in conjunction with supportive nursing care.

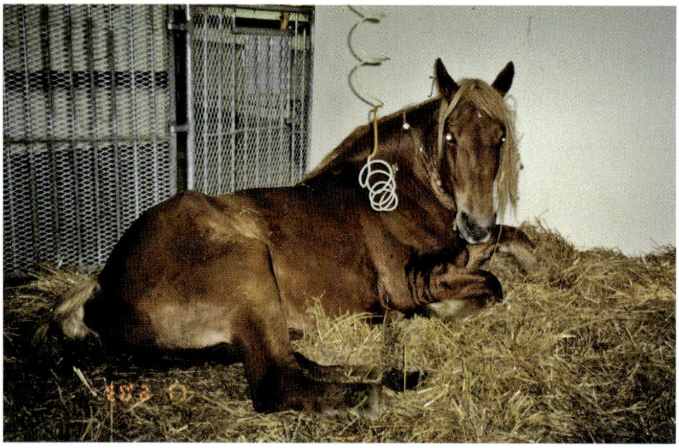

Figure 4.37 Tetraplegia in a horse affected with EHV-1.

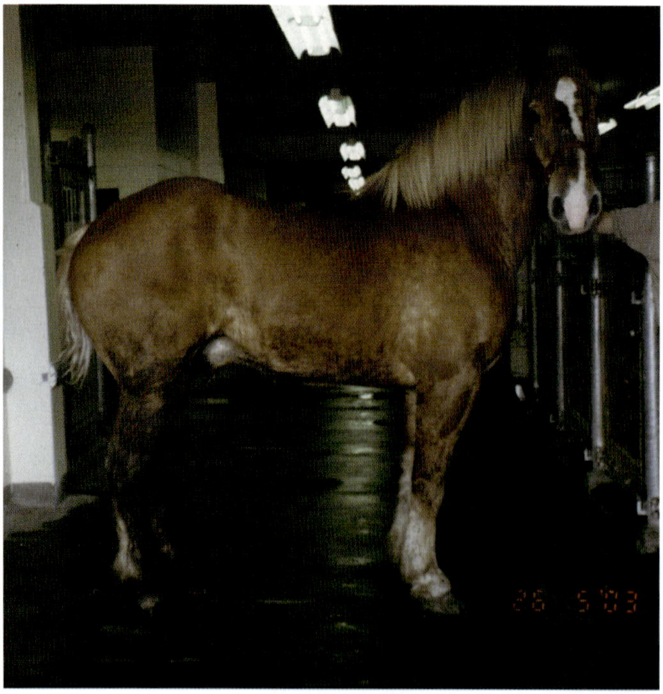

Figure 4.38 Urinary incontinence and urine scalding in a horse affected with EHV-1.

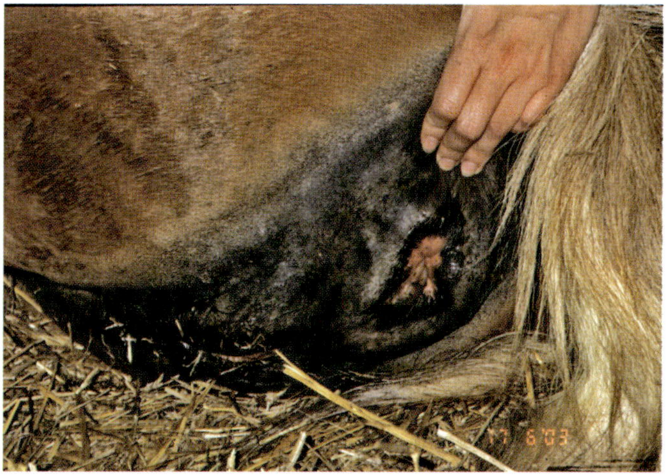

Figure 4.39 Flaccid anus and tail in a horse affected with EHV-1.

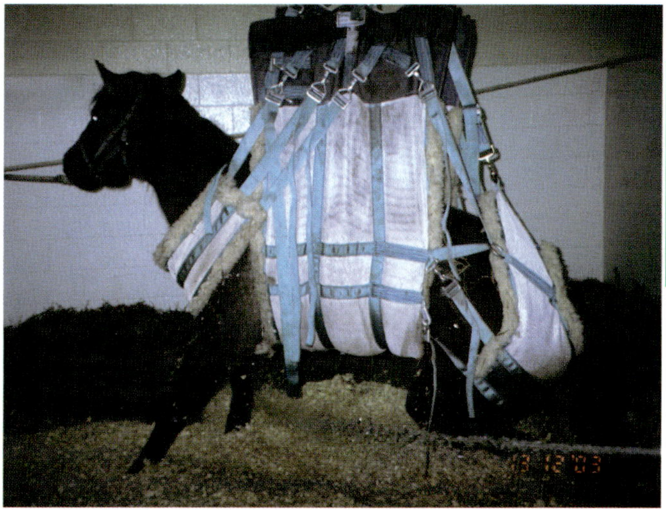

Figure 4.40 An adult horse affected with equine herpes myeloencephalitis due to equine herpes virus (EHV)-1. The hind limbs are more affected than the front limbs.

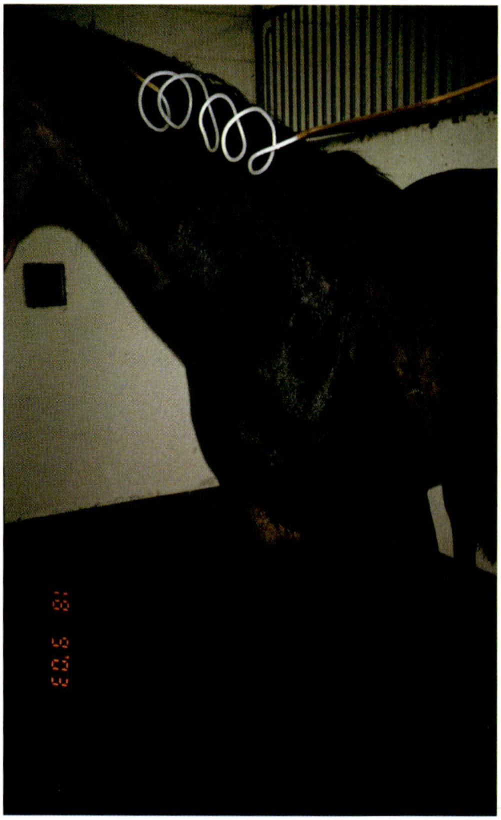

Figure 4.41 Patchy sweating in a horse affected with EHV-1.

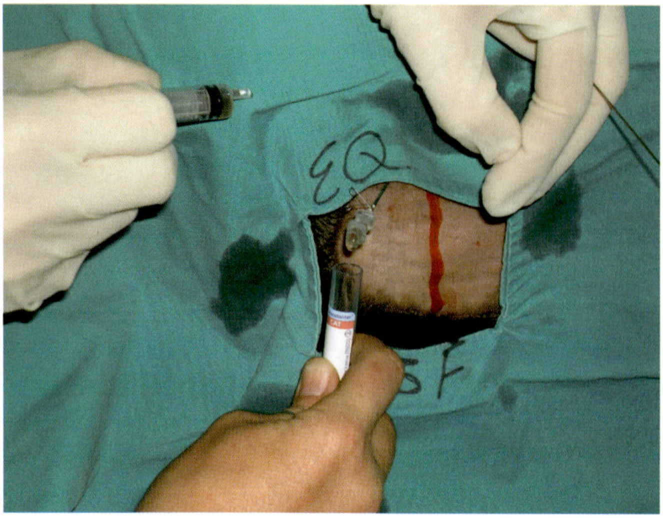

Figure 4.42 Atlanto-occipital centesis of cerebrospinal fluid.

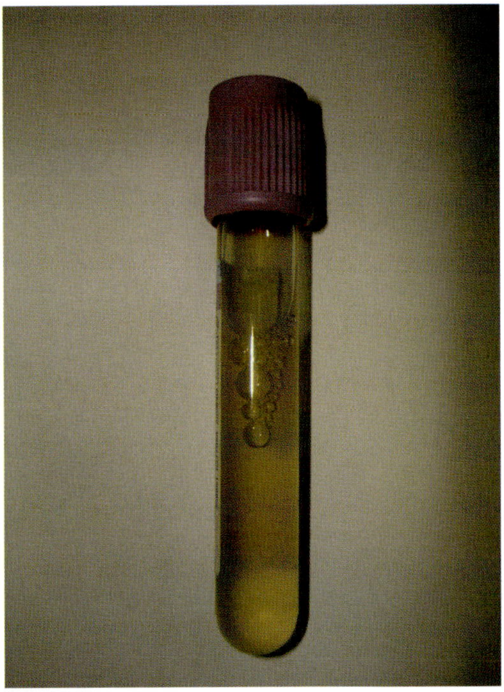

Figure 4.43 Cerebrospinal fluid from a horse affected with EHV-1. Note the xanthochromia.

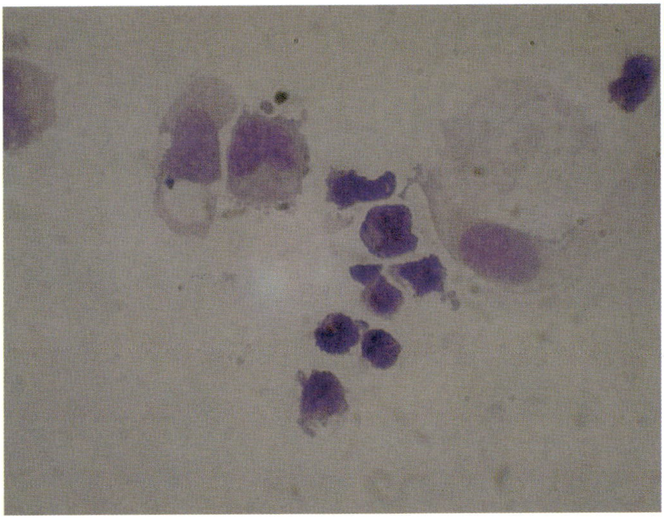

Figure 4.44 A photomicrograph of cerebrospinal fluid from a horse affected with EHV-1 showing a mononuclear pleocytosis (Diff-Quick stain).

Equine Protozoal Myeloencephalitis (EPM)

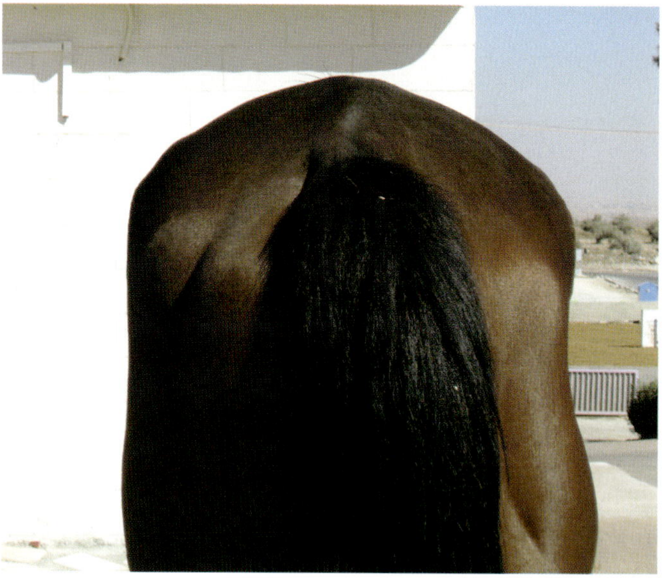

Figure 4.45 An adult horse suspected to be affected by equine protozoal myeloencephalitis (EPM). Note the atrophy of the gluteal muscles. Equine protozoal myeloencephalitis is an asymmetrical, multifocal, progressive disease of the central nervous system (CNS) caused by infection with *Sarcocystis neurona*. The parasite causes inflammation and necrosis of the CNS. This organism has the most unusual life cycle for any species of *Sarcocystis*. Unlike other species of *Sarcocystis*, *S. neurona* has a wide host range for its intermediate hosts. Opossums are the definitive (reservoir) host for this parasite and the horse is considered an aberrant host. Lesions are multifocal and asymmetrical. Onset of clinical signs is variable. Clinical signs include muscle atrophy, gait abnormality (ataxia, tetraparesis—fig. 4.46), knuckling, circumduction, crossing over). Head tilt, facial paralysis (fig. 4.47), circling, nystagmus, dysphagia, tongue paralysis (fig. 4.48), and blindness can be seen. Asymmetrical muscle atrophy is one of the known clinical signs of EPM.

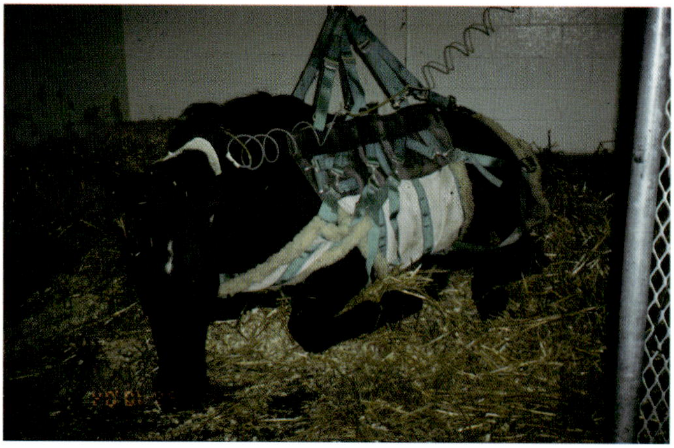

Figure 4.46 An adult horse affected by EPM. The horse had tetraparesis.

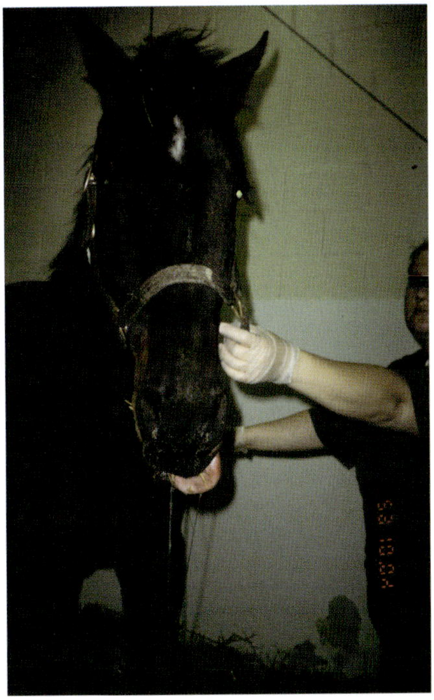

Figure 4.47 An adult horse affected by EPM. Note the droopy lips due to a damaged facial nerve.

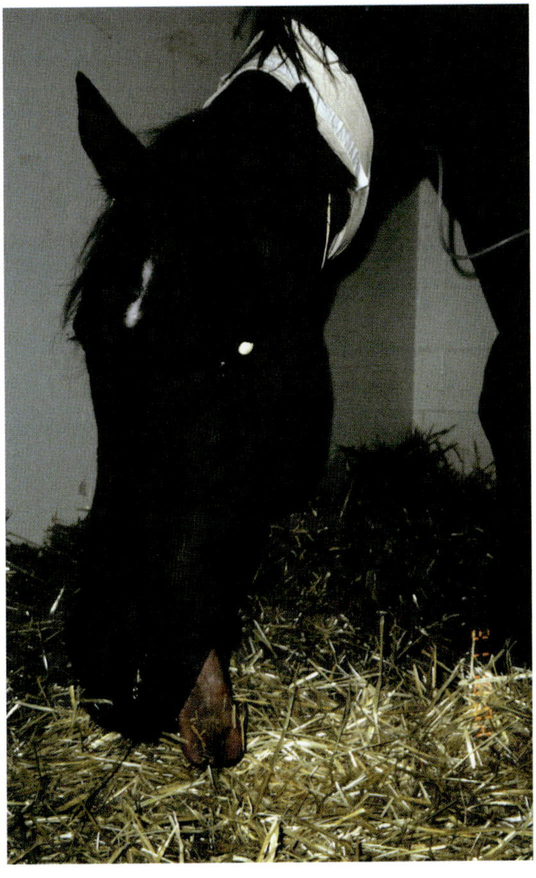

Figure 4.48 An adult horse affected by EPM. Note the tongue paralysis.

Equine Wobbler Syndrome (Cervical Vertebral Stenosis/Instability, Cervical Vertebral Malformation, Cervical Spinal Cord Compression)

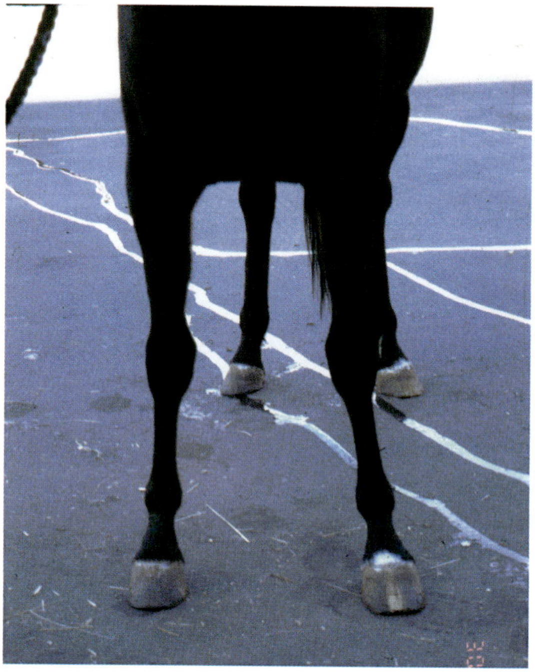

Figure 4.49 An adult horse affected with equine wobbler syndrome. Note the wide-base stance. The horse was ataxic in all four limbs. Equine wobbler syndrome is a developmental disease that is mainly seen in young Thoroughbred, quarter horse, and warm blood breeds. Male horses tend to be overrepresented. The disease has two types of compressive spinal cord lesions: excessive bone production (cervical static stenosis) and excessive movement of vertebrae during neck flexion (cervical vertebral instability). Clinical signs include ataxia (general proprioceptive dysfunction) with the signs most pronounced in pelvic limbs, spasticity, knuckling, stumbling, toe scuffing (fig. 4.50), incomplete limb protraction, crossing over, and pelvic swaying. Affected horses may fail to replace the limbs to normal position when limbs are placed in abnormal positions (fig. 4.51). Diagnosis is based on history, signalment, and clinical signs. The disease is confirmed by plain radiography and myelography of the cervical spinal cord. The cervical spine should be evaluated in relaxed (nonflexed) and flexed positions. See Chapter 6, Diseases of the Muscles.

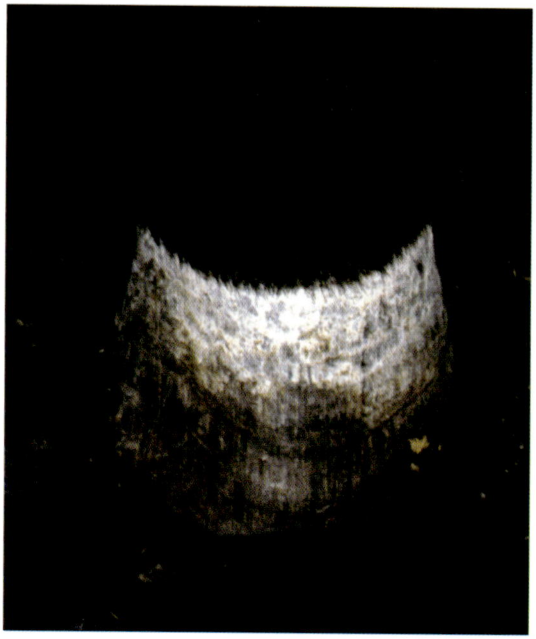

Figure 4.50 Toe scuffing in an adult horse affected with equine wobbler syndrome.

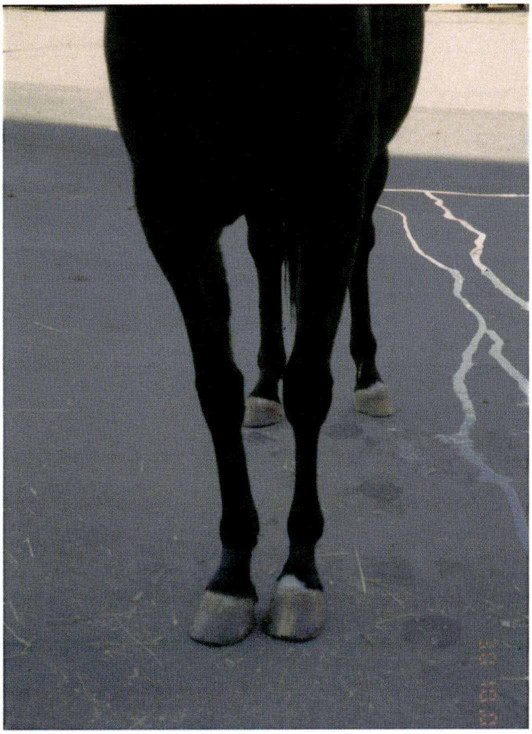

Figure 4.51 An adult horse affected with equine wobbler syndrome. The horse failed to replace the limbs to a normal position when the limb was placed in abnormal position.

Equine Motor Neuron Disease (EMND)

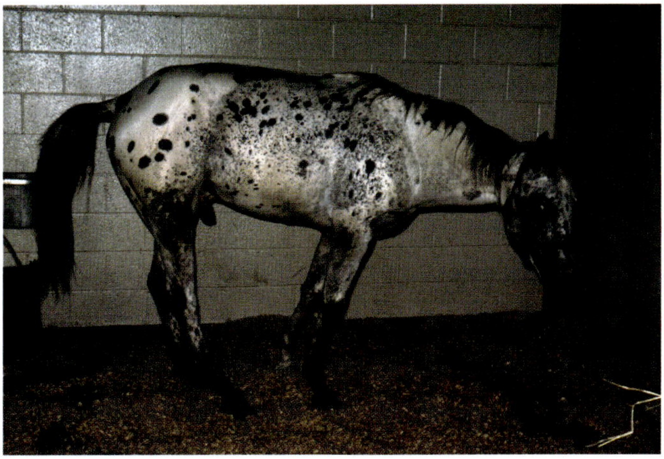

Figure 4.52 An adult horse affected with equine motor neuron disease (EMND). EMND is an acquired, progressive, neurodegenerative disease associated with low dietary vitamin E and lack of access to pasture. It is similar to amyotrophic lateral sclerosis (ALS or Lou Gehrig's disease) in people. Subacute infection of horses results in muscle fasciculation, trembling, increased periods of recumbency, a short-strided gait, shifting of weight, abnormal sweating, and low head carriage. Appetite remains good. Signs of chronic disease are characterized by muscle wasting, elevated tail carriage, and all four feet close together (fig. 4.52). Regions of the CNS that are usually affected include the ventral horn cells (lower motor neurons) of spinal cord grey matter and nuclei of cranial nerves V, VII, XII, and nucleus ambiguous. Oral vitamin E supplementation at 5,000–7,000 IU daily may provide some improvement if the disease is recognized early. Horses without access to green forage are at risk and preventive vitamin E supplementation should be instituted.

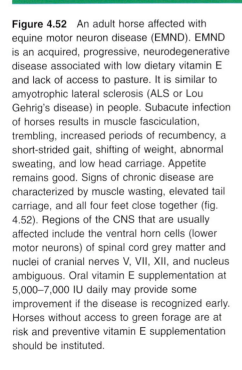

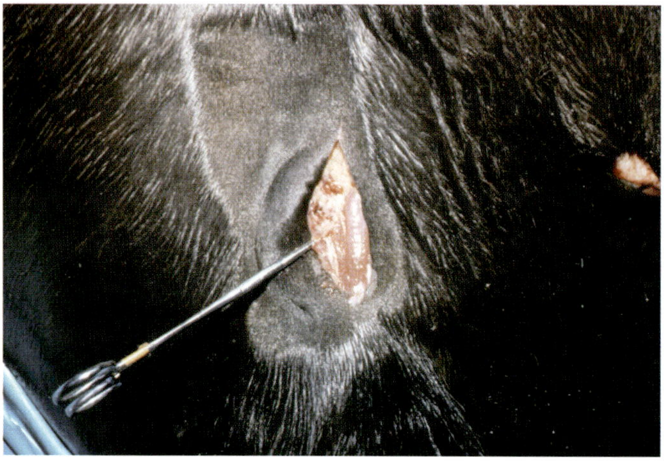

Figure 4.53 Diagnosis can be made based on clinical signs, previous cases on the premises, low serum vitamin E levels, sometimes elevated muscle enzyme levels and presence of lipofuscinlike, and patchy pigmentation in the retina. Biopsy of spinal accessory nerve or sacrocaudalis dorsalis muscle (fig. 4.53) can be done to confirm the diagnosis. (Image courtesy of Dr. D. Sellon and Dr. D. Zimmel.)

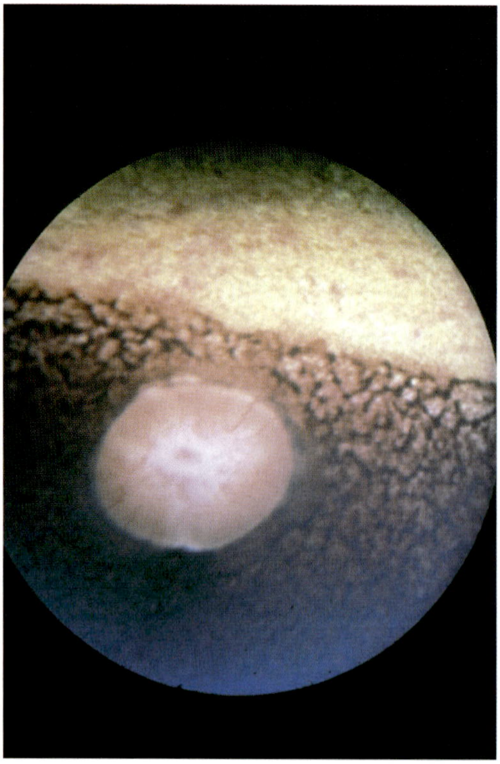

Figure 4.54 Lipofuscinlike pigment in the tapetal fundus of retina. (Image courtesy of Dr. D. Sellon and Dr. D. Zimmel.)

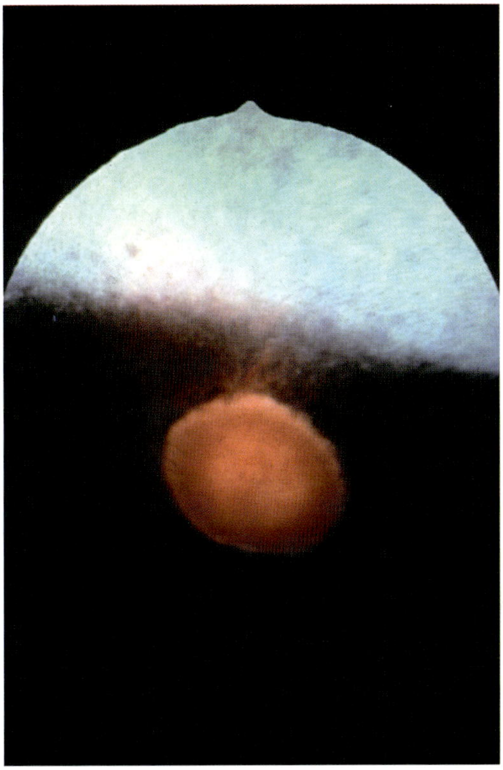

Figure 4.55 Fundus of a normal horse. (Image courtesy of Dr. D. Sellon and Dr. D. Zimmel.)

Rabies

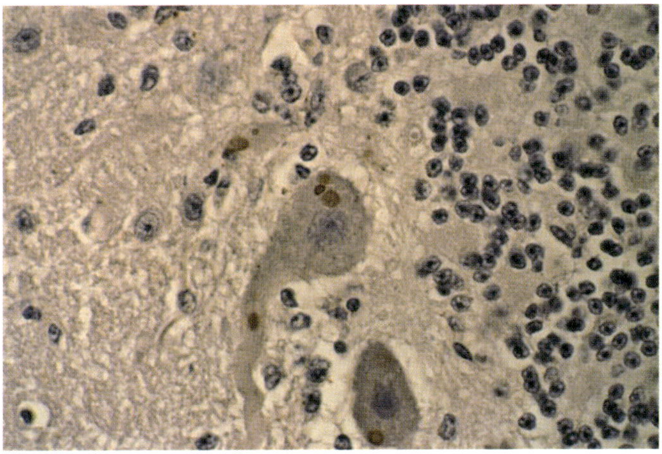

Figure 4.56 Histological examination, with immunoperoxidase stain, of the cerebellum of an animal affected with rabies. Note the brown-staining Negris bodies in Purkinje cells. Rabies is a rapidly progressive fatal neurologic disease that affects most warm-blooded animals. Affected horses can have two forms; dumb and paralytic. Common clinical signs in horses include fever, recumbency, hyperesthesia, tail and anal paralysis, ataxia, and paraplegia. Indirect fluorescent antibody testing, mouse inoculation studies, and histological observation of nonsuppurative encephalitis and Negri bodies can be done to confirm the diagnosis.

Stringhalt

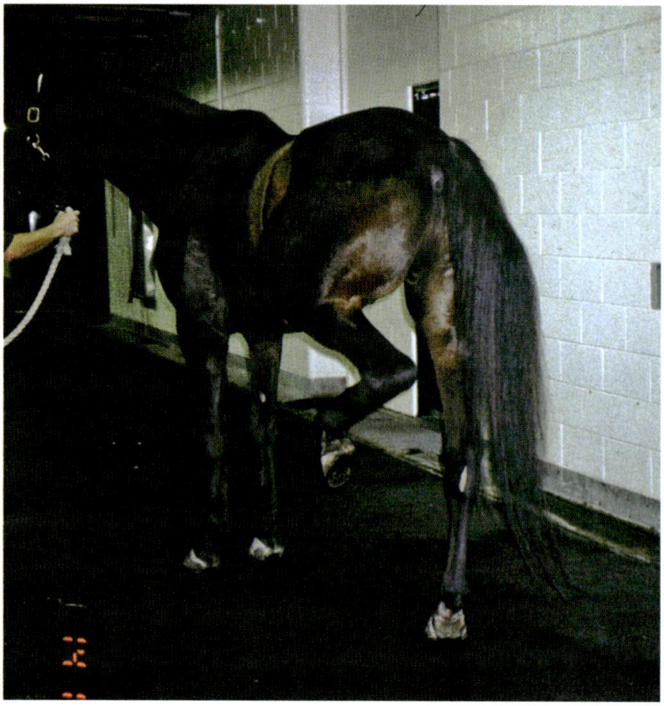

Figure 4.57 An adult horse affected with stringhalt. Note the hyperflexion of the hock joint. Stringhalt is a disease of unknown etiology that is characterized by hyperflexion of one or both hock joints. The disease may occur in both sporadic and epidemic forms (Australian stringhalt). Horses appear normal at rest but have a characteristic hyperflexion of the tarsocrural joint when moving. It can be unilateral or bilateral. Clinical signs worsen on turning or backing. Sporadic cases rarely recover spontaneously, and need surgical treatment. Most horses in the epidemic form recover in weeks to months without treatment when removed from pasture.

Tetanus (Lockjaw)

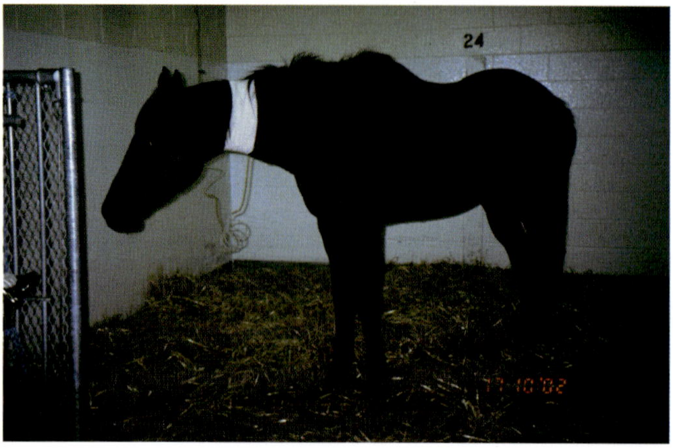

Figure 4.58 An adult horse affected with tetanus. Note the stiff posture of the horse with head and neck extended. Tetanus is an infectious neuromuscular disease characterized by muscular rigidity and death due to respiratory arrest. The disease is caused by *Clostridium tetani*. In horses, puncture wounds of the foot or soft tissues are the most common source of infection. Clinical signs are characteristic and include colic; vague stiffness; lameness that progresses to generalized spasticity; stiff gait with an extended head posture; "sawhorse" stance, elevated tail, excessive facial muscle tone, trismus (lockjaw) (fig. 4.59), prolapsed third eyelid (fig. 4.60), dysphagia and inability to swallow, and profuse frothy salivation (fig. 4.61). Horses that do not respond to treatment become recumbent and die (fig. 4.62).

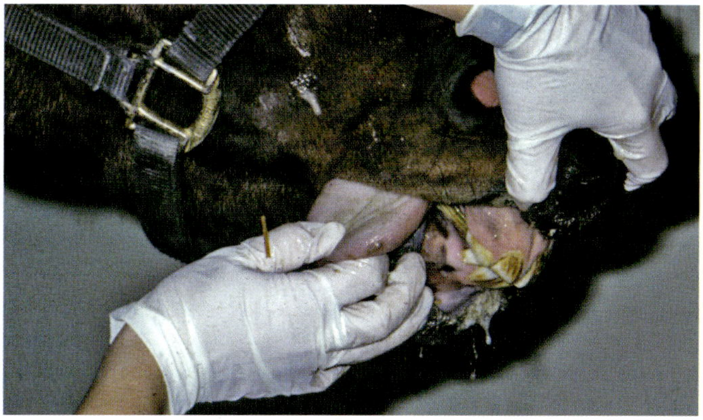

Figure 4.59 An adult horse affected with tetanus. Note the trismus (lockjaw).

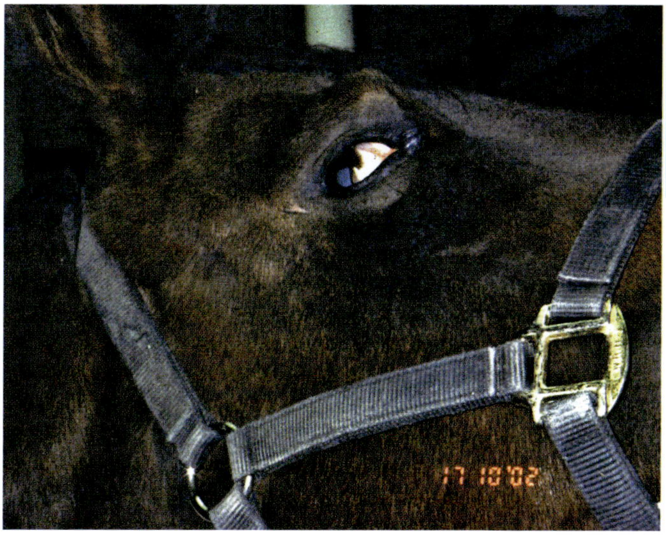

Figure 4.60 An adult horse affected with tetanus. Note the prolapsed third eyelid.

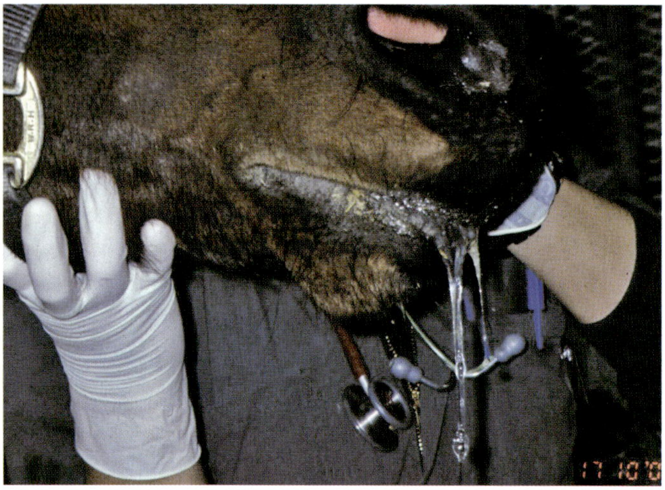

Figure 4.61 An adult horse affected with tetanus. Note the profuse frothy salivation.

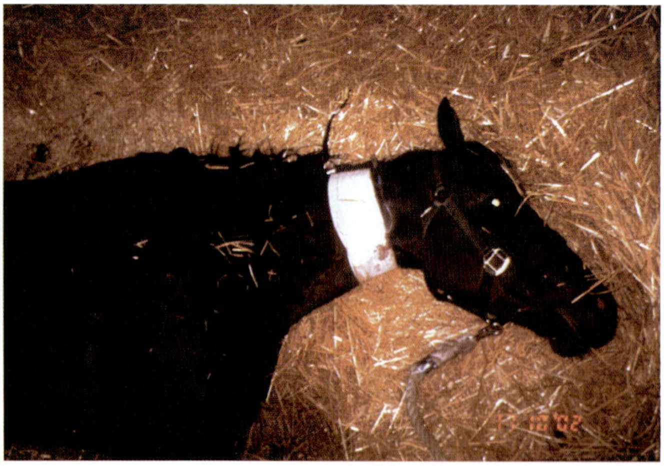

Figure 4.62 An adult horse affected with tetanus. The horse did not respond to treatment and became recumbent and died.

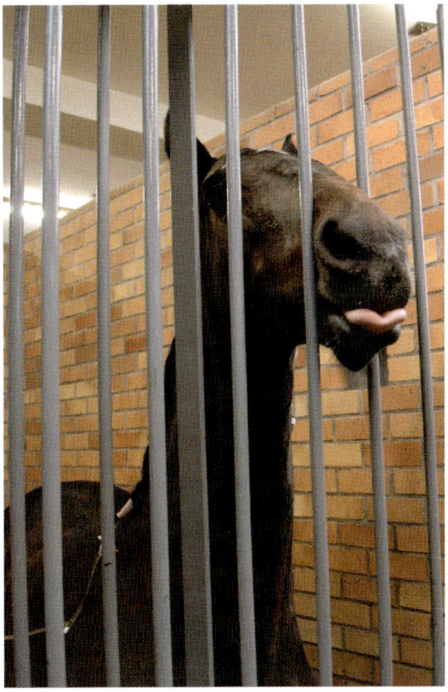

Figure 4.63 A horse with acute lead intoxication following oral ingestion of lead solders (fig. 4.63). Note the tongue paralysis (fig. 4.64) and resultant dysphagia. Clinical signs of lead toxicity in horses include altered mentation (depression or manic behavior), weight loss, laryngeal and pharyngeal dysfunction, aspiration pneumonia due to dysphagia, and ataxia. Diagnosis of lead poisoning is based on measuring lead concentration in blood/kidney/brain/liver or bone, and concentration of blood aminolevulinic acid and porphyrins. In acute poisoning, lead may be identified on postmortem (fig. 4.65). Treatment should include identifying and removing the lead source preventing reexposure, and chelation therapy using calcium disodium EDTA.

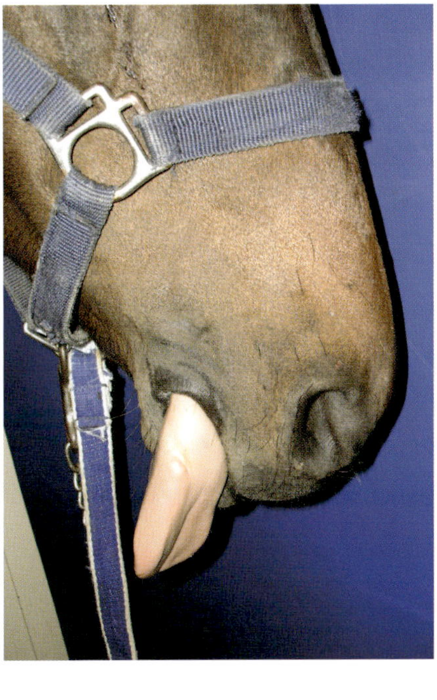

Figure 4.64 Tongue paralysis and dysphagia in a horse with acute lead poisoning.

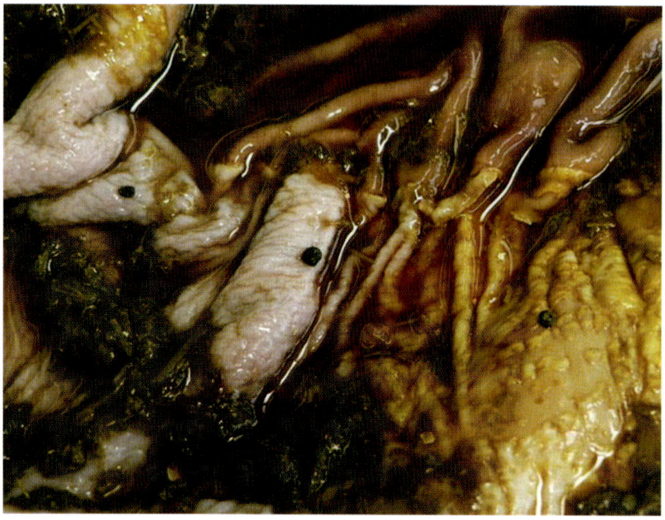

Figure 4.65 Lead pellets (2,614 ppm) found in the stomach of a horse with acute cerebral dysfunction. (Image courtesy of the Section of Pathology, Faculty of Veterinary Science, University of Pretoria.)

Cholesterol Granuloma (Cholesteatomas)

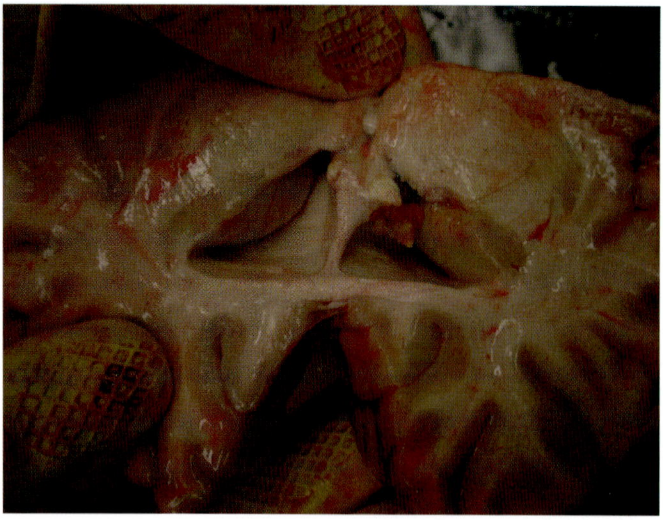

Figure 4.66 Postmortem examination of the brain of a horse affected with cholesterol granuloma (cholesteatomas). Cholesterol granulomas are found in the choroid plexuses of about 15% of old horses. Most of these masses do not cause any clinical signs unless they grow large enough to compress brain tissue. Clinical signs usually are intermittent and asymmetric, and indicate cerebral cortical dysfunction.

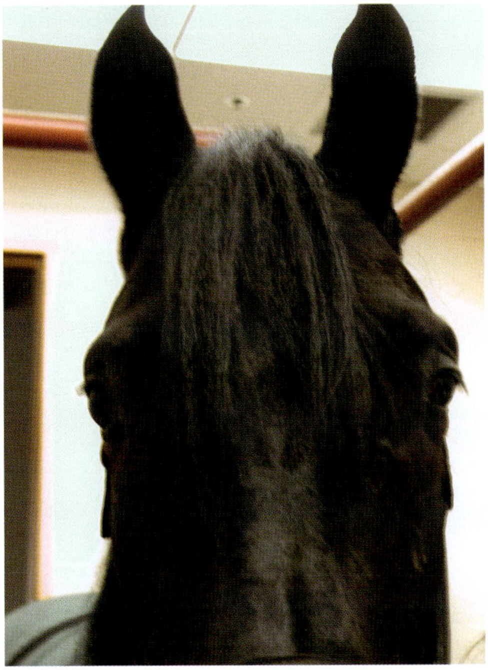

Figure 4.67 An adult horse affected with Horner's syndrome. Note the droopy left eyelid (ptosis). Horner's syndrome usually results from injury of the vagosympathetic trunk fibers or the cranial cervical ganglion as they pass through the neck, or over the caudodorsal aspect of the guttural pouches, respectively. The disease may occur in guttural pouch mycosis, traumatic lesions of the basisphenoid area, cervical trauma, space-occupying lesions in the anterior aspect of the thorax, periorbital mass, following IV injection. Clinical signs include miosis, enophthalmos, ptosis, regional hyperthermia, and sweating of face and neck (ipsilateral side). (Image courtesy of Dr. Maureen Wichtel, AVC, University of Prince Edward Island.)

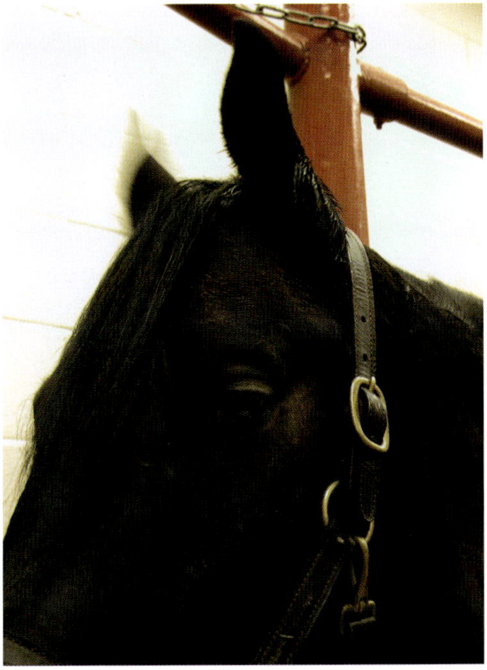

Figure 4.68 An adult horse affected with Horner's syndrome. Note the sweating at the base of the ear. (Image courtesy of Dr. Maureen Wichtel, AVC, University of Prince Edward Island.)

Otitis Media-Interna (Temporohyoid Osteoarthropathy)

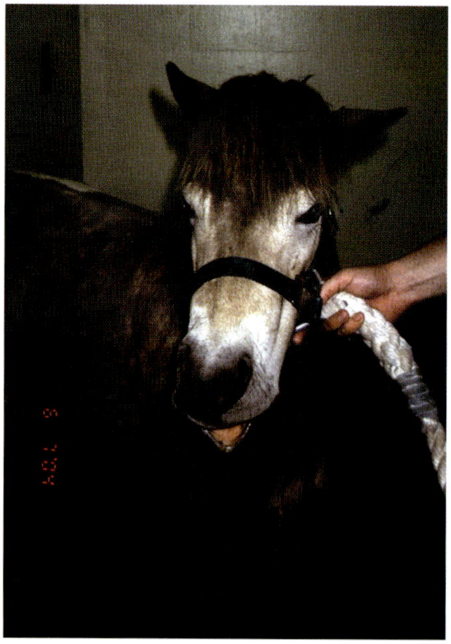

Figure 4.69 A horse affected with otitis media-interna (temporohyoid osteoarthropathy). Note the unilateral facial paralysis. In cases of otitis media-interna, the inflammatory process may localize to the petrous temporal bone and cause vestibular signs and dysfunction of CNs VII and VIII. However, sometimes inflammation extends outward into the temporohyoid joint and stylohyoid bone and lead to fusion of the joint and fracture of the petrous temporal bone. Affected horses may shake or rub ear for 2–3 weeks before onset of vestibular signs. Clinical signs include leaning, circling toward side of lesion; ipsilateral head tilt (fig. 4.70) and facial nerve paralysis; drooped ear/lips; drooling of saliva; ptosis (fig. 4.71) and exposure keratitis on ipsilateral side of lesion (fig. 4.72); deviation of nasal philtrum toward opposite side of lesion; nystagmus (rapid phase is away from the side of the lesion). Diagnosis is based on clinical signs, skull radiographs (fig. 4.73), and endoscopic examination of the guttural pouches (fig. 4.74). Transtympanic lavage (figs. 4.75 and 4.76), magnetic resonance imaging; and computed tomography (fig. 4.77) can also be done to diagnose temporohyoid osteoarthropathy.

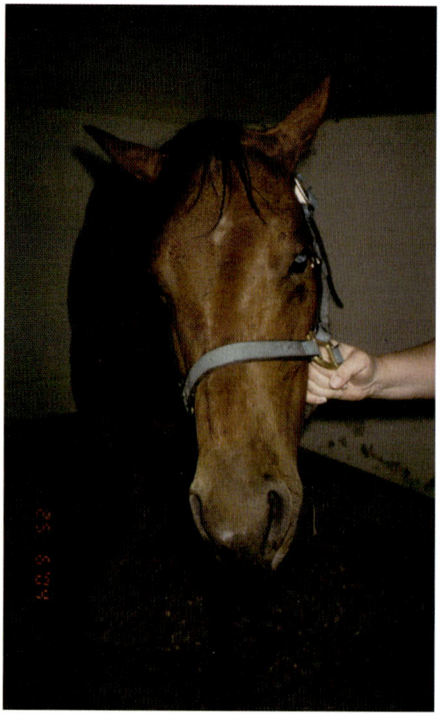

Figure 4.70 Head tilt in a horse affected with otitis media-interna.

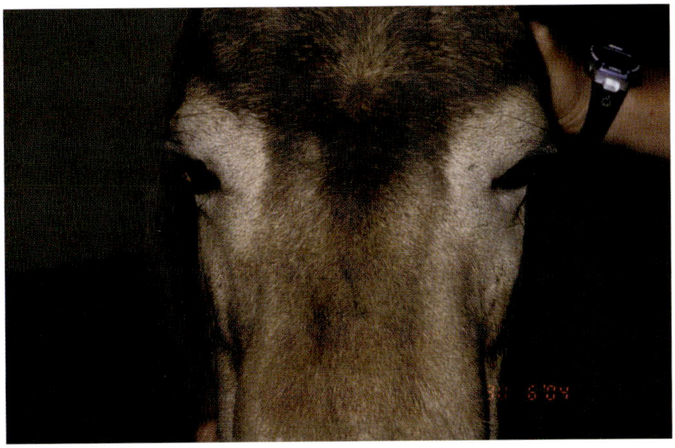

Figure 4.71 Ptosis (droopy eyelid) in a horse affected with otitis media-interna.

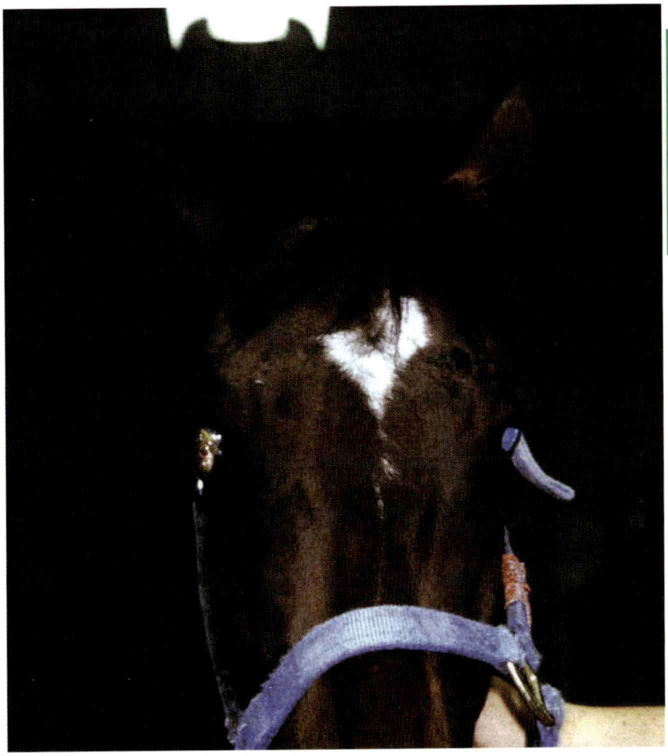

Figure 4.72 Keratitis and severe endopthalmitis in a horse affected with otitis media-interna.

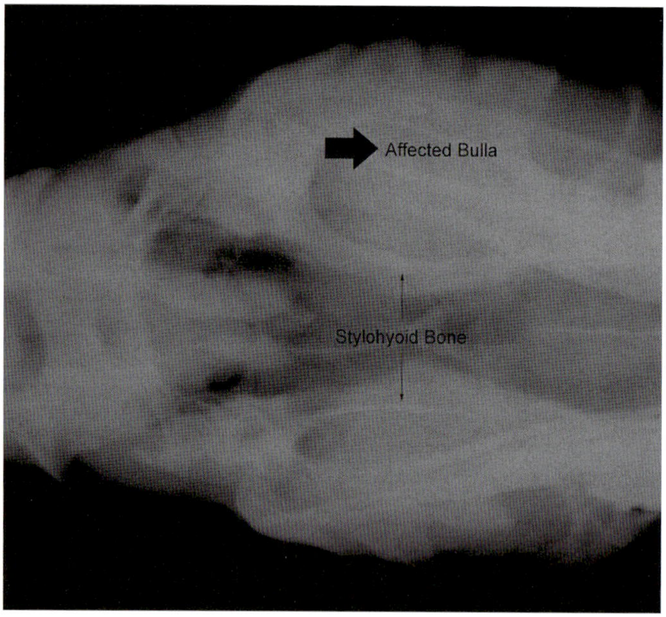

Figure 4.73 Ventrodorsal skull radiograph of a horse affected with otitis media-interna (temporohyoid osteoarthropathy), note the unilateral thickening of the stylohyoid bone. There is bony proliferation of the proximal stylohyoid and petrous temporal bones (affected bulla).

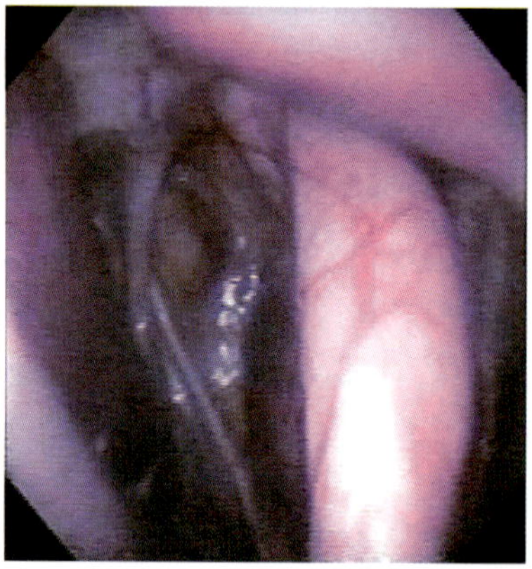

Figure 4.74 Endoscopic view of the guttural pouch in a horse affected with otitis media-interna. Note the thickened stylohyoid bone. (Image from Abutarbush SM and Carmalt JL, Endoscopy and arthroscopy for the equine practitioner. Made Easy Series. Jackson, WY: Teton NewMedia, 2008.)

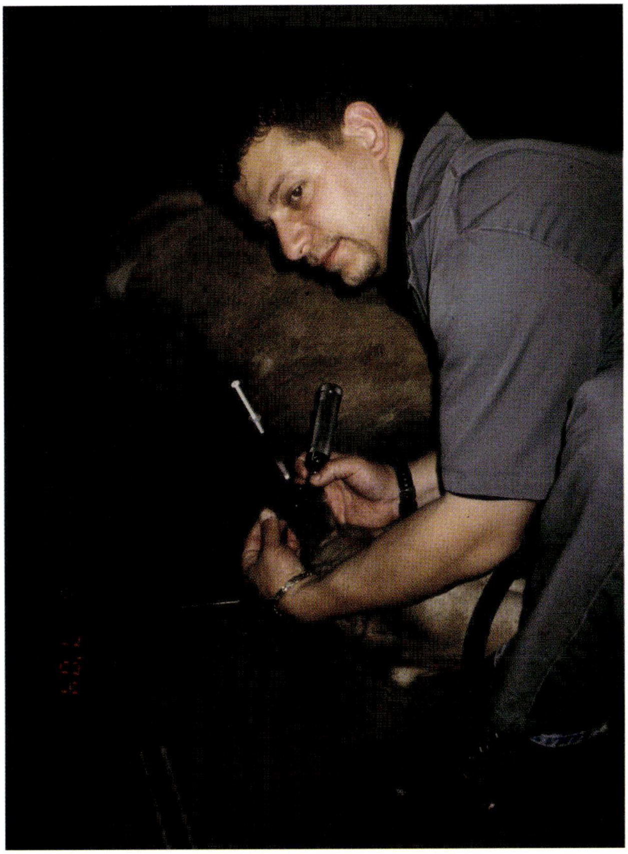

Figure 4.75 Transtympanic lavage in a horse affected with otitis media-interna. Although difficult, transtympanic lavage can be done to diagnose otitis media-interna in horses. The fluid obtained from the lavage can be sent for cytological examination and culture.

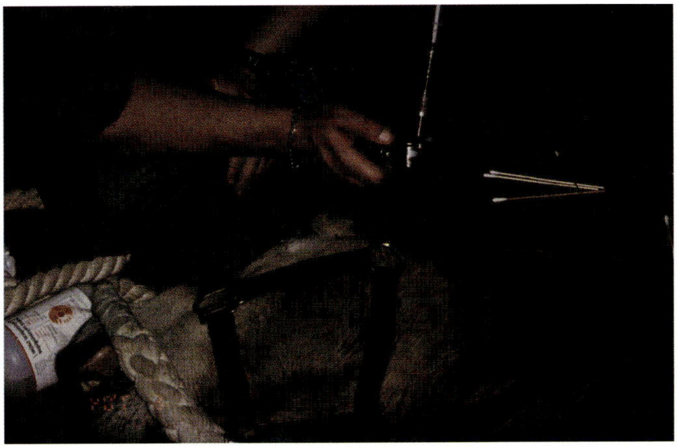

Figure 4.76 Close-up view of fig. 4.75.

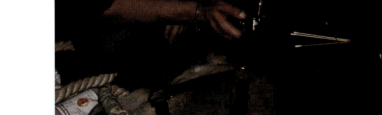

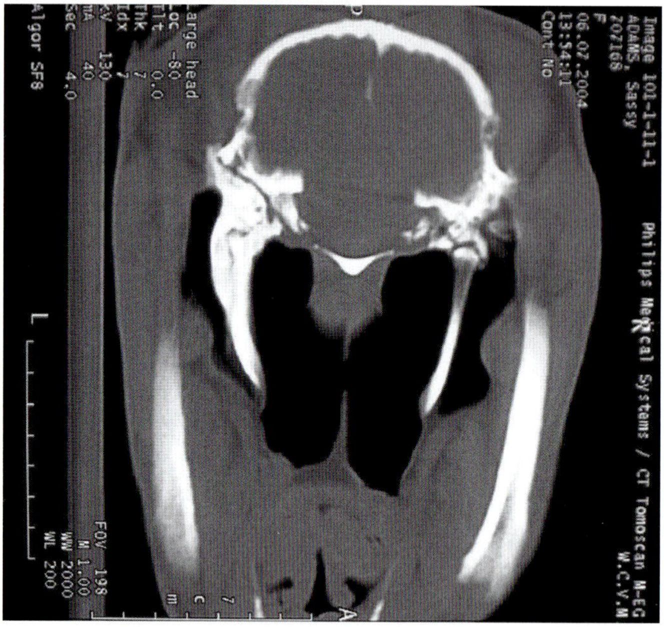

Figure 4.77 Computed tomography in a horse affected with otitis media-interna. Note the thickened stylohyoid bone.

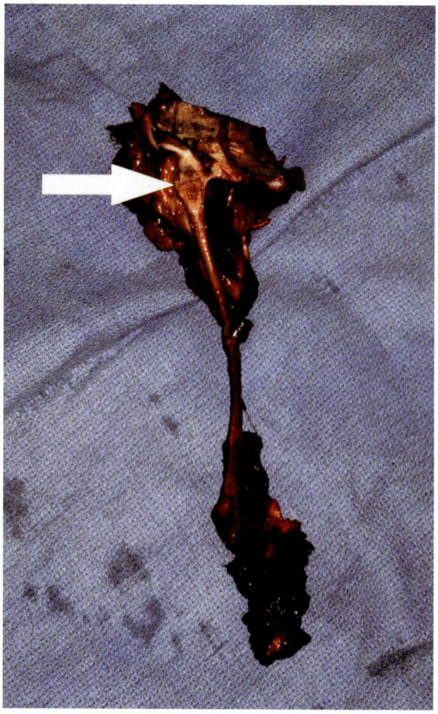

a

Figures 4.78a,b Postmortem examination of the stylohyoid bones (left and right) in a horse affected with unilateral otitis media-interna (temporohyoid osteoarthropathy). Fig. 78a is a photograph of the normal stylohyoid bone (arrow) compared to the affected one (arrow) in fig. 4.78b. Note the thickened stylohyoid bone in fig. 4.78b.

Figures 4.78a,b *Continued*

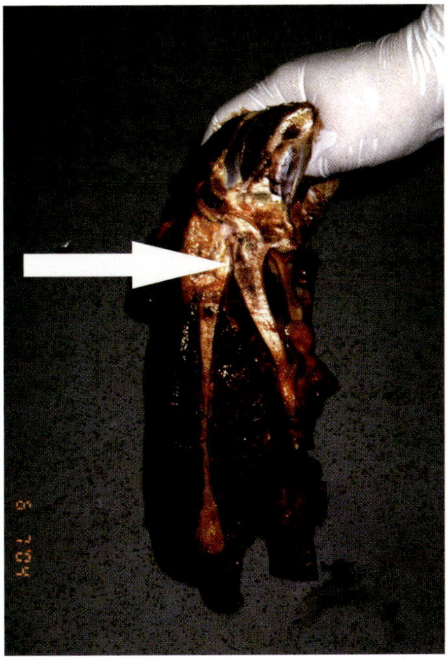

b

Radial Nerve Paralysis

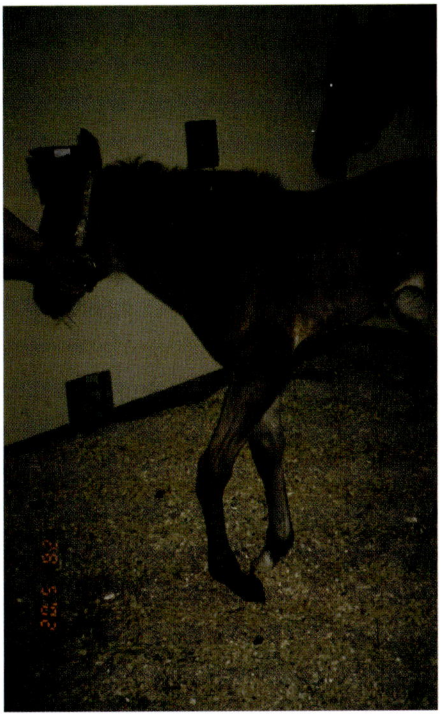

Figure 4.79 A foal with radial nerve paralysis. Note the dropped elbow and flexion of all distal limb joints. Radial nerve courses over the lateral aspect of the elbow joint and is susceptible to injury.

Facial Nerve Trauma

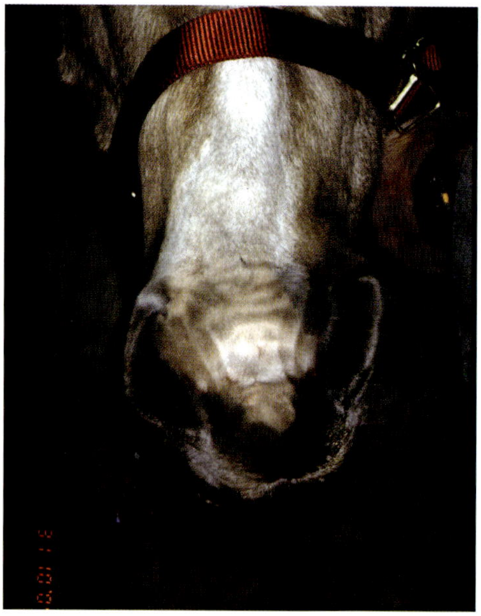

Figure 4.80 A horse affected with facial nerve trauma during an episode of severe colic. Not the unilateral facial paralysis that is manifested by right lip deviation and reduced flaring of the right nostril. Facial nerve damage can occur at the proximal or distal part. Proximal facial nerve damage occurs in petrous temporal bone fracture and otitis media-interna (temporohyoid osteoarthropathy). See otitis media-interna section above. Distal facial nerve damage is usually caused by a blow or lateral recumbency. The nerve gets damaged as it crosses the mandible or the zygomatic arch.

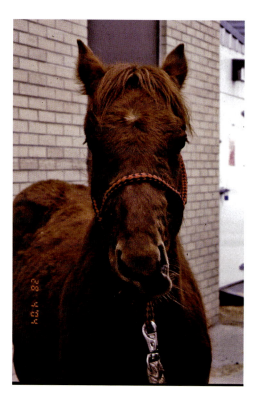

Figure 4.81 A horse affected with distal facial nerve trauma after lateral recumbency. Note that the lip and nostril are affected while the eyelid and ear are normal.

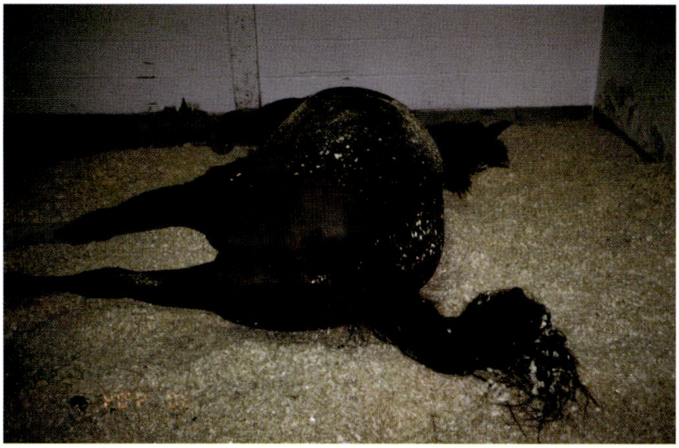

Figure 4.82 An adult horse affected with meningitis. The horse became recumbent after it had several behavioral changes. Meningitis is much more common in foals than adult horses. It is caused usually by a hematogenous spread of bacteria to the meninges, penetrating skull trauma, or extension of suppurative process in and around the head.

References

Abutarbush, SM, O'Connor, BP, Clark, C, Sampieri, F, Naylor, JM. Clinical West Nile virus in 2 horses in western Canada. Canadian Veterinary Journal 45(4):315–17, 2004.

Leighton, FA, Abutarbush, SM. The West Nile virus epidemic in North America: 1999–2002. Large Animal Veterinary Rounds 3(1): 2003.

Mayhew, IG. Large animal neurology: a handbook for veterinary clinicians. Philadelphia: Lea & Febiger, 1989.

Radostits, OM, Gay, CC, Blood, DC, et al. Diseases of the alimentary tract-1 veterinary medicine: a textbook of the diseases of cattle, sheep, pigs, goats and horses. 9th ed. London: WB Saunders, 2000.

Reed, SM, Bayly, WM, Selon, D. Equine internal medicine. Philadelphia: WB Saunders, 1253–89, 2004.

Smith, BP. Large animal internal medicine. 3rd ed. St. Louis: Mosby, 2002.

5 Diseases of the Integumentary System

Diseases of the Integumentary System
- Acquired Leukotrichia
- Actinobacillosis
- Atheroma
- Aural Plaques
- Bacterial Folliculitis
- Burns
- Bursitis (Shoe Boil and Fistulous Withers) and Pressure Sores
- Calcinosis Circumscripta (Tumoral Calcinosis)
- Cushing's Syndrome
- Cutaneous Habronemiasis
- Cutaneous Lymphosarcoma
- Dermatophilosis (Rain Scald)
- Dermatophytosis (Ringworm)
- Dermoid Cyst
- Hyperelastosis Cutis (Ehler Danlos Syndrome)
- Insect Bite Hypersensitivity (Queensland Itch, Sweet Itch)
- Lethal White Syndrome
- Lice (Pediculosis)
- Melanoma
- Nodular Necrobiosis (Eosinophilic Collagen Necrosis)
- Onchocerciasis
- Pemphigus
- Photosensitization
- Sarcoids
- Sarcoidosis
- Scalding (Urine, Serum, Chemical)
- Scratches (Greasy Heel, Pastern Dermatitis)
- Sporotrichosis
- Squamous Cell Carcinoma
- Stud Crud (Idiopathic Cannon Keratosis)
- Sunburn
- Telogen Defluxion
- Temporal Teratoma (Dentigerous Cyst, Ear Tooth, Heterotrophic Polydontia)
- Phaeohyphomycosis (Blackgrain Mycetoma, Maduromycosis)
- Tick Infestation
- Urticaria
- Vasculitis (Immune-mediated or Photoactive)
- Arabian Fading Syndrome
- Vitiligo

Warts (Papillomatosis)
Winter Atopy
Cutaneous Drug Reactions (Drug Eruption)
Food Hypersensitivity
Anhydrosis
Epizootic Lymphangitis (Histoplasmosis)
Junctional Epidermolysis Bullosa (JEB)

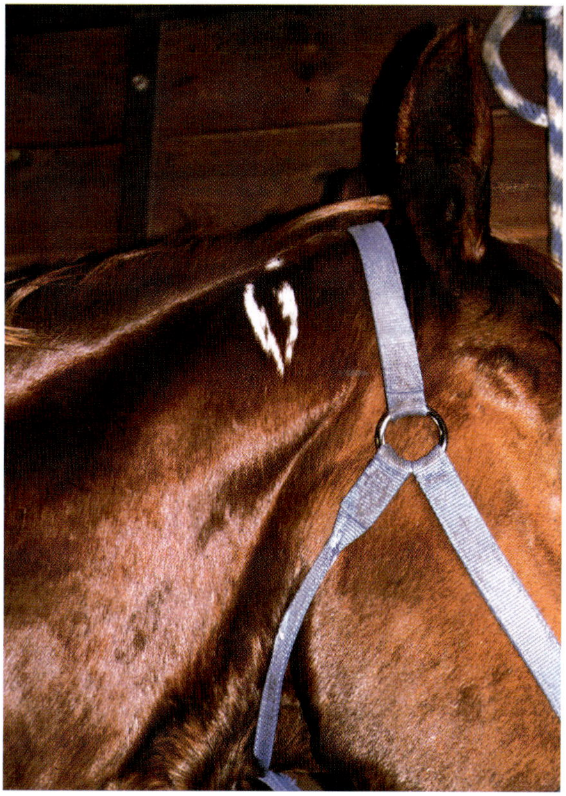

Figure 5.1 A depigmentation of hair, due to a variety of causes such as trauma, infection, or pressure (bandaging or cribbing straps). This condition is usually not progressive and in some cases is reversible. The picture is of a mature quarter horse. Note the wide area of white hair in the proximal region of the neck. This horse wore a cribbing strap. It is important to check this area during a prepurchase examination as horses that have this behavioral vice may not exhibit it during clinical examination.

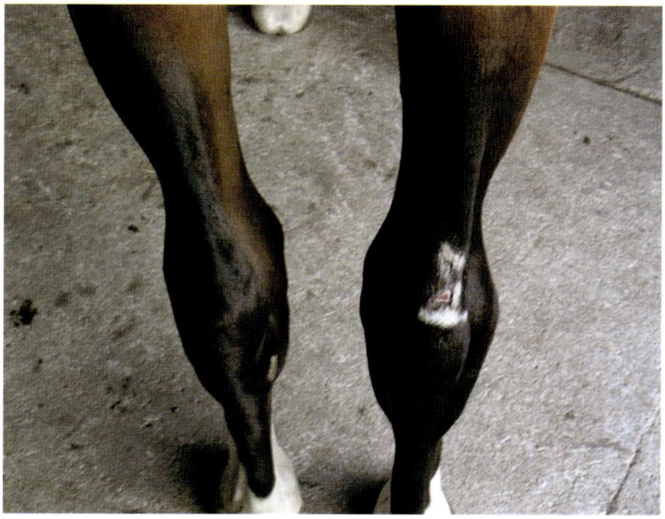

a

Figures 5.2a,b A mature quarter horse with acquired leukotrichia as a result of incorrect bandaging technique. In a show animal, this could result in more of a problem than the original injury for which the limb was bandaged.

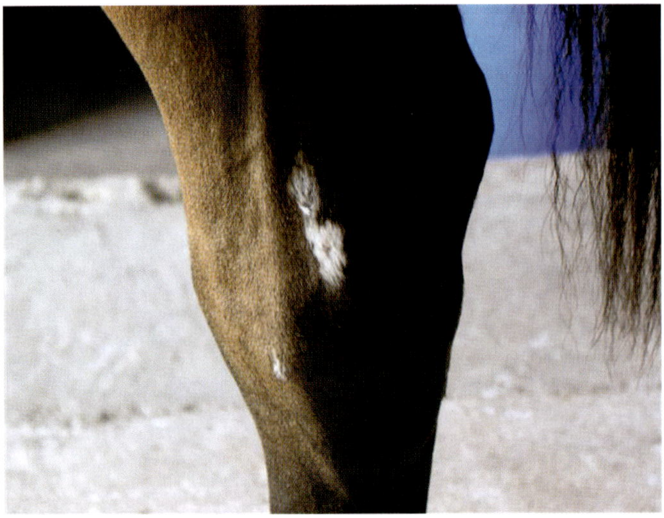

b

Figures 5.2a,b *Continued*

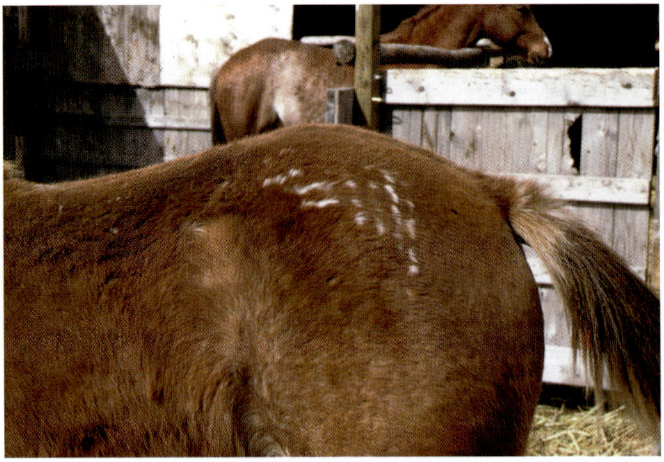

a

Figures 5.3a,b Reticulated leukotrichia in a young quarter horse. Reticulated leukotrichia is characterized by the development of crusty lesions that are eventually lost, followed by permanent depigmentation of the hair in a crosshatched pattern. Most commonly it affects the dorsal midline anywhere from tail to withers. It is considered to be a heritable familial trait in some quarter horses, Thoroughbreds, Standardbreds, miniatures, and Paso Finos, but can occur in other breeds. It has been described following vaccine reactions, erythema multiforme, and systemic disease, but it can develop with no known predisposing issue. As a coat color pattern it is known as "white lacing."

Figures 5.3a,b *Continued*

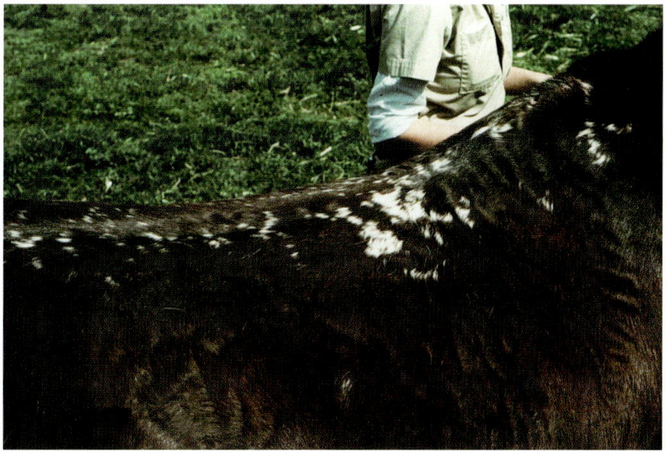

b

Actinobacillosis

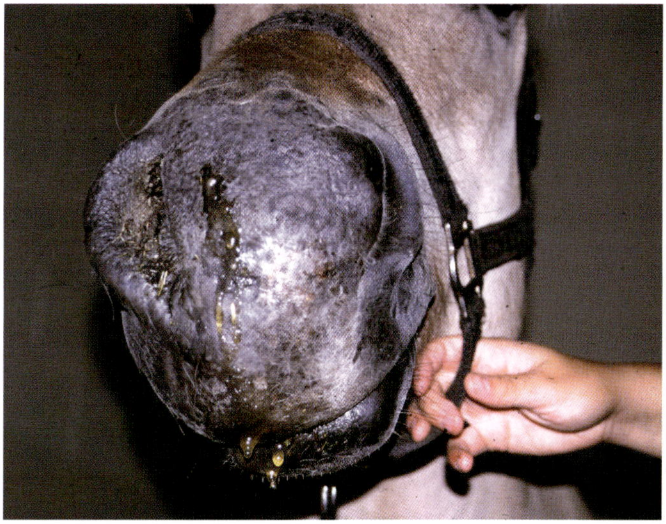

Figure 5.4 A rare soft-tissue infection of the muzzle, characterized by swelling, thickening, and fibrosis in a mature pregnant mare. Culture of tissue biopsy revealed a pure growth of Actinobacillus lignieresi. Treatment consisted of oral trimethoprim-sulfa and potassium iodide medication in addition to intravenous potassium iodide. Note the serum exudation.

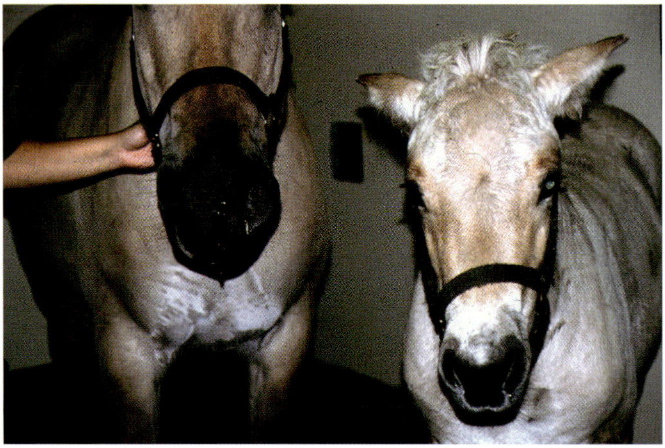

Figure 5.5 The same horse (postfoaling) after treatment.

Atheroma

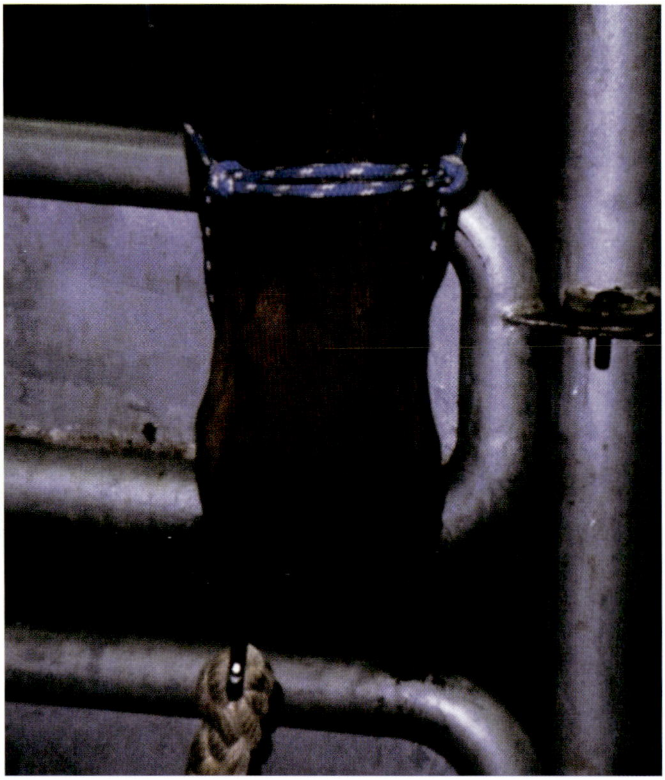

a

Figures 5.6a,b The pictures are of a weanling Arabian filly presented with a soft to semifirm swelling midway between the muzzle and the nose-band. This is an atheroma, usually present at the base of the false nostril. False nostril cysts are actually epidermal inclusion cysts and not true atheromas (sebaceous cysts). They can be seen occasionally in any sex or breed of horse at the area of the nasomaxillary notch. They are nonpainful, firm to fluid, well-circumscribed swellings in the apex of the false nostril. They can be unilateral or bilateral. They are present at birth but usually not visible. They tend to enlarge as the animal matures and can reach a size of 2–5 cm diameter. The contents are thick and creamy appearing. The lining of the cyst is epithelial in nature and contains no hair follicles or sebaceous glands.

Figures 5.6a,b *Continued*

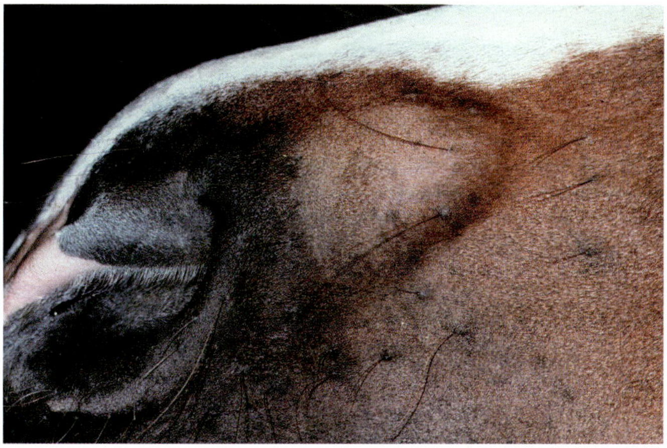

b

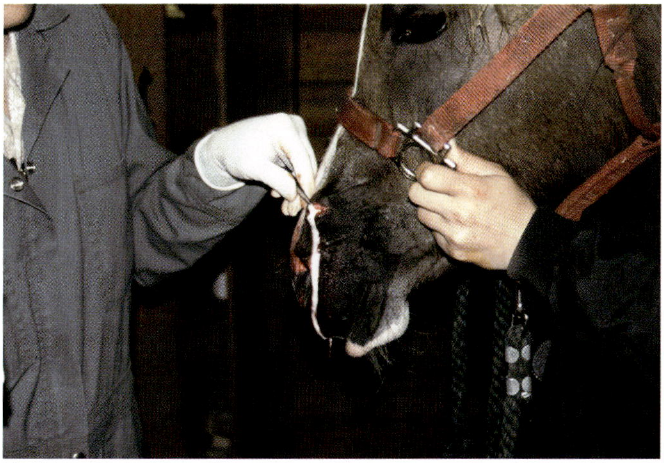

Figure 5.7 Atheroma is usually harmless. Usually they are of no consequence and can be left alone. If they get large enough to interfere with airway or tack, or for cosmetic reasons, they can be surgically removed. Complete surgical excision is the treatment of choice. However, intralesional injection using buffered formalin has also been reported. In this picture, the cyst has been approached directly from the dorsolateral aspect of the nostril rather than from within the nares. This has the potential to result in a less-cosmetic final result. Additionally, the lining of the cyst has been compromised, which is to be avoided.

Aural Plaques

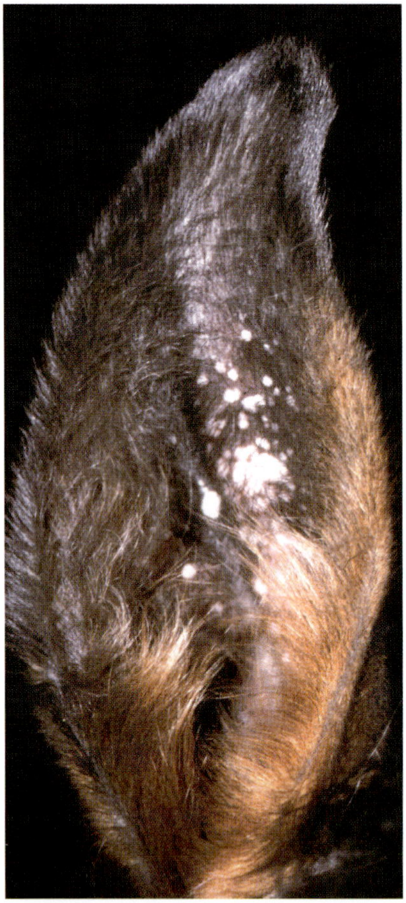

a

Figures 5.8a,b Common problem: Etiology is either fly-bite irritation or papilloma virus involvement. Generally, it begins as small raised depigmented spots becoming raised, white, hyperkeratotic plaques. Usually it is not painful if left alone. These rarely regress spontaneously. Figure 5.8a shows some early lesions peripherally and chronic lesions centrally.

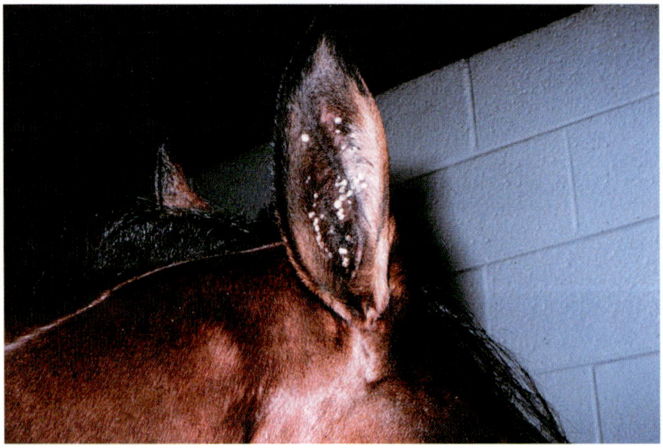

b

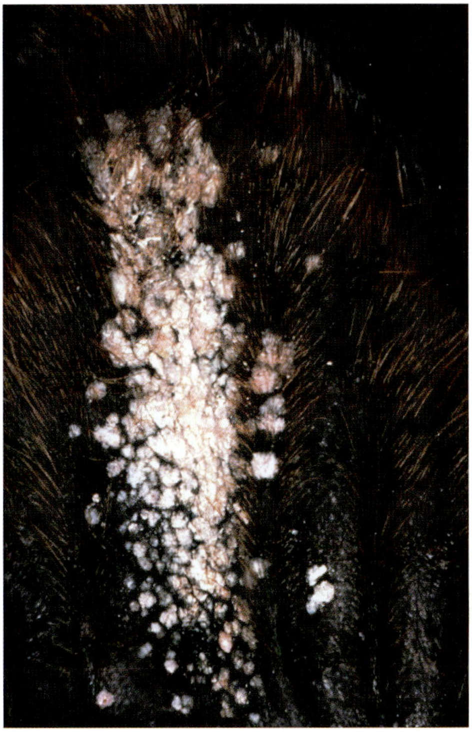

Figure 5.9 This pinna has suffered chronic irritation and in this case the horse was presented for head-shaking.

Bacterial Folliculitis

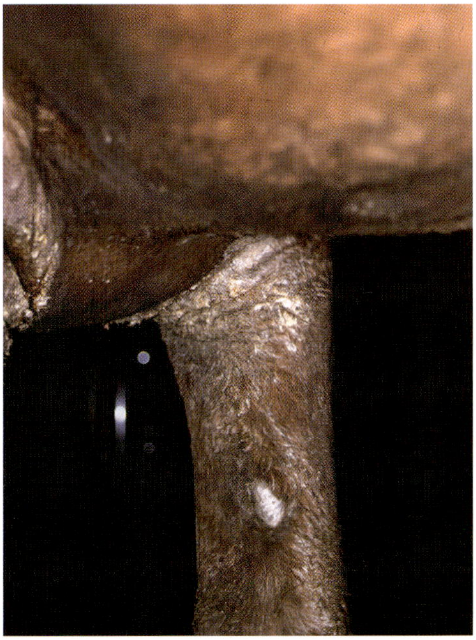

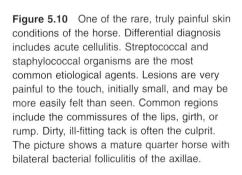

Figure 5.10 One of the rare, truly painful skin conditions of the horse. Differential diagnosis includes acute cellulitis. Streptococcal and staphylococcal organisms are the most common etiological agents. Lesions are very painful to the touch, initially small, and may be more easily felt than seen. Common regions include the commissures of the lips, girth, or rump. Dirty, ill-fitting tack is often the culprit. The picture shows a mature quarter horse with bilateral bacterial folliculitis of the axillae.

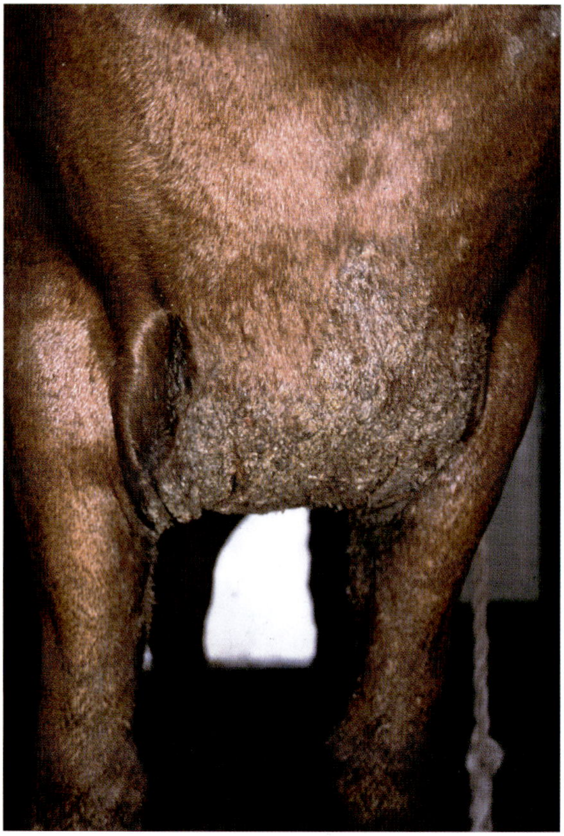

Figure 5.11 The same horse as in fig. 5.10 with extension of the lesion over the pectoral region.

Burns

Horses most commonly are burned in barn, bush, or grass fires. The prognosis depends on a combination of variables such as the extent and depth of skin involved, smoke inhalation causing respiratory compromise, and whether or not vital structures such as coronary bands, joints, eyes, and mouth are involved. Full extent of the damage to the skin may not be apparent on initial evaluation. Superficial burns are painful, but have the best prognosis for healing provided the area involved is not too extensive. Individuals are unlikely to survive if more than 50% of the body surface is involved, especially if the burns are deep. Involvement of more than 20% of the body surface area affects cellular and humoral immunity and depresses cardiac function. Areas of full depth burns are not painful. Fluid, electrolyte, and protein loss require supportive systemic care. Infections are a major risk and topical antibiotic dressings are required.

Figures 5.12a–c Postmortem pictures of a mature horse caught in a barn fire. There is extensive blistering and epithelial loss. As with other species, epithelial loss can result in significant protein loss, pain, and secondary infection. In this case, the owner could not afford the protracted treatment period for this animal.

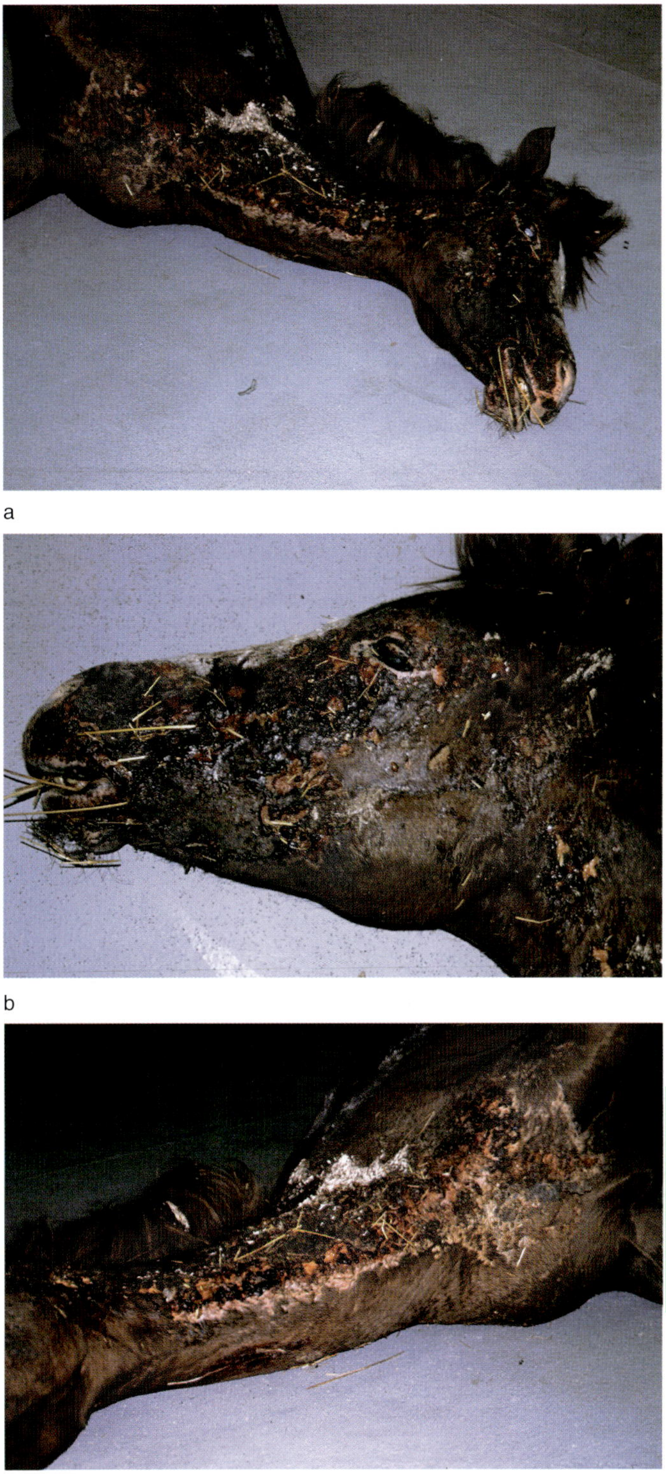

a

b

c

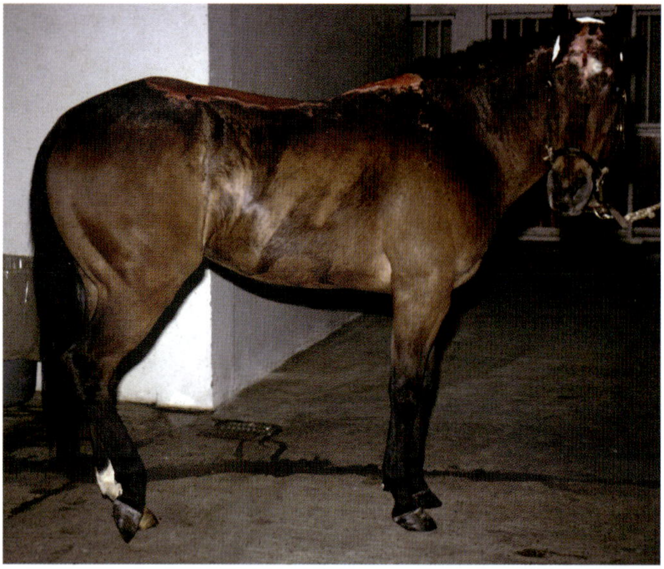

a

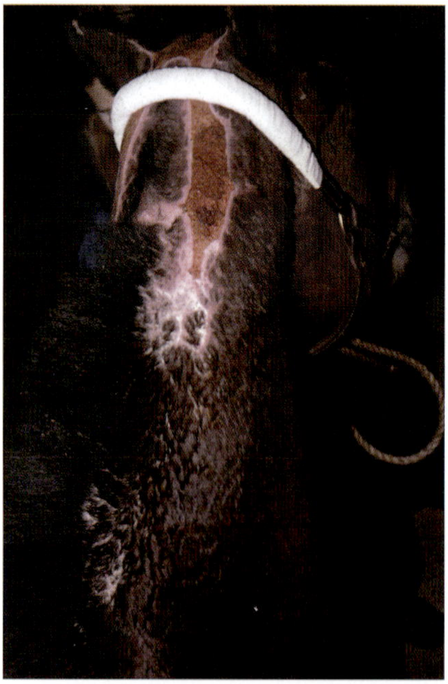

b

Figures 5.13a–f A through e are of a horse healing from burns sustained over the dorsum of his poll and back when a tractor exploded next to his stall. F is for a different horse after healing from burns sustained in a barn fire. The healed skin will not be as resilient as normal skin. This mare is fitted with a device that protects her withers skin from trauma when she rolls.

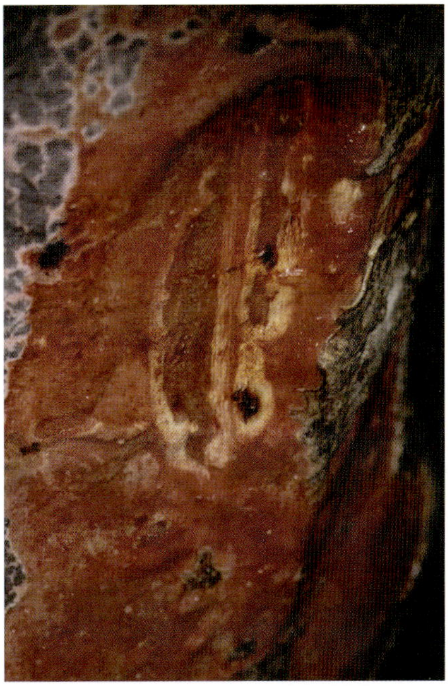

c

Figures 5.13a–f *Continued*

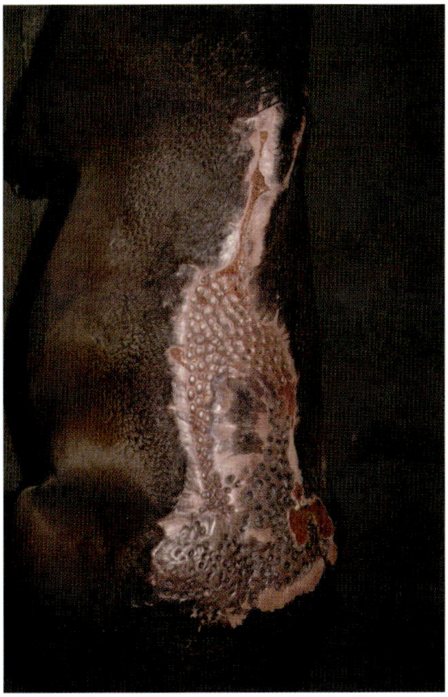

d

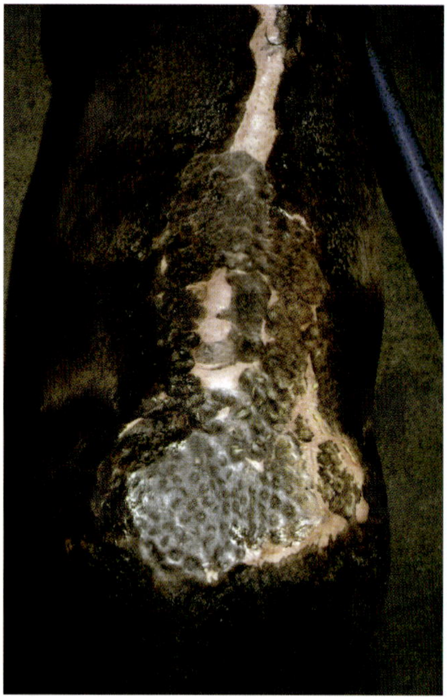

e

Figures 5.13a–f *Continued*

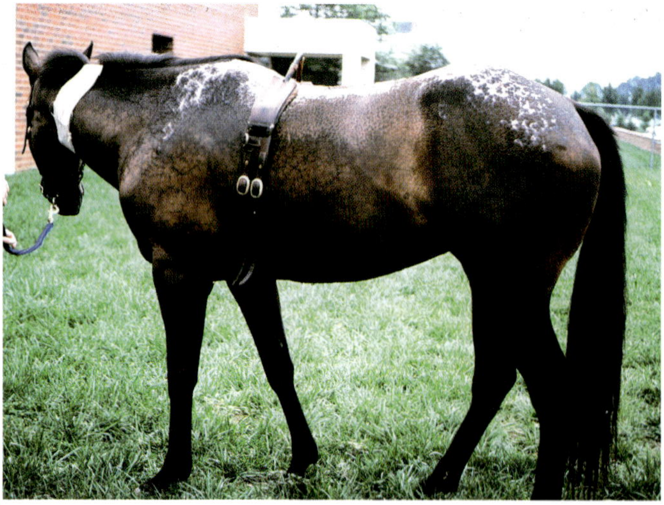

f

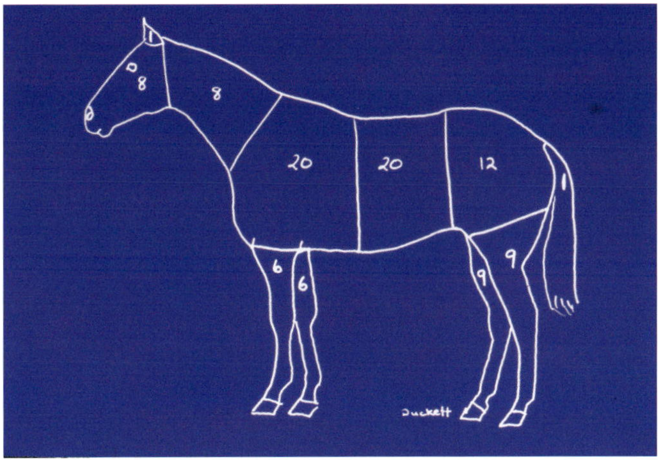

Figure 5.14a Estimated percentage body surface areas in adult horse.

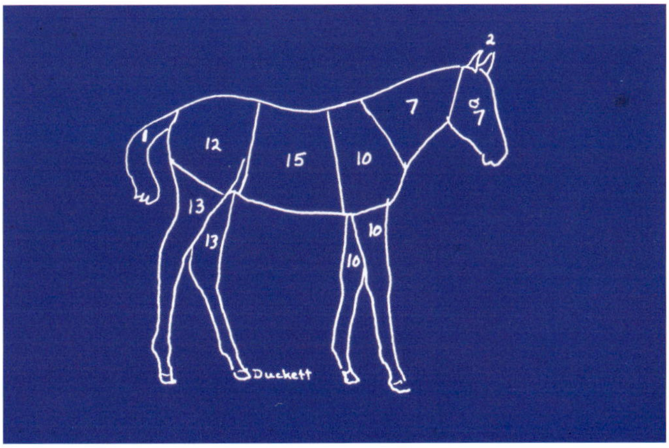

Figure 5.14b Estimated percentage body surface areas in foal.

Bursitis (Shoe Boil and Fistulous Withers) and Pressure Sores

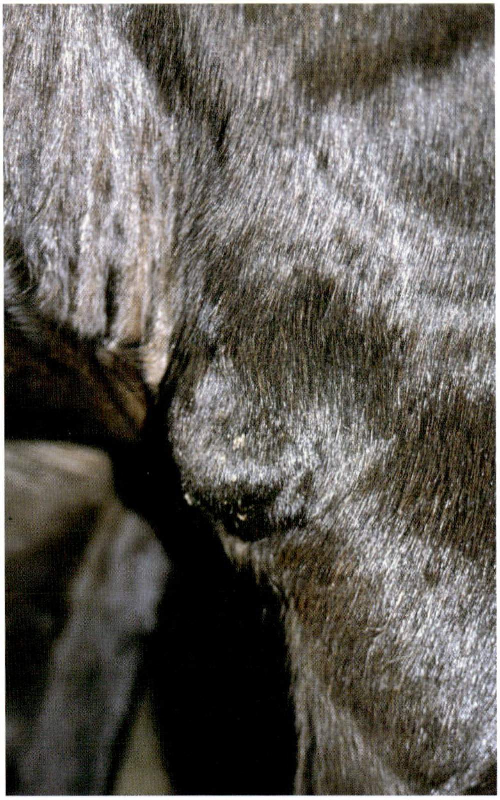

Figure 5.15 Inflammation of the subcutaneous bursa of the elbow region. Associated with chronic low-grade trauma from the heel-bulb region of the ipsilateral foot during sternal recumbency. It can present as a swelling in this region or, in advanced cases, as a draining tract, which may be purulent, swollen, and painful. The treatment is local or topical as well as the placement of a shoe-boil roll in the pastern region (see fig. 5.16).

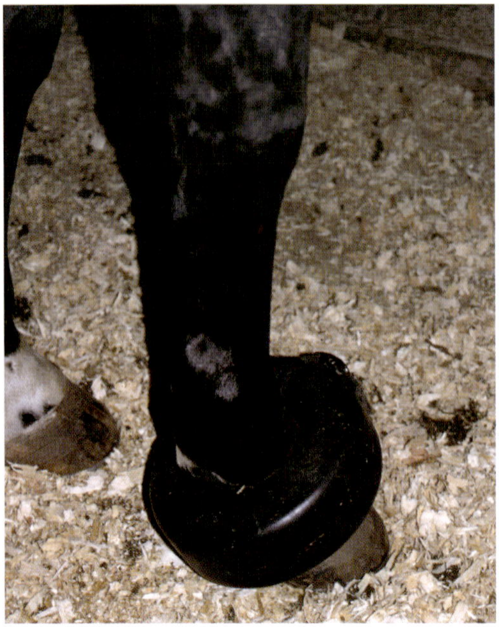

Figure 5.16 Placement of a shoe-boil roll in a case of cubital bursitis.

Figure 5.17 Inflammation of the supraspinous bursa is termed "fistulous withers." It is originally traumatic and then secondarily infected or primarily infected (brucellosis). Extensive surgical intervention is usually necessary. Note the midline swelling in the region of the withers in this mature horse.

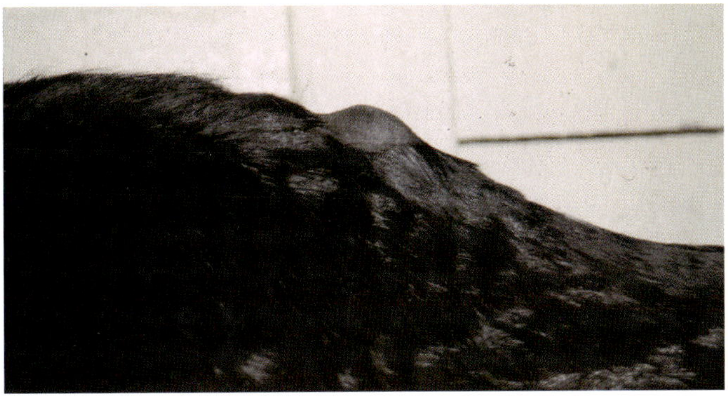

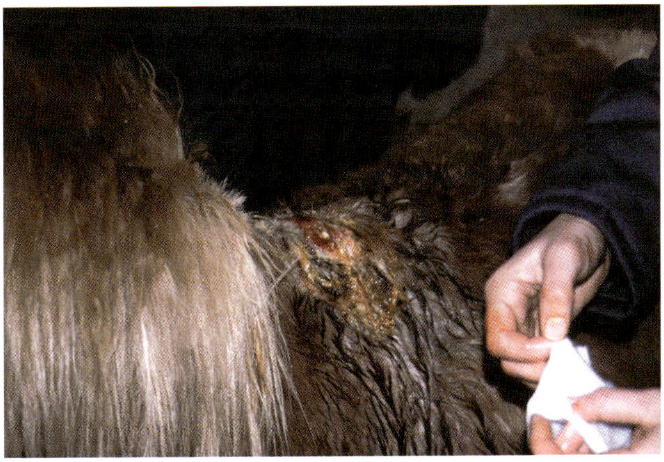

Figure 5.18 An old horse with fistulous withers. Note the purulent debris and rim of granulation tissue in this chronic case.

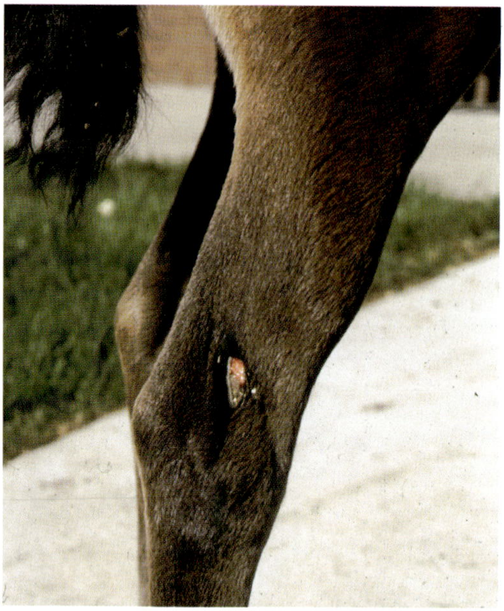

Figure 5.19 Pressure sores are common in foals due to a lack of bedding. Typical predilection sites include a vertical area immediately plantar to the lateral malleolus of the tibia in the region of the hock.

Calcinosis Circumscripta (Tumoral Calcinosis)

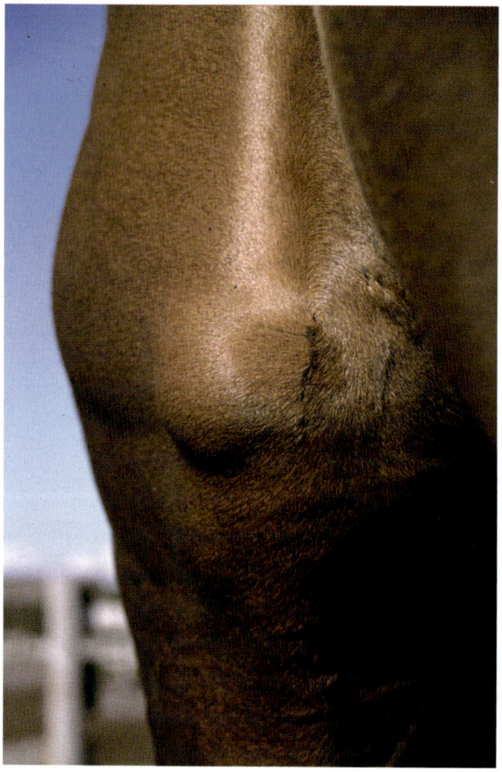

Figure 5.20 A rare developmental/congenital condition, predominantly of young male horses. It is characterized by local deposition of calcium salts in small nodules in subcutaneous tissues or tongue, or attached to tendons or joint capsules. Standardbred horses appear to be overrepresented. Lesions are typically in the lateral stifle region and in some cases are bilateral. In rare cases, the tarsus or carpus can be involved. The lesion is firm to the touch with no overlying skin damage. Often intimately attached to the underlying ligamentous tissue, muscle, or joint capsule, there is rarely a need to remove these. A craniocaudal view of a case of calcinosis circumscripta in a young racehorse.

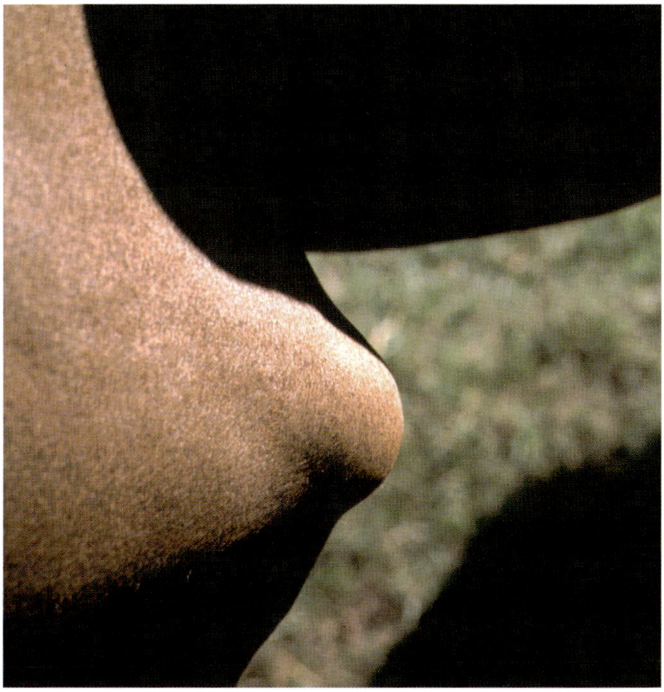

Figure 5.21 A lateromedial view of the same horse.

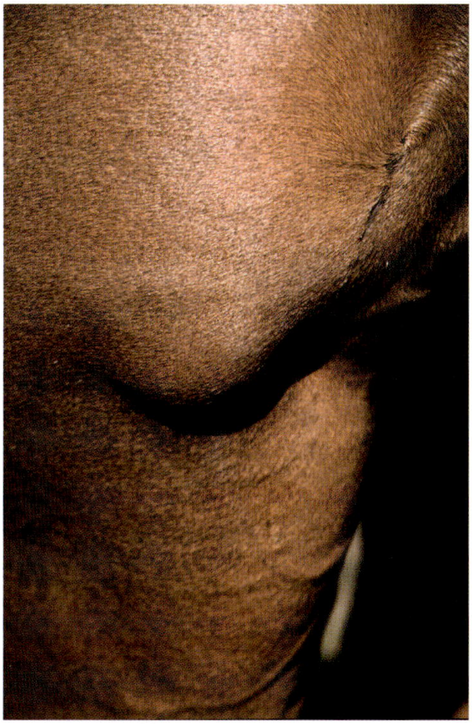

Figure 5.22 A dorsolateral view of the same horse.

Cushing's Syndrome

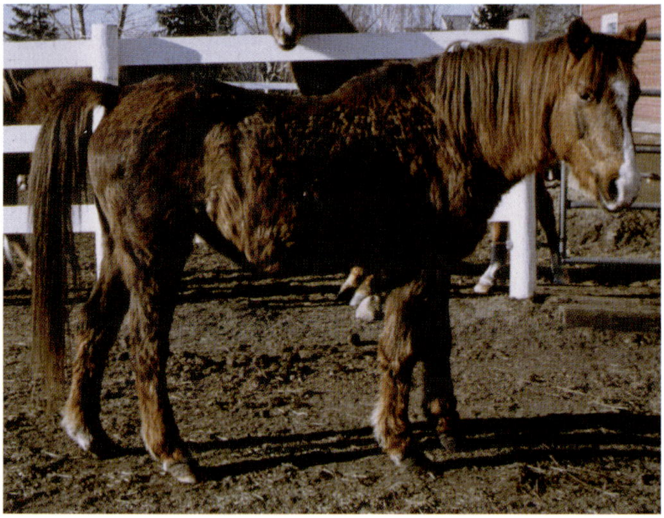

Figure 5.23 Hyperadrenocorticism or Cushing's syndrome. In the majority of cases the clinical signs in the horse are due to a functional pars-intermedia pituitary adenoma. There is a single case report of the clinical signs being associated with an adrenal tumor. Hirsutism and hyperhydrosis (sweating) in addition to muscle wasting, weight loss, laminitis, and in some cases polyuria and polydipsia can be seen. The picture is of an aged pony presented with the classic symptoms of hirsutism, potbellied (muscle wasting), swaybacked appearance and with evidence of past laminitic episodes on his feet; note the rings on the dorsal hoof horn. See also Chapter 9, Diseases of the Endocrine System.

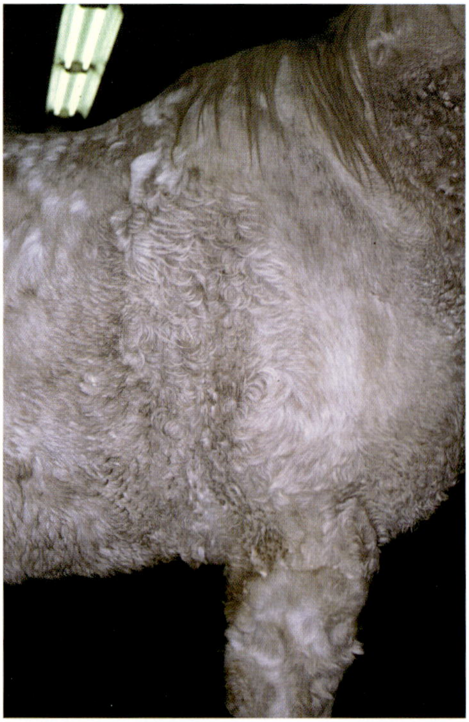

Figure 5.24 In this horse, note the matted hair coat suggestive of hyperhydrosis. This horse was wet to the touch and malodorous.

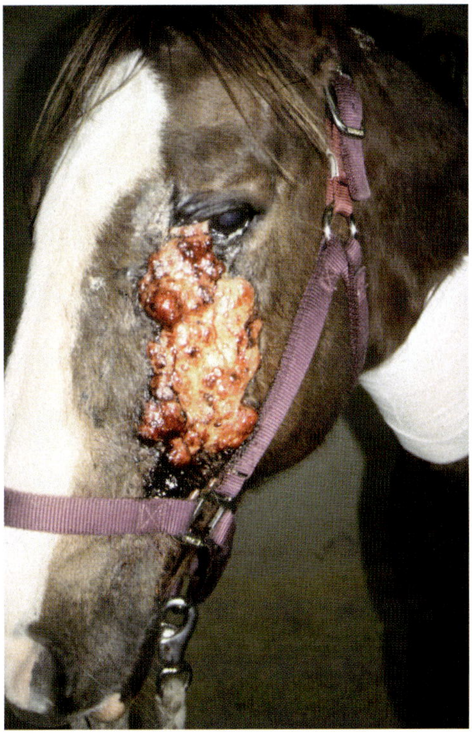

Figure 5.25 A helminth infection (*Habronema muscae*, *H. majus,* and *Draschia megastoma).* Adults reside within the stomach passing eggs and larvae via the feces into the intermediate host (housefly or stable fly). The host deposits infective larvae around the mouth of the horse, which are ingested to complete the life cycle. In open wounds or moist areas, such as conjunctiva of the eye with epiphora or prepuce, the infective larvae get deposited in error and incite a hypersensitivity reaction. Common differential diagnoses include fibroblastic sarcoid, exuberant granulation tissue, and squamous cell carcinoma. Unlike other diagnostic rule-outs, however, this disease is characterized by mild to moderate pruritis and the presence of yellow, caseous granules, appearing similar to rice grains, within the abnormal tissue. These represent foci of infection around nematode larvae. This picture is of a mature quarter horse with lachrymal habronemiasis. Note the extensive nature of the lesion.

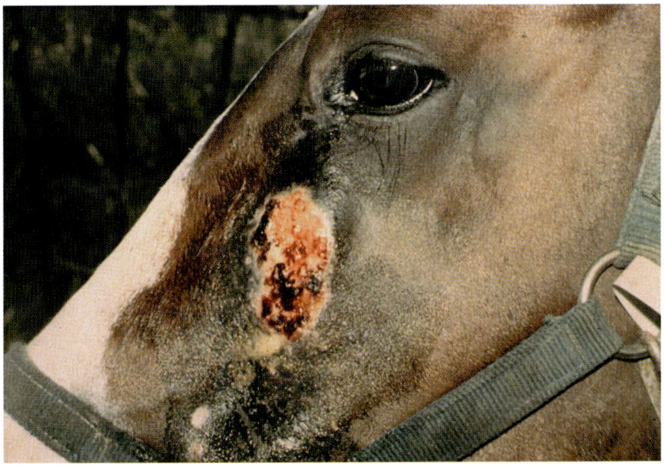

Figure 5.26 The same horse (fig. 5.25) after undergoing treatment. There are a multitude of different regimes cited for this condition, giving the reader an indication that any one may not be entirely successful. Systemic glucocorticoids alone or in addition to surgical debridement, cryotherapy, or oral parasiticides have been successful. Note that this is a seasonal disease with regression in the fall (autumn) as there is no overwintering of the larvae within the tissue.

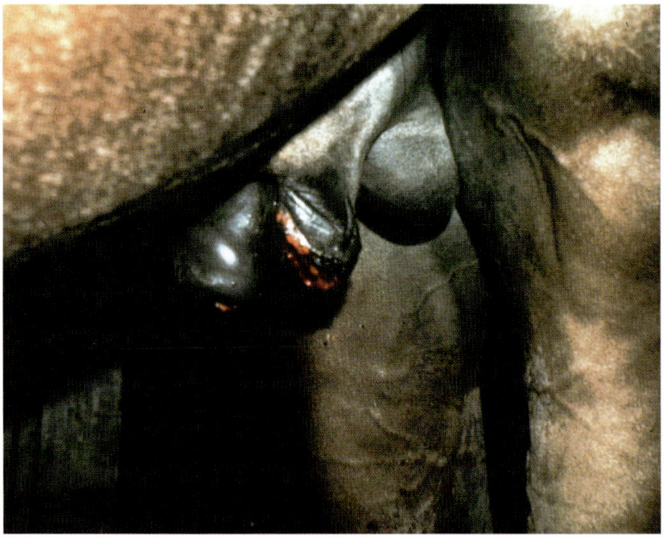

Figure 5.27a Preputial habronemiasis. Genital squamous cell carcinoma is an important differential diagnosis in this case.

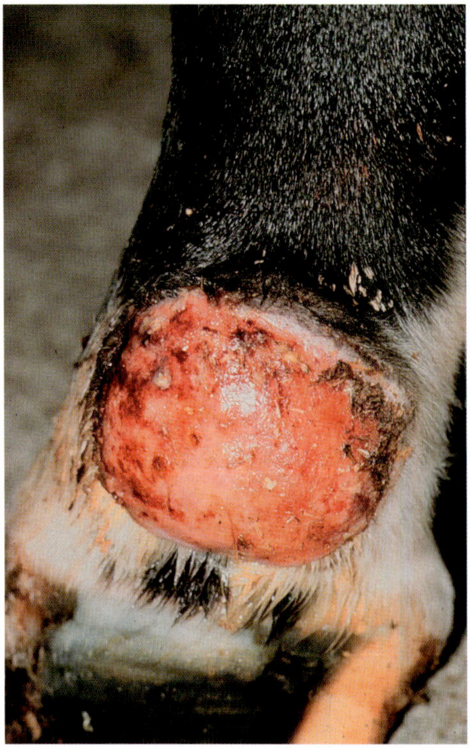

Figure 5.27b Cutaneous habronemiasis. Areas most affected are medial canthus of the eyes, lower limbs, and urethral process. Unlikely to be seen if horses are routinely dewormed with ivermectin. (Courtesy of J. P. Manning)

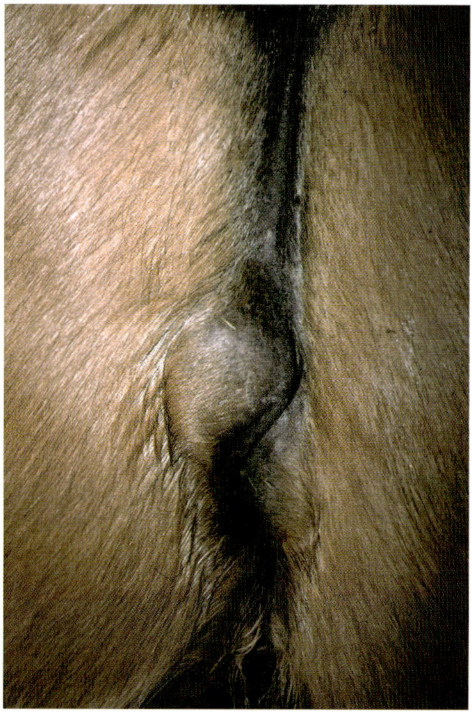

Figure 5.28 Cutaneous neoplasia, which occurs in 4%–35% of horses with lymphosarcoma. There are two distinct histological types giving rise to the clinical picture. Horses with epitheliotropic lymphosarcoma have generalized alopecia and scaling with distinct nodules or ulcerated regions. These may or may not be pruritic. More commonly, horses present with signs of nonepitheliotropic lymphosarcoma. These animals have systemic involvement that may manifest as anorexia, weight loss, and depression, as well as cutaneous signs. Skin lesions are usually firm, subcutaneous nodules that are not ulcerated. These tend to be found on the head, neck, trunk, and upper limbs. In some rare cases, large areas of thickened skin or urticarial lesions can be seen (fig. 5.30). This picture is of a mature gelding that presented with a large, firm mass in the ventral perineal region.

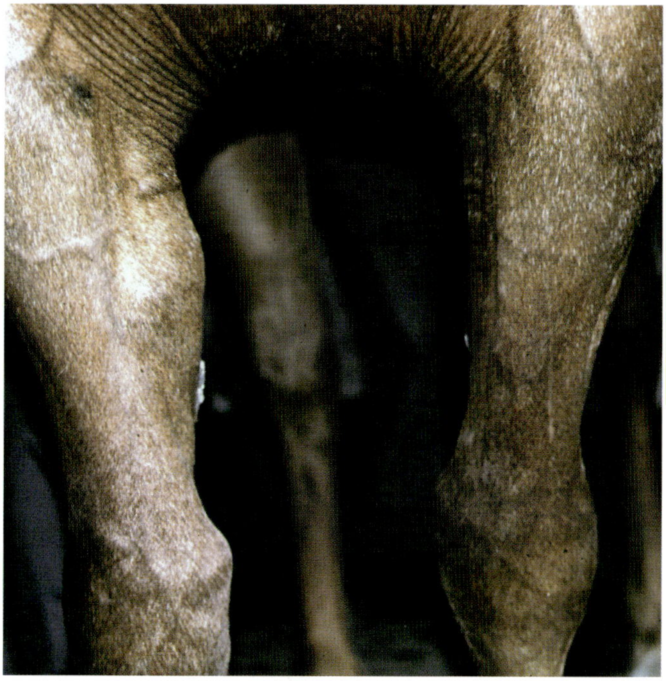

Figure 5.29 The horse in this picture presented with a firm subcutaneous mass on the proximomedial aspect of the right front leg.

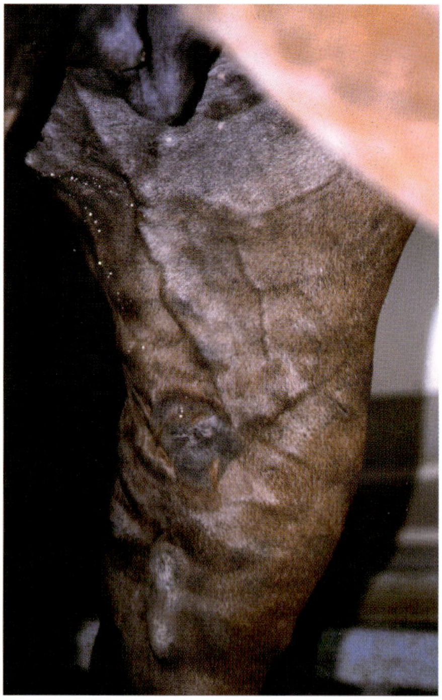

Figure 5.30 This mare presented with multiple, firm nodules on the proximomedial aspect of the left hind leg.

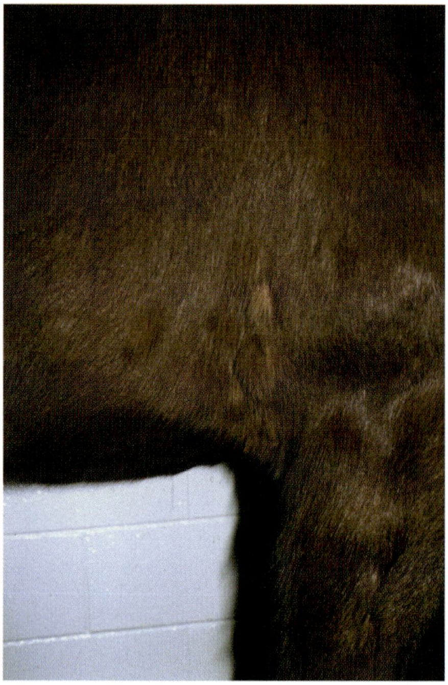

Figure 5.31 Note the "figure 8" shaped lesion immediately caudal to the elbow in this horse. This is an example of the urticarial type of lesion described above.

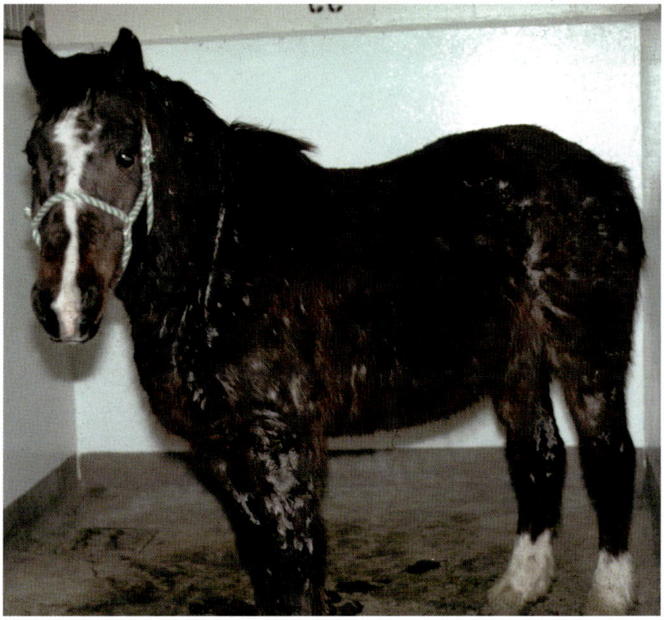

Figure 5.32 A common bacterial disease caused by *Dermatophilus congolensis,* which requires skin damage and moisture for infection. Horses can present with classic patterns of hair loss over the rump, sides of the neck, and flank. Typically, alopecia is the only clinical signs but some horses appear pruritic.

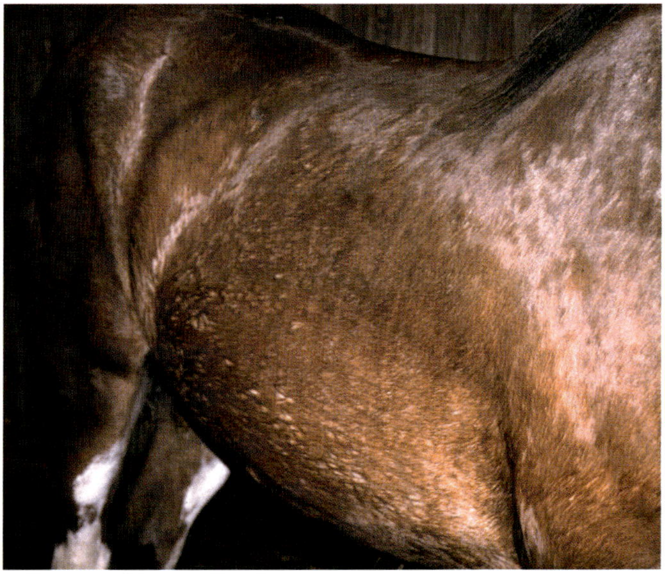

Figure 5.33a There are two seasonal forms, a wet exudative winter/fall form and a dryer form seen typically in those animals with a shorter summer coat. Exudation of serum results in matting of the hairs, which tend to stand proud of surrounding hair. This disease is an important rule out in any nonpruritic alopecia.

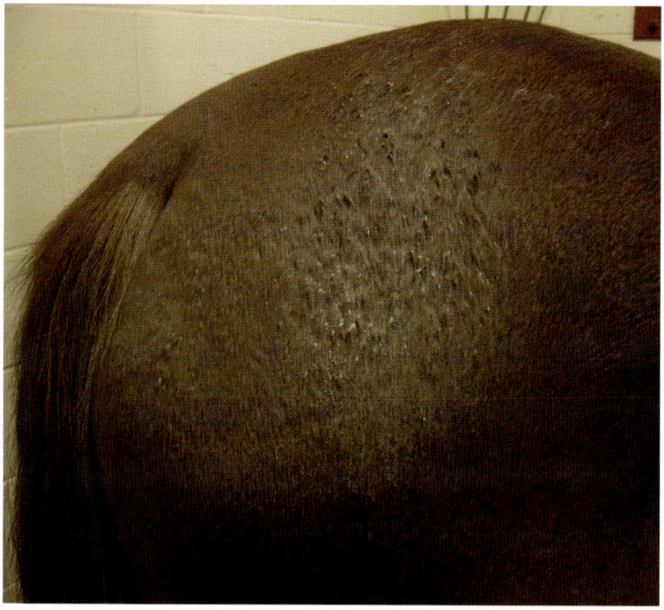

Figure 5.33b Epilating hair results in a number of hair shafts stuck within a crust of dried serum ("paint-brush" tufts). The underlying epidermis is abraded and contains a small pocket of purulent debris.

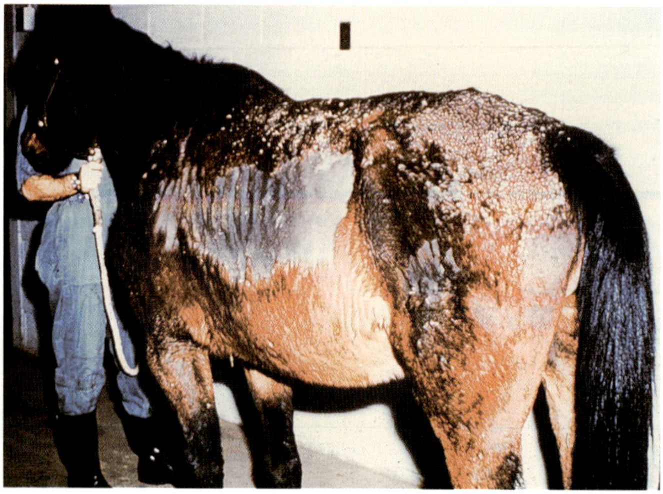

Figure 5.33c Severely affected animals may be depressed, anorexic, and pyrexic. Treatment involves the topical use of chlorhexidine (1%–4%) and, in some cases, systemic antimicrobials such as penicillin. Note the presence of multiple regions of "tufted hairs," which are standing proud of the skin in this horse. In many cases, lesions can be felt more easily than seen. (Fig. 5.33c courtesy of J. P. Manning.)

Figure 5.34 Lesions on the muzzle may resemble photosensitization or sunburn.

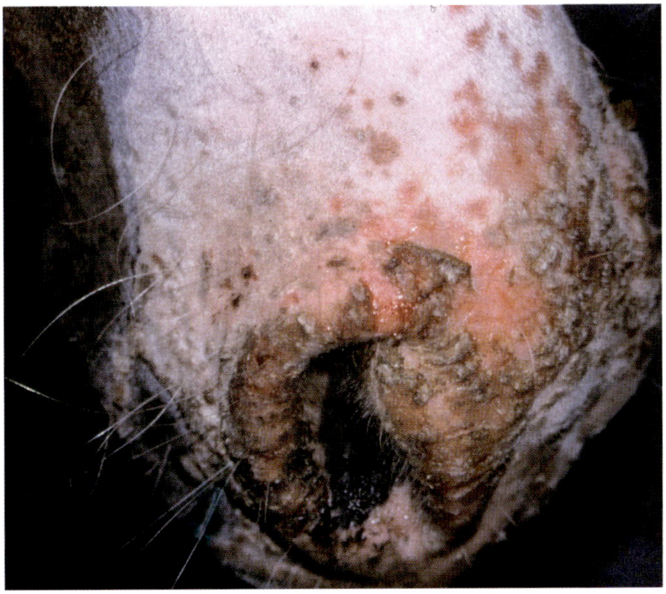

Dermatophytosis (Ringworm)

Figures 5.35a–c Common and contagious. *Trichophyton equinum var equi* and *Microsporum equinum* are the most common etiological agents. Clinical signs begin as small edematous plaques, usually on the girth, shoulder, chest, or face. It is nonpruritic but horses tend to resent picking of lesions. This disease can become generalized. In most cases, this is a self-limiting disease. Note the extensive hair loss in this yearling Thoroughbred horse. The lesion continued down the neck. This disease is one of the causes of rapid, progressive alopecia; differential diagnoses include pemphigus foliaceus or dermatophilosis.

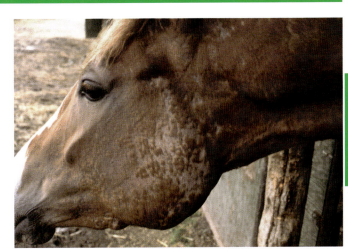

a

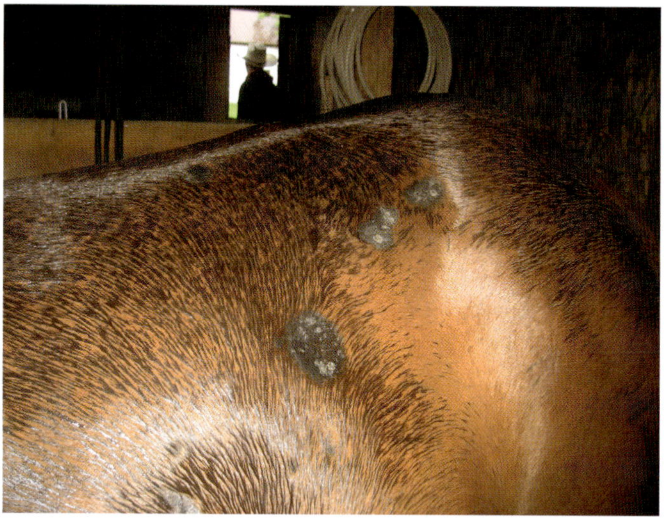

b

Figures 5.35a–c *Continued*

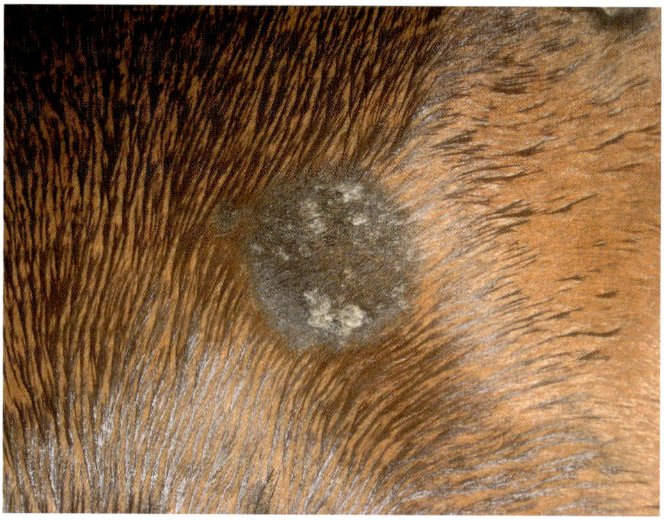

c

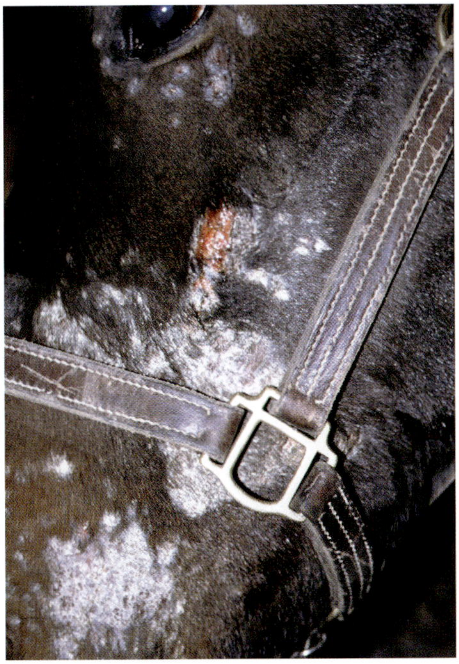

a

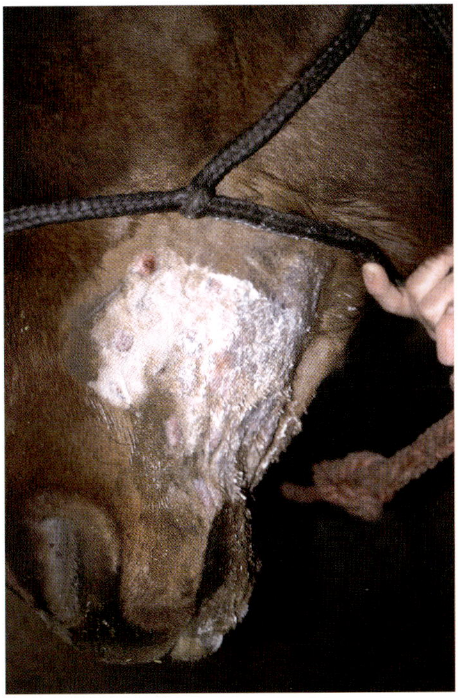

b

Figures 5.36a,b The overlying scab can be easily removed; the underlying epidermis is usually not damaged and has a mirrorlike surface. Any epithelial excoriation is usually a result of secondary trauma due to pruritis.

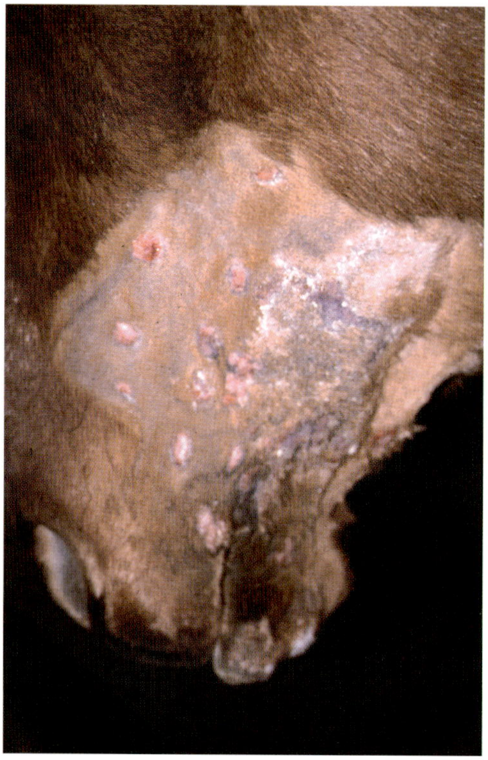

Figure 5.37 Self-limiting as mentioned above. Treatment options include topical therapy with an antifungal agent such as enilconazole. Note the improvement in epidermal skin following clipping, cleaning, and topical therapy.

Dermoid Cyst

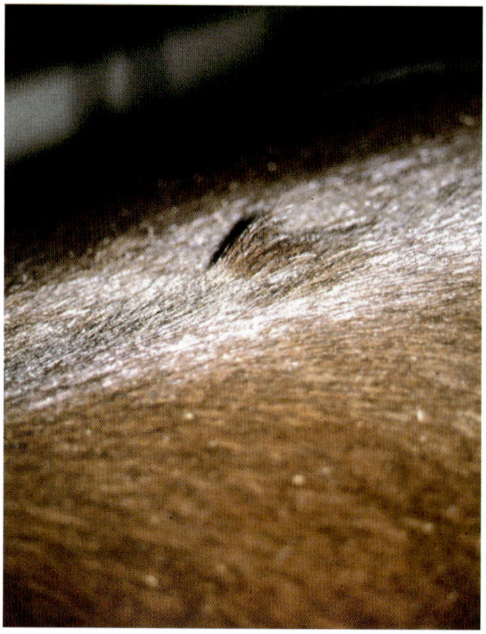

Figure 5.38 Relatively uncommon, these are developmental abnormalities that usually present on the dorsal midline. The cystic structure contains a grey/yellow caseous material with or without hair shafts. The elevation of the skin results in an obvious bump in the top line of the horse.

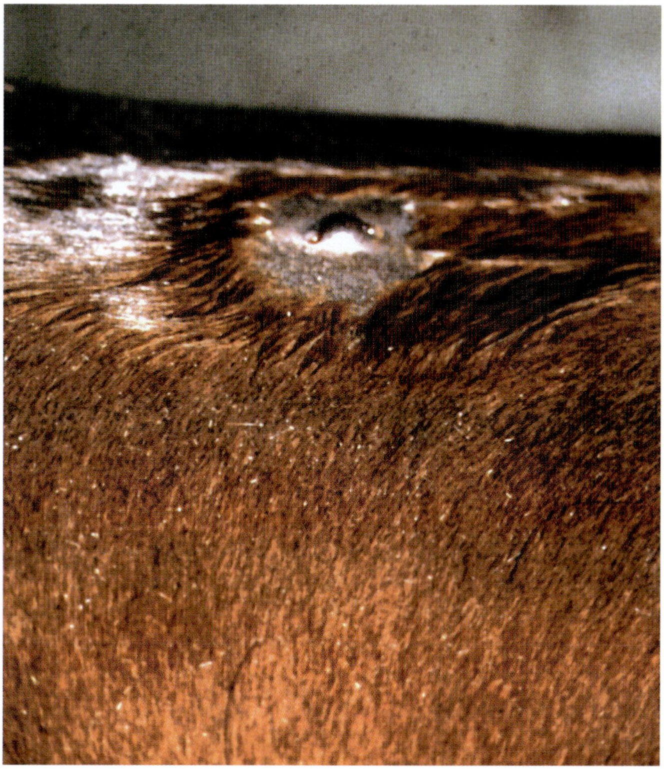

Figure 5.39 A dermoid cyst in another horse, clipped prior to expressing the contents.

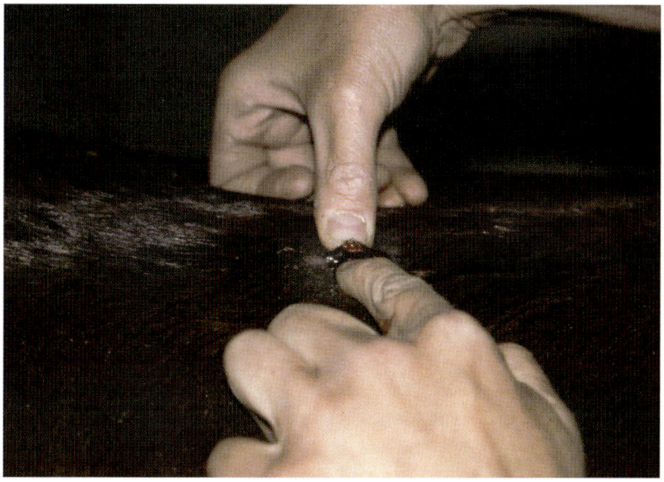

Figure 5.40 Expression of the contents manually. Using this technique, removal of the cyst lining is not undertaken; "painting" it with a strong iodine solution has been successful in preventing recurrence.

Hyperelastosis Cutis (Ehler Danlos Syndrome)

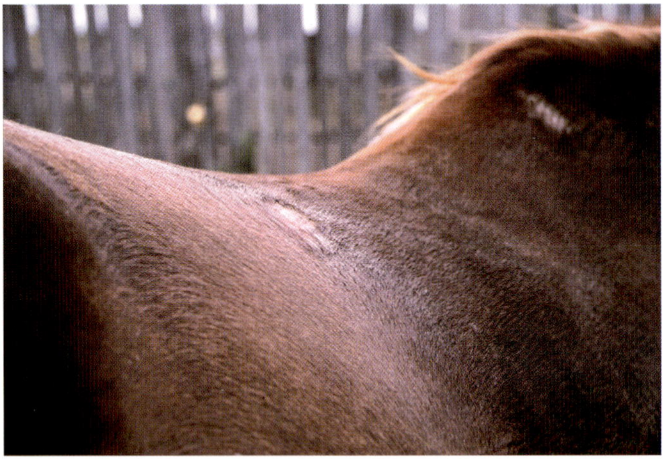

Figure 5.41 Hyperelastosis cutis in a 3-year-old cutting horse. Note the region of reduced pigmentation in the hair coat (withers and saddle region)). This is a genetic disorder of pre-pro-collagen formation. Normally constrained to regions of skin subject to shearing forces (under the saddle, girth, withers), this disease usually manifests as symptoms of pain/discomfort when saddled and, in some instances, by nonhealing or poorly healing skin wounds. It is usually seen in early "breaking" and training. Diagnosis is by clinical signs, investigation of the lineage of the horse, and, definitively, by biopsy. Wounds created during the biopsy may result in slow or nonhealing wounds.

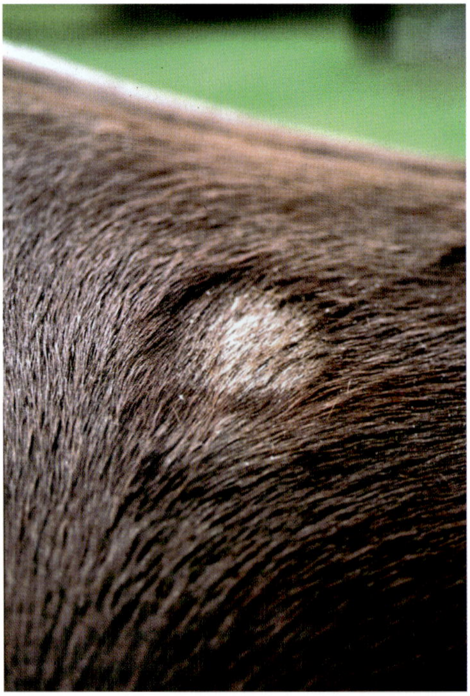

Figure 5.42 Hyperelastosis cutis in a 3-year-old cutting horse. Note the region of reduced pigmentation in the hair coat (withers).

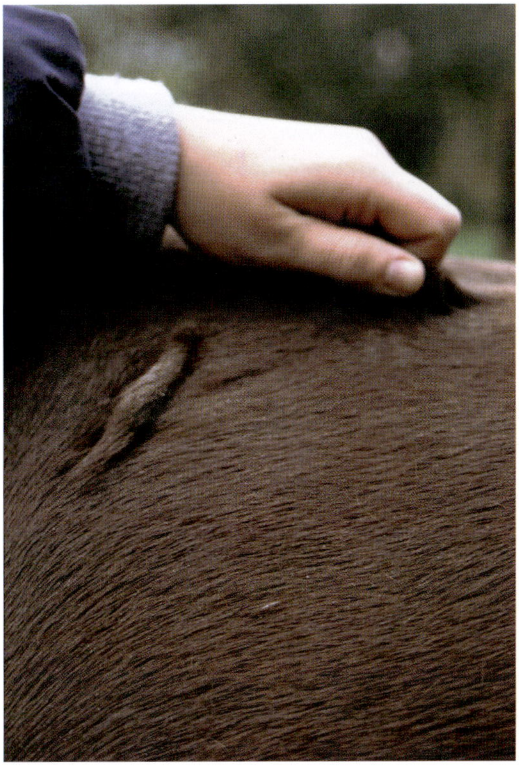

Figure 5.43 Note hyperelasticity of the skin.

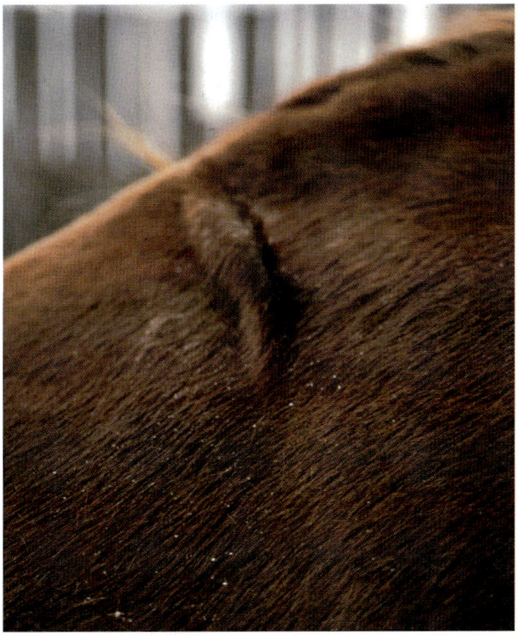

Figure 5.44 Prolonged skin tent time in this region (reduced elasticity). This picture was taken 45 seconds after skin tenting.

Insect Bite Hypersensitivity (Queensland Itch, Sweet Itch)

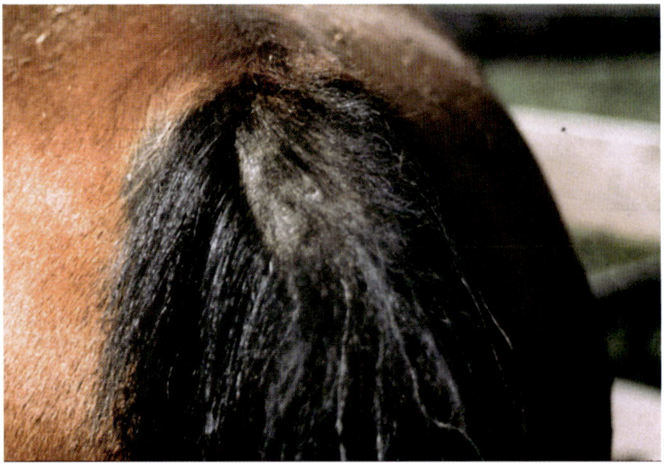

Figure 5.45 The most common skin disease in the horse. *Culicoides* and *Simulium* spp. are implicated. Clinical signs result from a combination of type I (immediate) and type IV (delayed) hypersensitivity reactions to the salivary antigens of these fly species. There is a strong seasonal occurrence corresponding to fly numbers. Affected horses tend to respond earlier in the season and with greater clinical response as they age. There are many species of *Culicoides,* each with preferential feeding sites on the horse. The resultant effect is that clinical signs may be seen on the dorsal or ventral midlines or on both. This picture is of the tail head of a mature horse. Note the alopecia, melanoderma, and thickening of this region due to repeated trauma associated with this condition. Differential diagnoses include lice, mange, *Oxyuris equi* infection, and food hypersensitivity. The fact that this horse was given anthelmintics regularly and the clinical signs occurred midsummer make a diagnosis of *Culicoides* hypersensitivity much more likely.

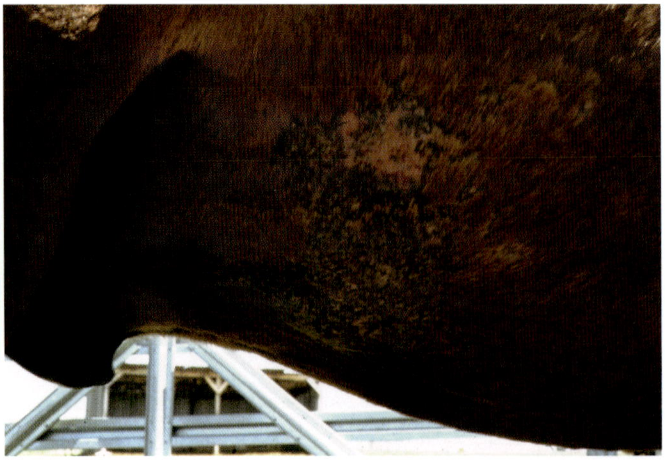

Figure 5.46a Initial cutaneous signs are rapidly eclipsed by the trauma associated with self-excoriation in this highly pruritic disease. Treatment options include systemic glucocorticoids as well as management changes such as stabling horses during dawn and dusk (peak feeding times for flies). Using fly sheets and masks as well as using fans within the stable facilities are also helpful. This picture is of a mature quarter horse gelding with *Culicoides* hypersensitivity. Self-excoriation has resulted in epidermal damage.

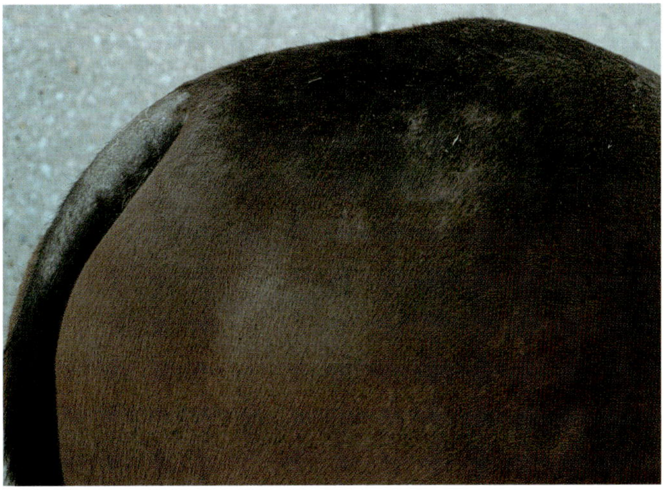

Figure 5.46b Hair loss and damage over the croup and tail due to rubbing.

Lethal White Syndrome

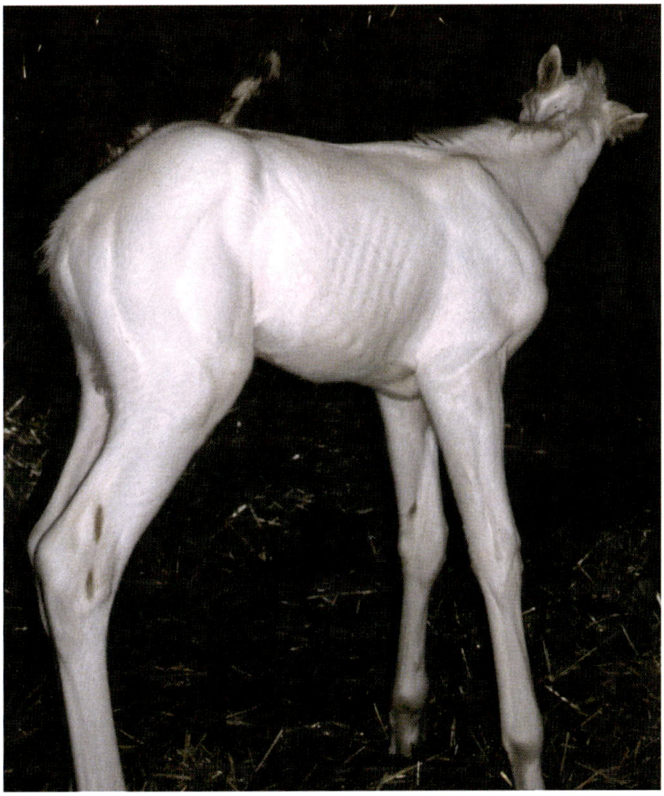

Figure 5.47 An autosomal recessive condition resulting from the breeding of two overo-paint horses.

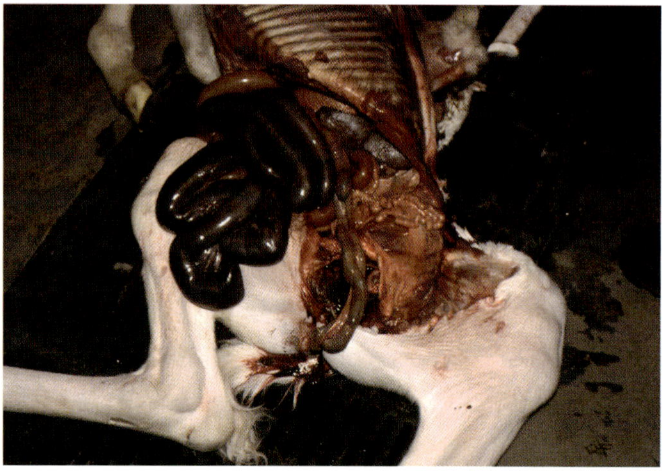

Figure 5.48 During embryological development an abnormality in the neural crest (responsible for the development of myenteric plexae as well as melanoblasts) results in a white foal with abnormalities in the ileum, caecum, and colons. The affected intestinal tract segments are atretic and narrowed. There is no effective treatment and these foals should be euthanized prior to the inevitable onset of fatal colic. This is a postmortem photograph showing a 4-day-old foal that was presented for colic. Note the distended, blackened small intestine.

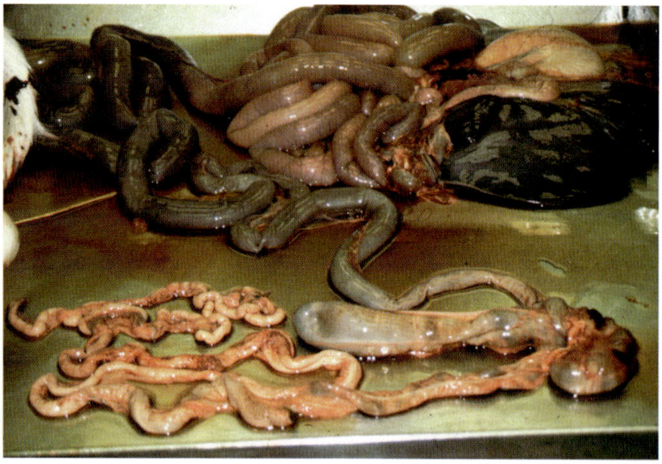

Figure 5.49 The gastrointestinal tract of the foal that was presented in fig. 5.48. Note the distended proximal gastrointestinal tract in the top of the picture. The distal gastrointestinal tract (cecum and colons, at the bottom of the picture) is hypoplastic and nonfunctional.

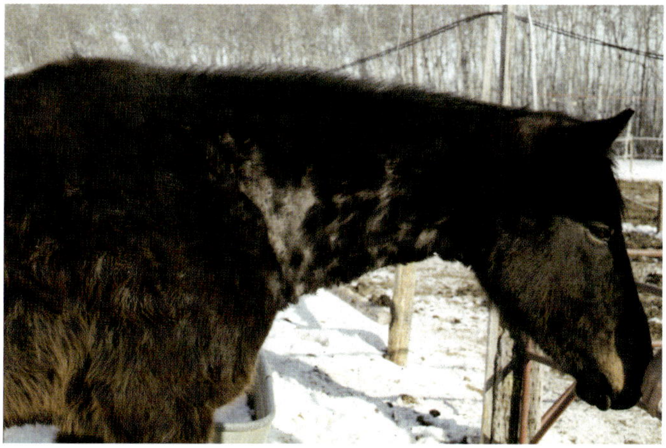

a

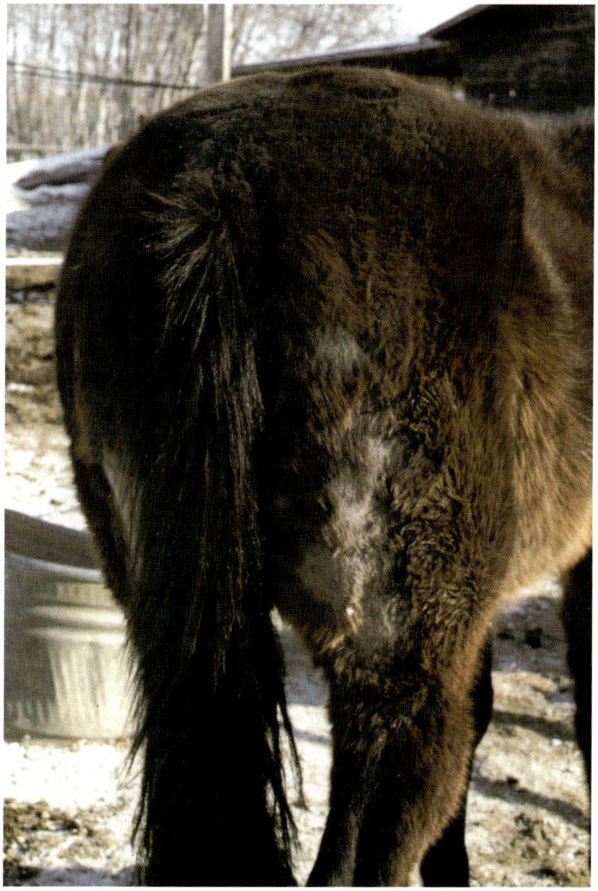

b

Figures 5.50a,b Very common: obligate parasites that are host specific. Ninety-nine percent of disease is caused by the biting louse (*Damalinia equi*), usually in the winter months. The other 1% is caused by the sucking louse (*Haematopinus asini*). Diagnosis is by clinical presentation of bilateral symmetrical alopecia. Any underlying epidermal excoriation is usually a result of trauma suffered during rubbing.

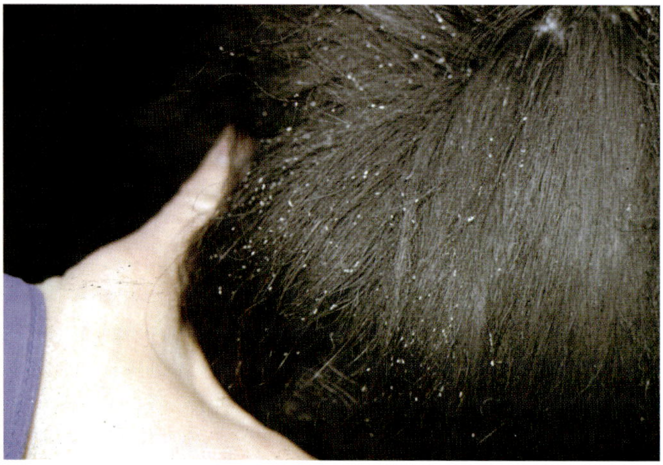

Figure 5.51 Diagnosis is by history (including time of year), clinical signs, and the identification of lice, as seen in this photograph.

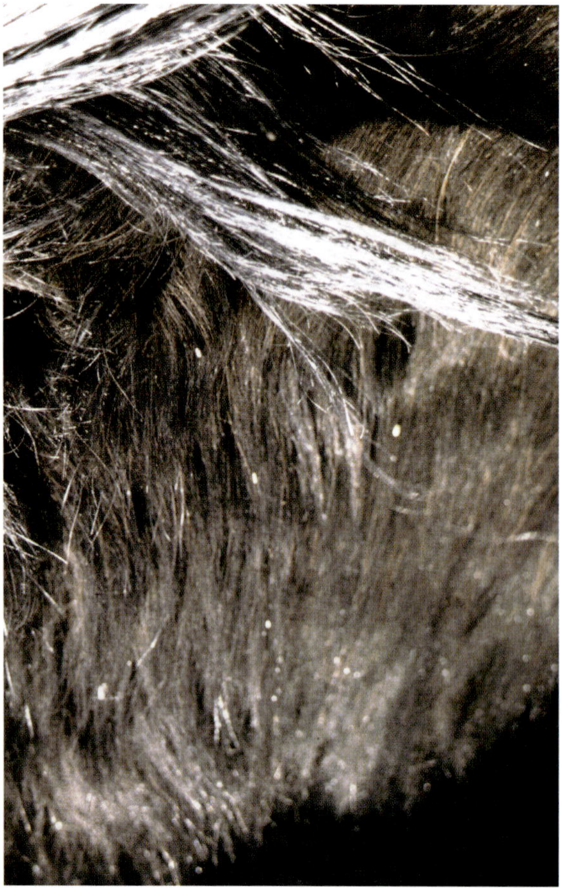

Figure 5.52 Diagnosis by identification of louse eggs attached to hair shafts.

5

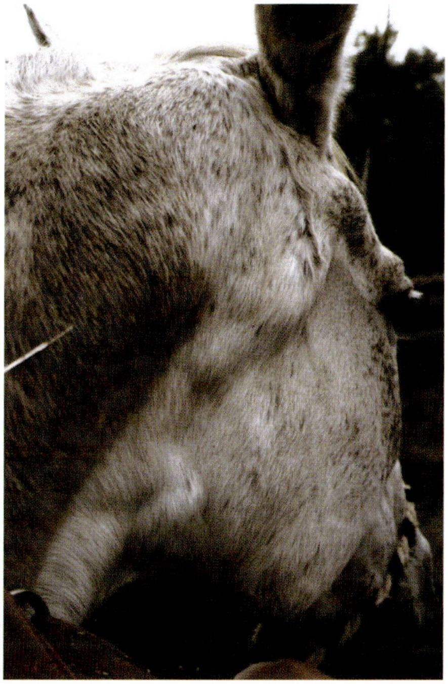

a

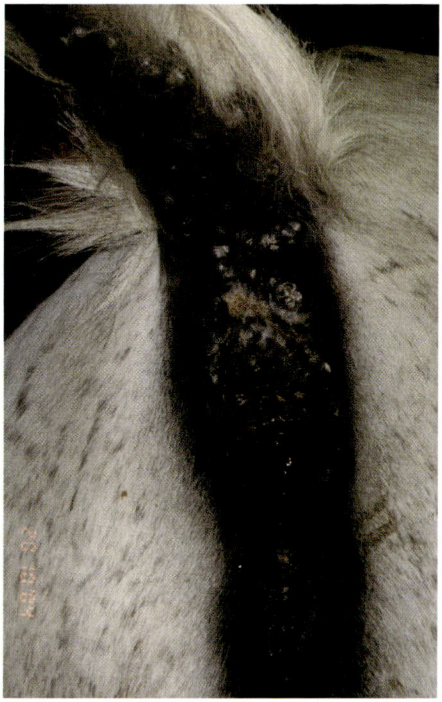

b

Figures 5.53a,b Commonly, but not exclusively limited to older grey horses. In most cases, these are benign and will not affect the longevity of the animal. In some cases, however, the melanomas may expand rapidly and metastasize. A, note the presence of a firm nodular mass in the parotid region of this aged grey mare. The abnormality was bilateral. B, perianal melanoma. In rare cases of perianal melanoma, metastasis to the caudal spinal cord can result in ataxia and recumbency.

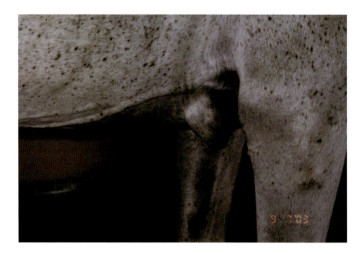

Figure 5.54 The mare presented in fig. 5.53b also had other regions of melanoma such as the swelling in the thoracic region caudal to the elbow.

Nodular Necrobiosis (Eosinophilic Collagen Necrosis)

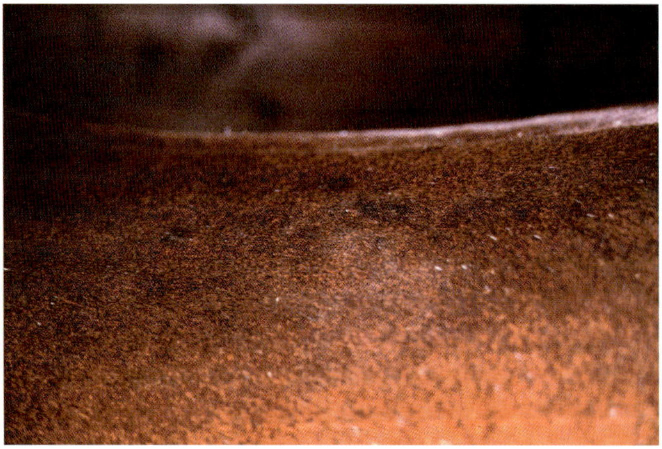

Figure 5.55 A condition of unknown etiology, however, it is likely to be associated with chronic low-grade trauma. Commonly seen in areas of "wear," under the saddle or saddle pad, girth, or withers. It can be more easily felt using gentle fingertip pressure than seen, but in some cases, as in this photograph, there are subtle hair-color changes. Note the multifocal regions of slight melanotrichosis in this chestnut horse.

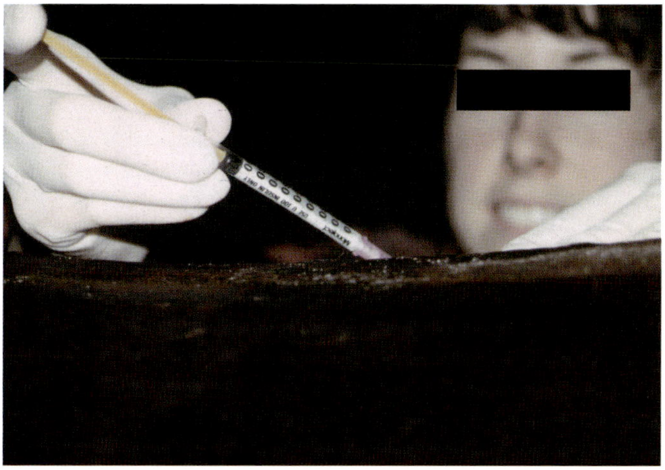

Figure 5.56 Affected regions may result in low-grade discomfort to the horse "under-saddle" and thus can be monitored or injected intralesionally using methylprednisolone. Resolution is usually complete.

Onchocerciasis

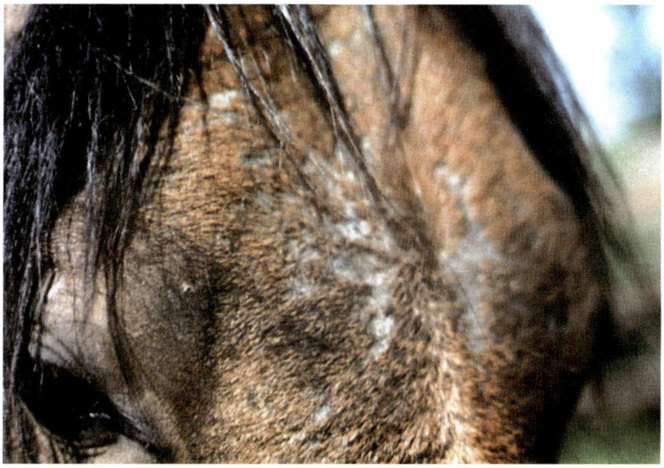

a

Figures 5.57a,b Skin lesions are associated with the microfilaria of the nematode *Onchocerca cervicalis.* The adult lives in the nuchal ligament and microfilaria migrate to the superficial skin especially of the face (a) and ventral midline (b). Not all animals with microfilaria manifest signs, so it is likely a sensitivity reaction that develops in some individuals that results in lesions characterized by alopecia, flaking, and depigmentation. The appearance of lesions is not seasonal. The intermediate host is *Culicoides* insects, so seasonal signs attributed to that vector may be present. Onchocerciasis is less prevalent since the introduction of and routine use of avermectin anthelmintics. Individuals with infestations may have transient ventral midline and facial swelling following administration of ivermectin or moxidectin, likely due to reaction from the dying microfilaria.

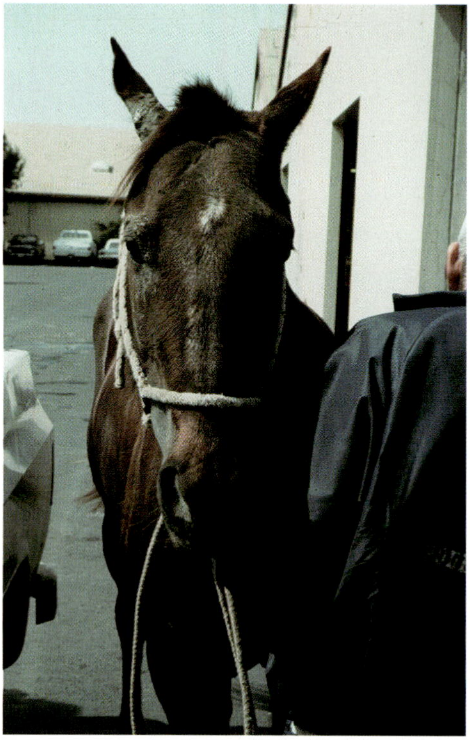

b

Figures 5.57a,b *Continued*

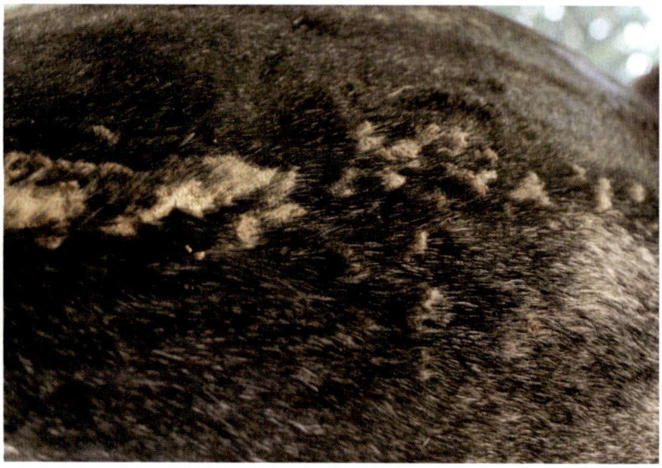

Figure 5.57c Patchy alopecia, crusting, and depigmentation of the ventral midline. (Image courtesy of J. P. Manning)

Pemphigus

Pemphigus foliaceus is an autoimmune disease of the epidermis. There are three recognized types of pemphigus in the horse; however, the most common is pemphigus foliaceus. Lesions usually begin on the face or legs but inguinal lesions also occur. The early signs of vesiculation are often missed and the horse presents to the clinician with erosions, crusting, oozing, and scaling. Half of horses with skin lesions will also present with distal limb edema without overlying disease. Definitive diagnosis is made from routine biopsy and histological identification of acantholysis of the epidermis. Do not clean or prepare the skin before biopsy as the characteristic lesions may be lost.

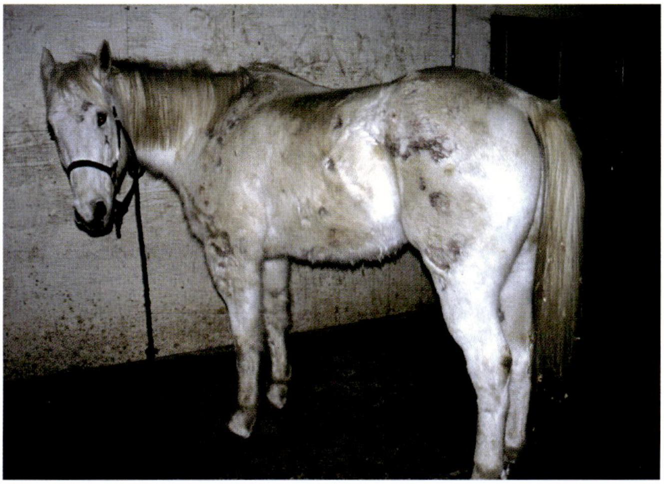

Figure 5.58a A horse of unknown age with alopecia and oozing—a case of pemphigus foliaceus.

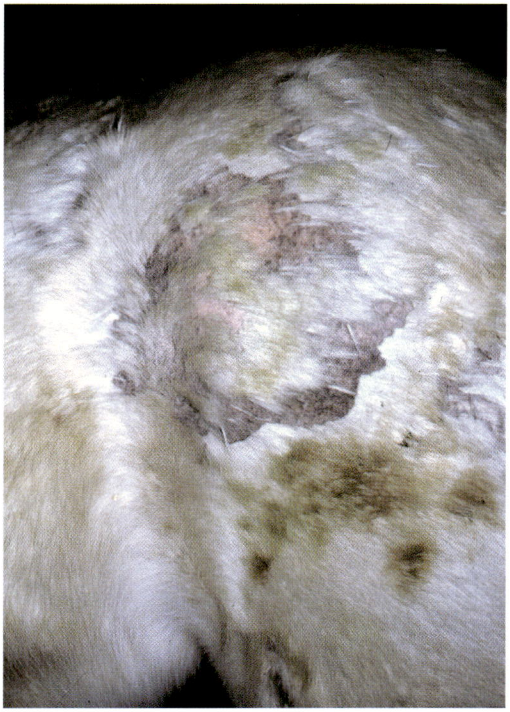

Figure 5.58b A close-up of the flank region in the horse from fig. 5.58a.

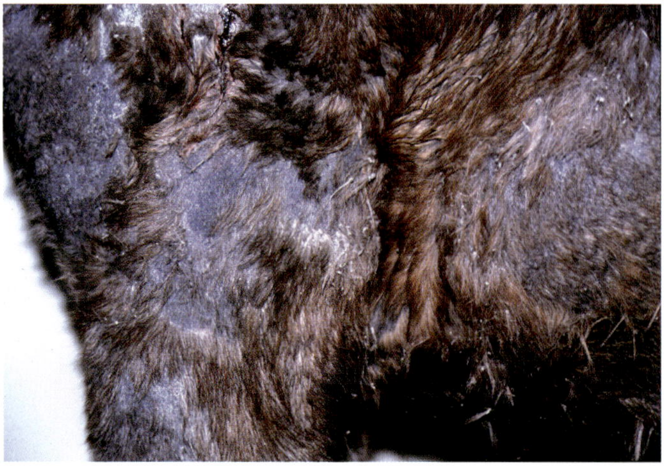

Figure 5.59a A photograph of the left upper forelimb of a quarter horse with alopecia, crusting, and secondary excoriation. Note the blood spot, upper midpicture in a case of pemphigus foliaceus.

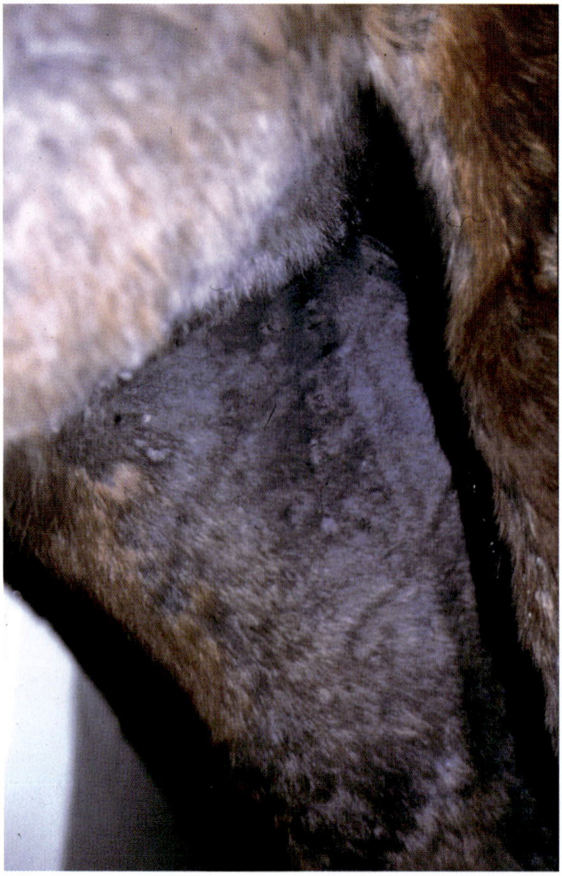

Figure 5.59b The same horse as in fig. 5.59a. Note the alopecia on the inside of the proximal hind limb and inguinal region.

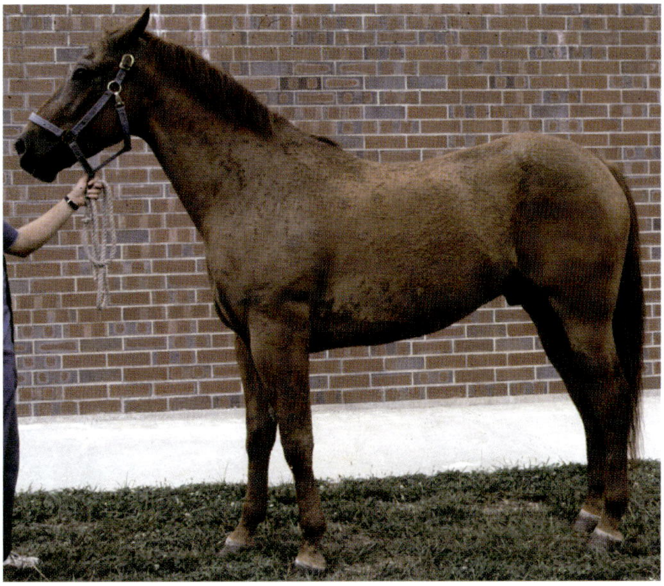

Figure 5.60a Pemphigus foliaceus in a horse. Lesions can be seen on the face, coronary bands, and ventrum and progress to total body involvement. It can be associated with pruritis and intense pain.

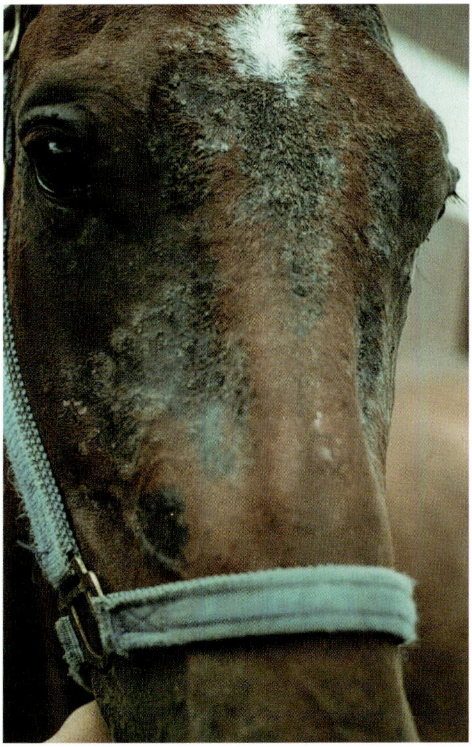

Figure 5.60b Face lesions.

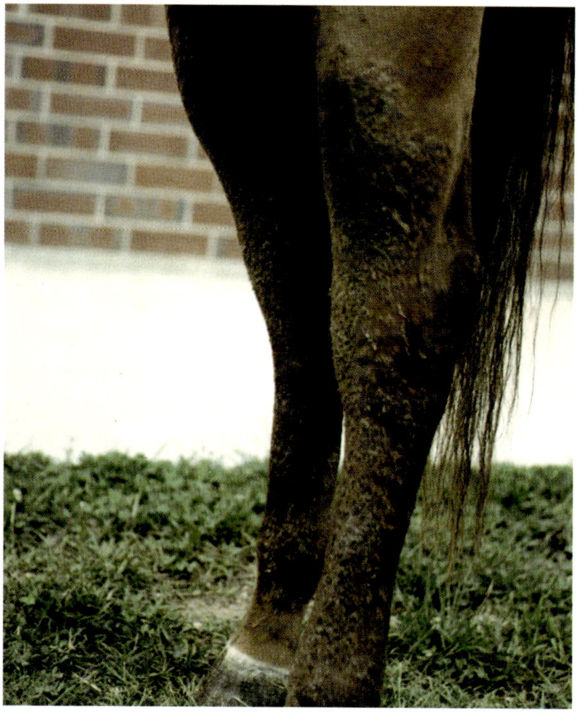

Figure 5.60c Hind limb lesions.

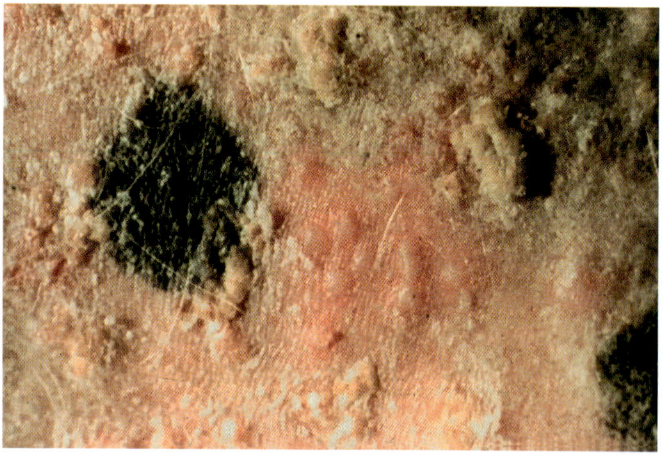

Figure 5.60d Early, transient blister formation. (Image courtesy of J. P. Manning)

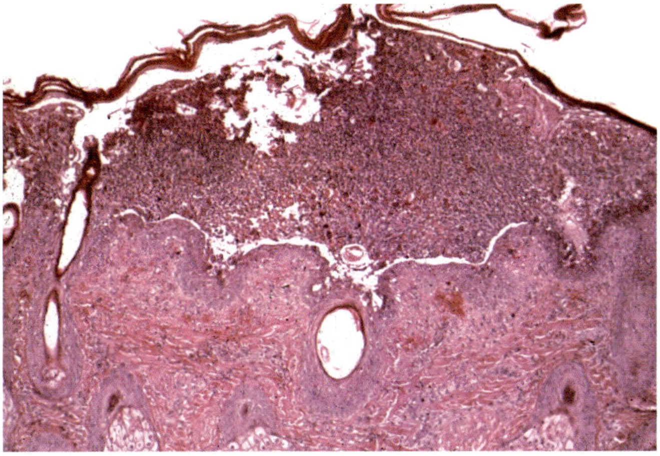

Figure 5.60e Histological section showing separation of the epidermis. (Image courtesy of J. P. Manning)

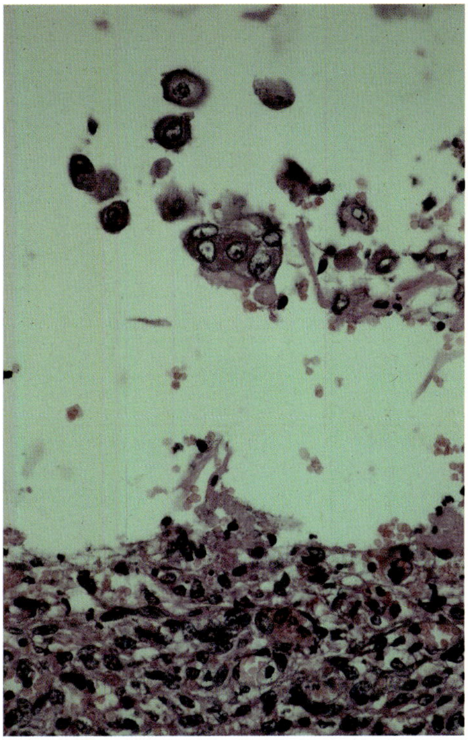

Figure 5.60f Characteristic round acantholytic cells on histological section. (Image courtesy of J. P. Manning)

Photosensitization

Photosensitization can be divided into primary (ingested, injected, or contact agents) or secondary (hepatogenous) causes. Others such as pigment synthesis abnormalities (porphyria) or idiopathic causes are less common in the horse. Usually it affects nonpigmented skin. This condition has also been recognized in cases of *Dermatophilus congolensis* infection (see Dermatophilosis above), which subsequently resolves after treatment for the primary condition. Some skin infections ("scratches") can result in a photoactive vasculitis subsequent to initial infection (see Vasculitis below).

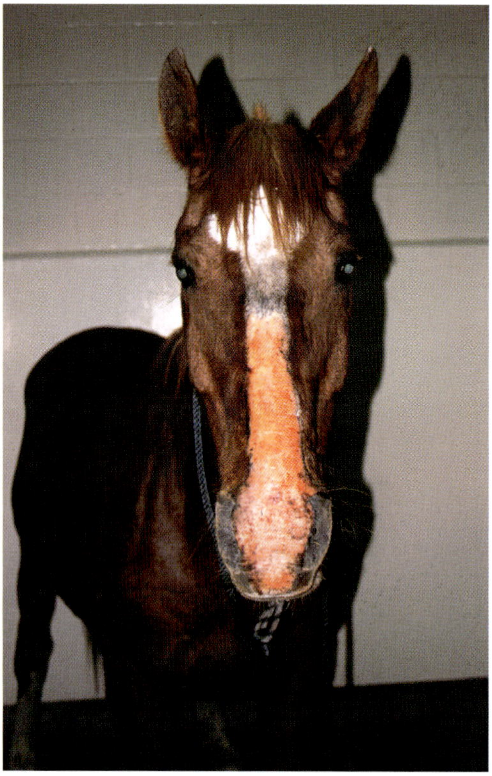

a

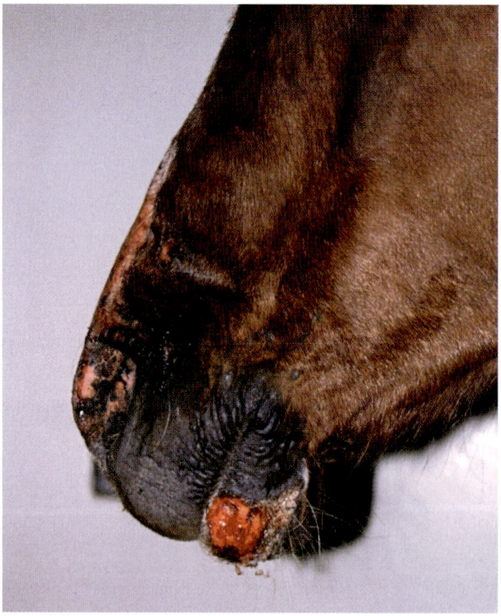

b

Figures 5.61a,b Photographs of the head of a mature quarter horse exhibiting idiopathic photosensitization. Lesions were present on all white areas of skin with encroachment into pigmented regions.

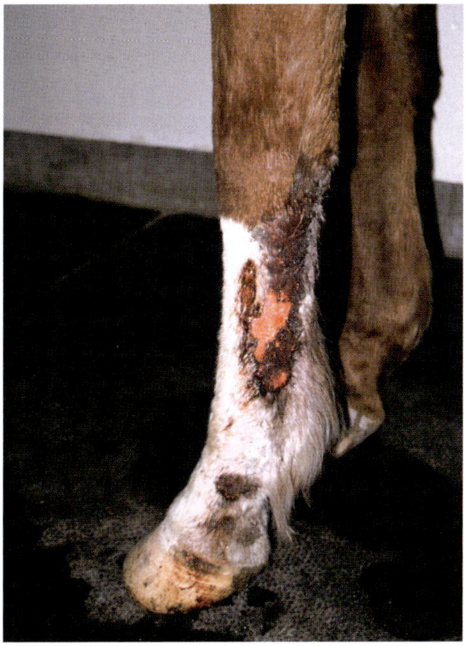

a

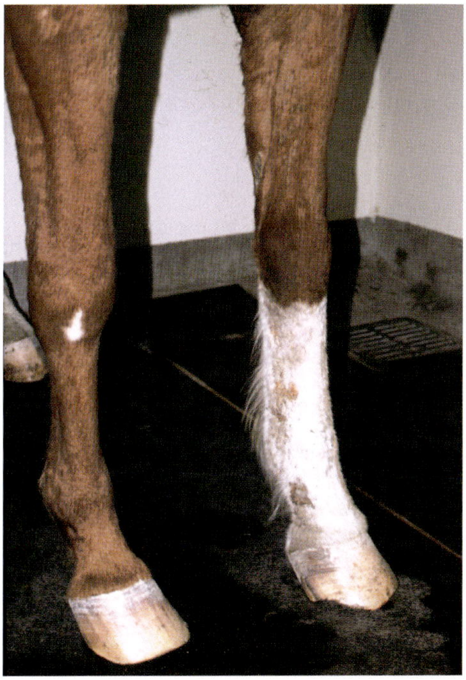

b

Figure 5.62a,b Photographs of the lateral and medial aspects of the left front leg in the same horse. Liver function tests were normal and *D. congolensis* was considered an etiological agent in this case. The horse responded to systemic glucocorticoids.

Sarcoids

Sarcoid is the most common skin tumor of the horse. A viral etiology (bovine papilloma virus) is proposed and outbreaks associated with heavy fly infestations can occur. Morphologically, lesions have been classified as occult, verrucous (warty), nodular, fibroblastic, malevolent, and mixed sarcoid. Treatment options (in order of success, highest first) include brachytherapy, chemotherapy (cisplatin), cryotherapy, cryotherapy with surgical resection, and surgical resection alone. It is important to take steps to reduce the incidence of autotransplantation if surgical excision is elected. Differential diagnoses should include granulation tissue, squamous cell carcinoma, cutaneous habronemiasis, melanoma, and dermatophytosis.

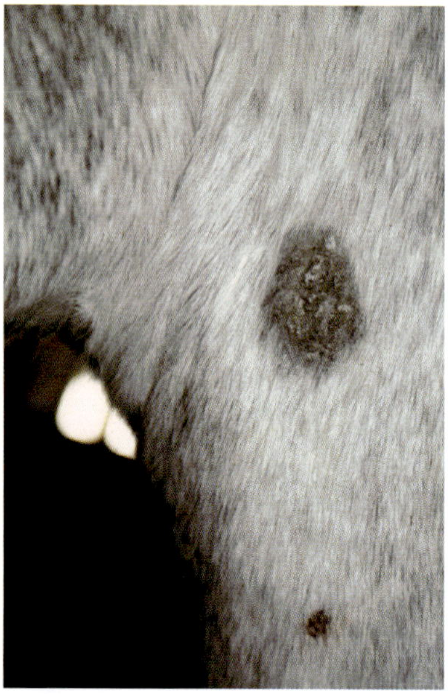

Figure 5.63a Photograph of a mature horse with a dry, flat sarcoid in the proximal cervical region.

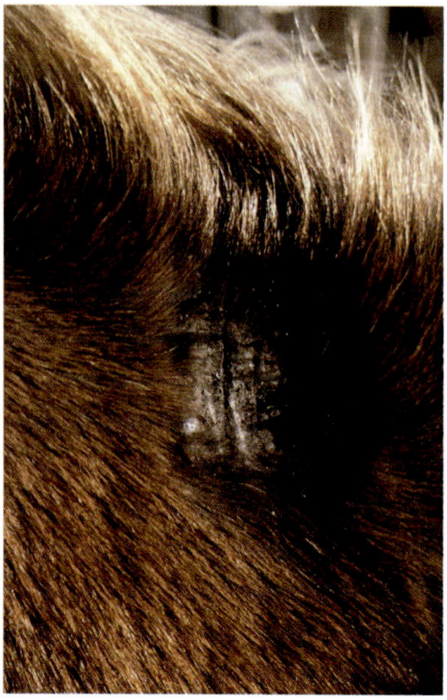

Figure 5.63b A flat sarcoid with alopecia at the base of the mane.

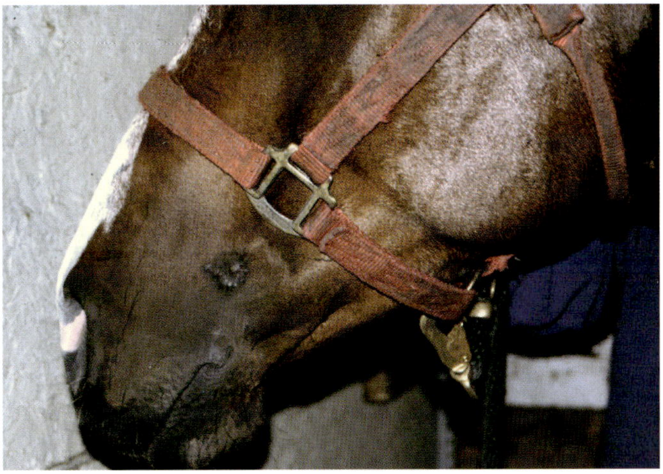

Figure 5.64 A nodular sarcoid dorsal and caudal to the commissure of the lip in a mature horse.

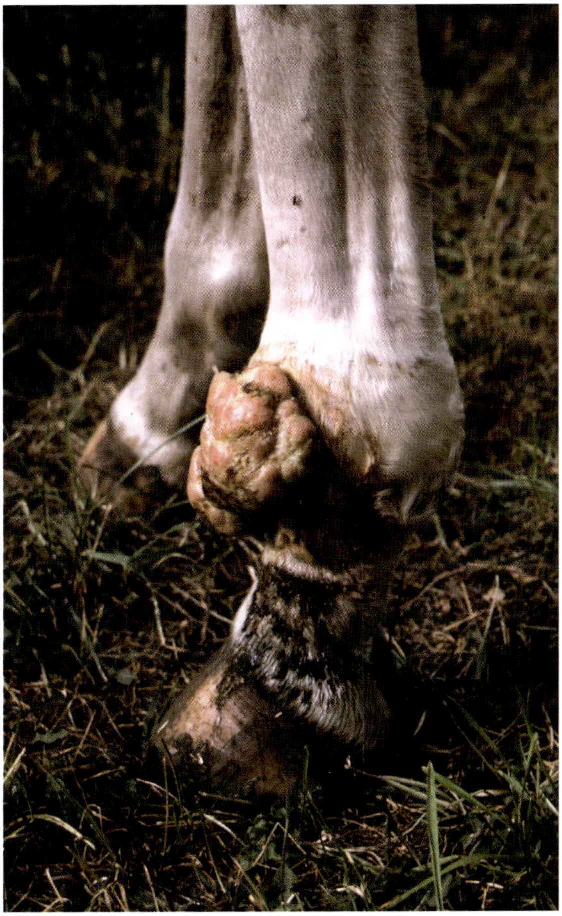

Figure 5.65a A fibroblastic sarcoid on the dorsolateral aspect of the left front fetlock.

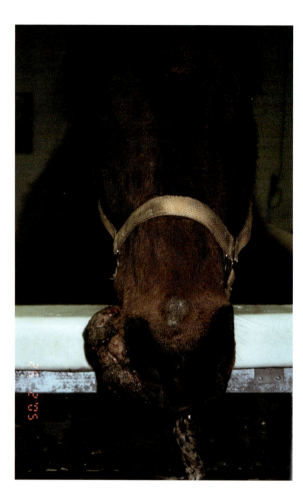

Figure 5.65b A fibroblastic sarcoid on the upper lip.

Sarcoidosis

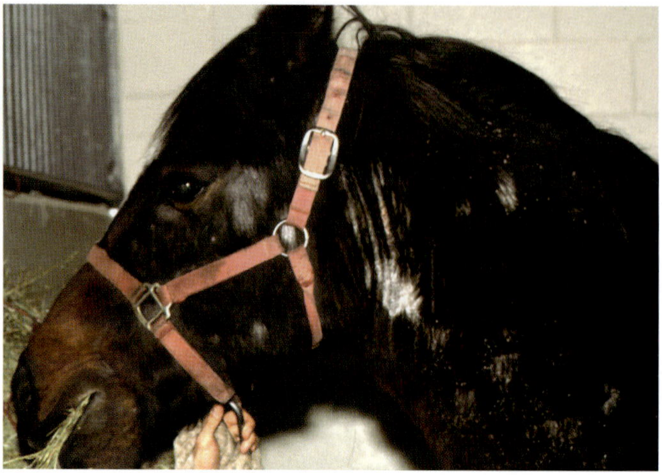

Figure 5.66 Sarcoidosis is a rare exfoliative dermatitis with unknown etiology. Signs of facial crusting and scaling tend to appear before generalized clinical signs. Systemic wasting disease is a common concurrent finding. Spontaneous regression can occur, however, progression of the disease to the point of euthanasia is more common. Shown here is a mature horse of undetermined age with generalized scaling and alopecia that was diagnosed with sarcoidosis.

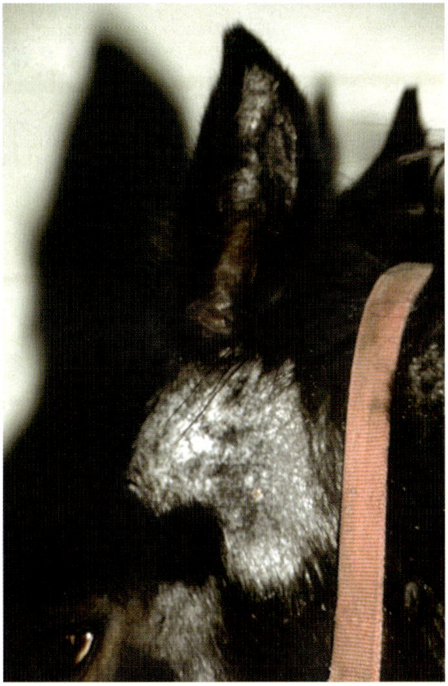

Figure 5.67 Progression of clinical signs in the above mentioned horse (fig. 5.66). Note this disease is not a manifestation of the common skin tumor sarcoid.

Scalding (Urine, Serum, Chemical)

The equine epidermis does not respond well to serum (draining wounds), urine (urine scalding), or chemicals, such as shampoos, that are not removed as per manufacturers' guidelines.

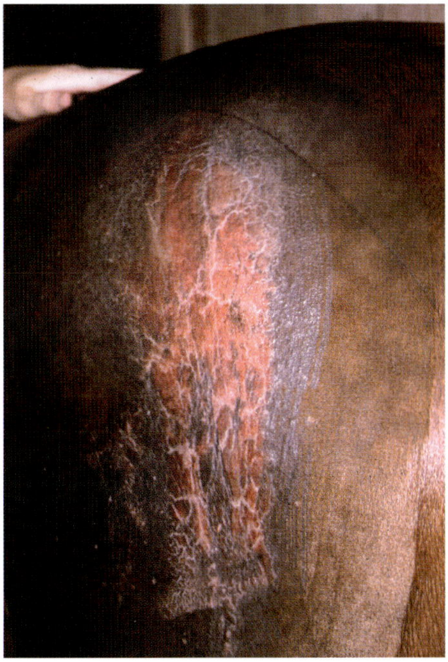

Figure 5.68a Serum scalding. This 10-year-old mare received intramuscular penicillin. There was severe serum exudation from the injection sites, which resulted in hair loss in this region. There was swelling, erythema, and significant pain associated with skin cracking, such that heavy intravenous sedation using a combination of acepromazine, detomidine, and butorphanol was required to clip and clean the region safely.

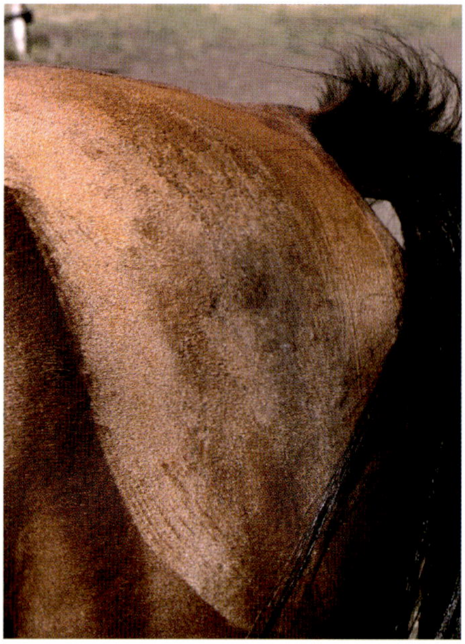

Figure 5.68b The same horse 10 days later. Note the early regrowth of hair and reduced erythema, and, clinically, the region could be palpated without obvious evidence of pain.

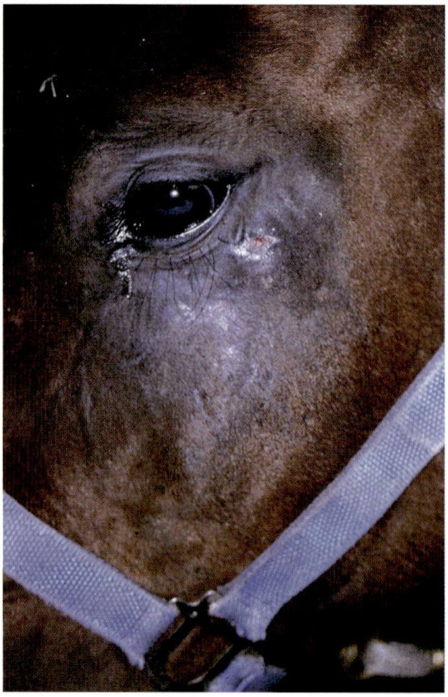

Figure 5.69a Serum scalding. Healing of serum scalding in a case of a periorbital foreign body (wood splinter). Note the region of alopecia along the drainage pathway.

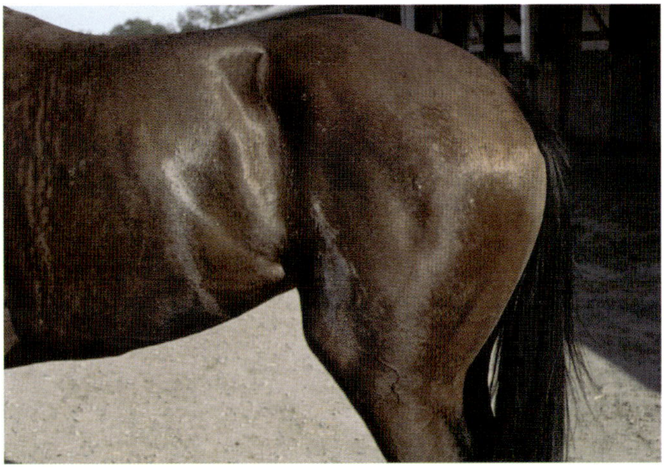

Figure 5.69b Serum scalding. Alopecia along a drainage pathway in a case of a proximal hind-limb wound.

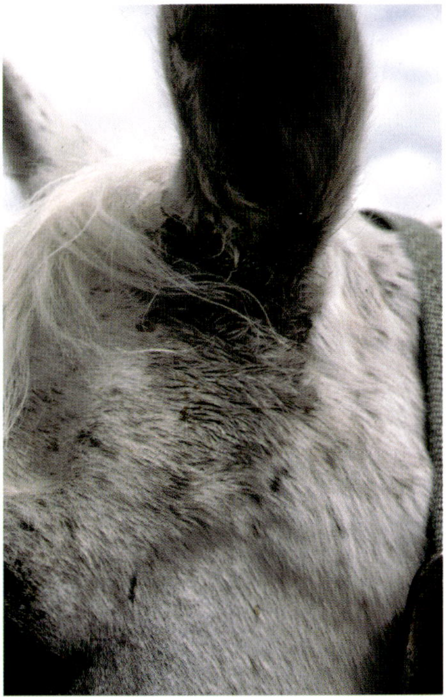

Figure 5.70a Chemical scalding. Periaural serum exudation in a mature horse associated with failure to remove shampoo following bathing.

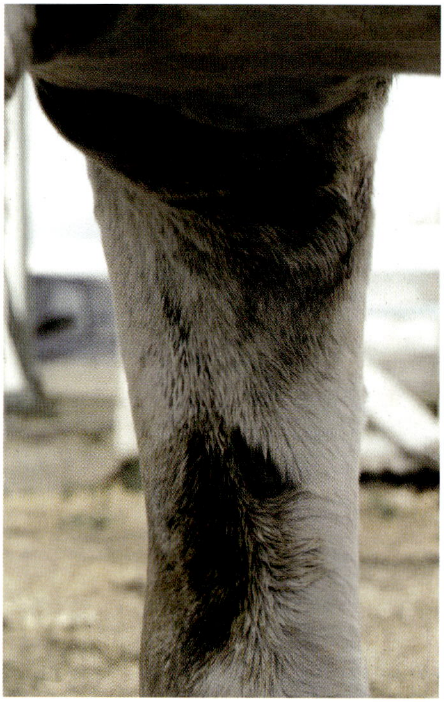

Figure 5.70b Chemical scalding. Axillary serum exudation in a mature horse associated with failure to remove shampoo following bathing.

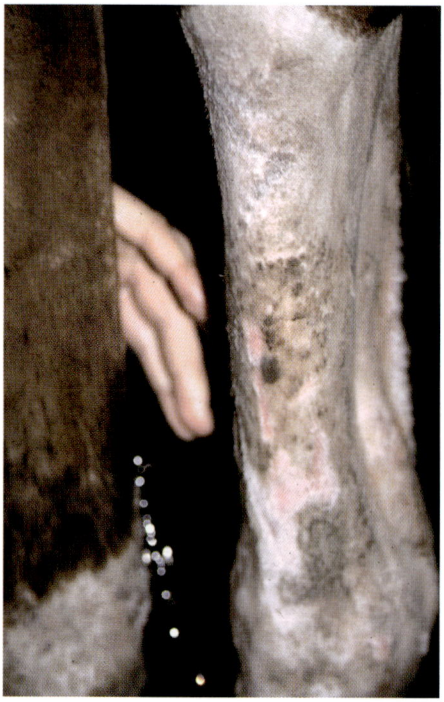

Figure 5.71 Chemical scalding. Alopecia and scaling associated with the use of an alcohol-based leg wrap in a mature horse.

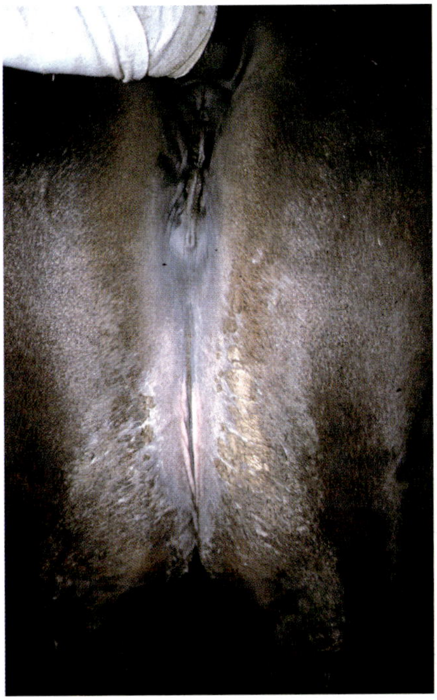

Figure 5.72 Urine scalding. Alopecia, erythema, and crusting in a mare with an abnormal contour of the vulvar lips resulting in urine contamination of the hind limbs.

Scratches (Greasy Heel, Pastern Dermatitis)

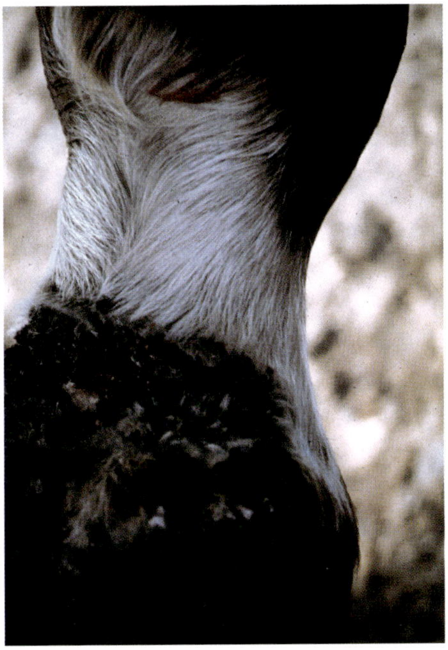

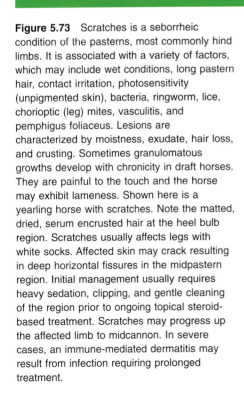

Figure 5.73 Scratches is a seborrheic condition of the pasterns, most commonly hind limbs. It is associated with a variety of factors, which may include wet conditions, long pastern hair, contact irritation, photosensitivity (unpigmented skin), bacteria, ringworm, lice, chorioptic (leg) mites, vasculitis, and pemphigus foliaceus. Lesions are characterized by moistness, exudate, hair loss, and crusting. Sometimes granulomatous growths develop with chronicity in draft horses. They are painful to the touch and the horse may exhibit lameness. Shown here is a yearling horse with scratches. Note the matted, dried, serum encrusted hair at the heel bulb region. Scratches usually affects legs with white socks. Affected skin may crack resulting in deep horizontal fissures in the midpastern region. Initial management usually requires heavy sedation, clipping, and gentle cleaning of the region prior to ongoing topical steroid-based treatment. Scratches may progress up the affected limb to midcannon. In severe cases, an immune-mediated dermatitis may result from infection requiring prolonged treatment.

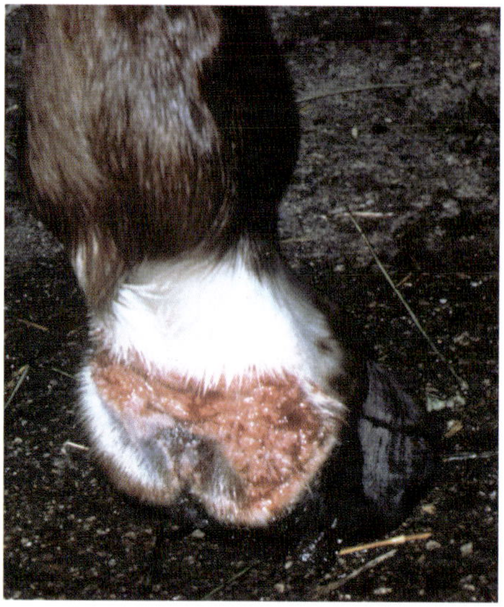

Figure 5.74 Scratches in a yearling horse (after initial cleaning and debridement).

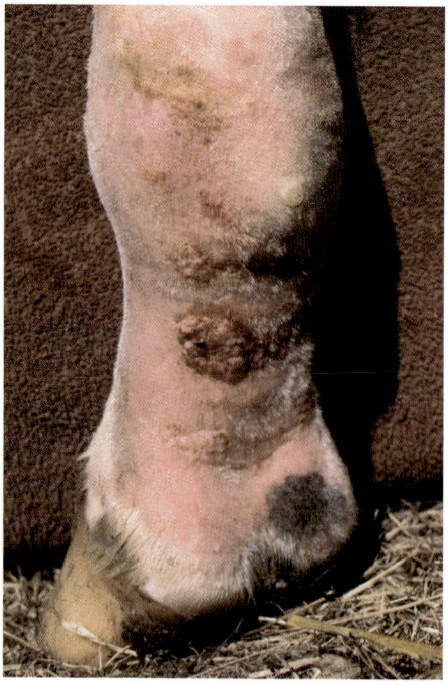

Figure 5.75 Scratches in a horse. Note the deep horizontal fissures in the midpastern region and the beginning of photoactive dermatitis (as below).

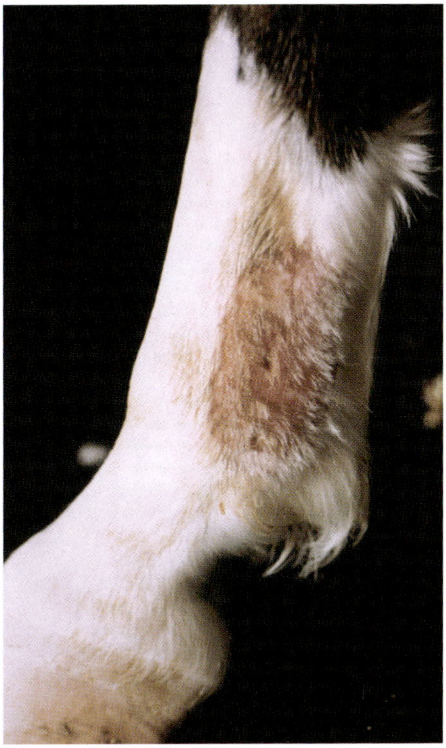

Figure 5.76 Photoactive vasculitis (an immune-mediated dermatitis) originating from pastern dermatitis (see Photosensitization and Dermatophilosis above, and Vasculitis below).

Sporotrichosis

Figures 5.77a–c A horse with cutaneolymphatic form of sporotrichosis (figs. 5.77a and b). This is a mycotic disease caused by the fungus *Sporothrix schenckii.* Affected horses may have cutaneous nodules (fig. 5.77c) on lower extremities, which extend proximally via the lymphatics resulting in "cording." These nodules may either be intact (fig. 5.78a) or become ulcerated and drain purulent material. Diagnosis is made by fine needle aspirate (fig. 5.78b) or biopsy and histopathological examination of a nodule (fig. 5.78c). Differential diagnosis of cutaneous nonulcerated nodules may be bacterial (*Corynebacterium* spp. and *Staphlococcus* spp.) or fungal (blastomycosis, coccidiomycosis, cryptococcus, and histoplasmosis). Treatment includes systemic iodides or griseofulvin.

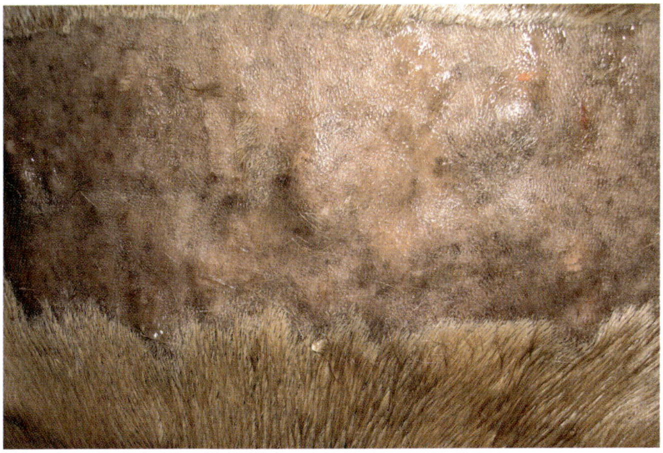

a

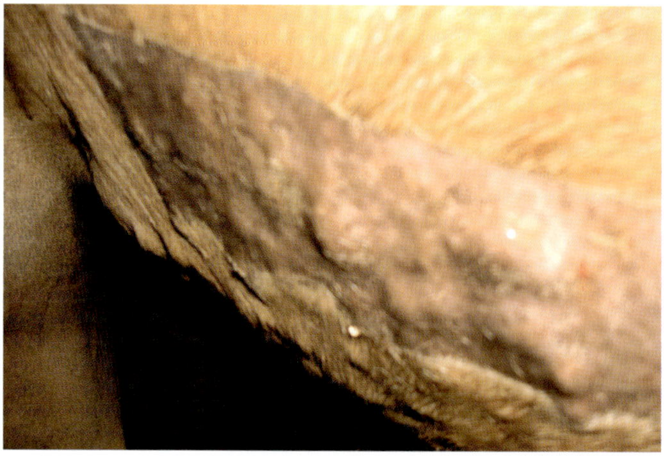

b

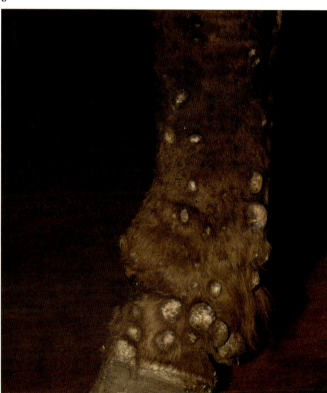

c

Figures 5.77a–c *Continued*

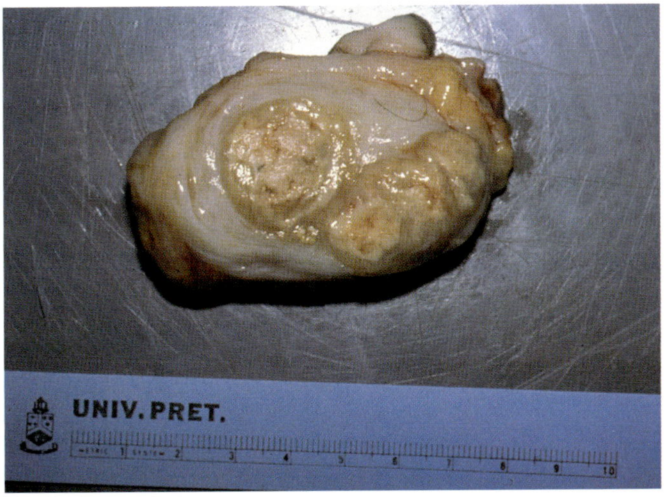

Figure 5.78a An excised fungal granuloma due to *Sporothrix schenckii*. (Image courtesy of the Section of Pathology, Faculty of Veterinary Science, University of Pretoria)

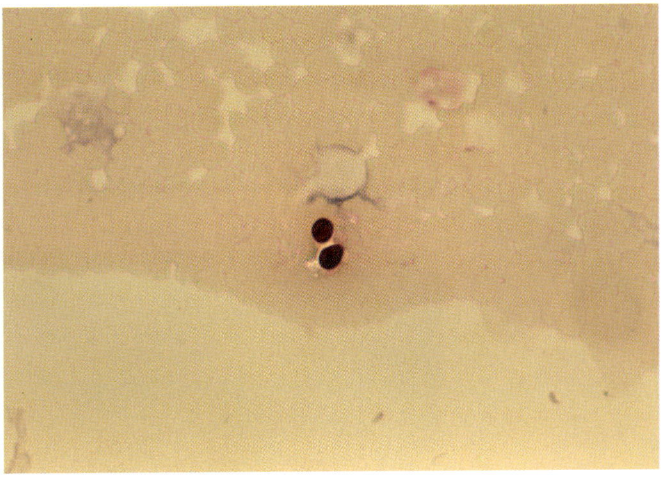

Figure 5.78b Photomicrograph of *Sporothrix schenckii* in an infected nodule showing yeastlike organisms following fine needle aspiration (Periodic acid-Schiff stain). (Image courtesy of the Section of Pathology, Faculty of Veterinary Science, University of Pretoria)

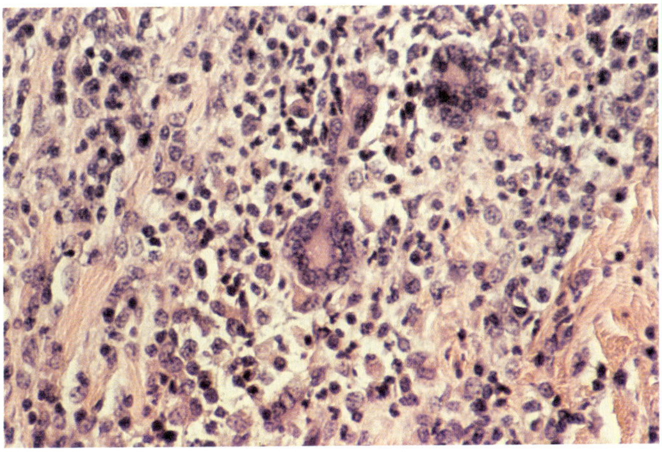

Figure 5.78c Photomicrograph of *Sporothrix schenckii* in an infected nodule showing multinucleated giant cells (hematoxylin and eosin stain). (Image courtesy of the Section of Pathology, Faculty of Veterinary Science, University of Pretoria)

Squamous Cell Carcinoma

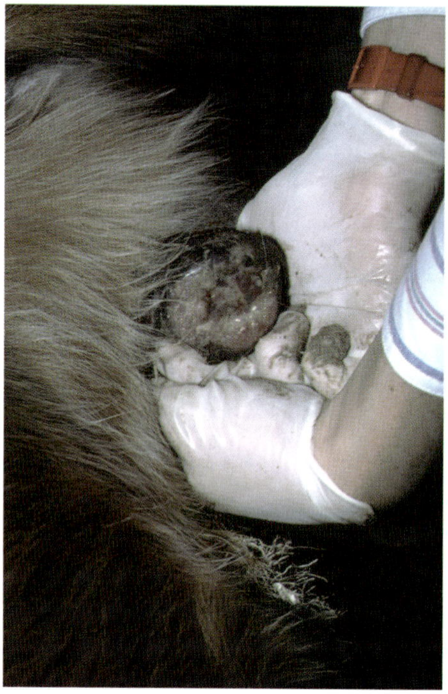

a

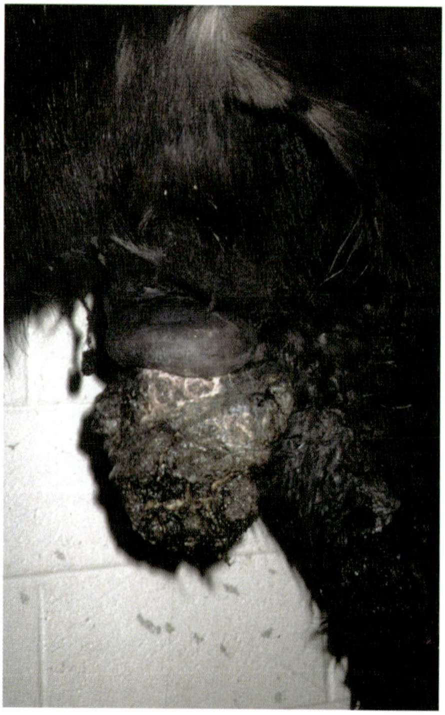

b

Figures 5.79a,b Squamous cell carcinoma is the most common malignant cutaneous neoplasm in the horse and is second only to sarcoid as the most common overall tumor. It is the most common tumor of the eyelids and genitalia. It is usually associated with previous sun damage and is preceded by shallow ulcerlike erosions. Chronic lesions can invade underlying bone in oral or pharyngeal cases. Preputial and penile squamous cell carcinoma is significantly more common in gelded than in intact horses. These images are of the distal end of the penis in a mature horse. Note the reddened, cauliflowerlike surface to the glans. See also Chapter 8, Diseases of the Reproductive System.

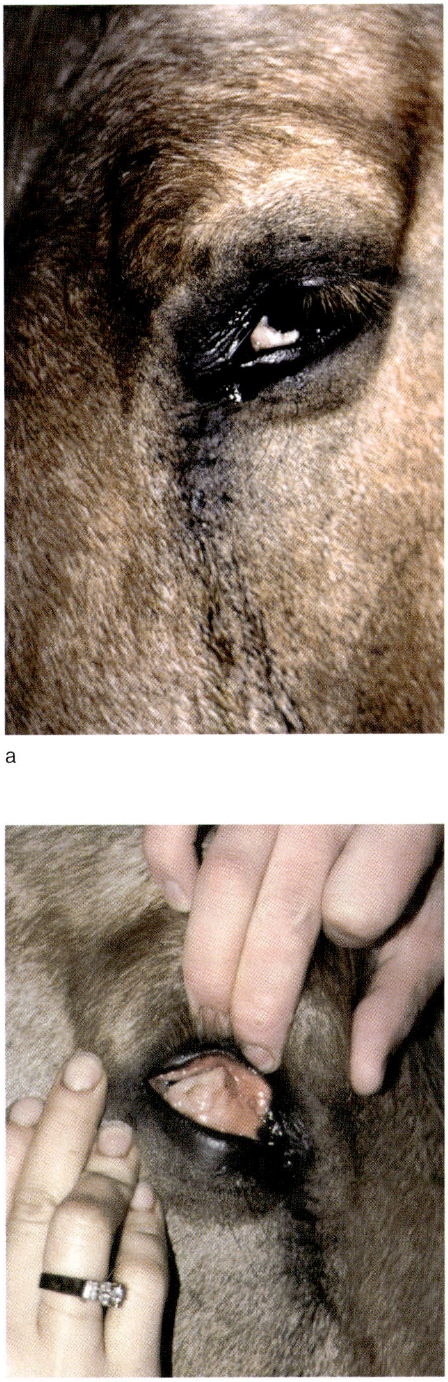

a

b

Figure 5.80a,b Epiphora (fig. 5.80a) in a horse that was presented for bilateral squamous cell carcinoma of the nictating membranes (fig. 5.80b).

Stud Crud (Idiopathic Cannon Keratosis)

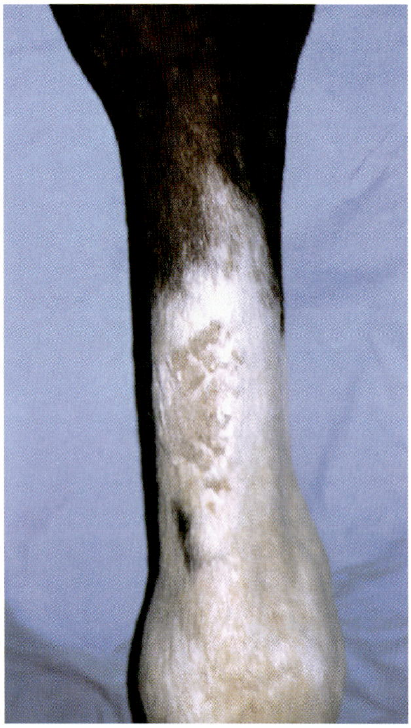

Figure 5.81 Relatively common dermatosis of unknown etiology. Seen almost exclusively on the hind limbs of horses where white and pigmented limbs are affected equally. It is not associated with urination on the dorsal aspect of the legs as it is seen in mares and fillies as well as male animals. Scaling and crusting with or without alopecia is the hallmark of this condition. This is more of a cosmetic than clinical problem. Crusts can be removed using water if desired, however, they will reappear.

Sunburn

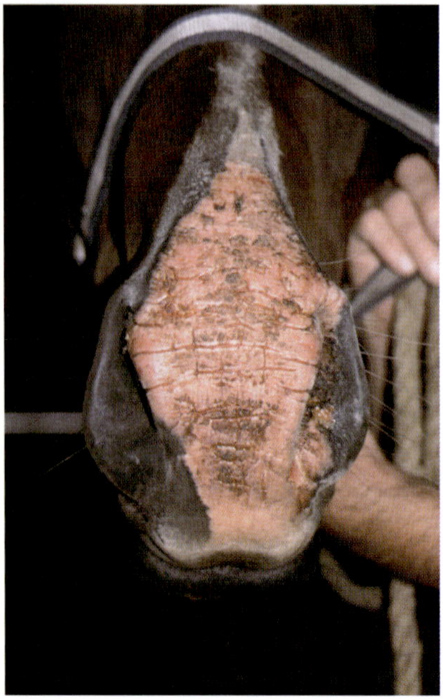

Figure 5.82 Sunburn is a common condition seen in equine practice. Differential diagnoses include photoactive vasculitis associated with *D. congolensis* infection and photosensitization. Treatment is with emollient creams and anti-inflammatory medications in the acute phase. Subsequent to this, the use of waterproof sunblock has been found to be useful.

Telogen Defluxion

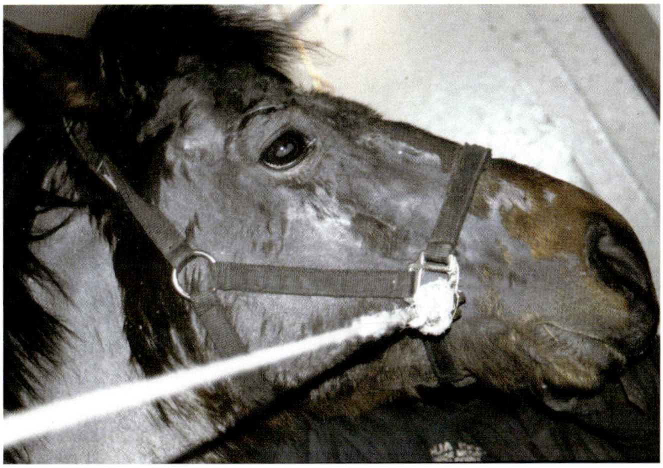

Figure 5.83 Telogen defluxion is a relatively rare condition associated with a systemic shock such as severe pyrexia or illness. The growth cycle of hair is terminated abruptly and follicles resynchronize into the resting or telogen phase. Hair shafts are easily epilated and severe alopecia occurs. This photograph is of the head of an old gelding with telogen defluxion. The owner had applied a blister to one of the legs 4 weeks previously.

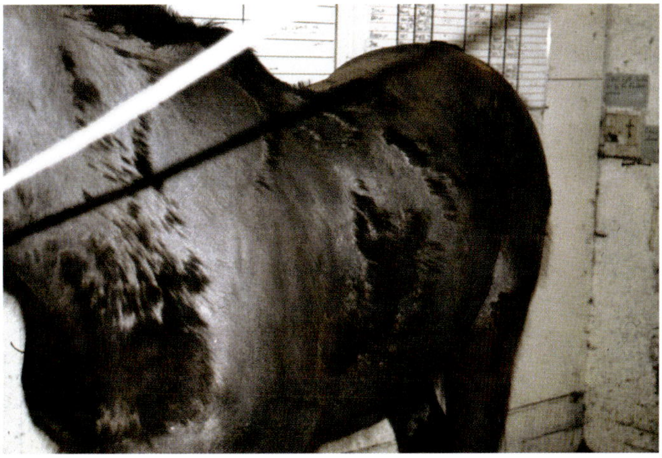

Figure 5.84 The same horse seen in fig. 5.83. Note the huge areas of hair loss with normal epidermis.

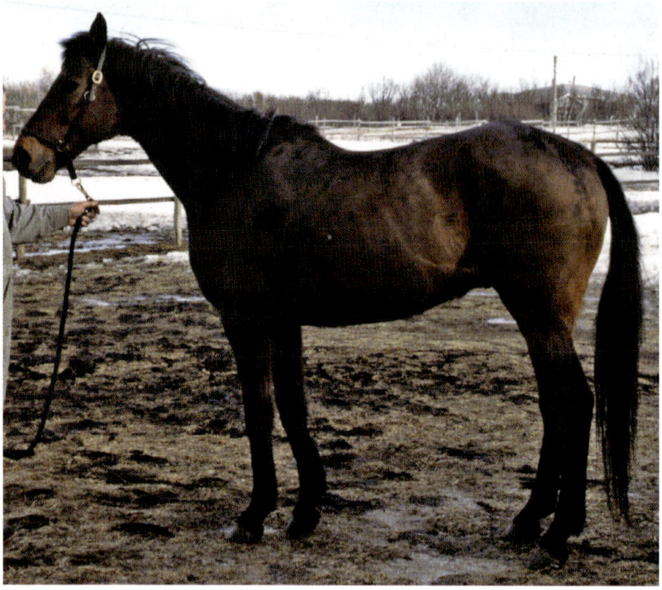

Figure 5.85 The same horse seen in fig. 5.83, 6 months later. Note the complete regrowth of the hair coat.

Temporal Teratoma (Dentigerous Cyst, Ear Tooth, Heterotrophic Polydontia)

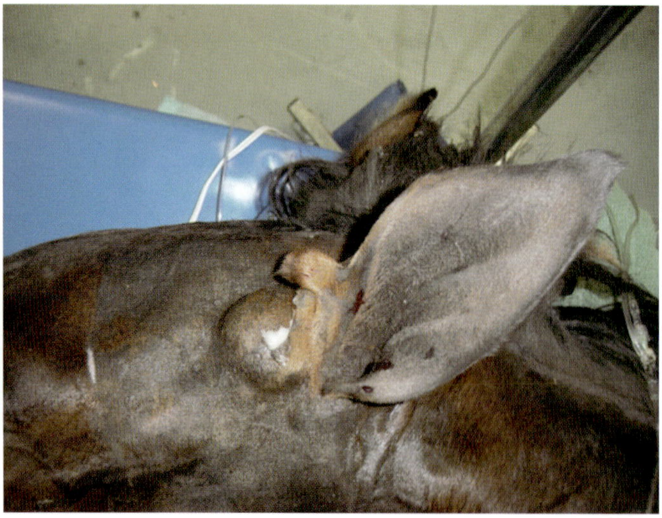

Figure 5.86 Temporal teratoma is a congenital condition associated with a first branchial arch defect. It results in the presence of a cystic cavity, which subsequently drains on the rostral border of the pinna or immediately rostral and ventral to the external ear canal. The tooth is often intimately attached to the temporal bone and develops according to the predetermined timetable. Thus, it may be small if approached early or contain a full mature cheek tooth if not removed prior to maturity. A large draining mass at the base of the left ear in a mature Thoroughbred mare. A complete cheek tooth was excised within the cystic structure.

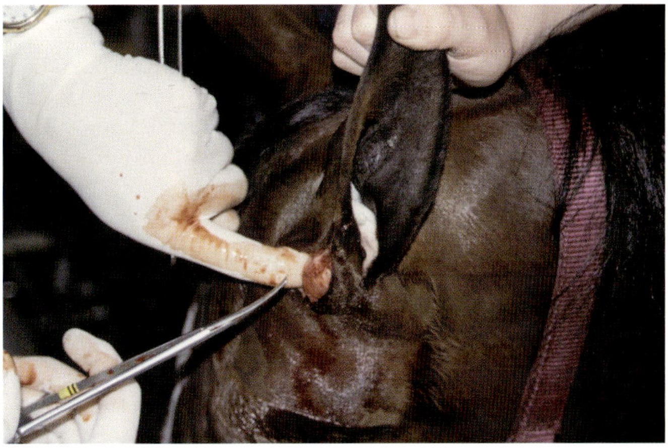

a

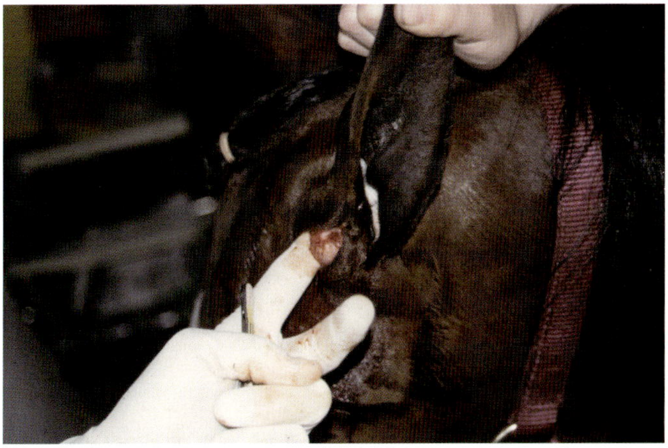

b

Figures 5.87a–e Surgical removal of temporal teratoma.

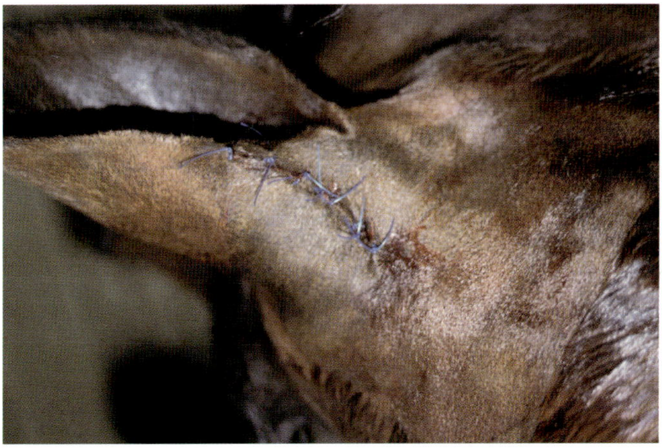

c

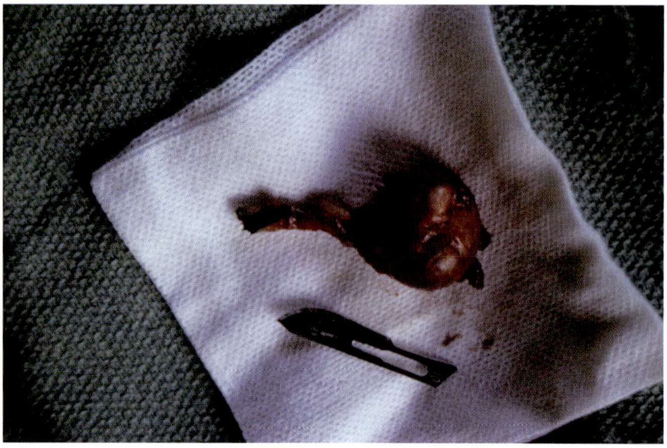

d

Figures 5.87a–e *Continued*

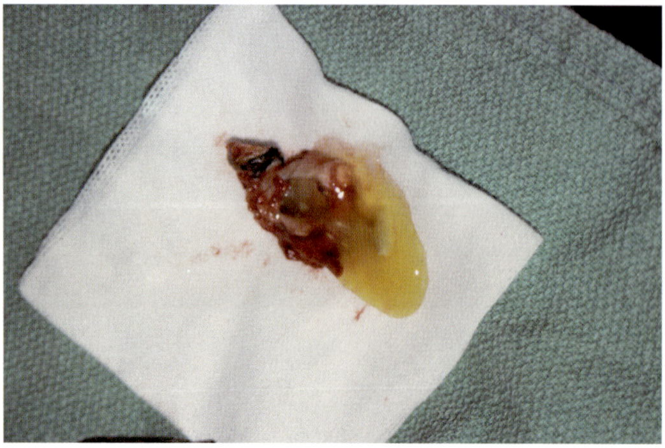

e

Phaeohyphomycosis (Blackgrain Mycetoma, Maduromycosis)

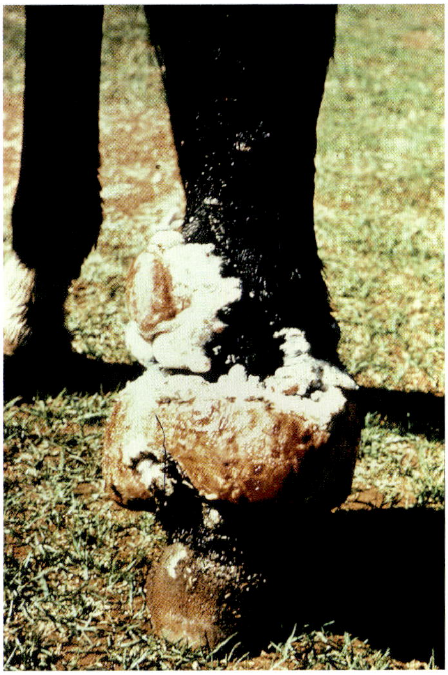

Figure 5.88a Nodular granulomatous dermatitis in a horse with phaeohyphomycosis. Numerous fungi have been previously incriminated and include *Alternaria*, *Aureobasidium*, *Cladophialophora*, *Dactylaria*, *Drechslera*, *Exserohilum*, *Exophiala*, *Fonsecaea,* and *Phialophora*. Clinical signs include multiple subcutaneous nodules that may involve the lymphatics and nasal granulomas. Diagnosis is reached by histopathological examination of a tissue biopsy obtained from the nodule (fig. 5.88b) and culture. Therapy includes surgical excision, and antifungal drugs. (Image courtesy of the Section of Pathology, Faculty of Veterinary Science, University of Pretoria)

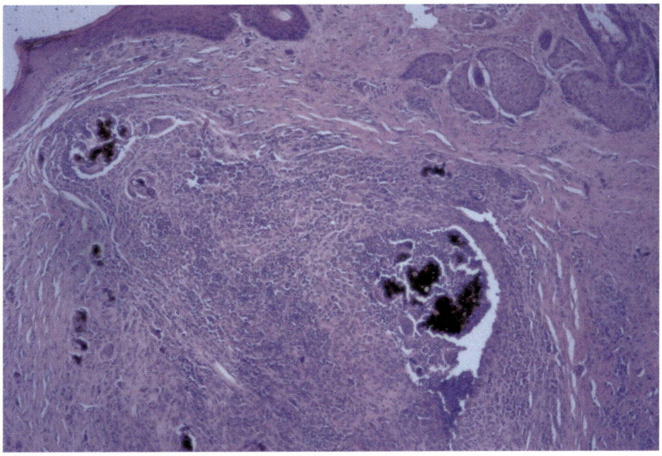

Figure 5.88b Photomicrograph of phaeohyphomycosis showing pigment-producing yeast organisms (hematoxylin and eosin stain). (Image courtesy of the Section of Pathology, Faculty of Veterinary Science, University of Pretoria)

Tick Infestation

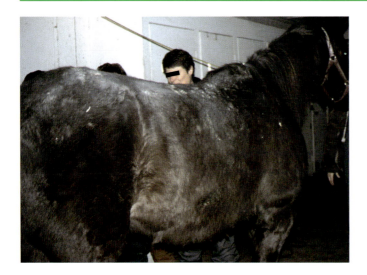

Figure 5.89 Tick Infestation is a common condition in the horse and usually not host-specific. This photograph is of a severe tick infestation in a mature horse. Note the alopecia and crusting limited to the dorsal midline.

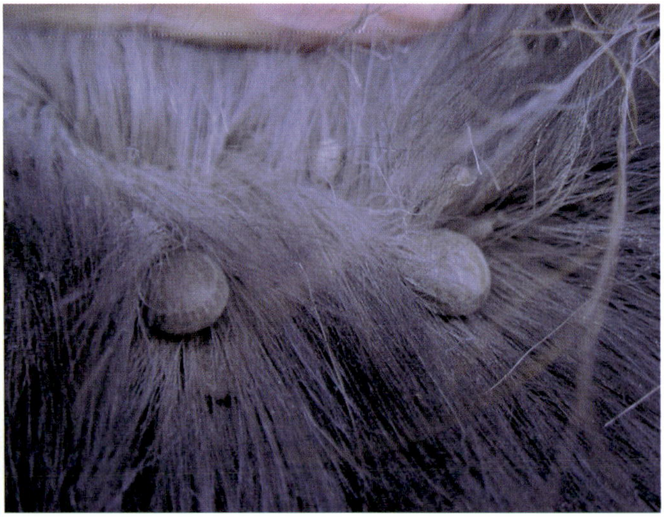

Figure 5.90a Multiple hard-bodied ticks (*Dermacentor albipictus*).

Figure 5.90b The number of ticks is easily appreciated using a tick comb.

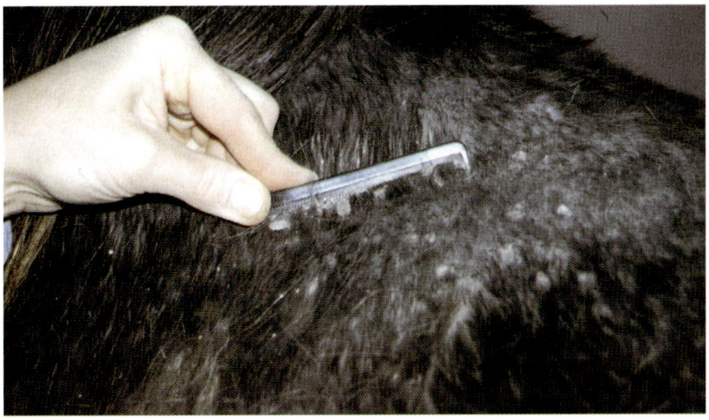

Urticaria

Figure 5.91 Urticaria is usually associated with mast cell degranulation. This may be due to a hypersensitivity reaction or other nonimmunologic stimuli. Wheals typically appear, which may be in a variety of shapes. Often, the inciting cause is not apparent but may include inhaled or topical allergens as well as pressure (dermatographia), heat, cold, exercise, stress, or chemical agents such as antibiotics. Note the diffuse, multifocal wheals (gyrate urticaria) in this mature Thoroughbred horse.

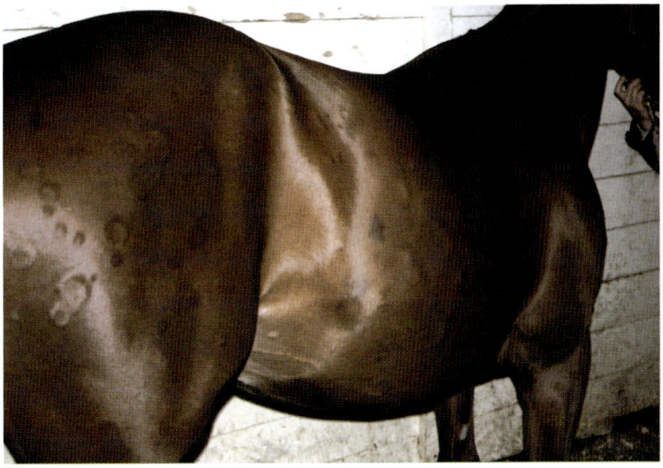

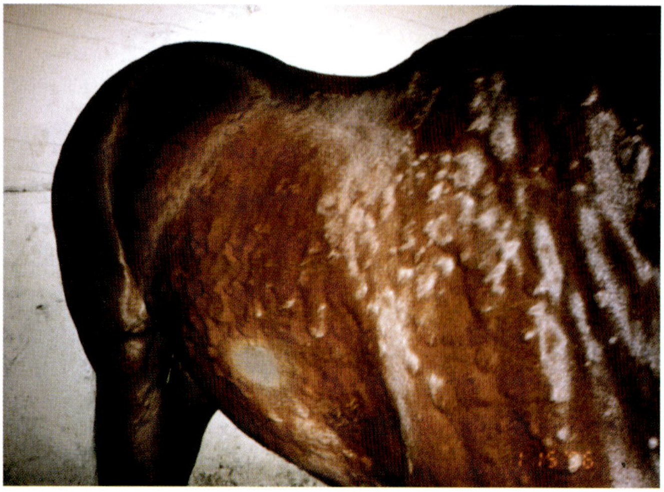

Figure 5.92 Conventional urticaria in this Thoroughbred. As with the horse in fig. 5.91, no inciting cause could be found and the horses were treated successfully using glucocorticoids.

Vasculitis (Immune-mediated or Photoactive)

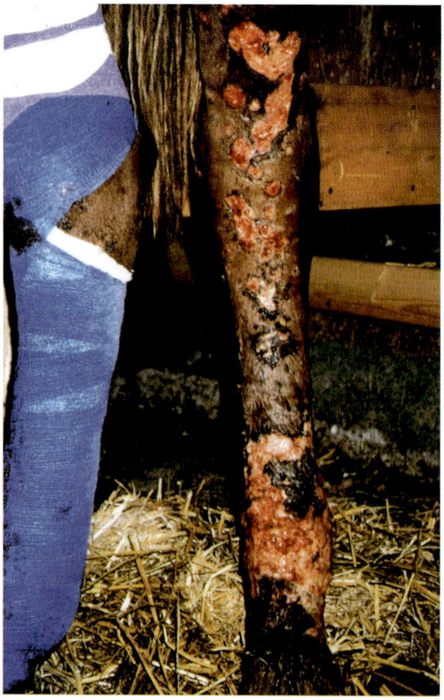

Figure 5.93 Immune-mediated vasculitis is the most common form in the horse and is typically associated with type III hypersensitivity reaction. Immune complex deposition results in the development of warm, painful edema. This is rapidly followed by serum exudation and if not resolved rapidly may result in a combination of epidermal splitting or severe serum scalding and loss of large areas of skin. *Streptococcus equi*–associated purpura hemorrhagica is a good example. Multifocal vasculitis may also develop in cases of septicemia (salmonellosis in foals) and can involve the tips of the pinnae and the lips. Note the multifocal regions of epidermal loss and serum exudation in this case of purpura hemorrhagica. The opposite hind limb is bandaged in an effort to limit swelling and provide protection to the underlying tissue. See also Chapter 2, Diseases of the Cardiovascular System.

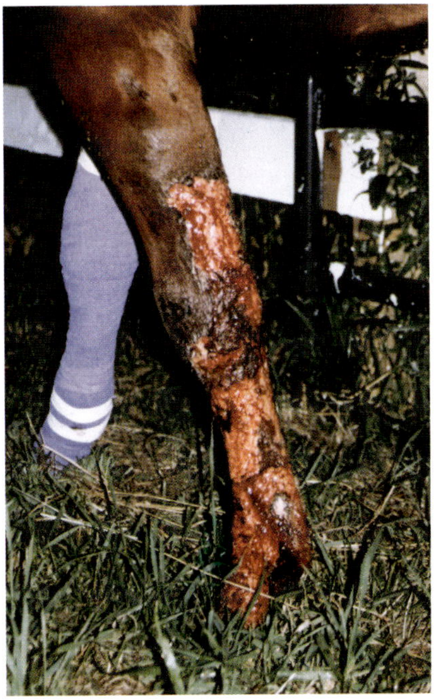

Figure 5.94 Another case of purpura hemorrhagica in which the forelimbs were affected the worst.

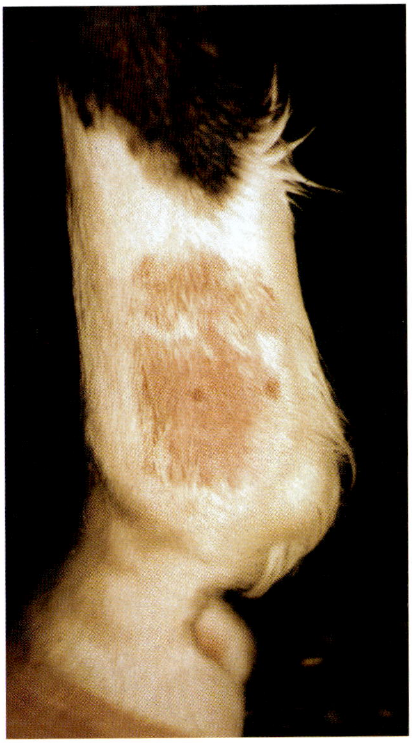

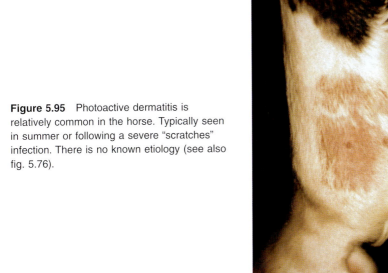

Figure 5.95 Photoactive dermatitis is relatively common in the horse. Typically seen in summer or following a severe "scratches" infection. There is no known etiology (see also fig. 5.76).

Arabian Fading Syndrome

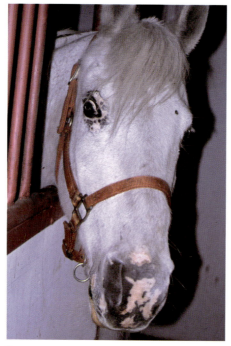

a

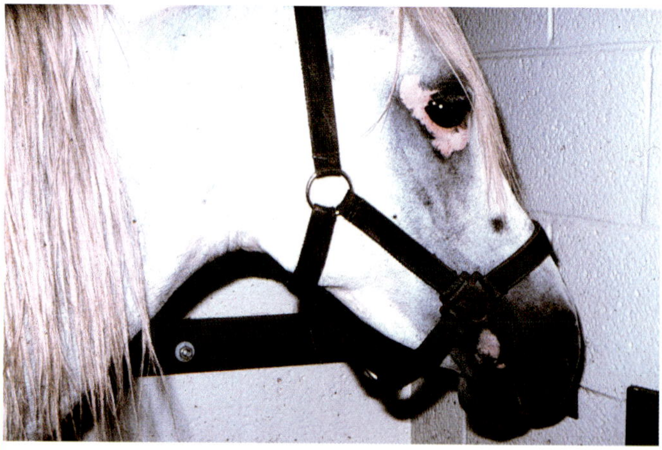

b

Figures 5.96a,b Arabian fading syndrome is also called pinky syndrome and Arabian leukoderma. Although it can occur in any breed, it is most common in young Arabian horses. The areas of skin affected may remain depigmented and may repigment, or the pigment may come and go. It is suspected to be hereditary. The skin is normal except for the loss of melanocytes and the main concern is often cosmetic appearance. The affected areas of skin are also more at risk to sunburn, photosensitization, and squamous cell carcinoma development. The areas most commonly affected are around the eyes, mouth, perineum, genitalia, and inguinal regions.

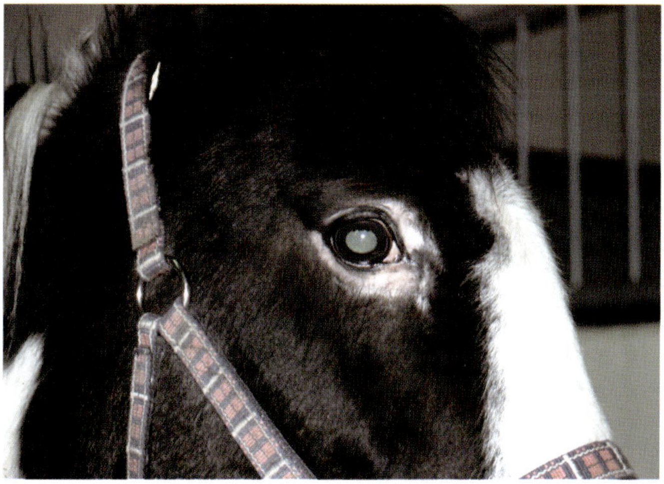

Figure 5.97 Vitiligo is depigmentation of skin. Etiology is unknown. It might be idiopathic or precipitated by primary melanocyte damage. It is usually seen in horses over 4 years old and may be heritable. Shown here is periocular depigmentation in a young paint horse.

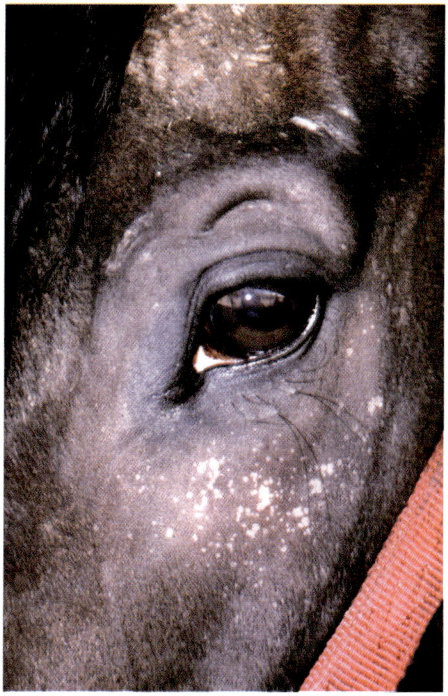

Figure 5.98 Acquired vitiligo of unknown origin in a mature quarter horse.

Warts (Papillomatosis)

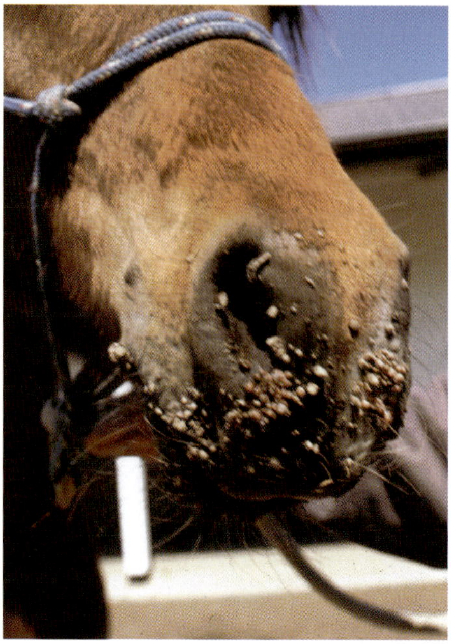

Figure 5.99 Common viral skin disease of young horses classically on the lips, muzzle, and periocular region. Spontaneous regression occurs. The picture shows a young Thoroughbred horse with multiple muzzle papillomas.

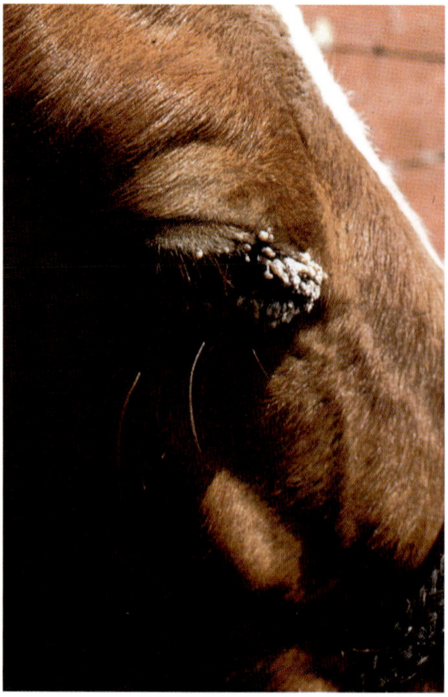

Figure 5.100 A young Thoroughbred horse with periocular papillomatosis.

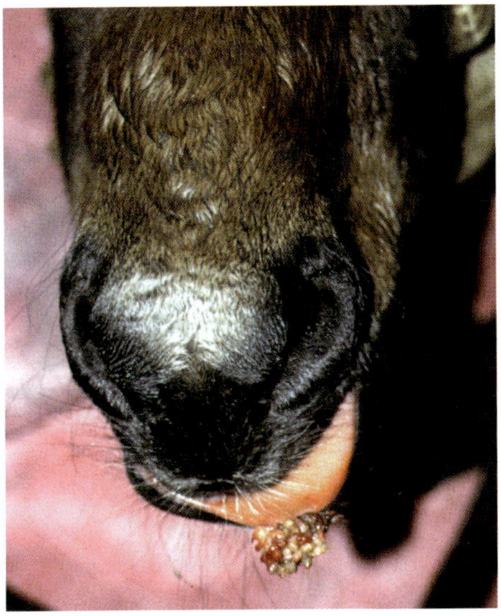

a

Figures 5.101a,b A congenital wart, epidermal nevi, on the tongue of a neonatal quarter horse foal before (a) and after (b) surgical removal.

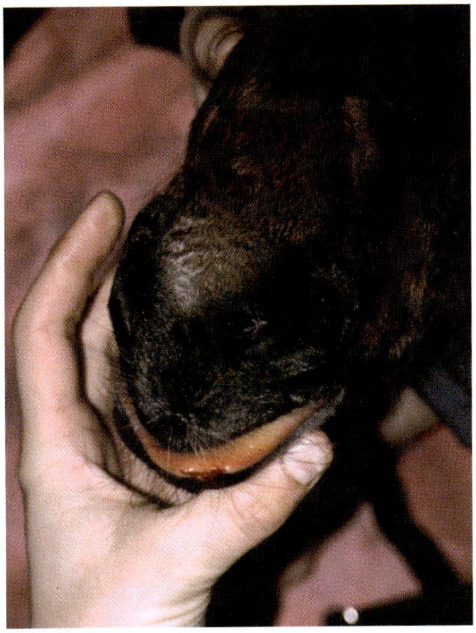

b

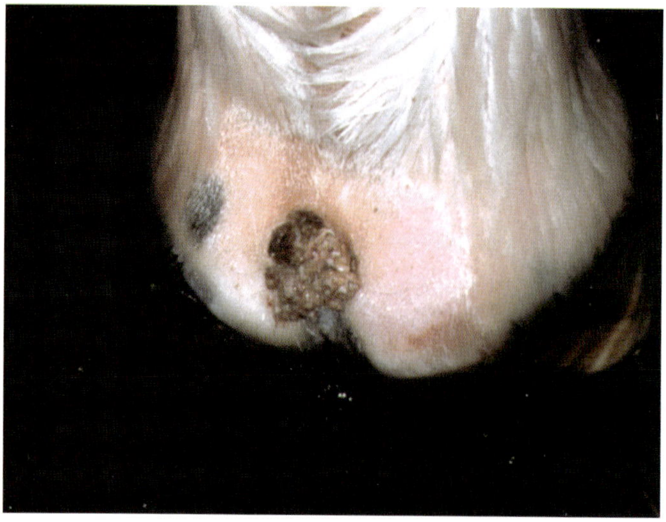

Figure 5.102a Another congenital wart (epidermal nevi) on the heel bulb of a quarter horse foal. This has been clipped prior to surgical removal.

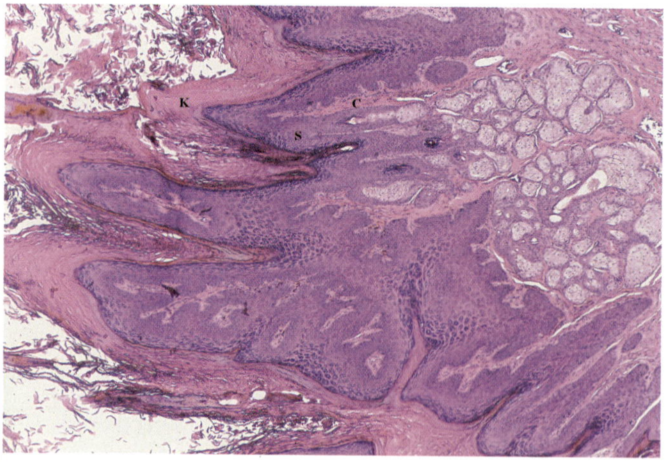

Figure 5.102b Photomicrograph of a papilloma showing squamous epithelium (S), stratum corneum (K), and a connective tissue stalk (C). There is marked epidermal hyperplasia and hyperkeratosis (hematoxylin and eosin stain).

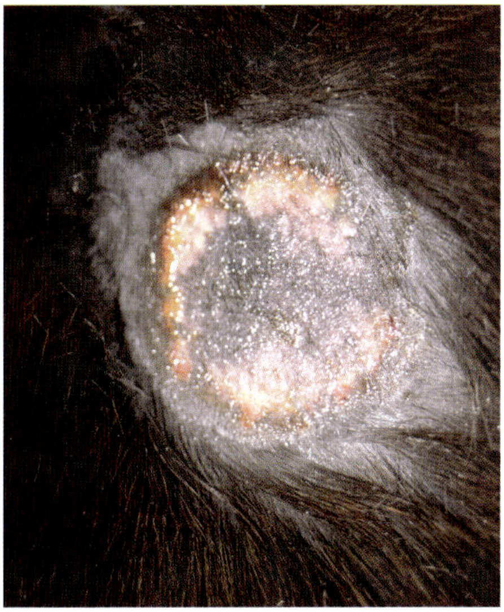

Figure 5.103 Winter atopy is thought to be associated with cold-induced mast cell degranulation. Lesions initially present as raised wheals with serum exudation. Crusting and alopecia follow. Affected regions are nonpainful but horses exhibit low-grade pruritis. This lesion is usually seen after the winter hair coat has grown, resulting in circular lesions of alopecia for the remaining winter. The summer coat develops normally. Lesions recur seasonally in affected horses. An early lesion in a mature horse is seen here. Note the alopecia and serum exudation.

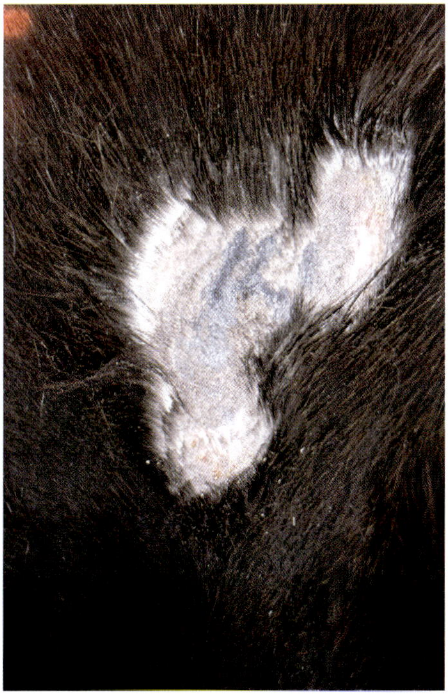

Figure 5.104 The same horse shown in the previous figure. In this photograph, the lesion has healed and an alopecic region remains.

Cutaneous Drug Reactions (Drug Eruption)

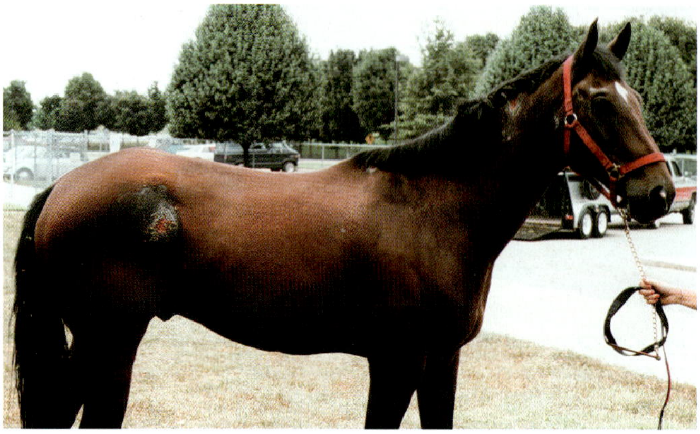

Figure 5.105 Cutaneous drug reactions are relatively uncommon but they can mimic any other skin diseases. This represents type IV hypersensitivity reaction. Skin lesions associated with drug eruption are extremely variable, but should appear immediately after the drug or vaccine has been administered. They may or may not be pruritic. A diagnosis requires an accurate and detailed history and biopsies to rule out other causes such as parasitic, infectious, or autoimmune diseases. This photograph is of a horse that was presented with non pruritic, bilaterally symmetrical alopecia and scaling skin lesions that had been on a course of oral phenylbutazone. Histological evaluation of the skin lesions was consistent with drug eruption.

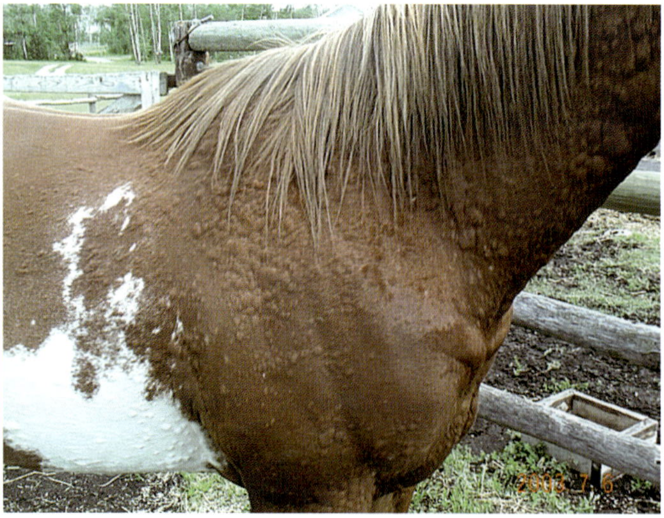

Figure 5.106 Drug eruption in a horse following vaccination. Note the urticaria (fig. 5.106) and severe dependant chest edema (fig. 5.107).

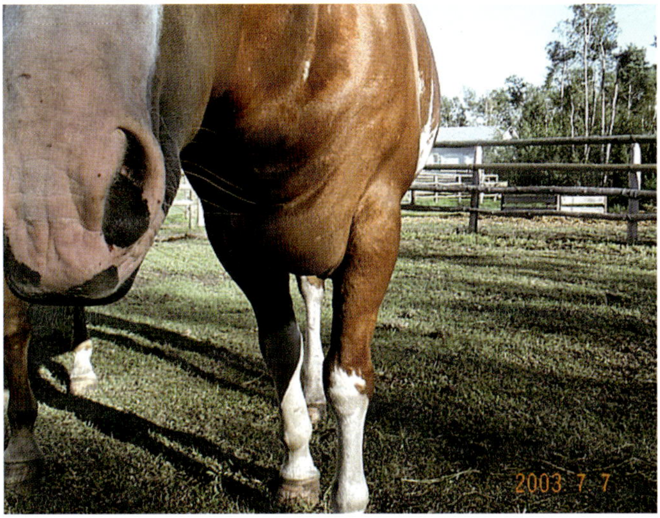

Figure 5.107 Drug eruption in a horse following vaccination. Note the severe dependant chest edema (fig. 5.107).

Food Hypersensitivity

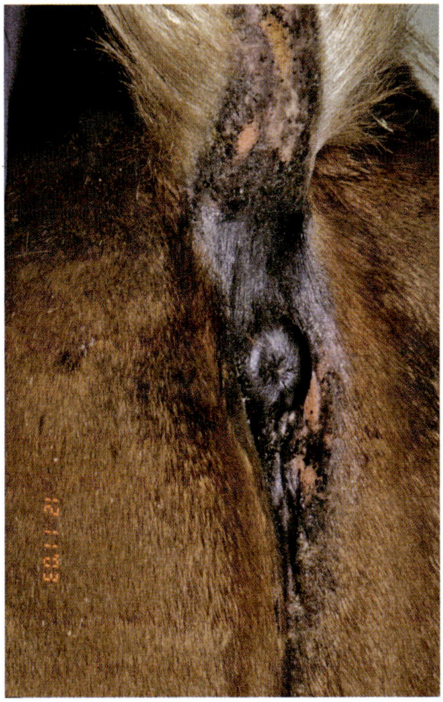

Figure 5.108 Food hypersensitivity is probably a complex type hypersensitivity reaction to certain feed types. Clinical signs include urticaria and pruritis, especially perineal pruritis. Differential diagnoses include insect hypersensitivity, lice, mange, and *Oxyuris equi* infection. These should be excluded before a diagnosis of food hypersensitivity can be established. Feed exclusion trials should be initiated. Good quality hay, which has never been given to the particular horse before, is given alone for 3 weeks. If the horse improves, this would confirm the diagnosis. This photograph is of a mature horse with perineal pruritis caused by feed hypersensitivity. This horse healed after changing the feed.

Anhydrosis

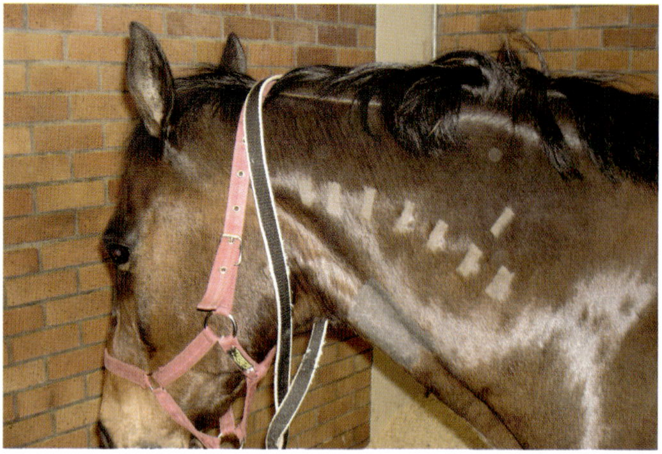

Figure 5.109 A horse evaluated for poor performance due to anhydrosis. The precise etiology is uncertain but down regulation of sweat gland β-2 receptors is suspected. Anhydrosis occurs in hot, humid regions and clinical signs include a decreased sweat response, dry skin, exercise intolerance, tachypnea at rest, and sustained postexercise hyperthermia. Diagnosis is based on clinical signs and intradermal injection of serial dilutions of adrenaline (figs. 5.110–5.112). Treatment includes correcting the hyperthermia using cold-water hosing or intravenous fluids, supplying oral electrolytes, and translocation of the horse to a more temperate region.

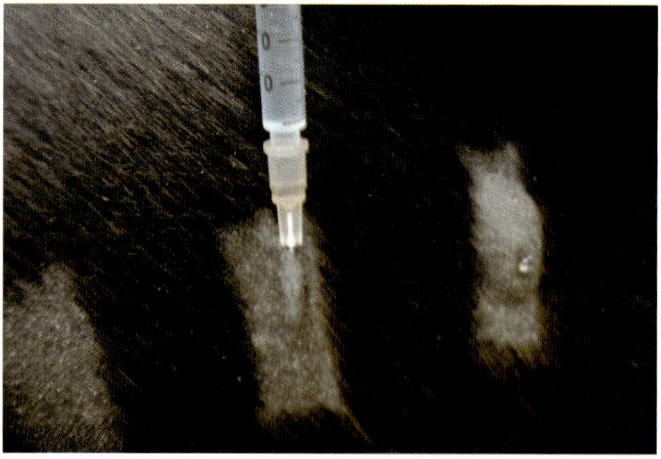

Figure 5.110 Intradermal injection of serial dilutions of adrenaline using a tuberculin syringe. Adrenaline at concentrations of $1:10^3$, $1:10^4$, $1:10^5$, and $1:10^6$, is injected intradermally at a dose of 0.5 ml each. In normal horses, sweating occurs over the injection sites, at all dilutions, within minutes. Affected horses respond only to the $1:10^3$ dilution, and then only after a period of 5 hours or more.

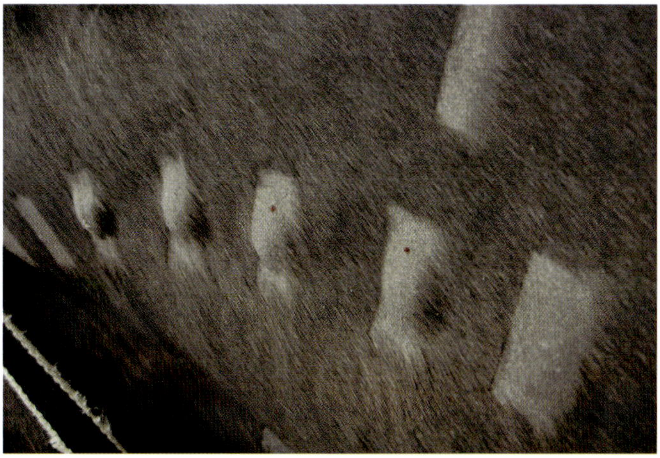

Figure 5.111 Intradermal injection of serial dilutions of adrenaline 3 minutes postinjection, in a horse affected with anhidrosis. No sweating noted.

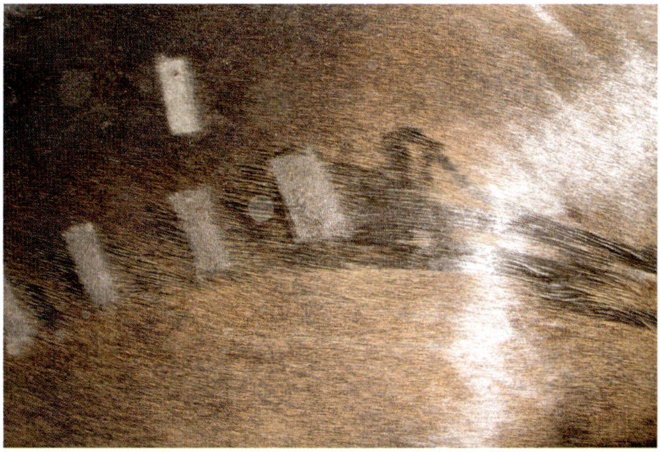

Figure 5.112 Sweating in response to intradermal injection of serial dilutions of adrenaline in the neck of an unaffected horse, 20 minutes postinjection.

Epizootic Lymphangitis (Histoplasmosis)

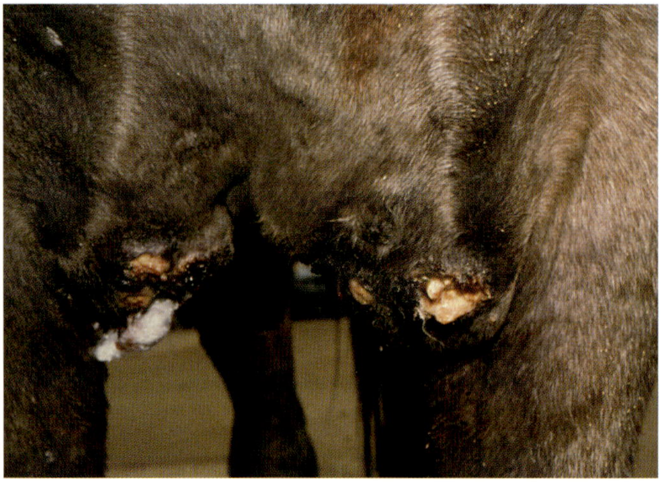

Figure 5.113 Multifocal, cutaneous, ulcerative fungal granulomas in the pectoral lymphatics of a horse with epizootic lymphangitis due to *Histoplasma capsulatum* var. *farciminosum.* The ulcerative granulomas were seen to be affecting the ventral abdomen and preputial sheath (fig. 5.114). This contagious fungal disease invades skin and enters lymphatics to cause cutaneous, ulcerative nodules that drain mucopurulent material. Definitive diagnosis is through a positive culture from affected tissues, cytology (fig. 5.115), or serology. Differential diagnosis includes sporotrichosis, ulcerative lymphangitis (*Corynebacterium pseudotuberculosis*), and farcy (*Burkholderia mallei*). Therapy may include the use of iodides, amphotericin B, or griseofulvin and a killed vaccine may be available in endemic regions. (Image courtesy of the Section of Pathology, Faculty of Veterinary Science, University of Pretoria)

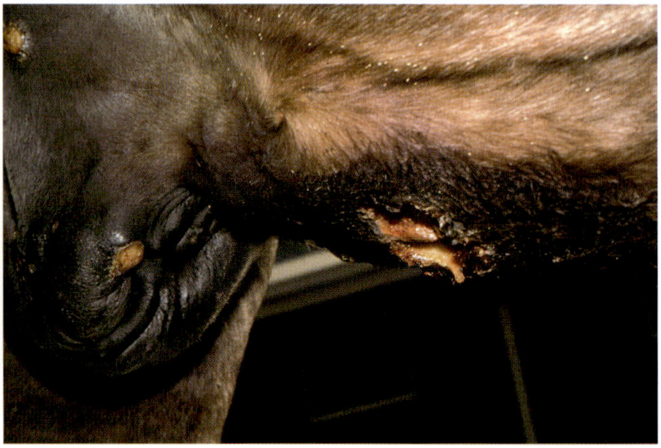

Figure 5.114 Cutaneous, ulcerative nodules along the ventral abdomen and preputial sheath of a horse with epizootic lymphangitis. (Image courtesy of the Section of Pathology, Faculty of Veterinary Science, University of Pretoria)

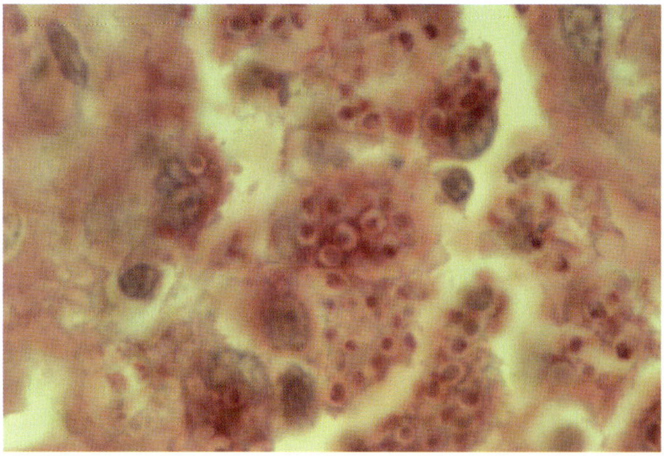

Figure 5.115 Photomicrograph of *Histoplasma capsulatum* var. *farciminosum* in an ulcerated nodule showing yeast organisms surrounded by clear halos (periodic acid-Schiff stain). (Image courtesy of the Section of Pathology, Faculty of Veterinary Science, University of Pretoria)

Junctional Epidermolysis Bullosa (JEB)

JEB is an inherited disease seen in Belgian and Belgian-cross foals. It is characterized by pressure sores, blistering, and sloughing of skin and hooves in newborn foals. Foals are born apparently normal and either succumb to infection or are humanely euthanized. Carrier animals have normal skin, but when bred, pass on the defective gene. Veterinary Diagnostic Laboratory at UC Davis offers a DNA test to identify carriers of the defective gene.

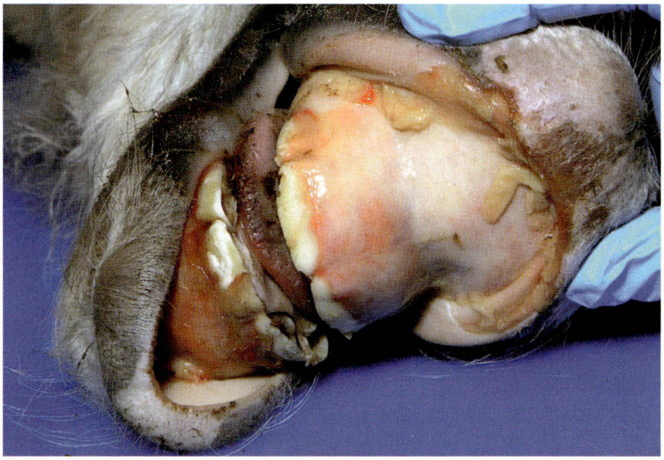

Figure 5.116 Blistering of gums and mucocutaneous junction of mouth.

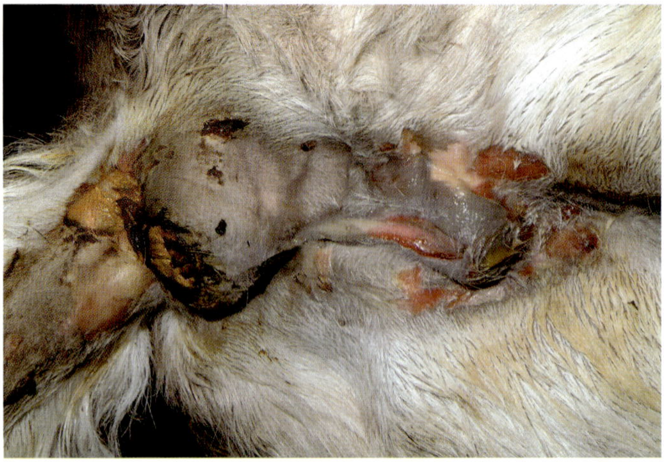

Figure 5.117 Blistering of perineal area.

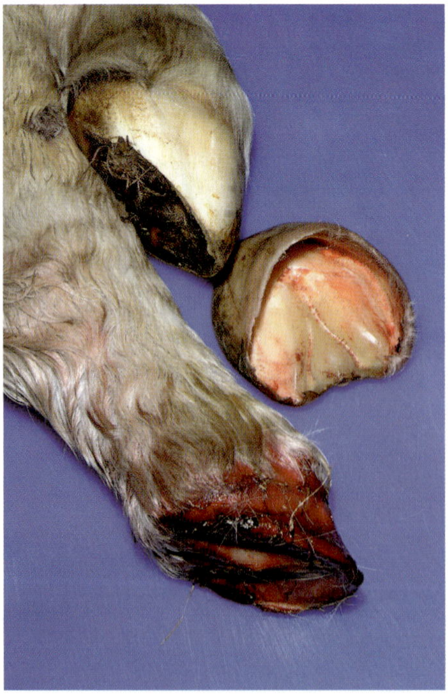

Figure 5.118 Sloughing of hoof or "red foot."

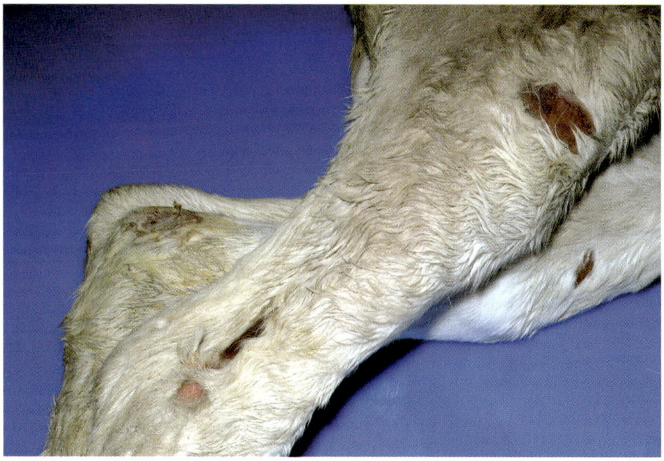

Figure 5.119 Pressure sores developing over bony protuberances.

Recommended Reading

Pascoe RR. Colour atlas of equine dermatology. Wolfe Publishing Ltd., 1990.
Pascoe RR, Knottenbelt DC. Manual of equine dermatology. London: Saunders, 1999.
Scott DW, Miller WH, Jr. Equine dermatology. St. Louis: Saunders, 2003.

6 Diseases of the Muscles

Diseases of the Muscles

- Hyperkalemic Periodic Paralysis (HYPP)
- Myopathies Associated with *Streptococcus equi* Infection
- Muscle Atrophy (Masseter Muscle)
- Sporadic Exertional Rhabdomyolysis (Tying Up, Monday Morning Disease)
- Polysaccharide Storage Myopathy (PSSM)
- Recurrent Exertional Rhabdomyolysis (RER)

Hyperkalemic Periodic Paralysis (HYPP)

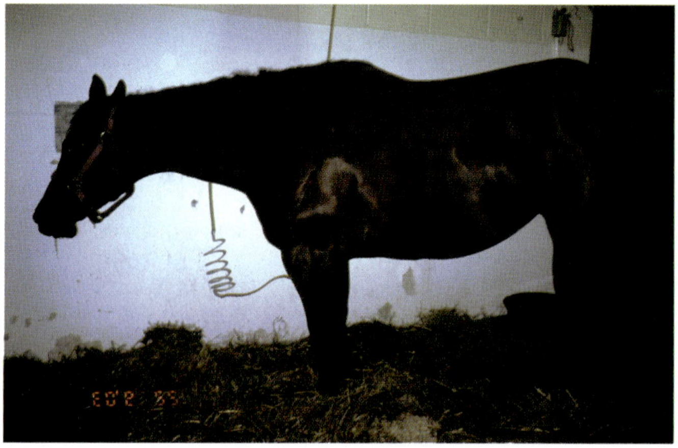

Figure 6.1 A quarter horse affected with hyperkalemic periodic paralysis. Note the sweating and muscle cramping. Hyperkalemic periodic paralysis is a disease that occurs in quarter horses, Appaloosas, and American paint horses. Affected horses are related to the quarter horse sire Impressive. The disease is inherited as an autosomal dominant trait. Clinical signs include episodes (usually 15–60 minutes) of sweating, muscle fasciculation and cramping, prolapsed third eyelid (fig. 6.2), myotonia, muscular weakness, dysphagia, and respiratory distress (fig. 6.3).

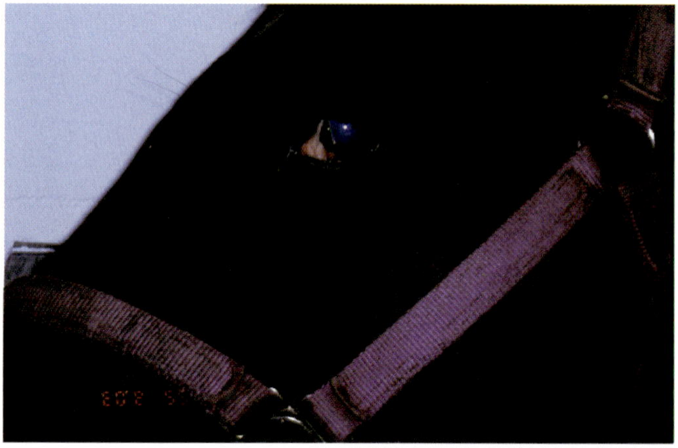

Figure 6.2 Prolapsed third eyelid in a horse affected with hyperkalemic periodic paralysis.

Figure 6.3 Respiratory distress and flaring of the nostrils in a horse affected with hyperkalemic periodic paralysis.

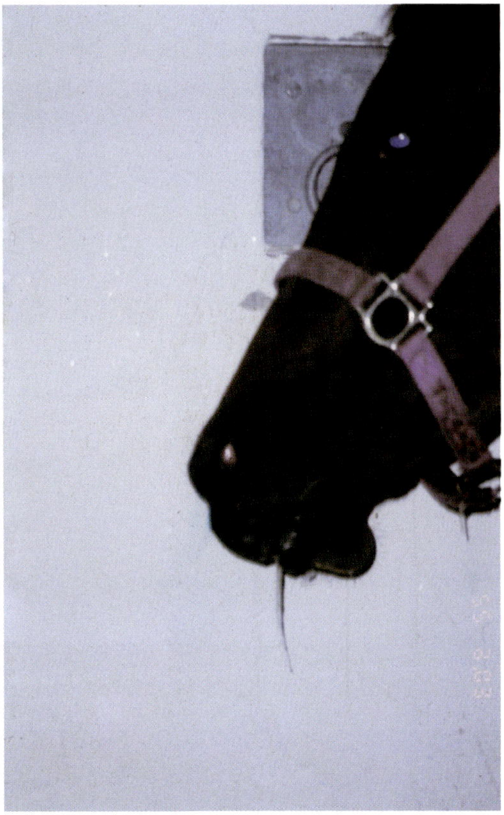

Myopathies Associated with *Streptococcus equi* Infection

Figure 6.4 An adult horse affected with *Streptococcus equi*–associated myositis. Note the severe muscle atrophy. In this case, clinical signs included malaise, rapid atrophy of the lumbar and gluteal muscles, fever, lethargy, elevated muscle enzymes, and low blood albumin concentration. Core biopsies of the gluteal muscles confirmed an antigen-associated myositis, believed to be *Streptococcus*. Treatment includes supportive care and corticosteroids administration. Relapse on subsequent exposure to *Streptococcus* antigen from both a vaccine and exposure to other horses is common.

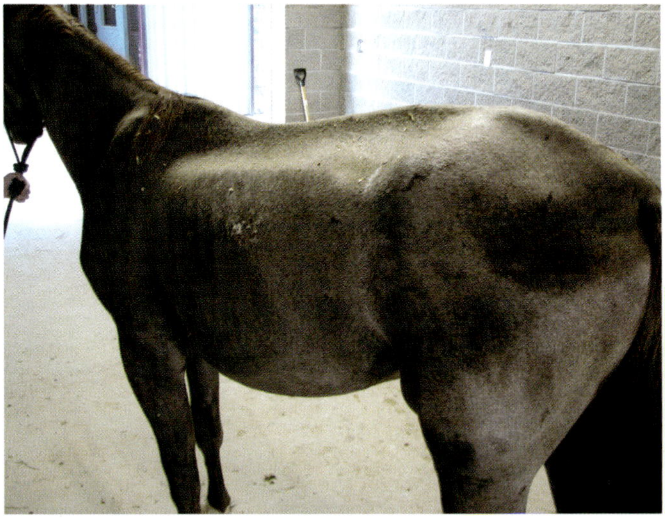

Muscle Atrophy (Masseter Muscle)

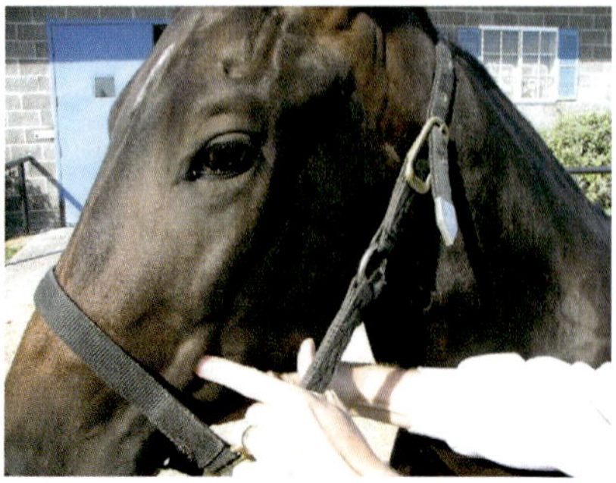

Figure 6.5 Masseter and temporal muscle atrophy in a 2-year-old quarter horse stallion. The atrophy occurred secondary to trauma during a trailer ride. Muscle atrophy is usually caused by denervation, disuse, malnutrition, cachexia, corticosteroid excess, and immune-mediated myositis.

Sporadic Exertional Rhabdomyolysis (Tying Up, Monday Morning Disease)

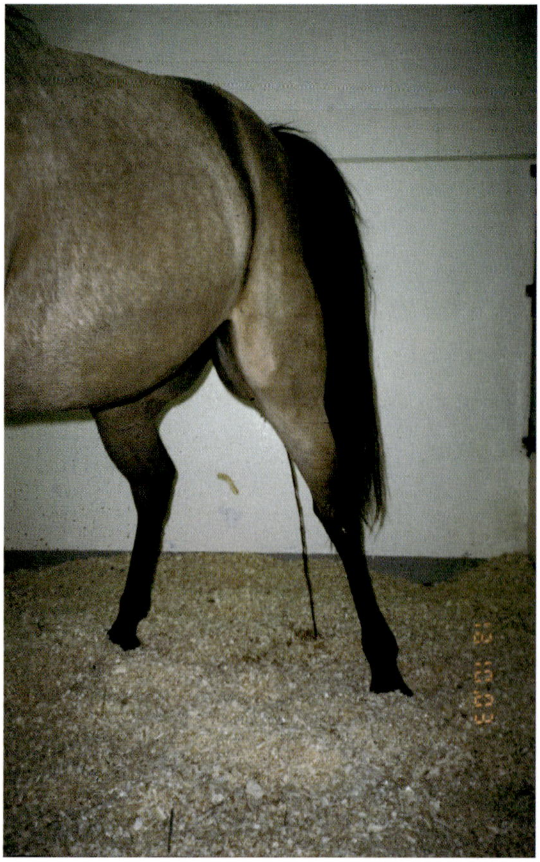

Figure 6.6 Myoglobinuria in a horse affected with sporadic exertional rhabdomyolysis (SER). SER is a multifactorial disease that is mainly caused by overexertion. Affected horses develop stiff, stilted gait, sweating, signs of colic, and reluctance to move.

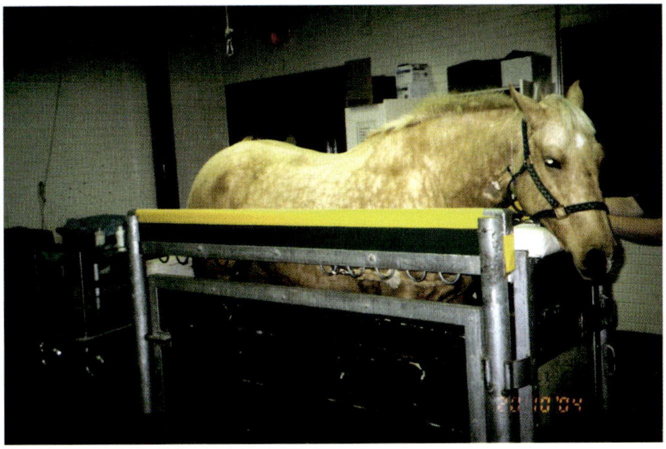

Figure 6.7 An adult horse affected with polysaccharide storage myopathy. PSSM is a glycogen storage disorder that is characterized by accumulation of abnormal polysaccharide and glycogen in the muscles. PSSM appears to be an inherited disease and affects Quarter horses, Paint, Appaloosa, Draft, and Warmbloods. Affected horses have numerous episodes of exertional rhabdomyolysis even after mild exercise. Diagnosis is based on histopathological examination of muscle biopsy (see figs. 6.8–6.12).

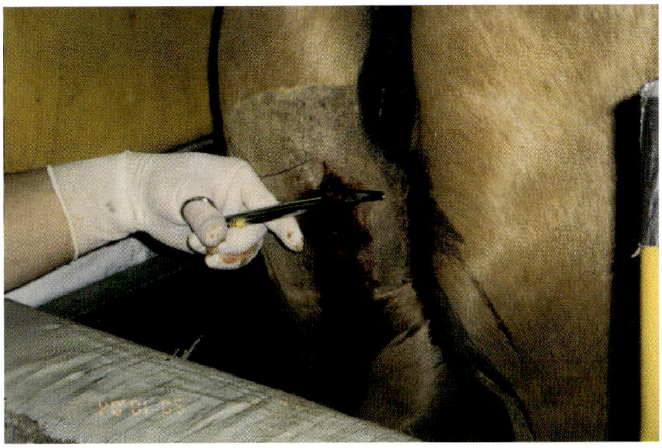

6.8

Figures 6.8–6.10 Semitendinosus/semimembranosus muscle biopsy obtained from the horse in fig. 6.7, and the biopsied muscle is mounted on a tongue depressor (fig. 6.10).

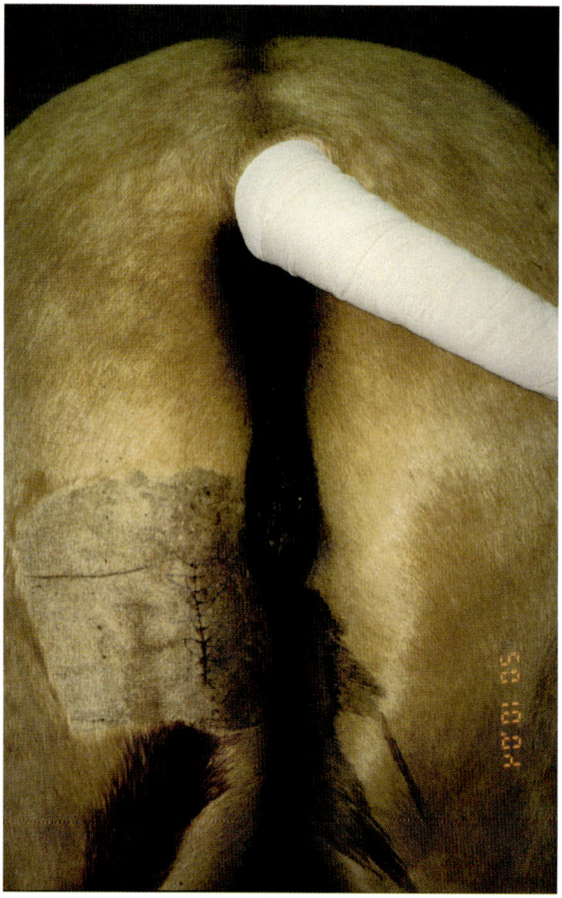

6.9

Figures 6.8–6.10 *Continued*

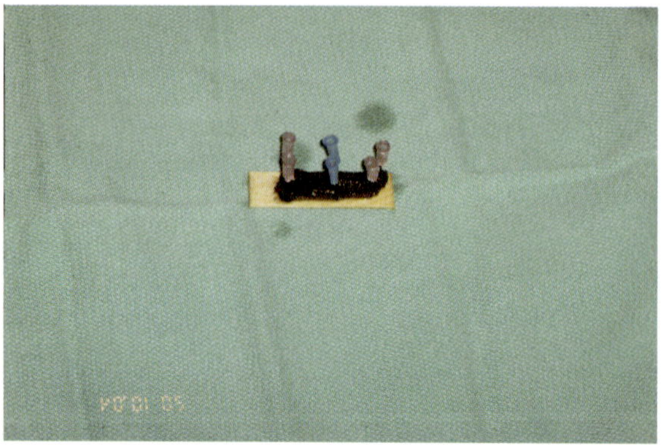

6.10

Figures 6.11–6.12 Periodic acid-Schiff stained slides for glycogen of muscles from a normal horse (fig. 6.11) and a horse affected with PSSM (fig. 6.12). Muscles affected with PSSM have dark stain and aggregates of intensely stained abnormal polysaccharides (fig. 6.12). (Images courtesy of Dr. S. Valberg, University of Minnesota)

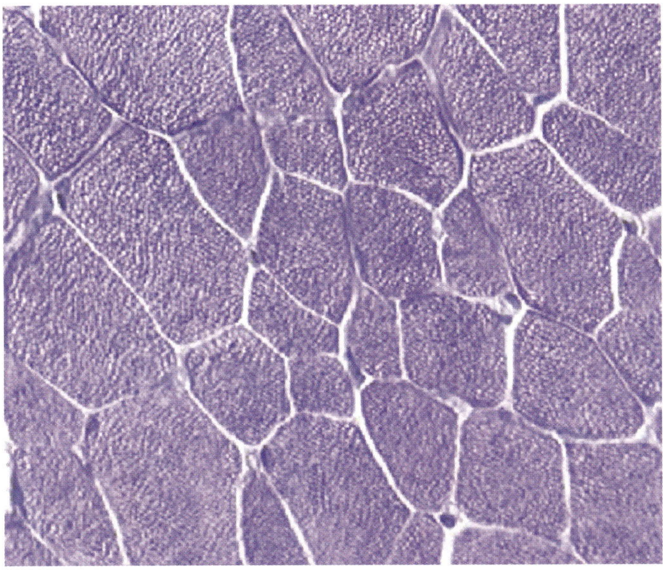

6.11

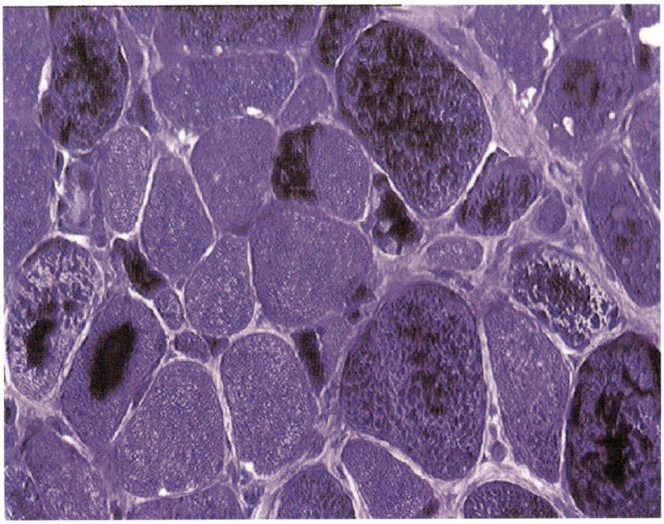

6.12

Recurrent Exertional Rhabdomyolysis (RER)

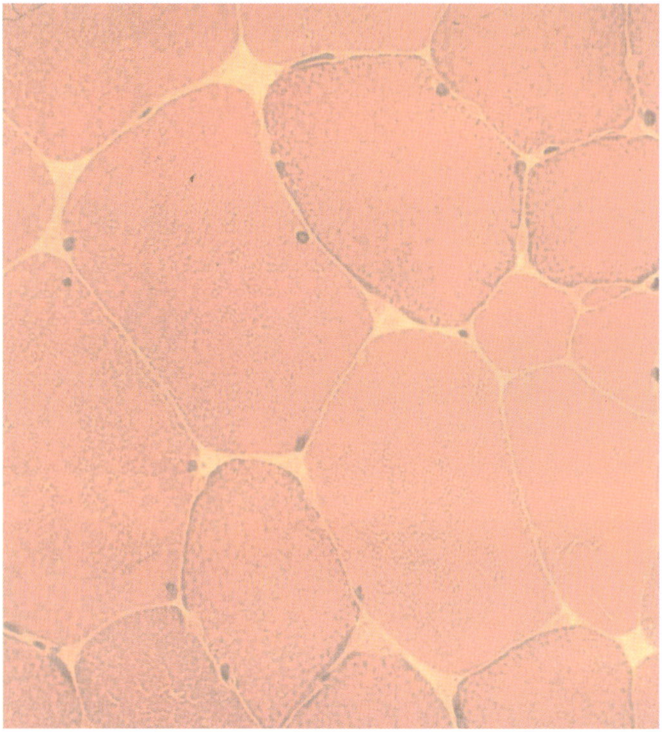

6.13

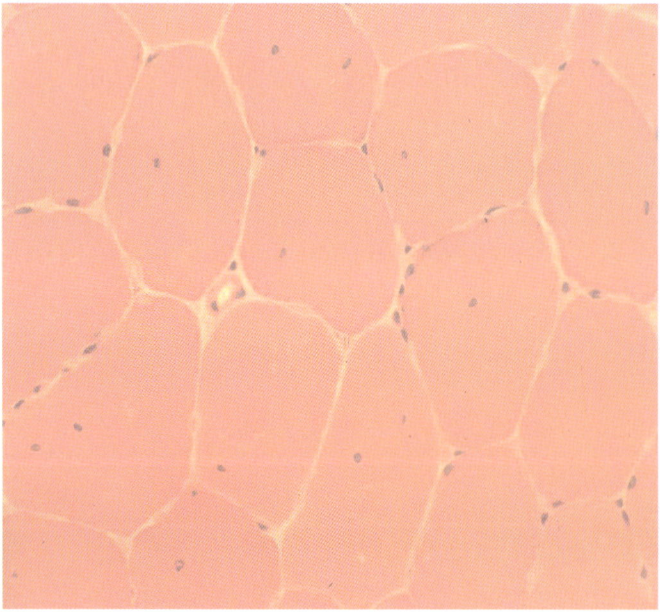

6.14

Figures 6.13–6.14 Hematoxylin and eosin stained slides of muscles obtained from a normal horse (fig. 6.13) and a horse affected with recurrent exertional rhabdomyolysis (fig. 6.14). Note the muscle fibers with numerous and centrally located nuclei (fig. 6.14). RER is a disease of racing Thoroughbreds, Standardbreds, and Arabian horses. Affected horses have recurrent episodes of muscle stiffness, sweating, and reluctance to move. Diagnosis is based on histopathological examination of muscle biopsy (fig. 6.14). (Images courtesy of Dr. S. Valberg, University of Minnesota)

Recommended Reading

Firshman AM, Valberg SJ, Bender J, Finno C. Epidemiologic characteristics and management of polysaccharide storage myopathy in quarter horses. Am J Vet Res. 64:1319–27, 2003.

Naylor JM, Nickel DD, Trimino G, Card C, Lightfoot K, Adams G. Hyperkalaemic periodic paralysis in homozygous and heterozygous horses: a co-dominant genetic condition. Equine Vet J. 31(2):153–59, 1999.

Valberg SJ. Diagnostic Approach to muscle disorders. In-depth muscle disorders. 52nd Proc American Assoc Equine Pract. 53:340–46, 2006.

Valberg SJ. Exertional rhabdomyolysis and polysaccharide storage myopathy in Quarter Horses. American Assoc Equine Pract. 228–30, 1995.

Valberg SJ, Geyer CJ, Sorum S, Cardinet GH, III. Familial basis of polysaccharide storage myopathy and exertional rhabdomyolysis in Quarter Horses and related breeds. Am J Vet Res. 57:286–90, 1996.

7 Diseases of the Bones, Joints, and Connective Tissues

The Navicular Bone
- Normal Radiographic Appearance of the Navicular Bone
- Navicular Bone Cysts, Enlarged and Abnormally Shaped Synovial Invaginations, and Enthesopathy
- Degenerative Change of the Navicular Bone
- Navicular Bone Fracture
- Nuclear Scintigraphic Imaging of the Navicular Bone

The Phalanges
- Osteoarthritis of the Proximal Interphalangeal Joint (High Ringbone)
- Osteoarthritis of the Distal Interphalangeal Joint
- Fracture of the Extensor Process of the Third Phalanx
- Nonarticular Fracture of the Wing of the Third Phalanx
- Articular Fracture of the Wing of the Third Phalanx
- Sagittal Fracture of the Third Phalanx
- Fracture of the Palmar Process of the Third Phalanx
- Osteomyelitis of the Third Phalanx
- Keratoma
- Ossification of the Accessory Cartilages of the Third Phalanx (Sidebone)
- Subchondral Cystic Lesion of the First Phalanx
- Subchondral Cystic Lesion of the Second Phalanx
- Subchondral Cystic Lesion of the Third Phalanx
- Complete Fracture of the First Phalanx
- Laminitis with Rotation and Laminar Separation
- Chronic Laminitis
- Assessment of the Third Phalanx Rotation

The Metacarpophalangeal and Metatarsophalangeal Joints (Fetlock Joint)
- Osteoarthritis
- Chronic Proliferative Synovitis
- Osteochondritis Dissecans (OCD)
- Sesamoiditis
- Septic Arthritis and Osteomyelitis
- Fracture of the Proximal Sesamoid Bone
- Fracture of the Proximal First Phalanx
- Fracture of the Third Metacarpus
- Fracture (Chip) of the Dorsoproximal First Phalanx
- Osseous Fragmentation of the Lateral Plantar Process of the First Phalanx
- Osseous Fragment Arising from the Plantar Margin of the First Phalanx

The Carpus and Metacarpus
- Soft Tissue Swelling of the Carpus
- Osteoarthritis
- Normal Third Carpal Bone and Third Carpal Bone with Mild Sclerosis of the Radial Facet
- Nuclear Scintigraphic Imaging of the Carpus
- Fracture of the Radial Carpal Bone
- Fracture of the Distal Radius
- Fracture of the Third Carpal Bone
- Ulnar Carpal Bone Cyst
- Radial Cysts
- Enchondroma and Enthesiophyte Formation at the Attachment of the Superior Check Ligament
- Metacarpal Periostitis ("Bucked Shin")
- Stress Fracture of the Third Metacarpus
- Avulsion Fracture of the Origin of the Suspensory Ligament
- Periostitis (Bony Reaction) at the Origin of the Suspensory Ligament
- Splint Exostosis ("Splint") of the Second Metacarpal Bone
- Fracture of the Fourth Metacarpal Bone with an Evidence of Osteomyelitis

The Tarsus and Metatarsus
- Osteochondritis Dissecans (OCD)
- Osteoarthritis (Degenerative Joint Disease, "Spavin")
- Fracture of the Talus
- Sequestration of the Calcaneus
- Fracture of the Fourth Metatarsal Bone
- Fracture and Osteomyelitis of the Fourth Metatarsal Bone
- Sequestrum Formation on the Third Metatarsal Bone

The Stifle and Tibia
- Subchondral Bone Cyst
- Osteochondritis Dissecans (OCD)
- Osteoarthritis of the Stifle Joint
- Cranial Cruciate Ligament Injury
- Fracture of the Patella
- Calcinosis Circumscripta (Tumoral Calcinosis)
- Tibial Stress Fracture

The Spine
- Normal Cervical Spine
- Malalignment and Compression of the Spinal Canal
- Articular Facet Reaction (Bone Proliferation)
- Cervical Vertebral Malformation Instability (Wobbler's Syndrome)
- Osteomyelitis of the Third Cervical Vertebra

The Head
- Anatomy of the Skull
- Sinusitis
- Sinus Cyst
- Ethmoid Hematoma
- Normal Dental Structures
- Tooth Root Abscess

Anatomy of the Pharynx and Guttural Pouches (Auditory Diverticula)
Guttural Pouches Empyema
Normal Larynx and Aryepiglottic Fold Entrapment
Fracture of the Sphenoid Bone and Guttural Pouch Hemorrhage
Dental Tumor of the Mandible
Mandibular Osteomyelitis

Normal Radiographic Appearance of the Navicular Bone

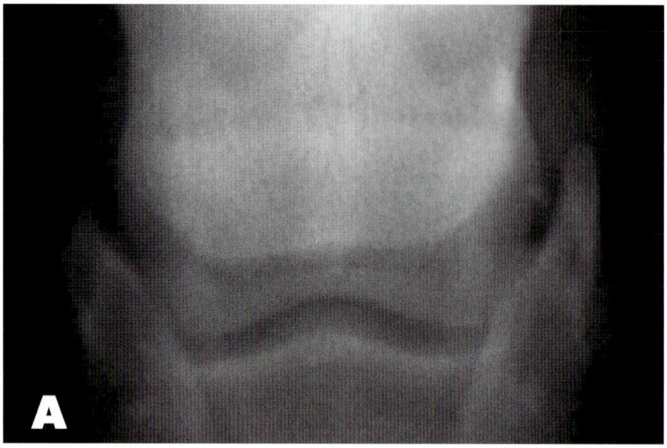

Figures 7.1a,b Dorsoproximal-palmarodistal oblique radiographic projections of the navicular bone of two horses. **Normal radiographic appearance of the navicular bone:** (A) There are no visible synovial invaginations along the distal border of the bone. (B) Several small triangular synovial invaginations are present on the distal border of the bone only. Both of these radiographic appearances are considered within the range of normal.

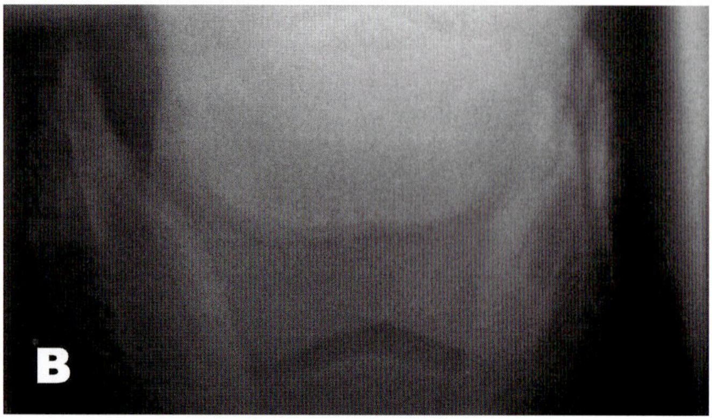

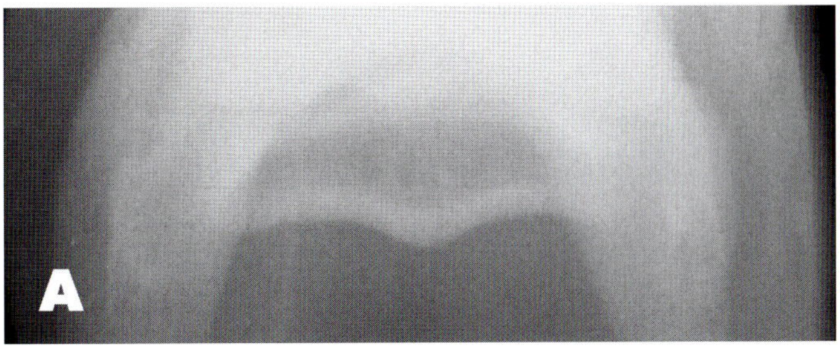

Figures 7.2a,b Palmaroproximal-palmarodistal oblique radiographic projections of the navicular bone of two horses. **Normal radiographic appearance of the navicular bone:** (A) Small synovial invaginations are barely visible within the medullary portion of the bone. (B) Two small, linear synovial invaginations are visible within the medullary portion of the bone. Normally, there should be no more than 5–7 of these invaginations and they should be tubular and narrow. Both of these radiographic appearances are considered within the range of normal.

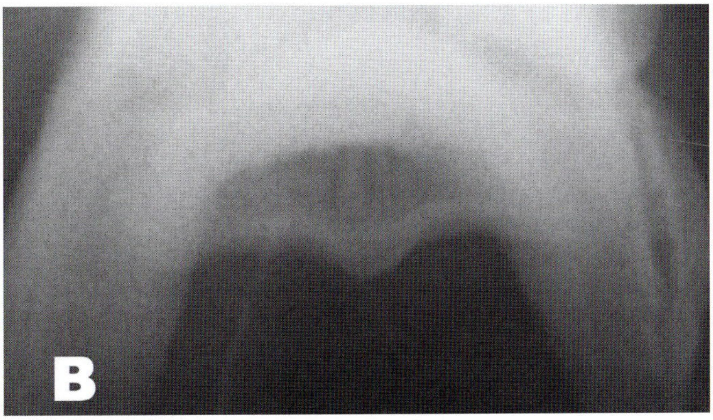

Navicular Bone Cysts, Enlarged and Abnormally Shaped Synovial Invaginations, and Enthesopathy

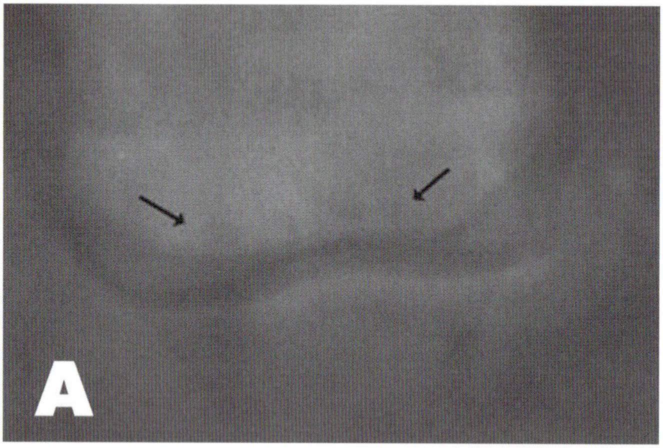

Figures 7.3a,b Dorsoproximal-palmarodistal oblique radiographic projections of the navicular bone of two horses. **(A) Enlarged and abnormally shaped synovial invaginations; (B) navicular bone cysts:** In (A) the synovial invaginations are increased in size and abnormally shaped (arrows). Several of them have a rounded appearance with a stalk extending to the margin of the bone; the term "lollipop" is often used to describe these lesions. The abnormal synovial invaginations are visible only on the distal border of the bone. In (B), several large round lucencies are present within navicular bone (arrows). This type of abnormal synovial invagination is often described as a cyst. Both of these radiographic appearances are considered evidence of navicular degeneration.

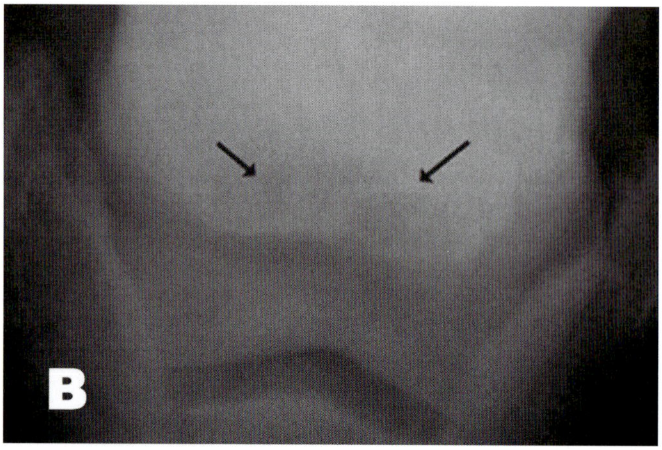

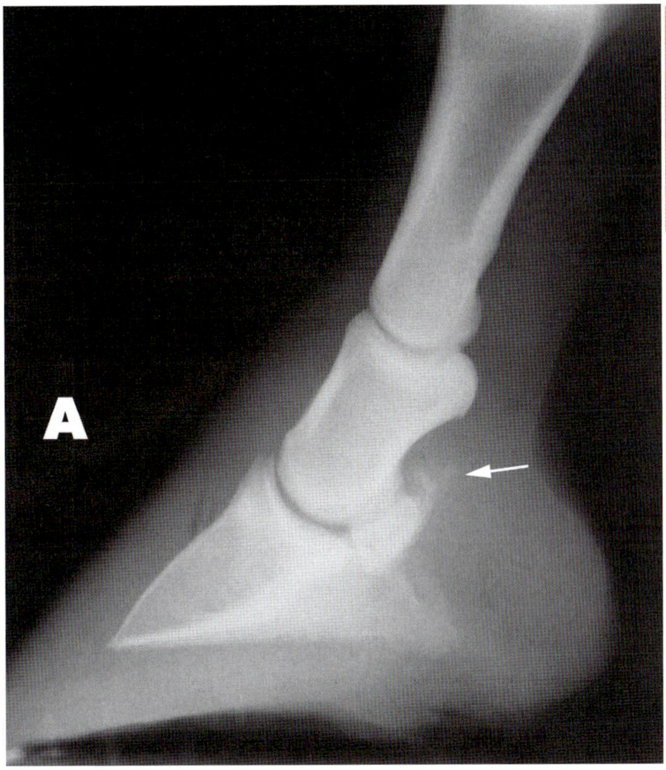

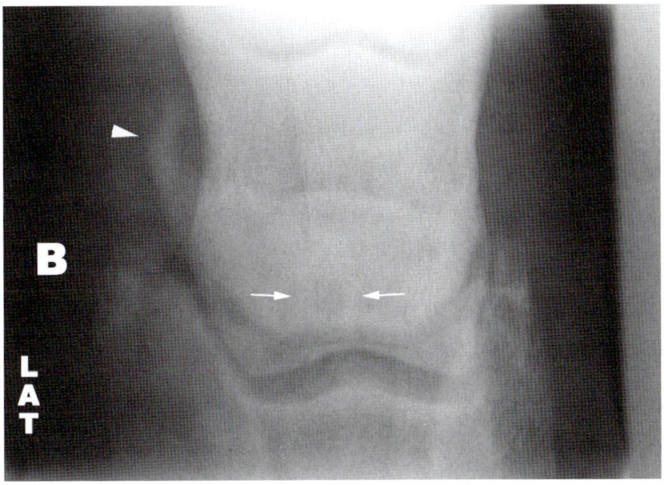

Figures 7.4a,b Lateral (A) and dorsoproximal-palmarodistal oblique (B) radiographic projections of the right forefoot of a 13-year-old quarter horse. **Navicular bone cyst with enthesopathy:** (A) In the lateral radiograph there is obvious bone production proximal to the navicular bone (arrow). The bone appears to arise from the proximal border of the navicular bone but the precise location cannot be determined with only a single view. (B) A dorsoproximal-palmarodistal oblique view of the same foot is used to show the proximal margin of the navicular bone. A large enthesophyte (arrowhead) is seen arising from the area of attachment of the lateral suspensory ligament of the navicular. Enthesophytes are considered evidence of abnormal tension on the suspensory apparatus of the navicular bone. A large cyst (arrow) is visible within the medullary cavity of the navicular bone.

Degenerative Change of the Navicular Bone

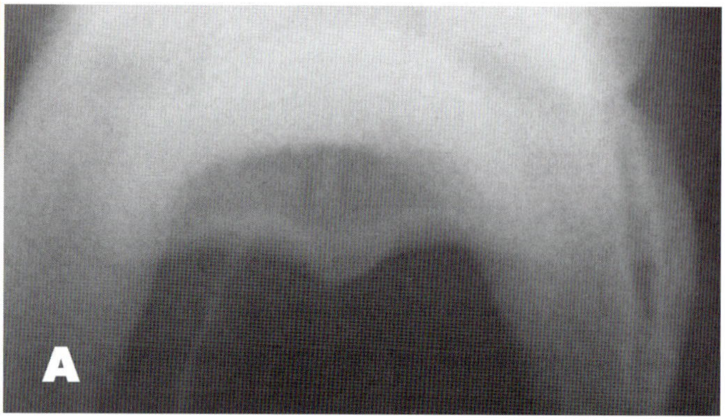

Figures 7.5a,b Palmaroproximal-palmarodistal oblique radiographic projections of the navicular bone of two horses. **(A) Normal radiographic appearance of the navicular bone; (B) degenerative change of the navicular bone:** In (B) there are several synovial invaginations visible within the medullary cavity. The synovial invaginations are not excessive in number but are enlarged—notice how "plump" they appear (arrows).

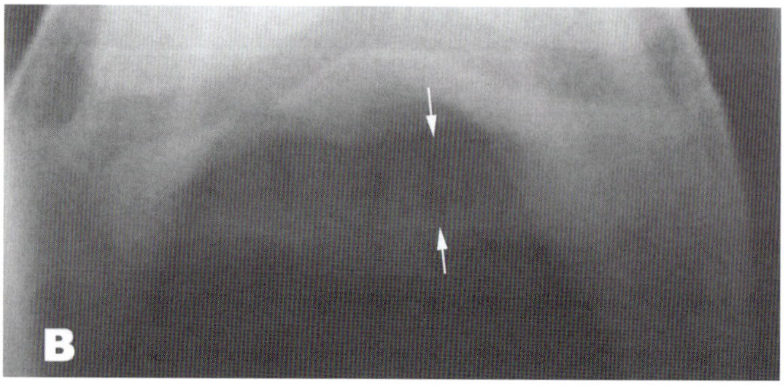

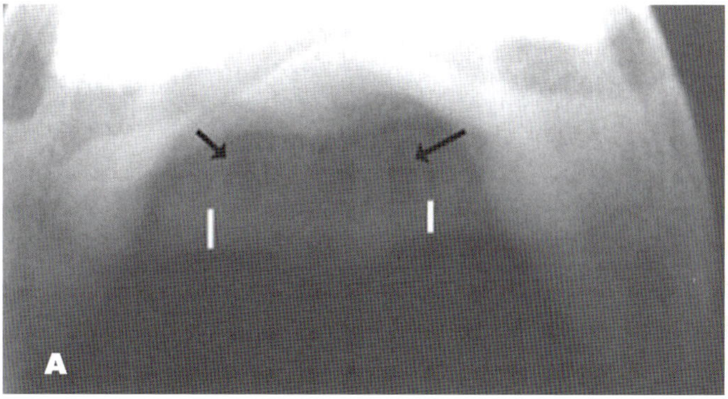

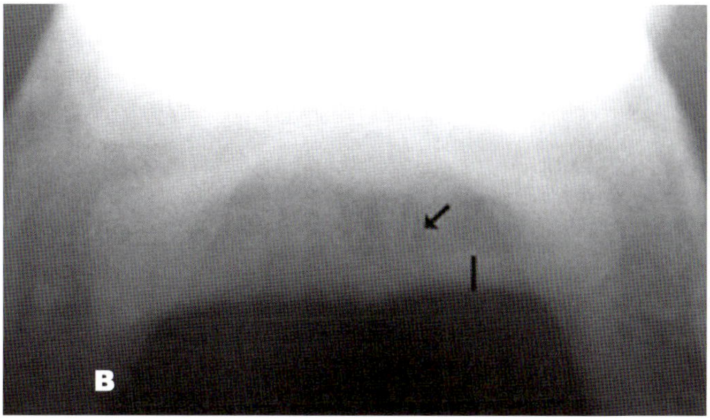

Figures 7.6a,b Palmaroproximal-palmarodistal oblique radiographic projections of the navicular bone of two horses. **(A) and (B) Degenerative change of the navicular bone:** Several changes are present within the navicular bone in (A). These include thickening of the flexor cortex with decreased distinction between the cortex and medulla of the navicular bone on the left side (white lines). Enlarged synovial invaginations are also present (arrows). In (B) sclerosis of the medullary cavity causes loss of the normal clear distinction between the cortical and medullary portions of the bone. This change is visible along the left side of this navicular bone. The black line indicates the normal flexor cortex. A large cyst is also faintly visible within the medullary cavity (arrow). The radiographic changes present in these navicular bones are evidence of severe navicular degeneration. These types of radiographic changes can be assessed only in the palmaroproximal-palmarodistal oblique radiographic projection, so it is important to include this view in the routine radiographic evaluation of the navicular bone.

Navicular Bone Fracture

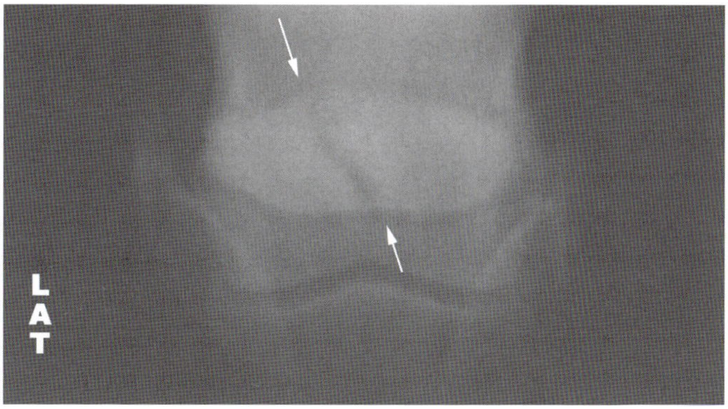

Figure 7.7 Dorsoproximal-palmarodistal oblique radiographic projection of a 6-year-old Standardbred. **Navicular bone fracture:** A fracture line is easily seen in the navicular bone. The fracture is wide and the margins are indistinct. These changes are typical of a chronic fracture. Most navicular bone fractures occur in navicular bones with significant underlying degenerative change; fracture of a normal navicular bone is extremely uncommon.

Nuclear Scintigraphic Imaging of the Navicular Bone

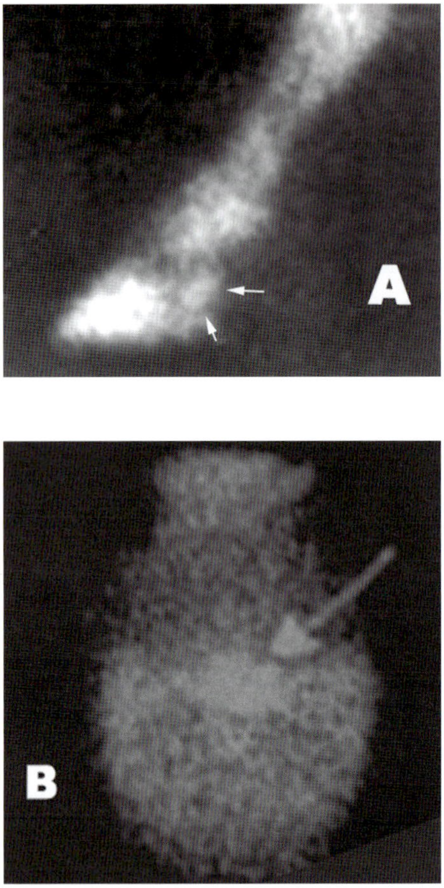

Figures 7.8a,b Lateral (A) and solar (B) views from the bone phase of a scintigraphic study of a 7-year-old quarter horse. **Moderate, diffuse isotope uptake in the navicular bone:** The navicular bone is not generally visible as a distinct structure in the bone phase of a scintigraphic study. In horses with navicular degeneration, bone activity is present and isotope uptake increases. The uptake in the navicular bone is visible at the palmar aspect of the distal interphalangeal joint (arrows) in the lateral view and at the caudal margin of the third phalanx (arrow) in the solar view.

Osteoarthritis of the Proximal Interphalangeal Joint (High Ringbone)

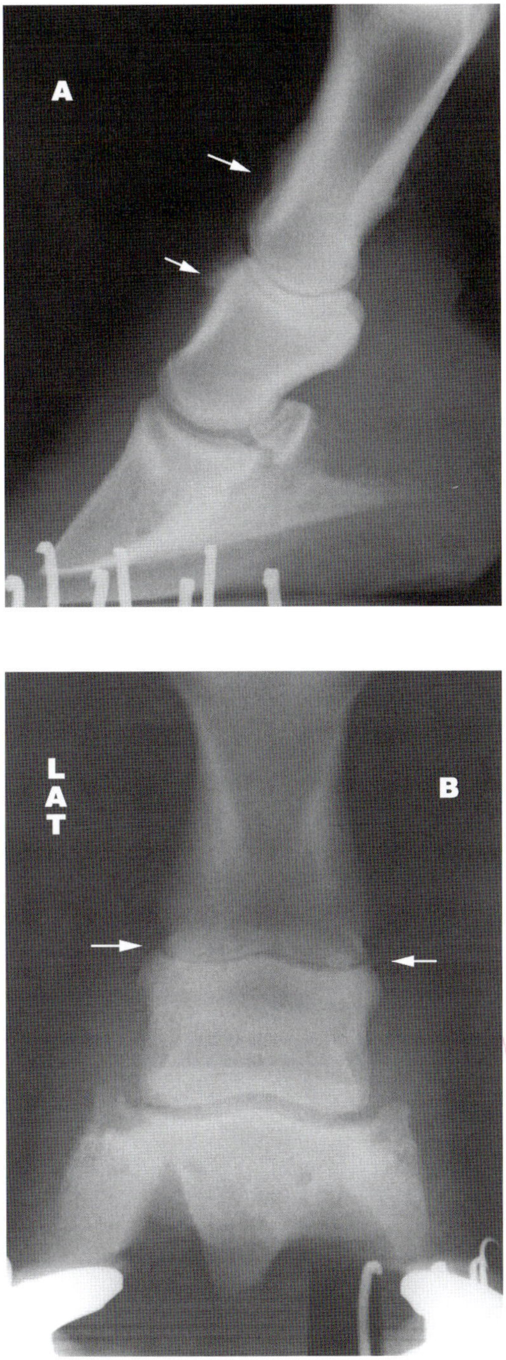

Figures 7.9a,b Lateral (A) and dorsopalmar (B) radiographic projections of the right proximal interphalangeal joint of a 13-year-old Appaloosa. **Osteoarthritis of the proximal interphalangeal joint (high ringbone):** Significant periosteal response is present on the dorsal margins of the proximal interphalangeal joint (white arrows). Notice that the periosteal response extends well away from the joint margins. This is often termed "extra-articular" ringbone. Narrowing of the proximal interphalangeal joint space (arrows) is present. With careful evaluation, subchondral lucencies can be seen in the distal surface of the proximal phalanx.

Osteoarthritis of the Distal Interphalangeal Joint

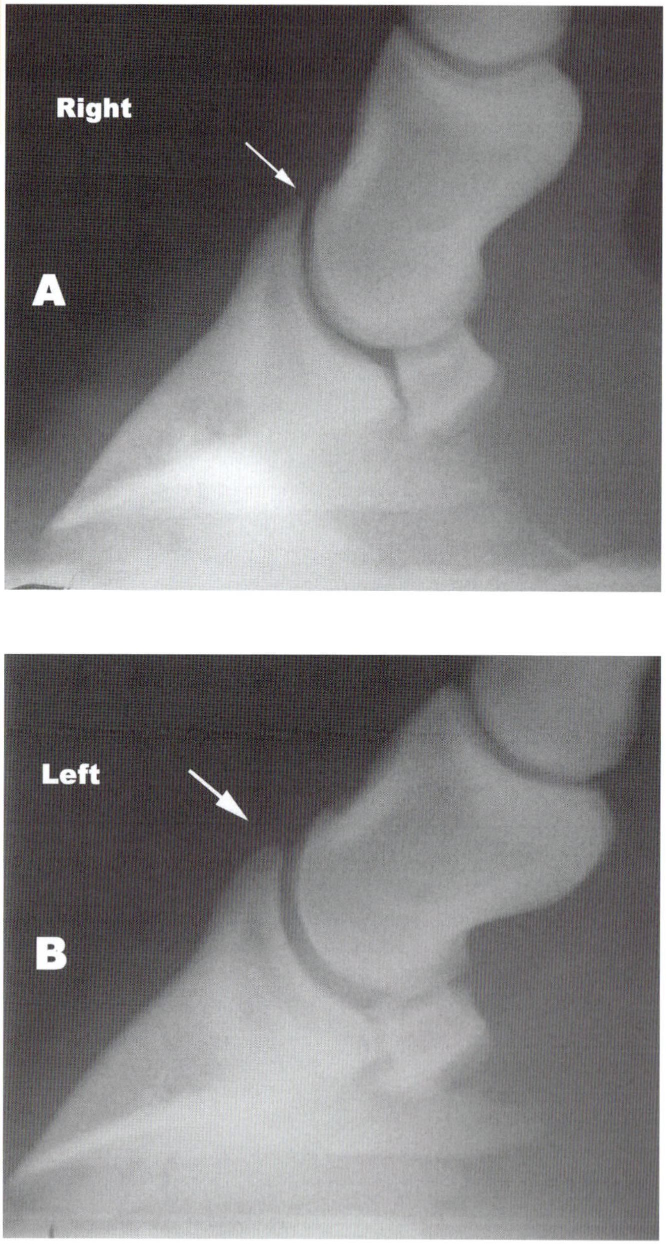

Figures 7.10a,b Lateral radiographic projections of the right (A) and left (B) distal interphalangeal joints of a 5-year-old quarter horse. **(A) Osteoarthritis of the right distal interphalangeal joint; (B) normal left distal interphalangeal joint:** Remodeling of the extensor process of the third phalanx has created a sharp dorsal extension of the bone (arrow). The dorsal aspect of the distal interphalangeal joint is narrow. The left distal interphalangeal joint is normal in appearance and was provided for comparison. There can be significant variation in the normal appearance of the extensor process but normal variation should be bilateral and is not in this case. Also, the extensor process is thought to be too sharply pointed to be within the range of normal anatomic variation.

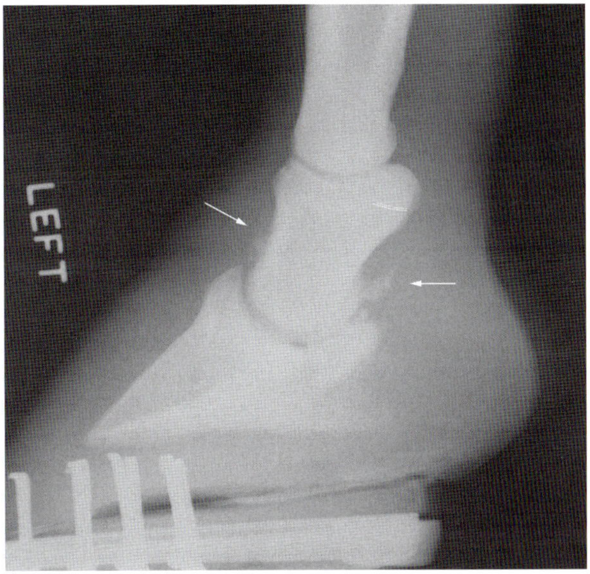

Figure 7.11 Lateral radiographic projection of the left distal interphalangeal joint of a 10-year-old Thoroughbred. **Osteoarthritis of the left distal interphalangeal joint:** Changes of osteoarthritis include remodelling of the extensor process of the third phalanx and proliferative new bone arising at the junction of the articular cartilage and distal interphalangeal joint capsule at the dorsal and palmar aspects of the joint (arrows). Subluxation of the distal interphalangeal joint "broken hoof-pastern axis" is also noted. Injury to the supporting ligamentous structures resulting in subluxation of the joint is suspected to be the underlying cause for the osteoarthritis.

Fracture of the Extensor Process of the Third Phalanx

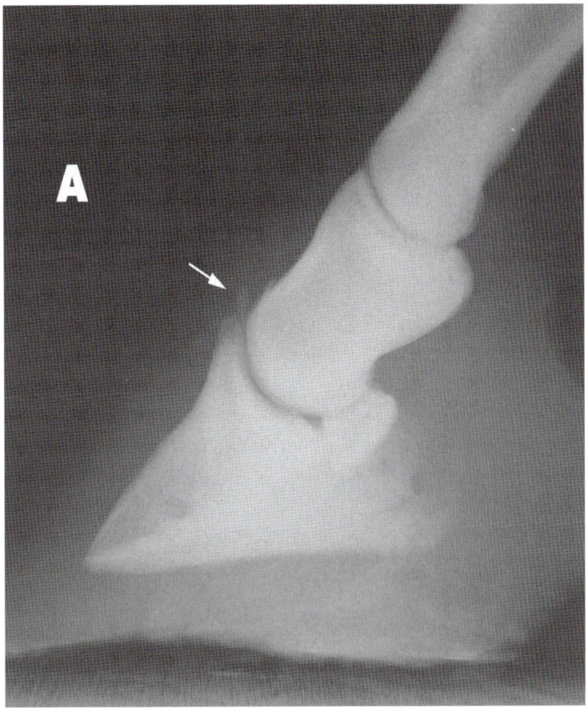

Figures 7.12a,b Lateral radiographic projections of the right distal interphalangeal joints of a 9-year-old (A) and a 7-year-old Hanoverian (B). **Fracture of the extensor process of the third phalanx:** In (A) the fracture fragment is small and has rounded margins (arrow). There is no evidence of osteoarthritis of the joint. The smooth margins of the osseous fragment and the lack of osteoarthritis suggest that this fracture is an incidental finding, not a cause of lameness. Intra-articular analgesia would be needed to determine the significance of this finding in a lame patient. In (B) the fracture fragment is very large and the fracture line is very wide and irregular (arrowhead). Marked sclerosis of the bone is present surrounding the fracture line. There is osteophyte formation on the extensor process (arrow) indicating that osteoarthritis is present. This is a chronic fracture of the extensor process; the fracture was known to have occurred 3 years previously. Remarkably enough this fracture was not a cause of lameness in this patient.

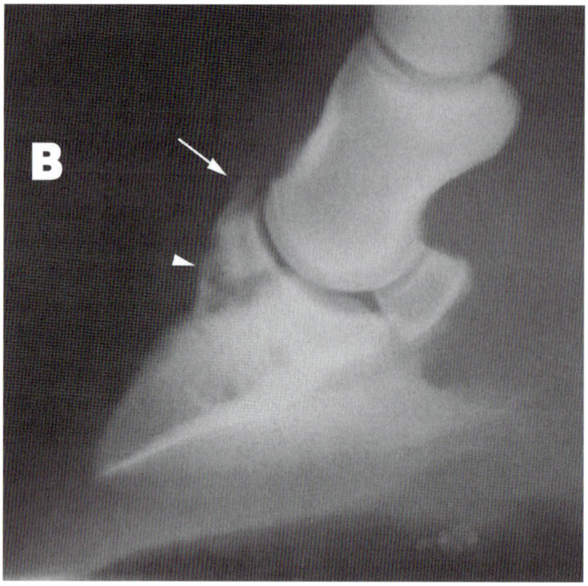

Figures 7.12a,b *Continued*

Nonarticular Fracture of the Wing of the Third Phalanx

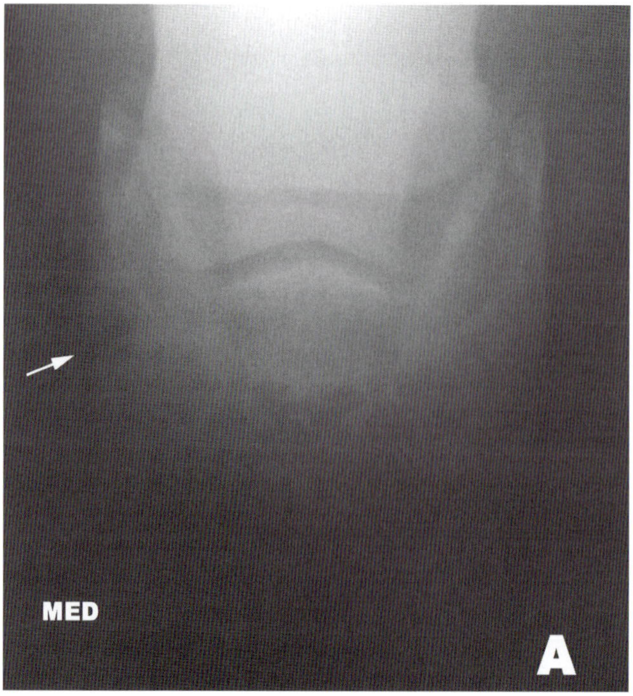

Figures 7.13a,b Dorsoproximal-palmarodistal oblique (A) and dorsoproximomedial-palmarodistolateral oblique (B) radiographic projections of the right fore third phalanx of a 6-year-old Hanoverian. **Nonarticular fracture of the medial wing of the third phalanx:** The fracture line is barely visible in the dorsoproximal-palmarodistal oblique view (arrow). Without careful assessment, this lucency might be mistaken for a normal vascular channel. In the dorsoproximomedial-palmarodistolateral oblique radiographic projection, the fracture line is much more distinctly seen (arrows). The fracture extends to the junction of the medial wing with the articular surface of the third phalanx. This is considered a nonarticular fracture or type 1 fracture of the third phalanx. This study demonstrates the importance of oblique radiographic projections if a fracture of the third phalanx is suspected.

Figures 7.13a,b *Continued*

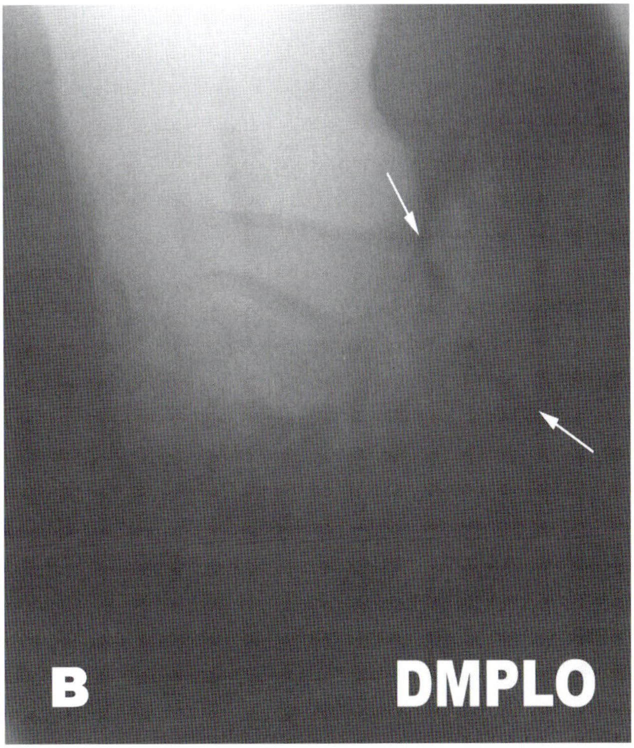

Articular Fracture of the Wing of the Third Phalanx

Figures 7.14a,b Dorsoproximal-palmarodistal oblique (A) and dorsoproximomedial-palmarodistolateral oblique (B) radiographic projections of the right fore third phalanx of a 3-year-old Standardbred. **Articular fracture of the medial wing of the third phalanx:** In this case the fracture line is much more visible in the dorsoproximal-palmarodistal oblique view (arrows). The fracture line appears wide and indistinct because it is not aligned exactly parallel to the X-ray beam. In the dorsoproximomedial-palmarodistolateral oblique view, the X-ray beam is parallel to the plane of the fracture and the fracture appears as a single line (arrows). The fracture extends to the articular surface and subtle malalignment of the articular surface is noted; this is often described as a "step" in the articular surface. This fracture is classified as a type 2 fracture of the third phalanx since it involves the articular surface.

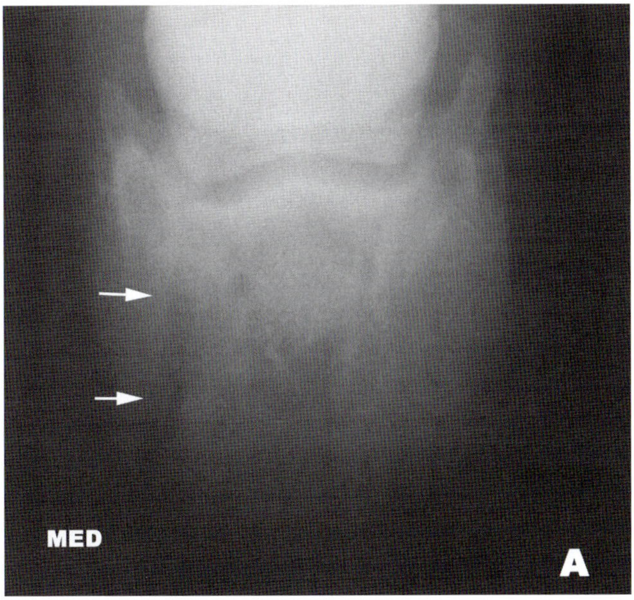

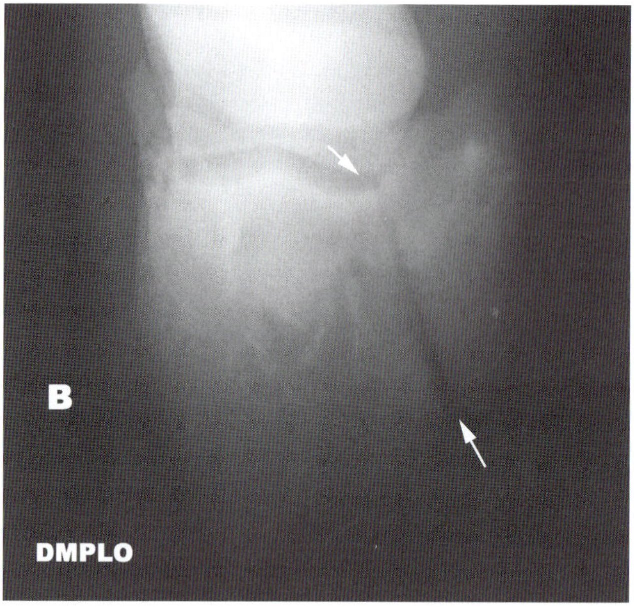

Figures 7.14a,b *Continued*

Sagittal Fracture of the Third Phalanx

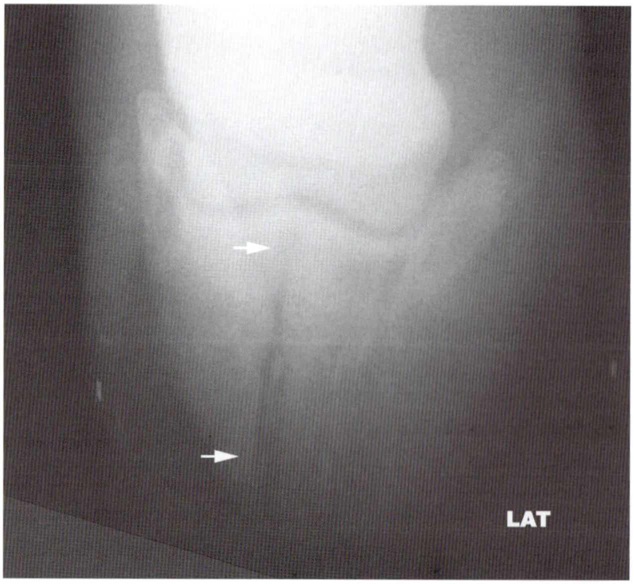

Figure 7.15 Dorsoproximal–palmarodistal oblique radiographic projection of the right fore third phalanx of a 10-year-old Morgan. **Sagittal fracture of the third phalanx:** This dorsoproximal-palmarodistal oblique radiographic projection is somewhat poorly positioned due to the patient's reluctance to bear weight. A fracture line is seen centrally in the third phalanx extending from the solar margin of the bone to the articular surface. A midsagittal fracture of the third phalanx is classified as a type 3 fracture.

Fracture of the Palmar Process of the Third Phalanx

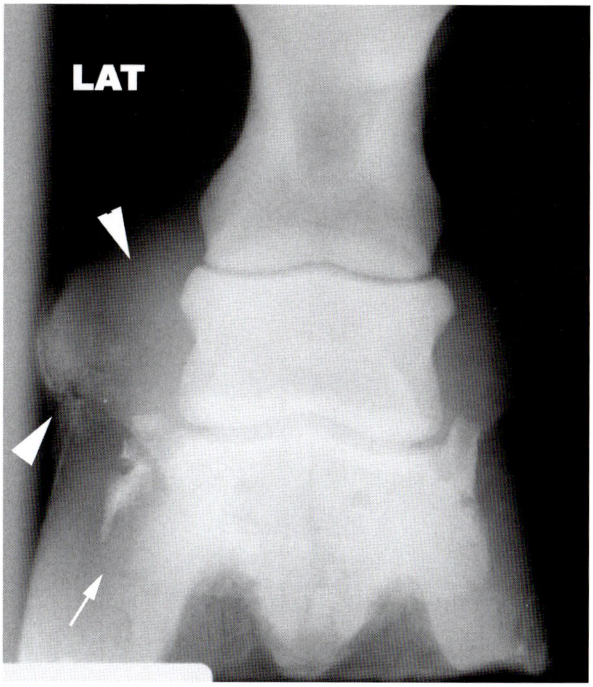

Figure 7.16 Dorsopalmar horizontal beam radiographic projection of the left forefoot in a 4-year-old Thoroughbred. **Fracture of the lateral palmar process of the third phalanx:** A portion of the lateral palmar process is separated from the third phalanx (arrow). There is marked thickening and irregularity of the soft tissues on the lateral aspect of the hoof in the area of the coronary band. The soft tissue changes are the result of a hoof abscess that migrated dorsally and drained at the coronary band. The fracture is likely secondary to osteomyelitis of the third phalanx. This is quite an unusual fracture configuration that was only visible in the dorsopalmar horizontal beam view. This view of the third phalanx is not routinely performed but can be useful in some cases.

Osteomyelitis of the Third Phalanx

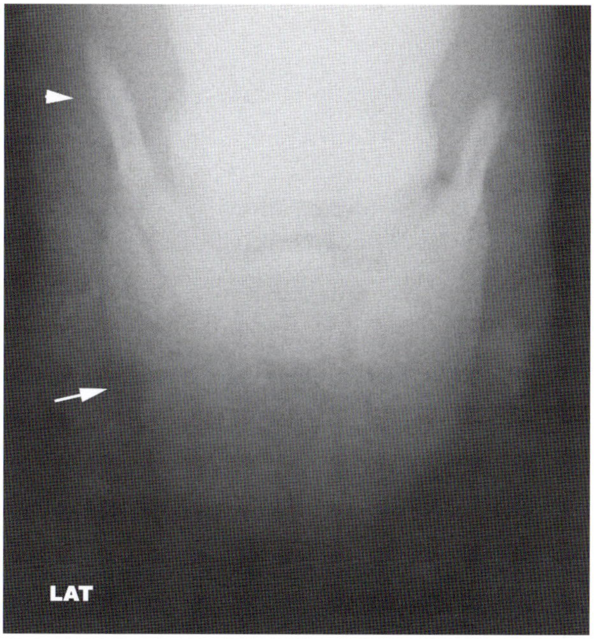

Figure 7.17 Dorsoproximal-palmarodistal oblique radiographic projection of the left fore third phalanx of a 9-year-old Hunter. **Osteomyelitis of the lateral margin of the third phalanx:** A focal lytic lesion is present on the lateral solar margin of the third phalanx (arrow). This is considered an evidence of osteomyelitis. Mineralization of the lateral accessory cartilage of the third phalanx, "sidebone," is also noted (arrowhead). This finding is usually of little clinical significance. Areas of mineral opacity in the hoof adjacent to the third phalanx are debris. Osteomyelitis of the third phalanx is relatively uncommon but can occur as a sequela to a sole abscess or solar penetration with a foreign object. In this case, the horse had been treated for a sole abscess for several weeks with no significant improvement; this history is a good indication for radiographic evaluation of the third phalanx.

Keratoma

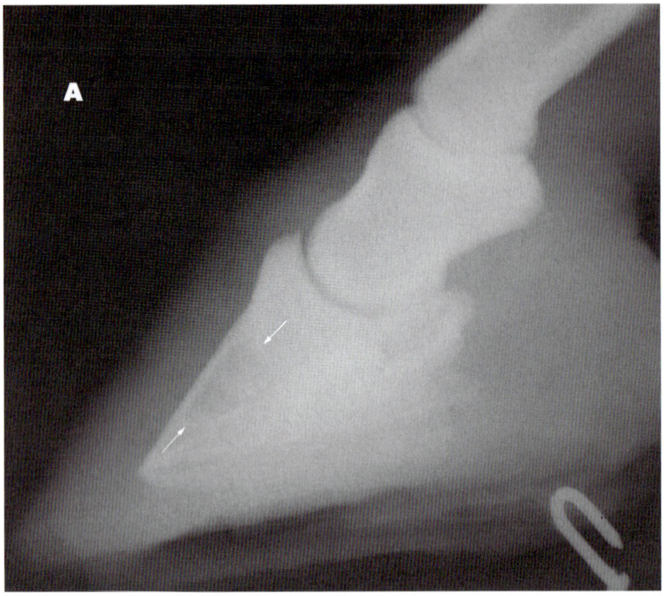

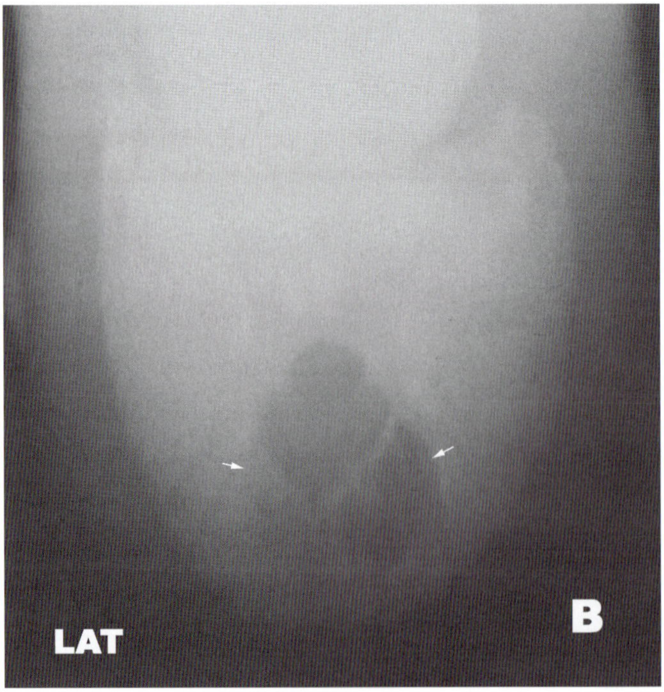

Figures 7.18a,b Lateral (A) and dorsoproximal-palmarodistal oblique (B) radiographic projections of the right hind foot of a 10-year-old Appaloosa. The nail in the lateral view was in an object that the horse was standing on. **Keratoma (soft tissue tumor) of the right hind foot:** These radiographic appearances are typical of keratoma. The area of bone resorption is visible in the lateral view (arrows) but is considerably more obvious in the dorsoproximal-palmarodistal oblique view (arrows). Although there is bone loss as in osteomyelitis, the large size of the lesion and the distinct margination make a diagnosis of osteomyelitis unlikely. Keratomas are relatively rare benign tumors that arise from the keratin-containing cells of the lamina of the hoof. The tumors grow as soft tissue masses within the hoof capsule. Because there is little room for expansion of the mass, resorption of the distal phalanx occurs as a result of pressure necrosis. Very rarely, other types of soft tissue tumors arising from the laminar tissue will create this radiographic appearance. Tumor types that have been reported in the literature include hemangioma, squamous cell carcinoma, and intraosseous mast cell tumor.

Ossification of the Accessory Cartilages of the Third Phalanx (Sidebone)

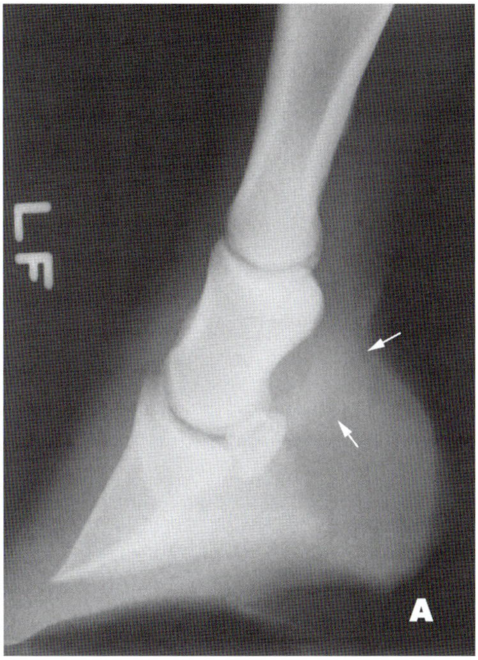

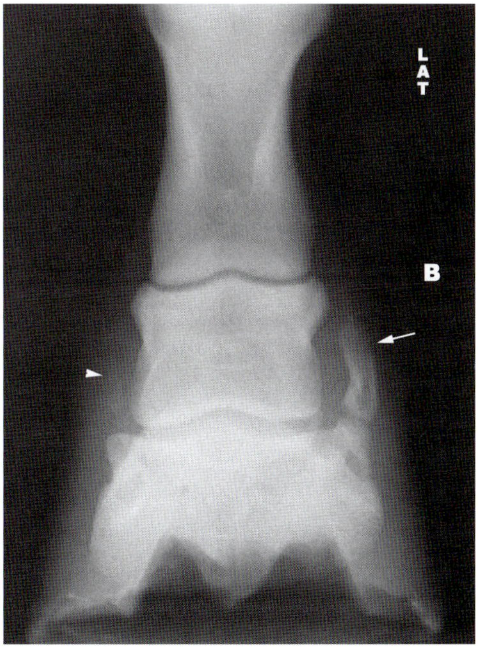

Figures 7.19a,b Lateral (A) and dorsopalmar horizontal beam radiographic projections of the left forefoot of a 12-year-old Thoroughbred cross. **Ossification of the accessory cartilages of the third phalanx (sidebone):** In the lateral view, the faint mineral opacity palmar to the middle phalanx (arrows) is the superimposed ossified lateral accessory cartilage. In the dorsopalmar view, the accessory cartilages are visible as mineralized structures extending proximally. The lateral cartilage (arrow) is large and well mineralized. The lucent line between the ossified cartilage and the remainder of the distal phalanx is an area of nonossified cartilage between the bone and the ossified cartilage, not a fracture line. The medial accessory cartilage has less-extensive mineralization (arrowhead). Ossification of the accessory cartilages of the distal phalanx occurs to some extent in most horses. It is only when the ossification is extensive that a clinical problem may arise. Excessive ossification is thought to be related to trauma to the cartilages as a result of concussion to the quarters of the hoof. The concussive force to this area may be worse in horses with poor conformation, as a result of poor shoeing or as a result of work performed on hard surfaces. Many horses with radiographic evidence of extensive cartilage ossification have no lameness related to it.

Subchondral Cystic Lesion of the First Phalanx

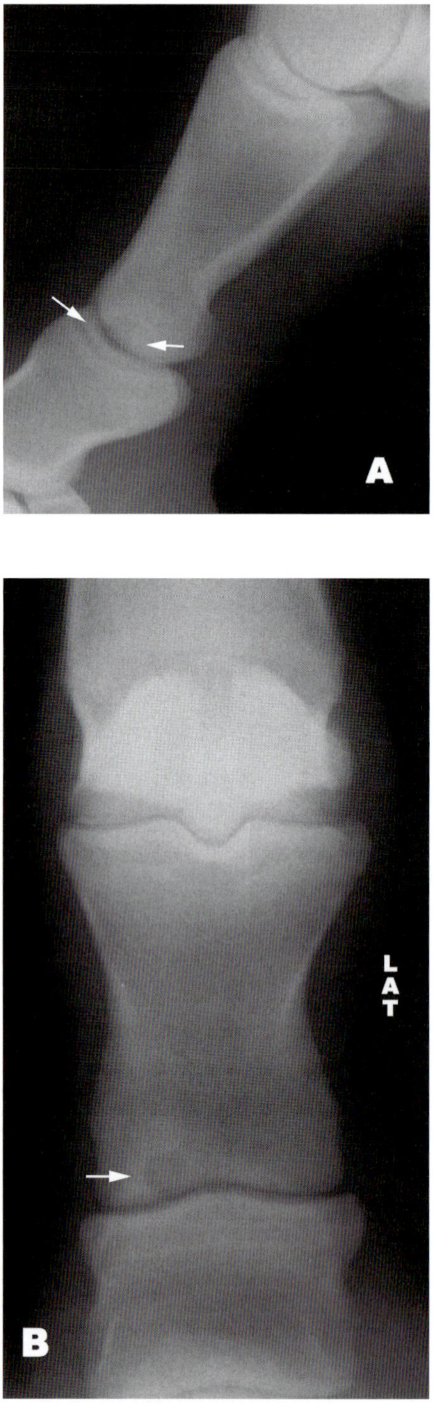

Figures 7.20a,b Lateral (A) and dorsopalmar (B) radiographic projections of the left forefoot of a 1-year-old Belgian. **Subchondral cystic lesion of the distomedial first phalanx:** The cyst is faintly visible in the lateral view (arrows). In the dorsopalmar view, the cyst is clearly visible (arrow). In both views, the cyst appears to communicate with the proximal interphalangeal joint space. Occasionally, subchondral bone cysts occur in the phalanges as a result of osteochondrosis, a developmental orthopedic disease. The cysts may occur adjacent to any joint but are most typically seen in the distal articular surface of the proximal phalanx, proximal articular surface of the middle phalanx, and at the articular surface of the distal phalanx.

Subchondral Cystic Lesion of the Second Phalanx

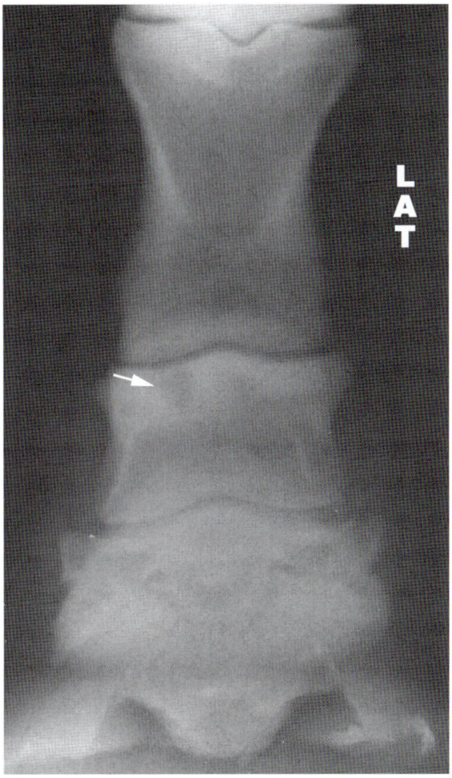

Figure 7.21 Dorsoplantar horizontal beam radiographic projection of the right rear foot of a 2-year-old Standardbred. **Subchondral cystic lesion of the proximomedial second phalanx:** The cyst is visible as an area of lucency at the proximal margin of the second phalanx (arrow). Visualization of the lesion is enhanced by a margin of sclerotic bone. A very subtle lucent area is visible in the distal first phalanx adjacent to the bone cyst. This appearance is created by extension of the cyst into the articular surface of the second phalanx, which superimposes with the distal first phalanx to give the false impression that the subchondral lesion extends across the joint.

Subchondral Cystic Lesion of the Third Phalanx

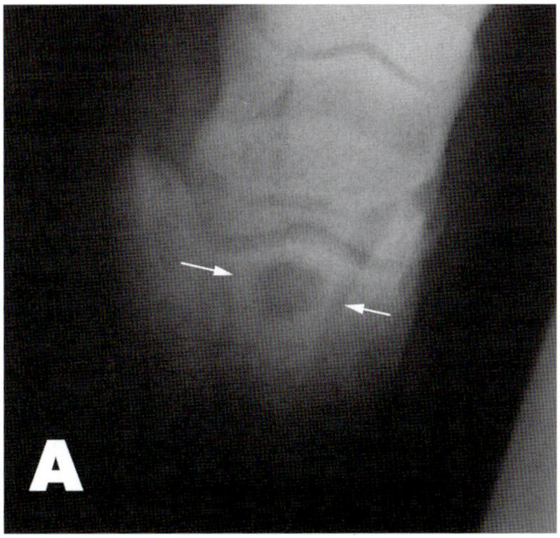

Figures 7.22a,b Dorsoproximal-palmarodistal oblique (A) and lateral (B) radiographic projections of the left forefoot of a 3-year-old Arabian. **Subchondral cystic lesion of the third phalanx:** In the dorsoproximal-palmarodistal oblique view, there is a very large, well-defined circular lucency (arrows) in the third phalanx, just distal to the extensor process. Sclerotic bone surrounds the cyst. In the lateral view, an ill-defined area of lucency is present distal to the extensor process (arrowhead) and the extensor process has undergone significant remodeling (arrow). In this case, it is not possible to define a clear communication between the cyst and the distal interphalangeal joint. However, based on the presence of osteoarthritis of the distal interphalangeal joint, it is extremely likely that the cyst and the joint space communicate.

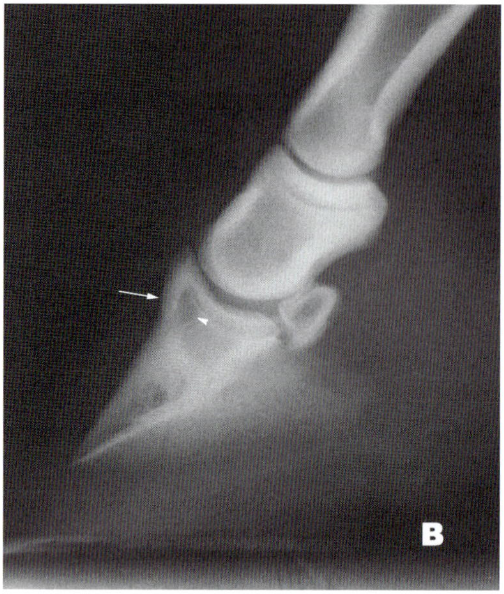

Figures 7.22a,b *Continued*

Complete Fracture of the First Phalanx

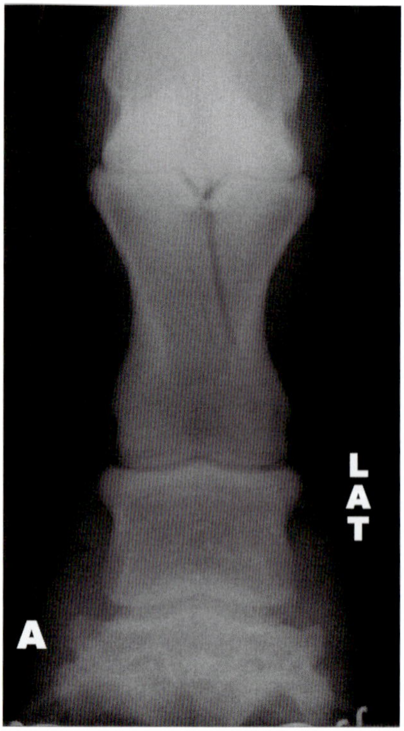

Figures 7.23a,b Dorsopalmar (A) and dorsolateral-palmaromedial oblique (B) radiographic projections of the left metacarpophalangeal joint of a 3-year-old Standardbred. **Complete fracture of the first phalanx:** In the dorsopalmar view, there appear to be two fracture lines in the first phalanx. Only one fracture is present but two lines are visible because the plane of the fracture is different in the dorsal and palmar cortices of the bone. The fracture extends to the proximal articular surface of the first phalanx. Although this was not apparent in the dorsopalmar view, evaluation of the dorsolateral-palmaromedial oblique view shows that the fracture line extends to the distal articular surface of the first phalanx as well (arrow). Involvement of both articular surfaces of the bone decreases the prognosis for return to athletic function. Evaluation of these two views provides some indication as to the complexity of this type of fracture. Complete radiographic evaluation is needed to help determine the location of all of the fracture lines. If available, computed tomography can be used to provide accurate assessment of the fracture for surgical planning.

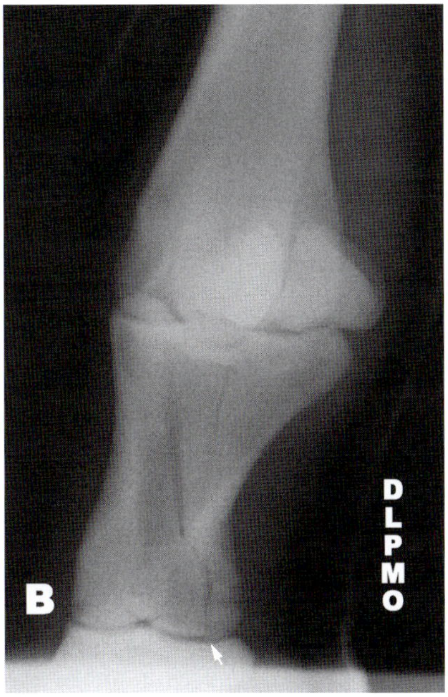

Figures 7.23a,b *Continued*

Laminitis with Rotation and Laminar Separation

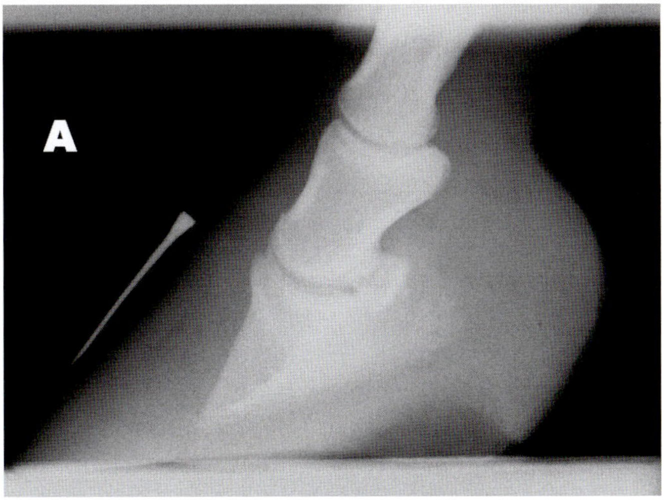

Figures 7.24a,b Lateral radiographic projections of the left forefoot of 6-year-old (A) and 8-year-old Morgans (B). **(A) Laminitis with rotation; (B) laminitis with rotation and laminar separation:** Both of these horses have evidence of laminar thickening and of significant rotation (palmar deviation) of the third phalanx. In (A), the laminar tissues of the hoof are thick but are otherwise normal in appearance. In (B), gas has dissected between the lamina from the sole of the hoof (arrow).

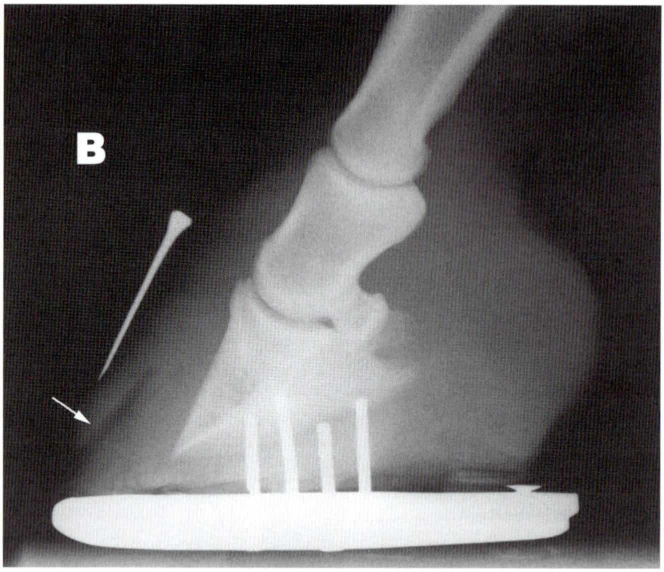

Figures 7.24a,b *Continued*

Chronic Laminitis

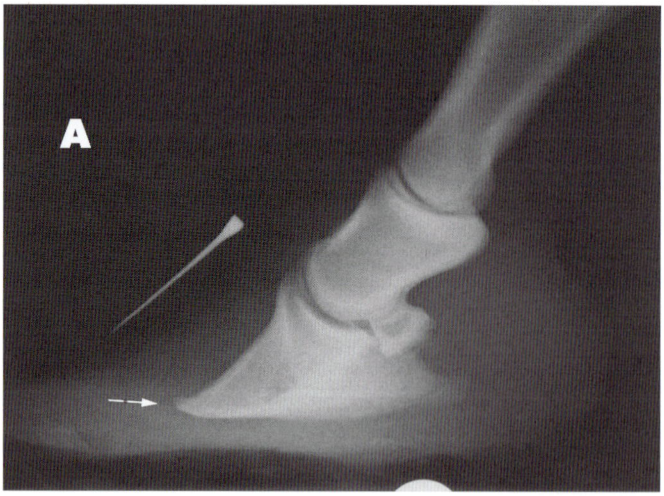

Figures 7.25a,b Lateral radiographic projections of the left forefoot of 12-year-old (A) and 10-year-old ponies (B) **with chronic laminitis:** Both patients show radiographic evidence of chronic laminitis. In A although the toe is excessively long, there is relatively good alignment of the third phalanx and the hoof wall. Remodeling of the dorsal solar margin has created a projection of bone (arrow). This is an indicator of chronic laminitis. The pony in (B) shows extreme changes of chronic laminitis. Abnormal growth of the hoof wall has caused formation of "founder rings" on the dorsal surface of the hoof wall. The toe of the hoof has grown excessively long and has been trimmed. Resorption of the peripheral portion of the third phalanx has occurred, and only the articular portion of the bone remains. The "lacy" appearance of the proximal sesamoid bones is evidence of disuse osteopenia, an indication that the patient bears very little weight on the limb.

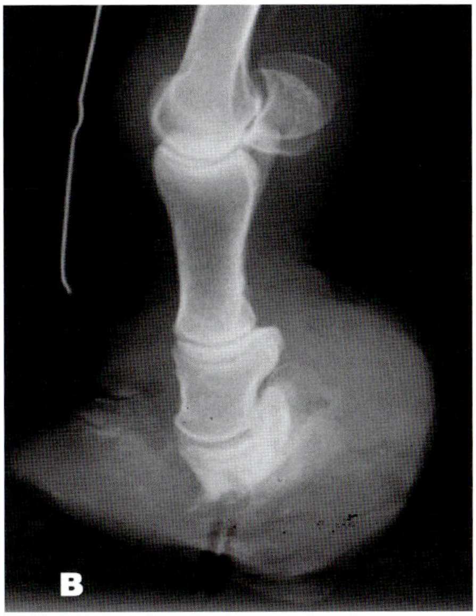

Figures 7.25a,b *Continued*

Assessment of the Third Phalanx Rotation

Figures 7.26a,b Lateral radiographic projection of a forefoot showing two methods of assessment for third phalanx rotation. **(A)** Lines are drawn along the dorsal aspect of the hoof wall and distal phalanx (red lines). A line is then drawn parallel to the ground surface of the hoof to intersect these two lines. The angles (1) and (2) are compared and in a normal horse should be approximately equal. If rotation is present, angle (2) will be greater than angle (1). In the example used here, angle (1) measured 58 degrees and angle (2) measured 60 degrees. **(B)** The distance between the dorsal surface of the hoof and the dorsal surface of the distal phalanx is measured at proximal, middle, and distal locations. The three measurements should be approximately equal. If rotation is present, the distal and/or middle measurements will be greater than the proximal ones. In the example used here, the measurements are proximal = 25 mm, middle = 25 mm, and distal = 28 mm.

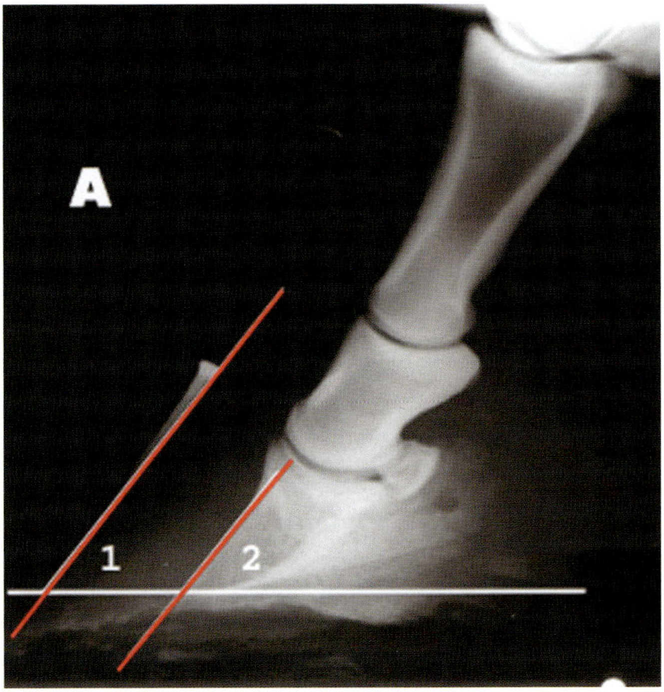

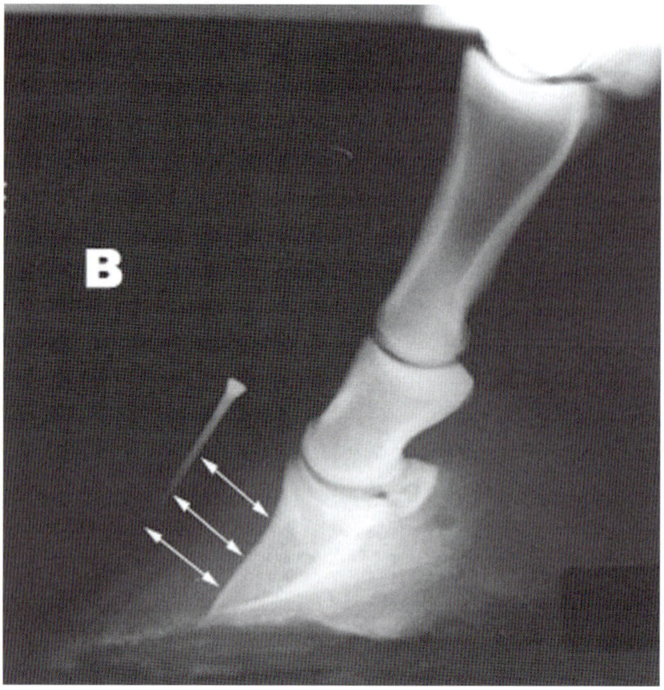

Figures 7.26a,b *Continued*

THE METACARPOPHALANGEAL AND METATARSOPHALANGEAL JOINTS (FETLOCK JOINT)

Osteoarthritis

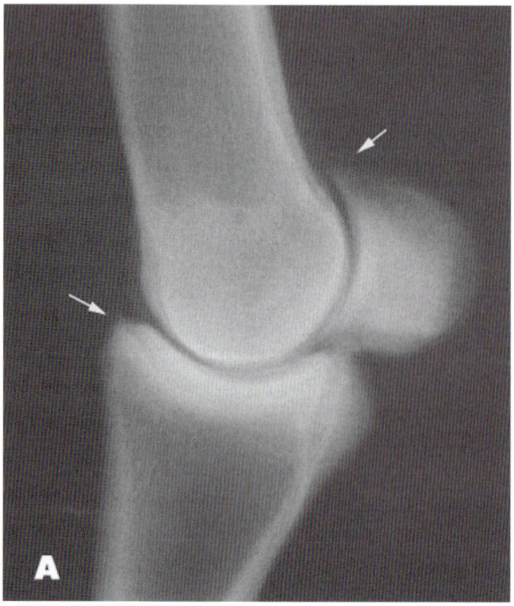

Figures 7.27a,b Lateral (A) and dorsolateral-palmaromedial oblique (B) radiographic projections of the right metacarpophalangeal joint of a 4-year-old Standardbred. **Mild osteoarthritis of the metacarpophalangeal joint:** In the lateral view, minimal osteophyte formation is present along the dorsal proximal margin of the first phalanx and on the proximal articular margin of a proximal sesamoid bone (arrows). Osteophytes are often most prominent along the dorsomedial and dorsolateral aspects of the metacarpophalangeal joint. In this case, osteophyte formation is much more evident (arrows) in the oblique radiographic projection. The oblique radiographic projections are of significant importance to completely evaluate this joint.

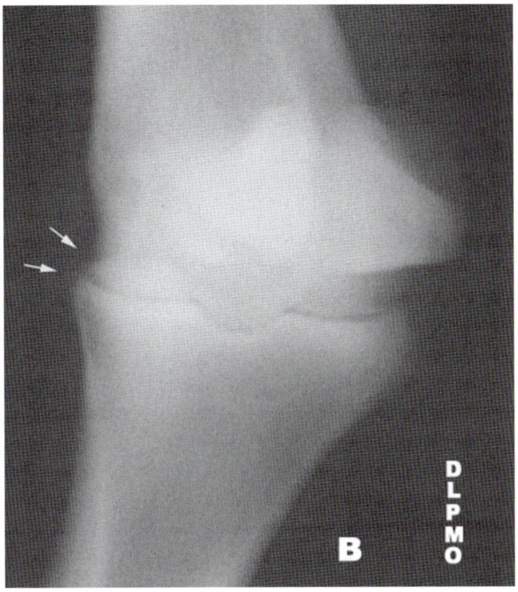

Figures 7.27a,b *Continued*

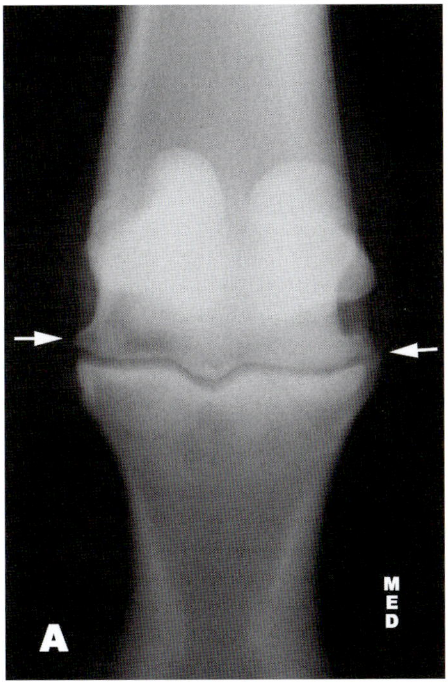

Figures 7.28a,b Dorsopalmar (A) and dorsolateral-palmaromedial oblique (B) radiographic projections of the right metacarpophalangeal joint of a 6-year-old Standardbred. **Moderate osteoarthritis of the metacarpophalangeal joint:** The osteophytes on the joint margin (arrows) in this example are easily seen. They are larger and are much more opaque. These osteophytes have had time to fully mineralize and are evidence of chronic degenerative joint diseases (DJD). Note that the articular surfaces of the joint are slightly irregular adjacent to the osteophytes. The degenerative process within the joint has caused degeneration and/or loss of the articular cartilage and changes are now occurring in the subchondral bone. This is an evidence of progression of DJD.

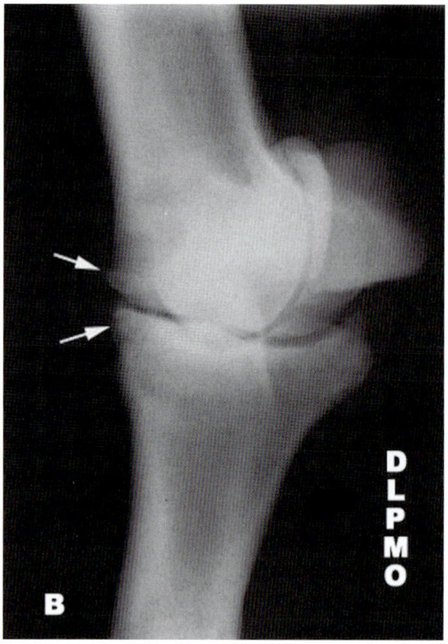

Figures 7.28a,b *Continued*

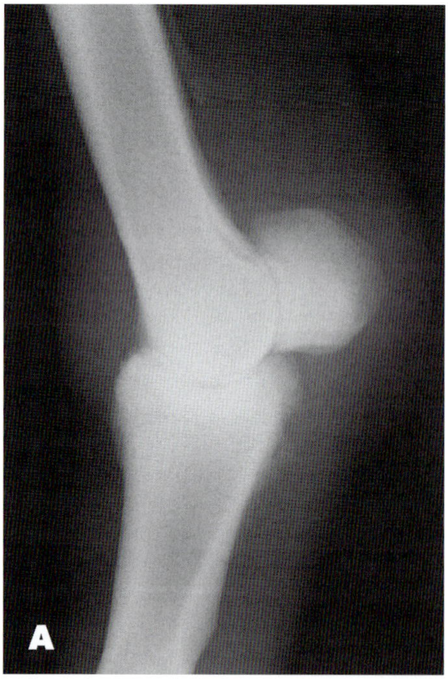

Figures 7.29a,b Lateral (A) and dorsopalmar (B) radiographic projections of the left metacarpophalangeal joint of a 2-year-old Standardbred. **Severe osteoarthritis of the metacarpophalangeal joint:** There is marked thickening of the metacarpophalangeal joint capsule. Irregular proliferative bone is present on the dorsal and palmar margins of the first phalanx in areas where the joint capsule and ligamentous structures attach. The joint space is narrower than normal but this appearance may be created by the angle of the X-ray beam. The dorsopalmar view confirms that narrowing of the joint space is present, particularly on the medial aspect of the joint. The proximal aspect of the first phalanx adjacent to the medial articular surface is increased in opacity. This is the result of thickening of the subchondral bone and is generally described as subchondral sclerosis. A large area of lucency (black arrows) is present within the area of sclerosis; this is an evidence of subchondral lysis. Irregular proliferative bone is present on the medial aspect of the proximal first phalanx in the area of joint capsular attachment. The severity of the joint space collapse, the degree of capsular distension present, and the large amount of bony reaction in areas of capsular attachments are all changes that suggest joint sepsis as the cause of the osteoarthritis.

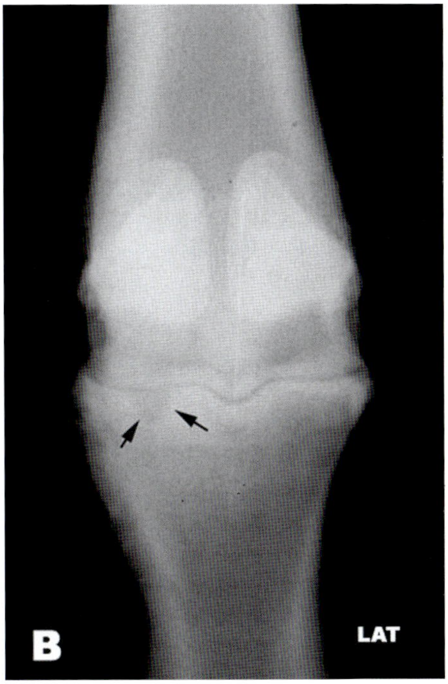

Figures 7.29a,b *Continued*

Chronic Proliferative Synovitis

Figures 7.30a,b Lateral radiographic projections of the right metacarpophalangeal joint of a 7-year-old Standardbred (A) and of the left metacarpophalangeal joint of a 9-year-old Standardbred (B). **Chronic proliferative synovitis of the metacarpophalangeal joint:** In (A) it is not possible to evaluate the soft tissue structures of the joint due to the technique used. There is a "scooped–out" appearance to the dorsal aspect of the third metacarpus (arrow) in the region of attachment of the joint capsule. A similar appearance is present at the palmar aspect of the third metacarpus immediately proximal to the condyles (arrowheads). The proliferative synovial tissues have caused pressure necrosis and resorption of underlying bone. In (B) the dorsal aspect of the third metacarpus is similar in appearance. In this case, chronic irritation/inflammation caused by synovial proliferation has caused periosteal new bone to form on the dorsal aspect of the third metacarpus (arrow) and proximal phalanx (arrowhead).

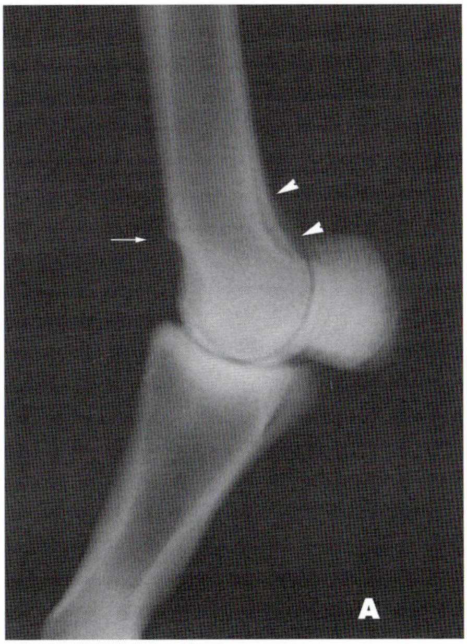

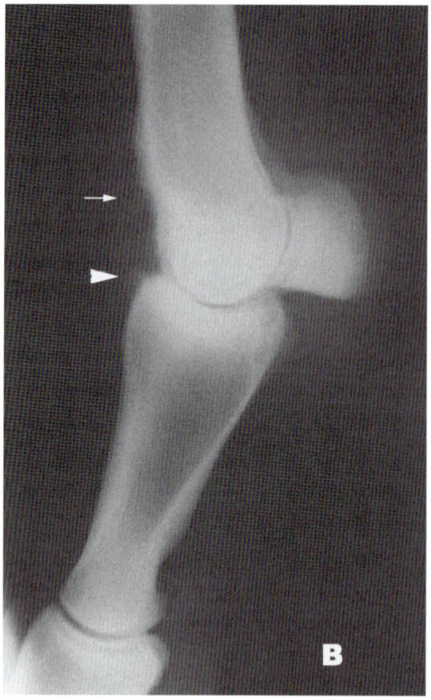

Figures 7.30a,b *Continued*

Osteochondritis Dissecans (OCD)

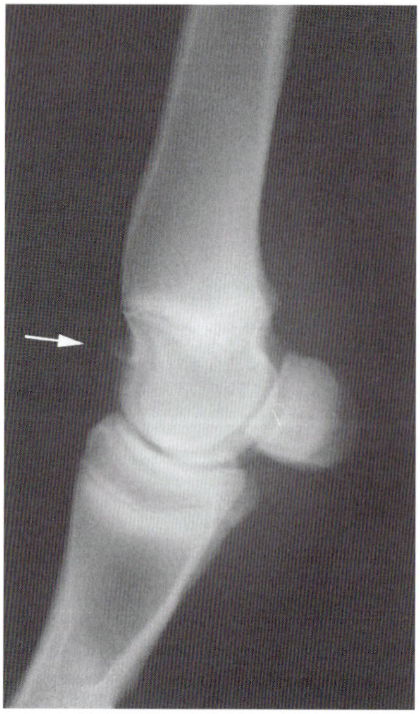

Figure 7.31 Lateral radiographic projection of the left metatarsophalangeal joint of a 6-month-old Belgian. **Osteochondritis dissecans (OCD) of the median sagittal ridge of the third metatarsal bone:** Several osseous fragments are visible (arrow). The largest fragment appears to be attached at the sagittal ridge. The smaller fragments may be adhered to the joint capsule. Note the large amount of intra-articular swelling associated with the OCD lesion.

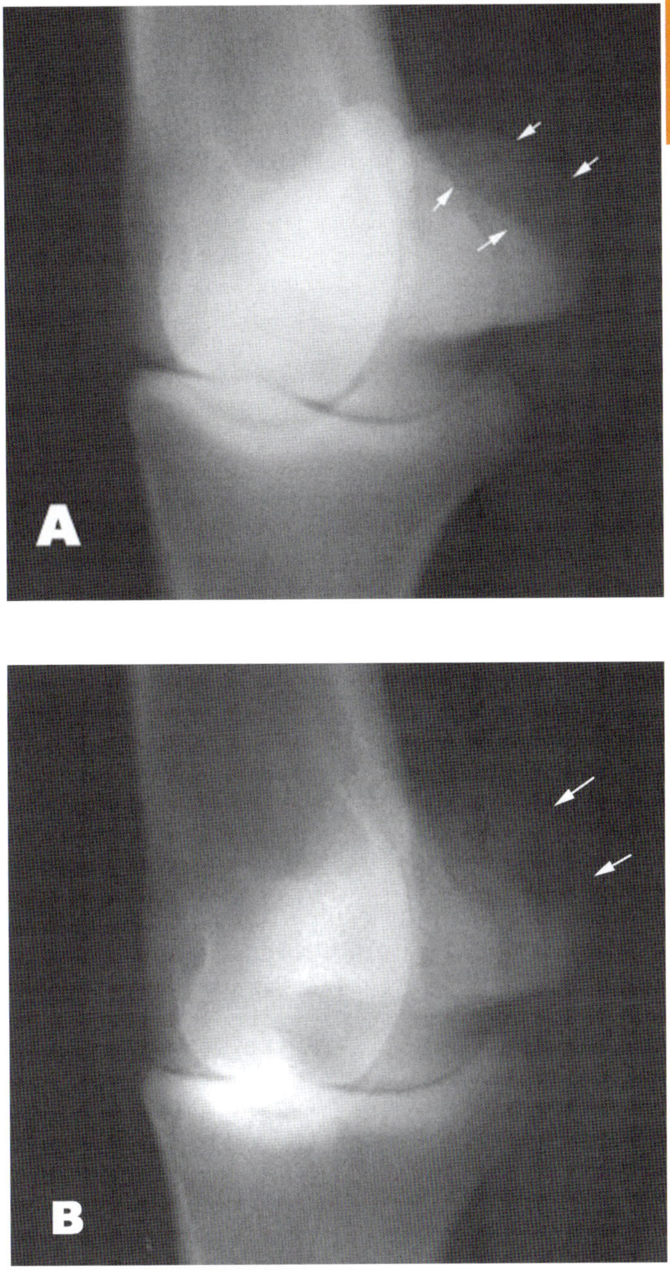

Figures 7.32a,b Dorsomedial-plantarolateral oblique radiographic projections of the left metacarpophalangeal joint of a 2-year-old Standardbred (A) and of the left metatarsophalangeal joint of a 4-year-old Standardbred (B). **(A) Type 2 sesamoiditis of the medial proximal sesamoid bone; (B) Type 3 sesamoiditis of the medial proximal sesamoid bone:** Sesamoiditis is described as a periostitis and osteitis affecting the abaxial surface of proximal sesamoid bones. One or both sesamoid bones in a joint may be affected and multiple joints may be affected. Sesamoiditis is a relatively common radiographic finding and may be a cause of lameness. It is most often seen in racehorses. Sesamoiditis has been classified into three categories based on the radiographic appearance of the sesamoid bone. Type 1 sesamoiditis is defined as less than three linear defects less than or equal to 1 mm in width. (A) Type 2 sesamoiditis is defined as three or more linear defects less than or equal to 1 mm in width. Five linear lucencies are present along the abaxial margin of the medial proximal sesamoid bone (arrows). Type 2 sesamoiditis may be present as an incidental finding; if a horse with type 2 sesamoiditis is lame, the lameness is generally due to concurrent soft tissue injury. (B) Type 3 sesamoiditis is defined as the presence of wide, abnormally shaped defects. Any linear defect over 1 mm in width or any defect with a shape other than linear would qualify as evidence of type 3 sesamoiditis. A very large circular defect is present along the abaxial margin of this sesamoid bone (arrows). Type 3 lesions are consistently associated with lameness and carry a poor prognosis for a return to function.

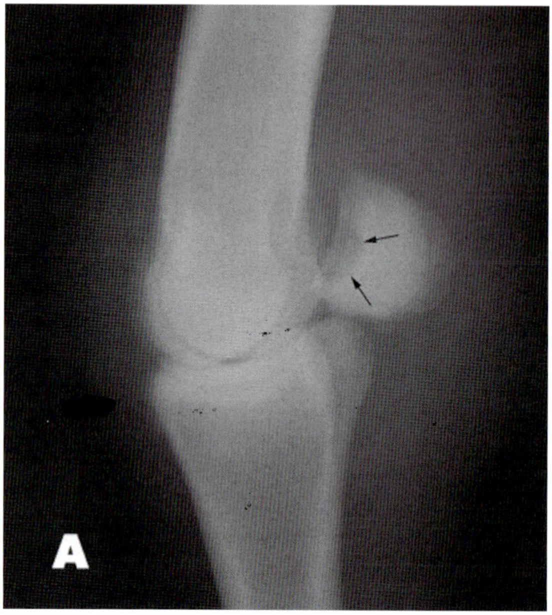

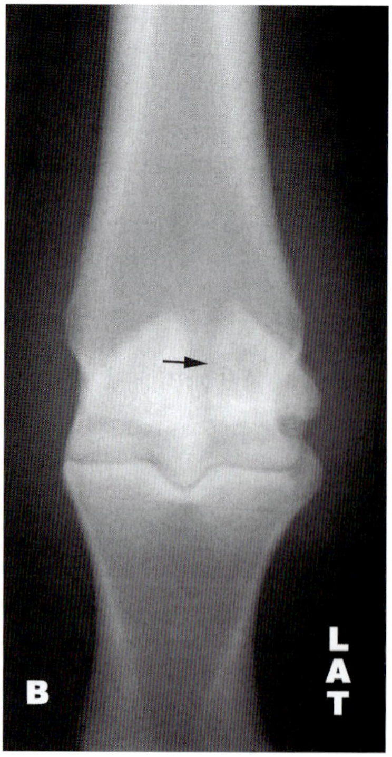

Figures 7.33a,b Lateral (A) and dorsoplantar (B) radiographic projections of the right metatarsophalangeal joint of a 4-year-old Standardbred. **Septic arthritis with osteomyelitis of the lateral proximal sesamoid bone:** There is massive distension of the fetlock joint capsule. Irregular proliferative response is present on the dorsal margin of the proximal part of the first phalanx (lateral view). A lucency is present in the articular surface of one of the proximal sesamoid bones (arrows) but with only a lateral view it cannot be determined if this is the lateral or medial sesamoid bone. In the dorsoplantar view, the lucency is present on the axial margin of the lateral sesamoid bone (arrows). Unlike sesamoiditis, the lesions of sesamoid osteomyelitis are present on the axial, articular margin of the bone. Sesamoid osteomyelitis typically occurs concurrently with septic tenosynovitis of the flexor sheath and/or septic arthritis of the fetlock joint. In this case, septic arthritis developed after joint injection. Horses with sesamoid osteomyelitis are generally severely lame and the prognosis is guarded.

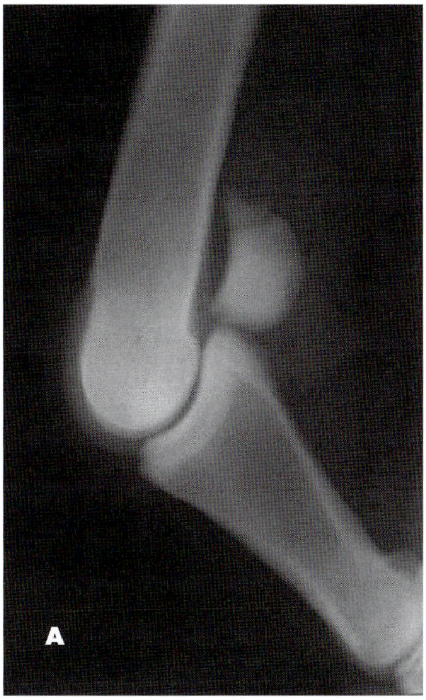

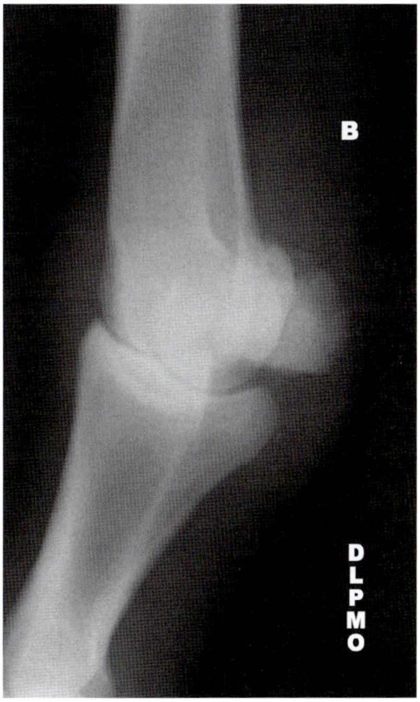

Figures 7.34a,b Lateral (A) and dorsolateral-palmaromedial oblique (B) radiographic projections of the right metacarpophalangeal joint of a 2-year-old Standardbred. **Apical fracture of the lateral proximal sesamoid bone:** The apical fracture is visible in the lateral view (A), but with only a lateral view, the exact location of the fracture cannot be determined. Oblique radiographs are needed to determine whether the lateral or medial proximal sesamoid bone is fractured. The fractured sesamoid is visible in the dorsolateral-palmaromedial oblique view (B) indicating that the fracture is in the lateral proximal sesamoid bone. Apical fractures involve the proximal one-third or less of the sesamoid bone and are the most common type of fracture. Surgical removal of the fracture fragment is the treatment of choice. Fracture of the apical portion of the sesamoid bone can disrupt the attachment of the suspensory branch and/or cause ligamentous injury. Ultrasound evaluation of the contralateral suspensory branch may be indicated in horses with apical sesamoid bone fractures.

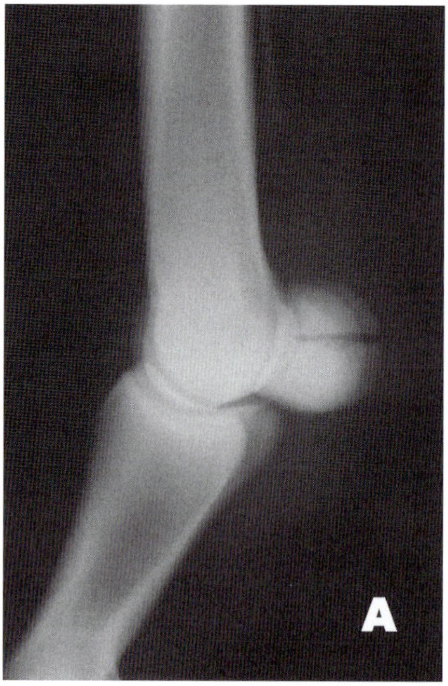

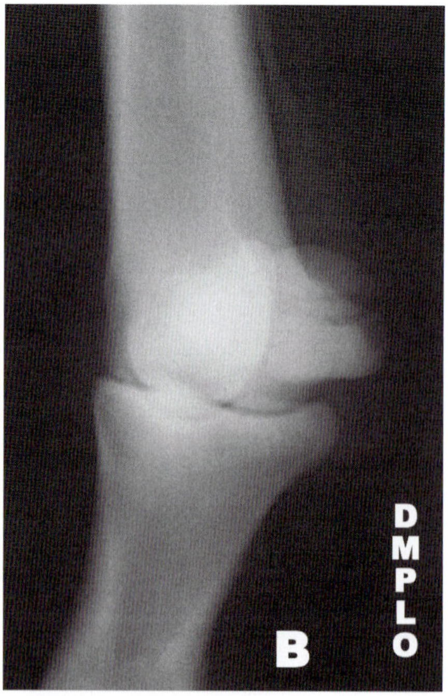

Figures 7.35a,b Lateral (A) and dorsomedial-palmarolateral oblique (B) radiographic projections of the right metacarpophalangeal joint of a 2-year-old Standardbred. **Midbody fracture of the medial proximal sesamoid bone:** The midbody fracture is visible in the lateral view (A), but with only a lateral view, the exact location of the fracture cannot be determined. Oblique radiographs are needed to determine whether the lateral or medial proximal sesamoid bone is fractured. The fractured sesamoid is visible in the dorsomedial-palmarolateral oblique view (B) indicating that the fracture is in the medial proximal sesamoid bone. In the oblique view, there appears to be two fracture lines; this appearance is the result of obliquity of the X-ray beam, which makes the axial and abaxial margins of a single fracture appear as two lines. Midbody sesamoid fractures are uncommon and carry a relatively poor prognosis for return to function.

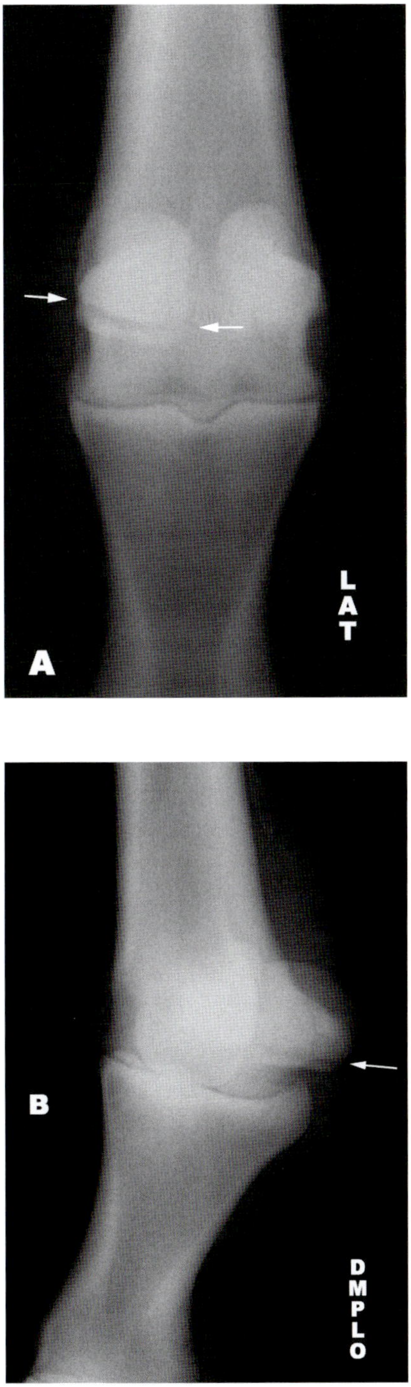

Figures 7.36a,b Dorsopalmar and dorsomedial-palmarolateral oblique radiographic projections of the left metacarpophalangeal joint of a 4-year-old Standardbred. **Basilar fracture of the medial proximal sesamoid bone:** Fracture of the distal one-third or less of the proximal sesamoid bone is considered a basilar fracture. This fracture is essentially an avulsion fracture of the attachment of the distal sesamoidean ligaments. The fractured sesamoid is visible in the dorsopalmar view (A—arrows) and in the dorsomedial-palmarolateral oblique view (B—arrow). Basilar sesamoid fractures are uncommon and carry a relatively poor prognosis for return to function.

Fracture of the Proximal First Phalanx

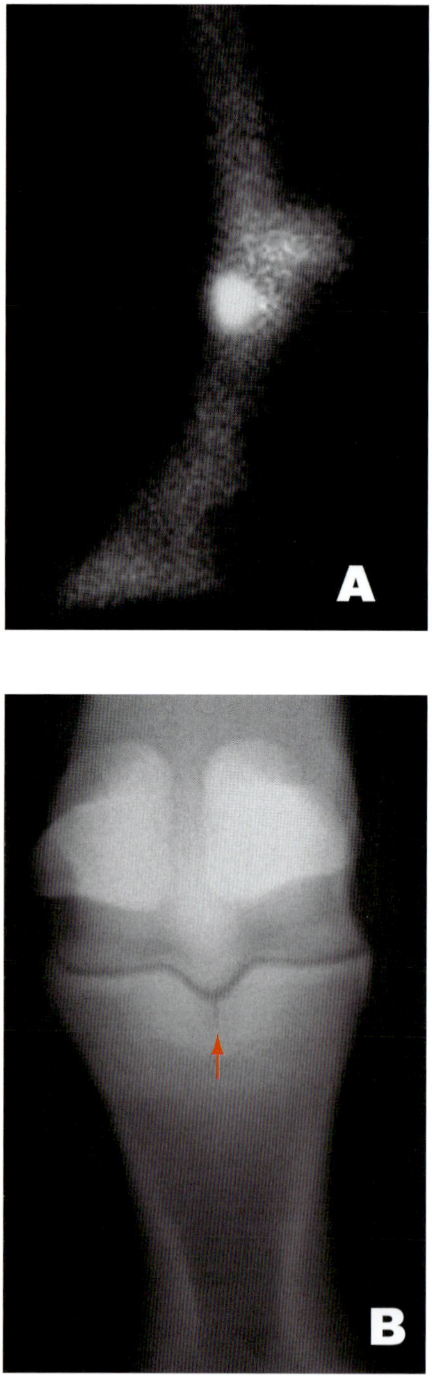

Figures 7.37a,b Nuclear scintigraphic image (A) and dorsoplantar radiographic projection (B) of the metatarsophalangeal joint of a 3-year-old Standardbred. **Incomplete sagittal fracture of the proximal first phalanx:** The scintigraphic study shows a focal intense area of isotope uptake in the dorsoproximal first phalanx. The intensity of the uptake is consistent with the presence of a fracture. In the dorsoplantar radiograph, a linear lucency is seen extending into the proximal phalanx from the sagittal groove (arrow). These fractures are usually only visible in the dorsopalmar (or dorsoplantar) radiograph. In the acute phase, the fracture line may be difficult to impossible to visualize. Within 7–10 days, bone resorption will occur along the margins of the fracture making the fracture line wider. Sclerosis of the surrounding bone may create increased opacity around the fracture. These changes allow the fracture line to be more easily seen. Because these fractures can be difficult to diagnose with radiography in the acute stages, nuclear scintigraphy is often used if such a fracture is suspected.

Fracture of the Third Metacarpus

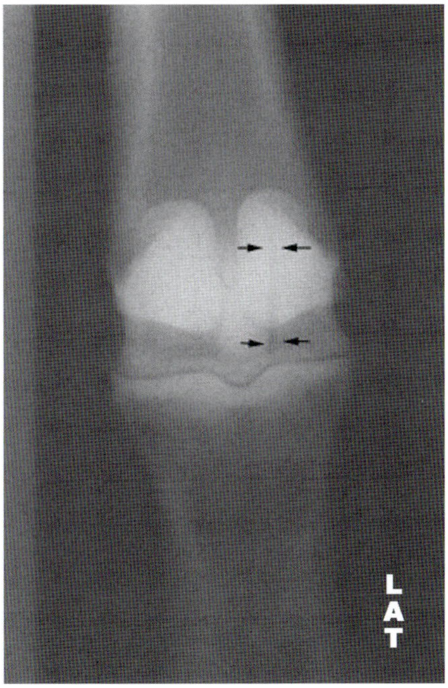

Figure 7.38 Dorsopalmar radiographic projection of the left metacarpophalangeal joint of a 4-year-old Standardbred. **Lateral condylar fracture of the third metacarpus:** There is an incomplete nondisplaced fracture of the lateral condyle (arrows). Fractures occur in the condyles of the third metacarpal and third metatarsal bones, almost always in racehorses. In Thoroughbreds, the third metacarpal bone is affected twice as often as the third metatarsal bone; in Standardbreds the distribution is more even between the fore and hind limbs. These fractures are visible in a well-exposed dorsopalmar (plantar) view. Oblique views are taken to completely evaluate the fracture. It is imperative to take a complete series of radiographs of the entire bone since condylar fractures often spiral proximally into the cannon bone. A flexed dorsopalmar (plantar) view of the fetlock joint is used to evaluate the palmar condylar surface for small fracture fragments and the sesamoid bones for concurrent axial fractures.

Fracture (Chip) of the Dorsoproximal First Phalanx

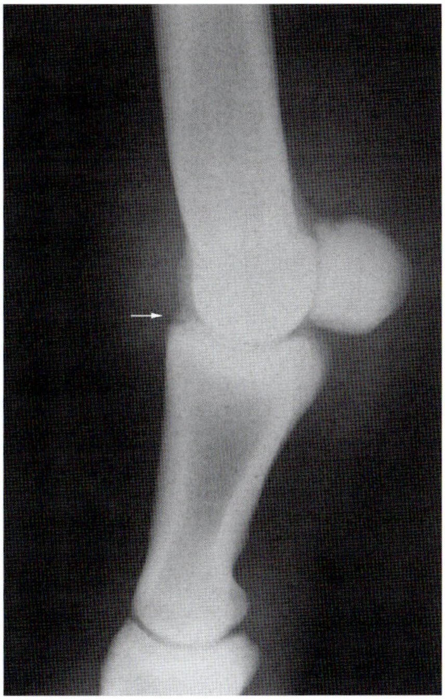

Figure 7.39 Lateral radiographic projection of the left metacarpophalangeal joint of a 6-year-old warmblood. **Fracture (chip) of the dorsoproximal first phalanx:** There is a large fracture fragment arising from the dorsoproximal articular margin of the first phalanx (arrow). Also note the large degree of distension of the metacarpophalangeal joint capsule. Fracture fragments in this location are not always associated with lameness. In some cases, the fragments are small and do not cause any inflammatory response within the joint. In this case, the fracture fragment is relatively large and there is evidence of significant synovial inflammation. This fracture is most likely a cause of lameness.

Osseous Fragmentation of the Lateral Plantar Process of the First Phalanx

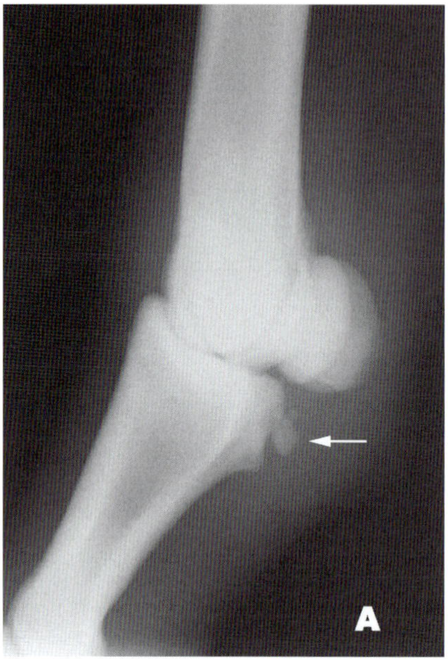

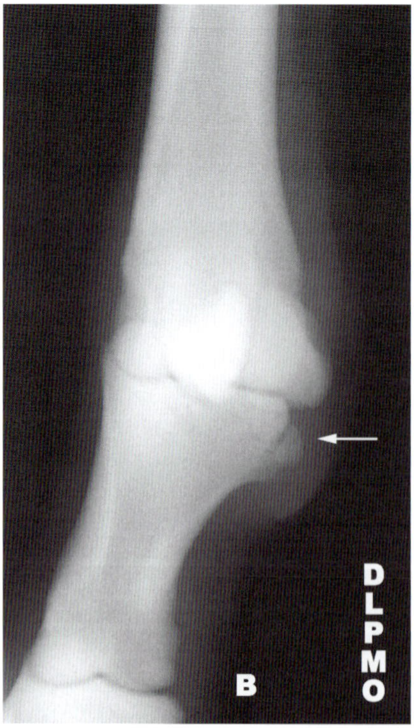

Figures 7.40a,b Lateral (A) and dorsolateral-palmaromedial oblique (B) radiographic projections of the left metatarsophalangeal joint of a 3-year-old Standardbred. **Osseous fragmentation of the lateral plantar process of the first phalanx:** Several osseous fragments are present arising from the margin of the lateral plantar process (tubercle) of the first phalanx (arrows). Fragments are present within the joint capsule but do not affect the articular surface. Notice the intracapsular soft tissue swelling that is associated with the fragment (lateral view). There is controversy as to whether these fragments represent a development lesion (osteochondrosis/separate center of ossification) or fracture of the bone.

Osseous Fragment Arising from the Plantar Margin of the First Phalanx

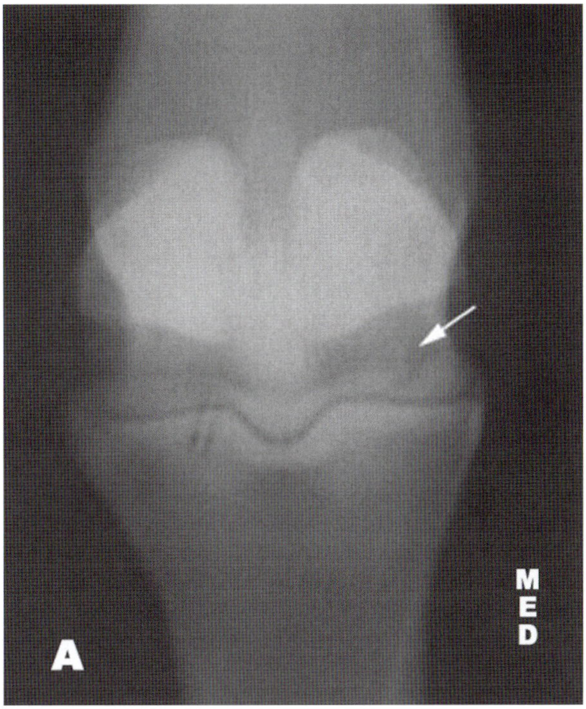

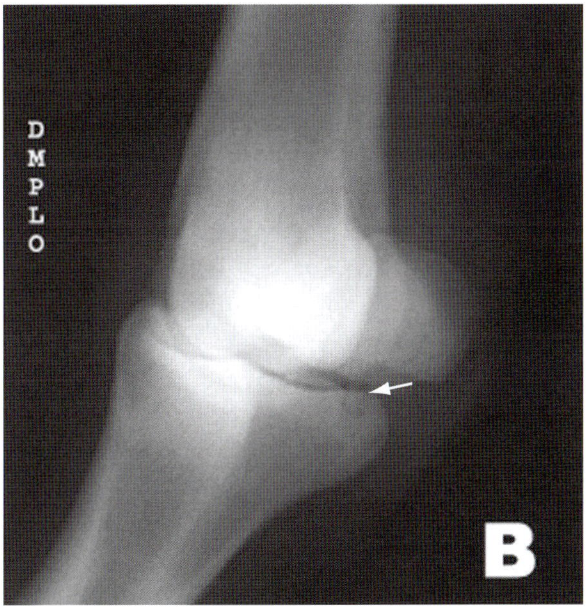

Figures 7.41a,b Dorsoplantar (A) and dorsomedial-plantarolateral oblique (B) radiographic projections of the left metatarsophalangeal joint of a 3-year-old Standardbred. **Osseous fragment arising from the plantar margin of the first phalanx:** In the dorsoplantar radiograph, the osseous fragment is visible in the medial aspect of the joint (arrow). The dorsomedial- plantarolateral oblique radiograph confirms the plantaromedial location of the bone fragment (arrow). There is some controversy as to whether these fragments are developmental (osteochondrosis) or avulsion fractures at the attachment of the distal sesamoidean ligaments. These fragments are very common in the hind limbs of Standardbreds. In a large proportion of Standardbreds, there is no lameness associated with the presence of these fragments.

Soft Tissue Swelling of the Carpus

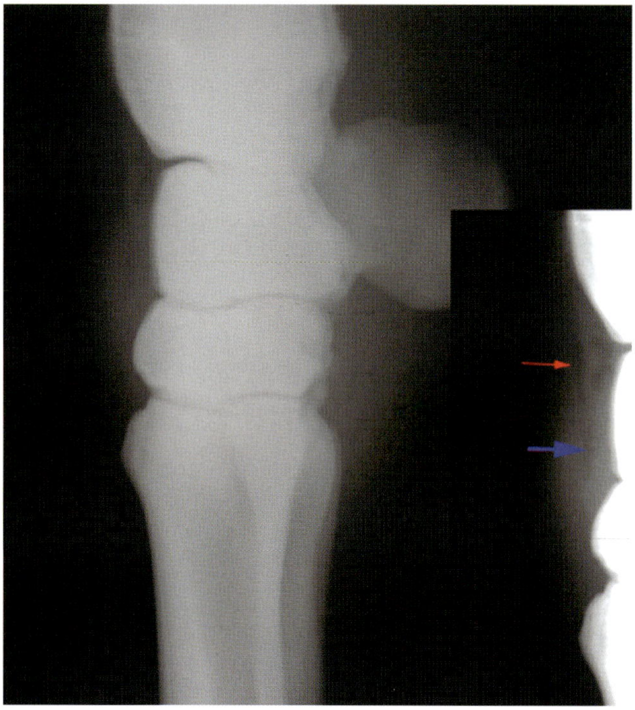

Figure 7.42 Lateral radiographic projection of the left carpus of a 3-year-old Standardbred. **Soft tissue swelling of the carpus:** Evaluation of the dorsal soft tissues will help to determine if the swelling is intracapsular in location (see inset). Two linear lucencies are present on the dorsal aspect of the antebrachiocarpal joint (red arrow), these are fat pads that are normally present on either side of the extensor tendon. Only a single linear lucency is present on the dorsal aspect of the middle carpal joint and located more dorsally than normal (blue arrow). Displacement and/or compression of the normal fat pads are evidence of distension of the middle carpal joint. Fat pads are not normally present dorsal to the carpometacarpal joint so this cannot be used for evaluation of the joint effusion.

Osteoarthritis

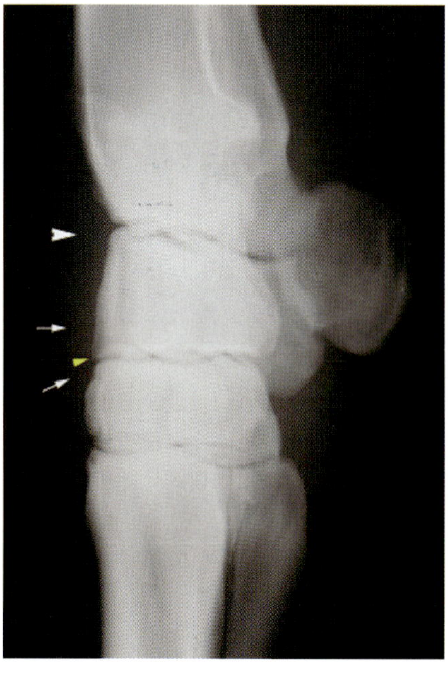

Figure 7.43 Dorsolateral-palmaromedial oblique radiographic projection of the right carpus of a 4-year-old Standardbred. **Mild osteoarthritis of the antebrachiocarpal joint:** In this radiograph the fat pad of the antebrachiocarpal joint is normal (large arrowhead) but the fat pad of the middle carpal joint has been compressed by distension of the joint capsule (arrows). Mild rounding and subchondral lucency is present at the distal dorsomedial aspect of the radial carpal bone (small arrowhead) These changes are the earliest evidence of bone remodeling. The early osseous changes of osteoarthritis often occur on the dorsomedial and dorsolateral joint surfaces of the carpus. This is why oblique radiographic projections are such an important part of a complete radiographic examination of the joint.

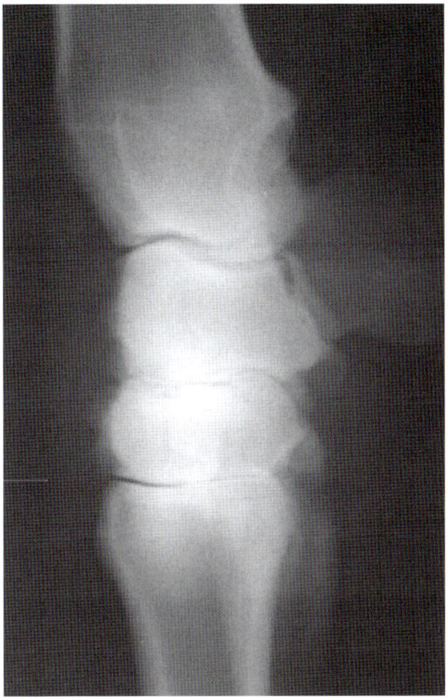

A

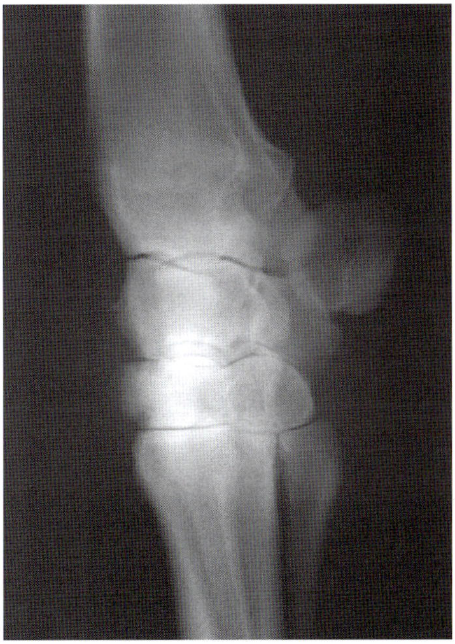

B

Figures 7.44a,b Lateral (A) and dorsolateral-palmaromedial oblique (B) radiographic projections of the left carpus of a 6-year-old Standardbred. **Moderate osteoarthritis of the middle carpal joint:** In the lateral view, there is significant osteophyte formation on the dorsal margin of the distal radial and proximal third carpal bone. In the oblique view, the osteophyte formation extends to the dorsomedial margin of the radial and third carpal bones.

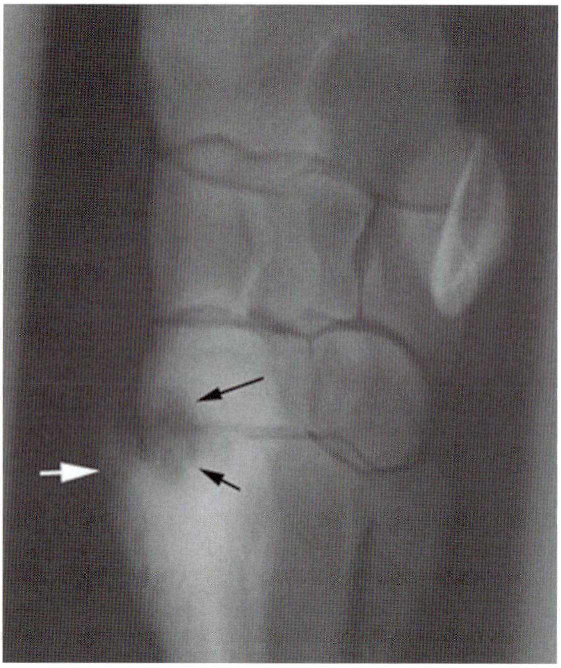

A

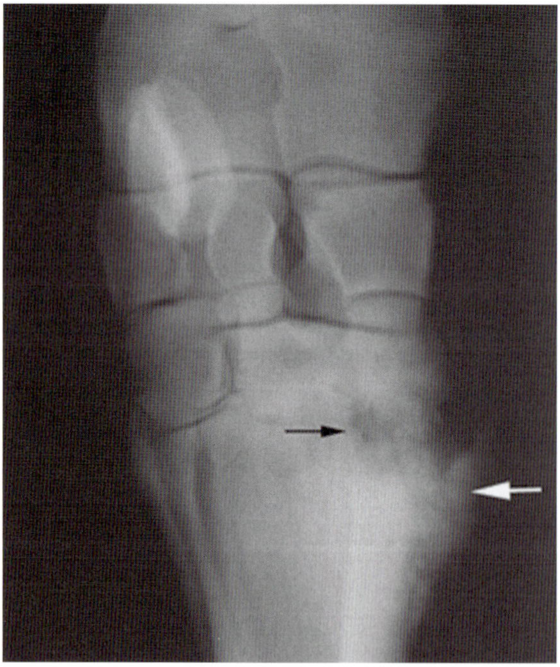

B

Figures 7.45a,b Lateral (A) and dorsolateral-palmaromedial oblique (B) radiographic projections of the left carpus of a 7-year-old quarter horse. **Severe osteoarthritis of the carpometacarpal joint:** There is marked irregular proliferative bone on the dorsal and dorsomedial aspect of the carpometacarpal joint (white arrows). A large area of bone lysis is seen centered at the joint and extending into the third carpal and metacarpal bones (black arrows). The degree of bone destruction and the "exuberant" appearance of the proliferative response suggest that joint sepsis is present.

Normal Third Carpal Bone and Third Carpal Bone with Mild Sclerosis of the Radial Facet

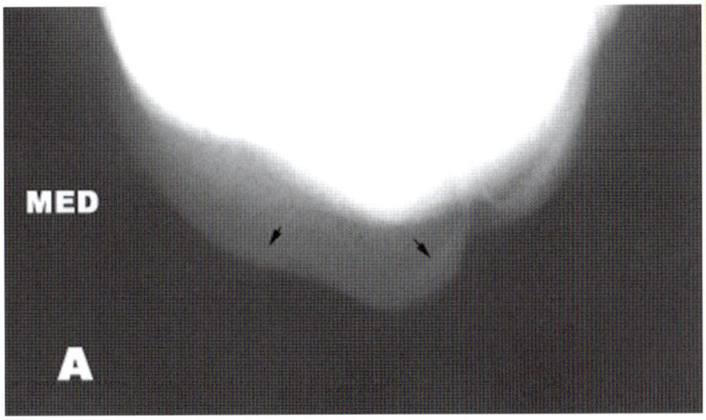

Figures 7.46a,b Dorsoproximo-dorsodistal oblique ("skyline") radiographic projections of the distal row of carpal bones. **(A) Normal third carpal bone; (B) Third carpal bone with mild sclerosis of the radial facet:** In the normal third carpal bone, it is possible to differentiate the cortex of the bone from the medullary cavity—the cortex is visible as an outer margin of opaque bone (arrows); the medullary cavity is more lucent. Remodeling of the third carpal bone occurs as a normal response to the rigors of training in young race horses. Radiographically, the area of bone remodeling appears to be of increased opacity and it is no longer possible to distinguish the cortex and medulla of the bone (arrows). This change occurs first in the radial facet (the medial aspect of the bone) and may eventually involve the intermediate facet (the lateral aspect of the bone) as well. Mild sclerosis of the third carpal bone is present in almost all horses early in training as an incidental finding.

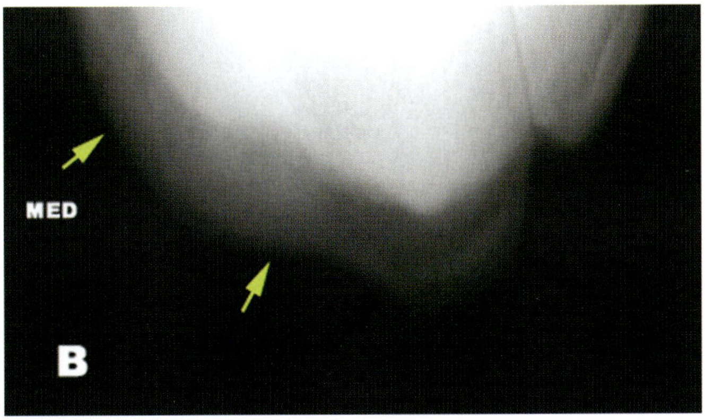

Nuclear Scintigraphic Imaging of the Carpus

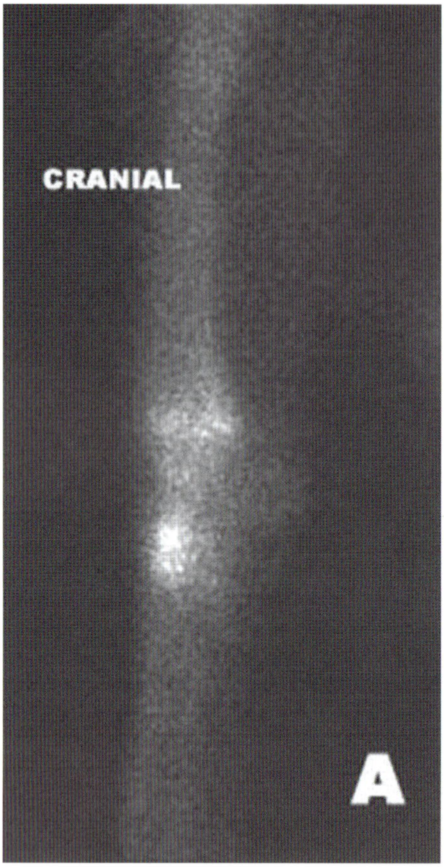

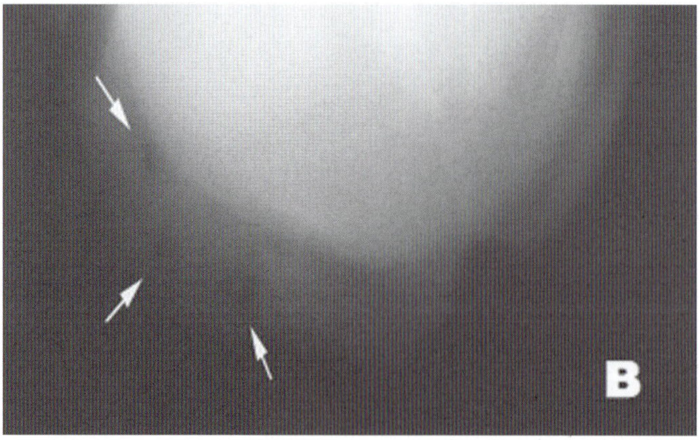

Figures 7.47a,b Nuclear scintigraphic image (A) and dorsoproximo-dorsodistal oblique ("skyline") (B) radiographic projection of the distal row of carpal bones of a 3-year-old Standardbred. **(A) Isotope uptake in the dorsal aspect of the distal carpal row; (B) Sclerosis of the radial and intermediate facets of the third carpal bone:** There is moderately intense isotope uptake in the dorsal aspect of the distal row of carpal bones (white area). This corresponds to significant bone activity in the area of the third carpal bone. In the radiograph, there is severe sclerosis of the radial facet of the third carpal bone and moderate sclerosis of the intermediate facet. Several areas of lucency are present within the region of sclerosis (arrows). This finding is evidence of lysis of the subchondral bone, which suggests that significant cartilage damage is also present (remember, cartilage is not visible in radiographs).

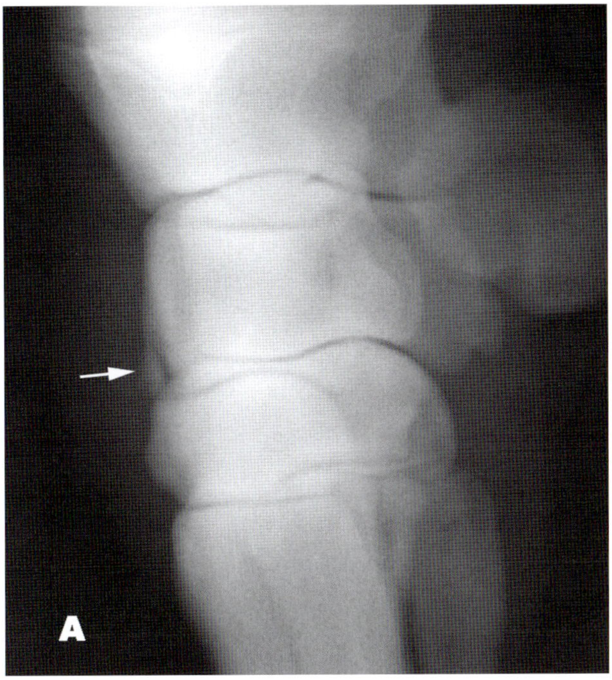

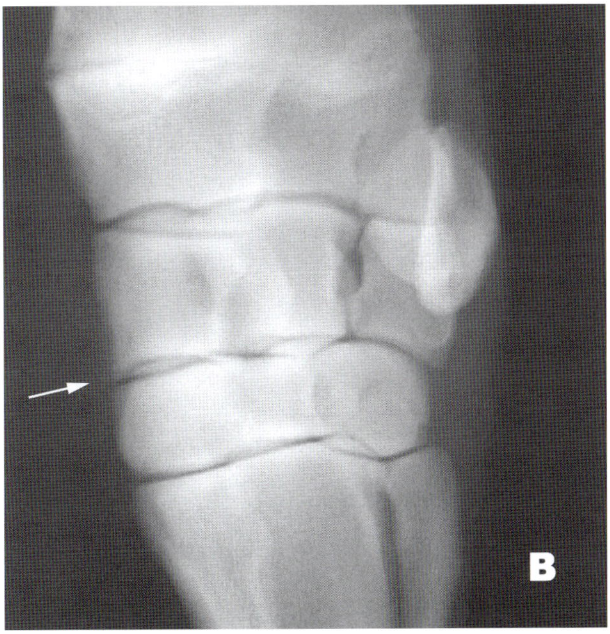

Figures 7.48a,b Lateral (A) and dorsolateral-palmaromedial oblique (B) radiographic projections of the right carpus of a 2-year-old Standardbred. **Fracture of the distal margin of the radial carpal bone:** The lateral view is slightly obliqued so that the dorsomedial aspect of the radial carpal bone is highlighted. The fracture fragment is clearly seen in this view (arrow). The DLPMO view is more dorsopalmar than it should be and the fracture fragment is not visible on the medial margin of the radial carpal bone. Subtle lucency and remodeling of the articular margin of the radial carpal bone is apparent (arrow).

Fracture of the Distal Radius

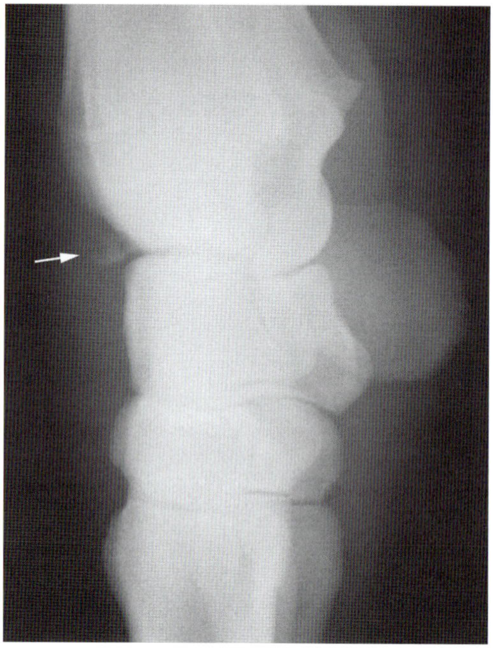

Figure 7.49 Lateral radiographic projection of the left carpus of a 2-year-old Thoroughbred. **Fracture of the distal radius:** A fracture fragment is seen at the dorsal margin of the antebrachiocarpal joint (arrow). The fracture appears to arise from the distal radius. A dorsoproximal-dorsodistal oblique (skyline) projection of the distal radius could be used to confirm the location of the fracture. This type of carpal fracture is more common in Thoroughbred and quarter horse racehorses. Hyperextension of the carpal joints during the stance phase of a gallop is thought to be the cause of this type of fracture.

Fracture of the Third Carpal Bone

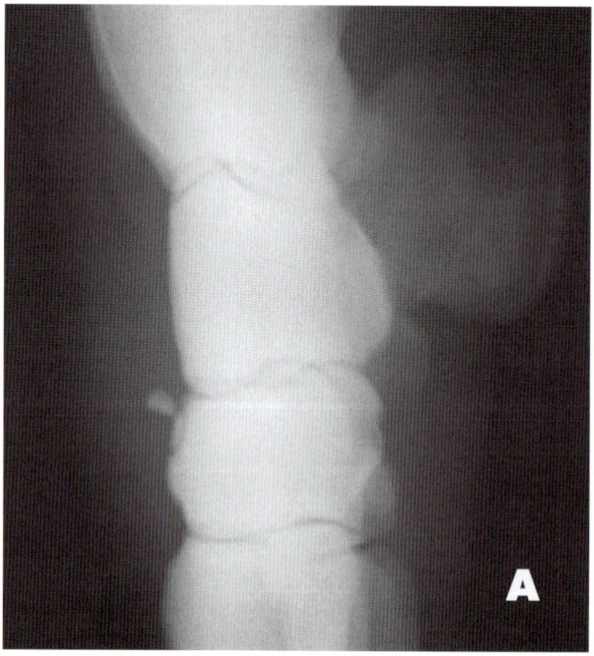

Figures 7.50a,b Lateral (A) and dorsolateral-palmaromedial oblique (B) radiographic projections of the right carpus of a 3-year-old Standardbred. **Fracture of the proximal dorsomedial margin of the third carpal bone:** In the lateral view (A), it is difficult to determine the origin of the fracture fragment. It could arise from the proximal margin of the third or fourth carpal bone. Also notice the large amount of capsular distension in the middle carpal joint. In the DLPMO view (B), the fracture is highlighted on the dorsomedial aspect of the joint. The third carpal bone is the dominant structure on the dorsomedial surface of the joint so the fracture must be in the third carpal bone.

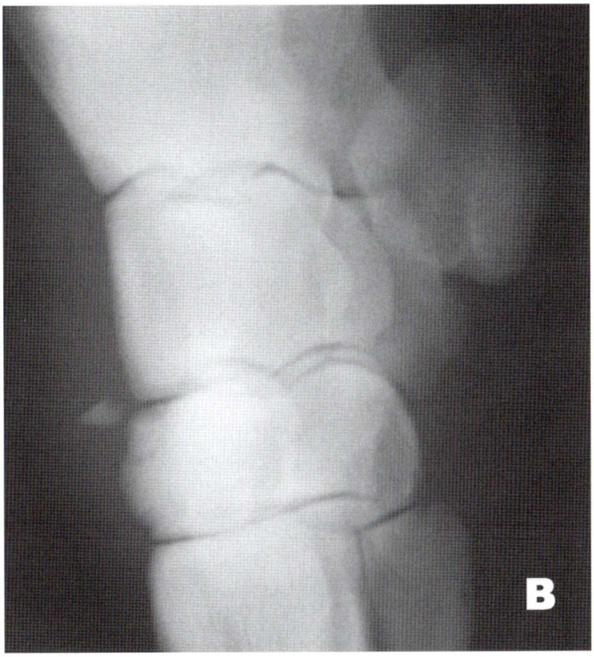

Figures 7.50a,b *Continued*

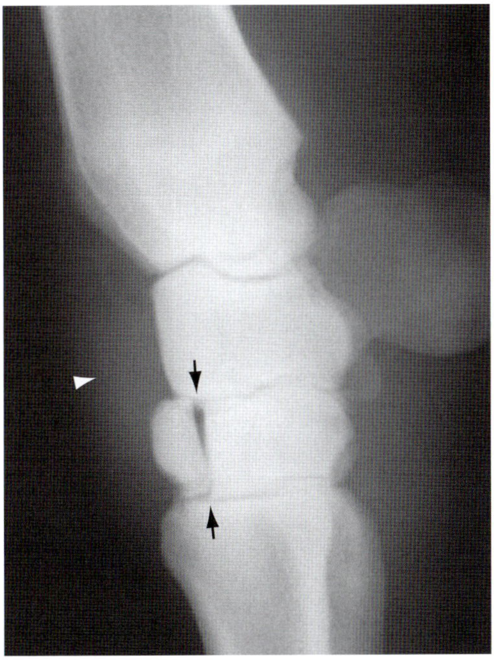

A

Figures 7.51a,b Lateral (A) and flexed lateral (B) radiographic projections of the left carpus of a 2-year-old Standardbred. **Slab fracture of the third carpal bone:** In the lateral radiographic projection, there is a large, cranially displaced fracture fragment. The fracture line (arrows) extends from the middle carpal joint to the carpometacarpal joint. The arrowhead indicates the rather marked degree of capsular distension that is present in the middle carpal joint. A slab fracture is, by definition, a fracture that extends through a bone from one articular surface to another articular surface. Many slab fractures are nondisplaced and are much more difficult to define in radiographs than this one. This flexed lateral radiographic projection is of the same carpus. Due to flexion of the joint, the fracture fragment is no longer displaced and the fracture line is barely visible (arrows).

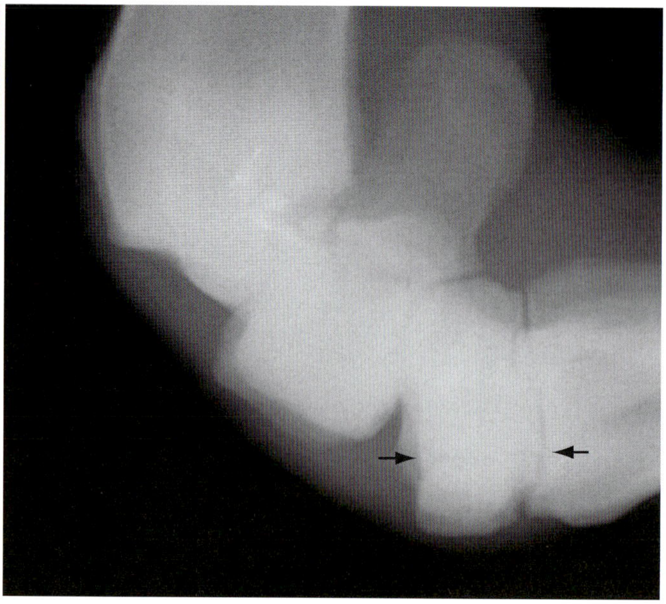

B

Figures 7.51a,b *Continued*

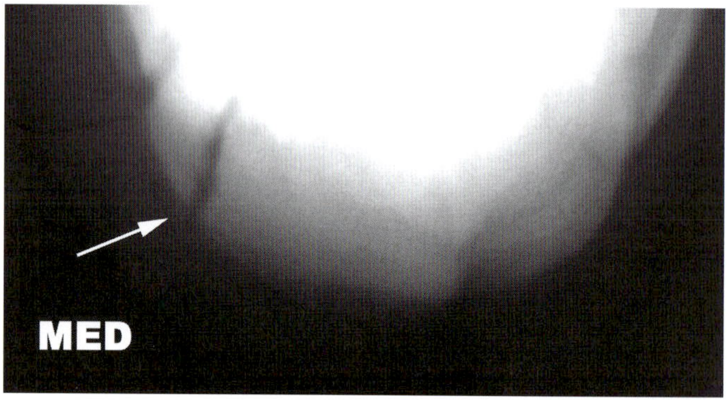

Figure 7.52 Dorsoproximal-dorsodistal oblique radiographic projection of the distal carpal row of the left carpus of a 5-year-old Standardbred. **Slab fracture (sagittal) of the third carpal bone:** This slab fracture is oriented along the sagittal plane of the limb and was only visible in the dorsoproximal-dorsodistal oblique view. This type of slab fracture is relatively uncommon, but this case shows the importance of obtaining dorsoproximal-dorsodistal oblique views of the carpus in racehorses.

Ulnar Carpal Bone Cyst

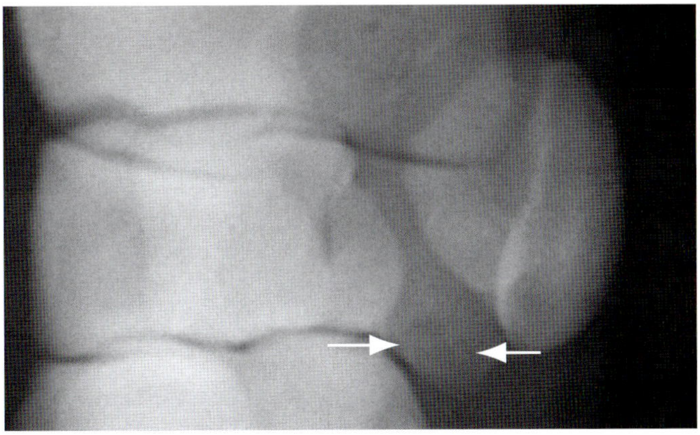

Figure 7.53 Dorsolateral-palmaromedial oblique radiographic projection of the left carpus of a 3-year-old Standardbred. **Ulnar carpal bone cyst:** Early reports of osteochondrosis lesions in the equine described cystlike lesions within the bones of the carpus and tarsus. This type of lesion is still occasionally seen, but the significance of this finding is often uncertain. In many cases, the lesion is considered incidental since either the horse is not lame or the lameness is isolated to a different area. This image shows just such a "cystlike" lesion in the ulnar carpal bone (arrows). In the past, these lesions have been considered to be a variant of osteochondrosis. However, a recent paper described lesions of this type as being the result of avulsion of the lateral palmar intercarpal ligament. Cases described had been examined arthroscopically and the evidence presented for ligamentous avulsion was convincing.

Radial Cysts

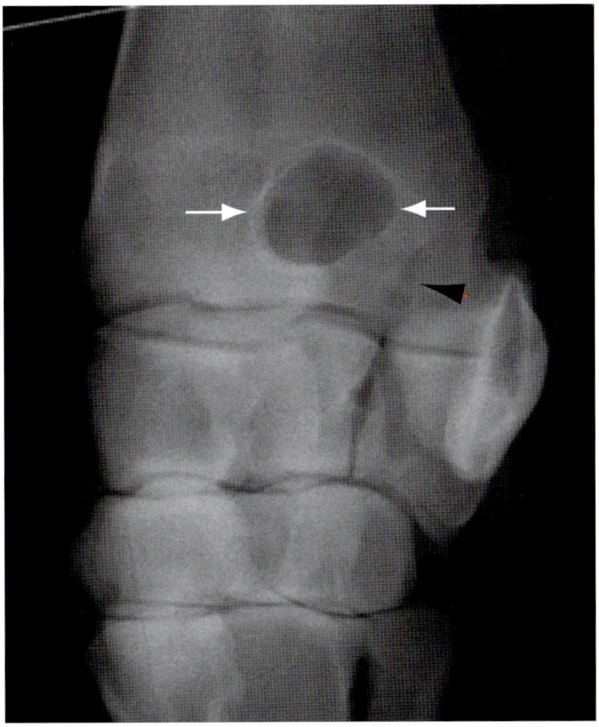

Figure 7.54 Dorsolateral-palmaromedial oblique radiographic projection of the left carpus of a 2-year-old Standardbred. **Radial cysts:** In this patient, an extremely large cyst (white arrows) and two smaller cysts (arrowhead) are visible in the distal radial epiphysis. There can be little doubt that these cysts are the result of osteochondrosis. Based on the location of the cysts, the lack of enchondral ossification likely occurred at the distal radial physis, not the articular cartilage, which would cause a subchondral bone cyst.

Enchondroma and Enthesiophyte Formation at the Attachment of the Superior Check Ligament

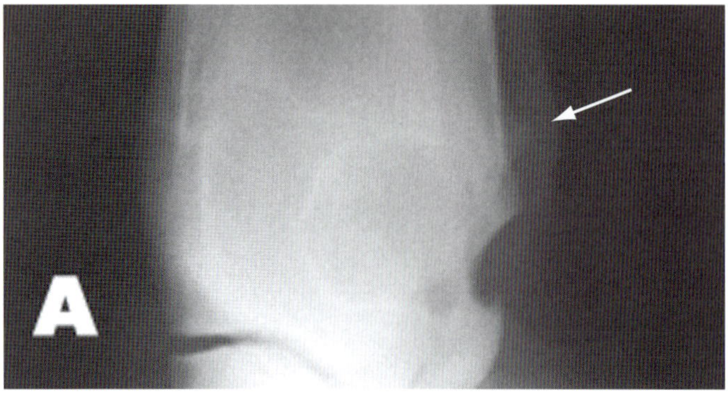

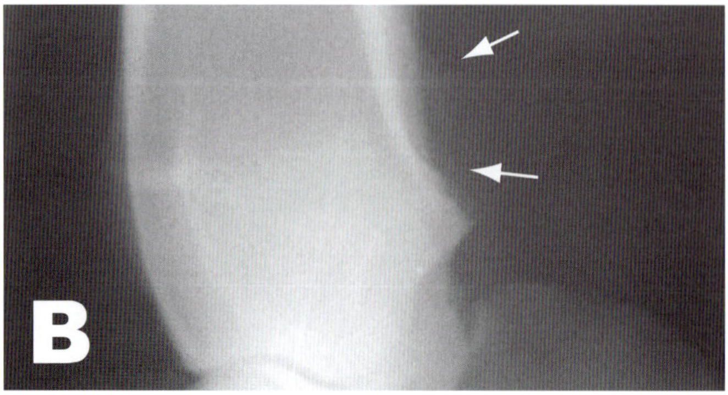

Figures 7.55a,b Lateral radiographic projections of the left carpus of a 2-year-old Standardbred (A) and a 6-year-old Standardbred (B). **(A) Enchondroma; (B) enthesiophyte formation at the attachment of the superior check ligament:** Enchondromas (arrow A) develop as cartilage-capped projections of bone at the level of physes. These exostoses increase in size until physeal closure occurs and then undergo remodeling. They are typically smooth in appearance and are often bilateral. Common locations in horses include the distal radial and distal tibial physes. They are most often incidental findings but may be a component in carpal canal syndrome. Enthesiophytes are areas of periosteal new bone at the attachment sites of ligaments, tendons, or joint capsules. Enthesiophyte formation at the origin of the superior check ligament (arrows B) tends to be more extensive and more irregular in appearance than an enchondroma. Enthesiophyte formation in this area is an indication of tension at the ligament attachment and may be seen in horses with superficial digital flexor tendonitis. However, it may also be seen as an incidental finding.

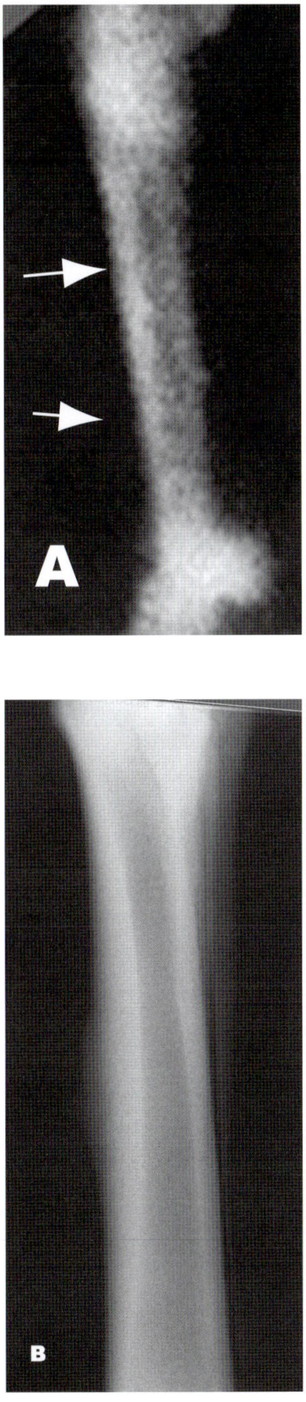

Figures 7.56a,b Nuclear scintigraphic image (A) and dorsolateral-palmaromedial oblique radiographic projection (B) of the left metacarpal region of a 2-year-old Standardbred. **Metacarpal periostitis ("bucked shin"):** The scintigraphic image demonstrates moderate increase in isotope activity along the entire length of the dorsal cortex of the third metacarpus (arrows). The radiograph demonstrates thickening of the dorsomedial cortex of the third metacarpus. The thickening is most prominent in the middle one-third of the bone. Metacarpal periostitis is the result of training at fast speeds. This training places compressive forces on the dorsal cortex of the metacarpal bone. As a response to these compressive forces, the cortical bone thickens. In the young horse, the region of greatest stress is the dorsomedial cortex.

Stress Fracture of the Third Metacarpus

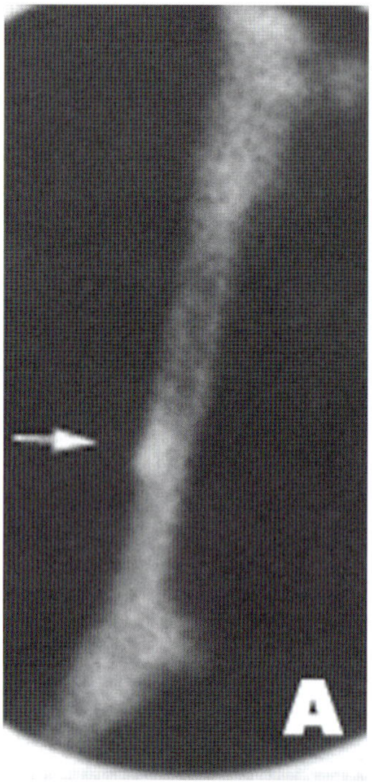

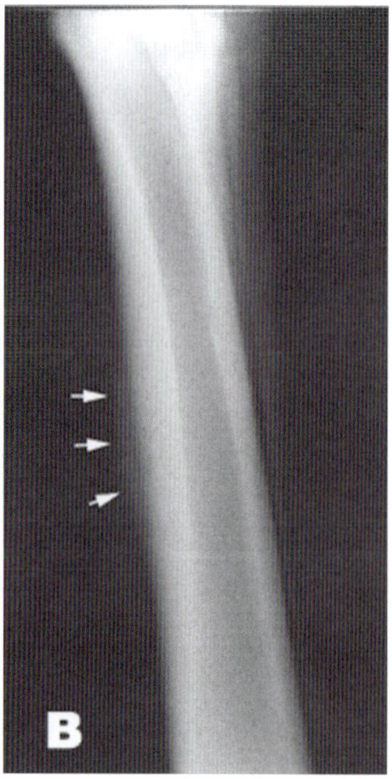

Figures 7.57a,b Nuclear scintigraphic image (A) and dorsomedial-palmarolateral oblique radiographic projection (B) of the left metacarpal region of a 3-year-old Thoroughbred. **Stress fracture of the dorsolateral cortex of the third metacarpus:** The scintigraphic image demonstrates intense isotope uptake focally on the dorsal cortex of the third metacarpus (arrow). The radiograph demonstrates thickening of the dorsal cortex of the third metacarpus and a smooth subperiosteal callus (arrows). The focal nature of the subperiosteal callus is an indication that a stress fracture has occurred and is now healing. Diffuse thickening of the dorsal cortex of the third metacarpus is the result of periostitis. Periostitis often precedes the development of a stress fracture. Metacarpal stress fractures are more common in Thoroughbreds than in Standardbreds and usually occur on the dorsolateral aspect of the bone.

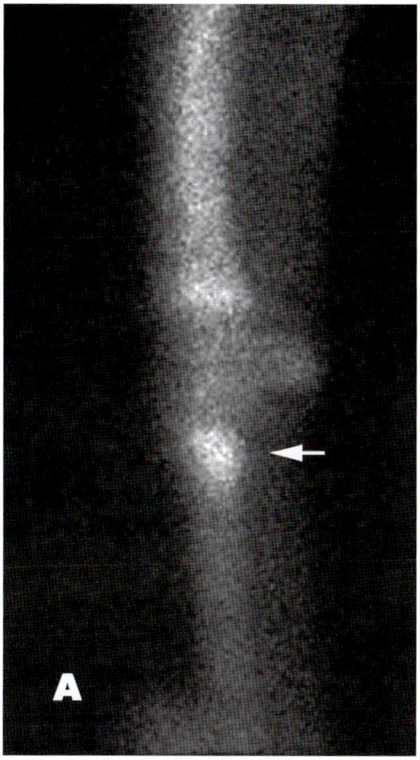

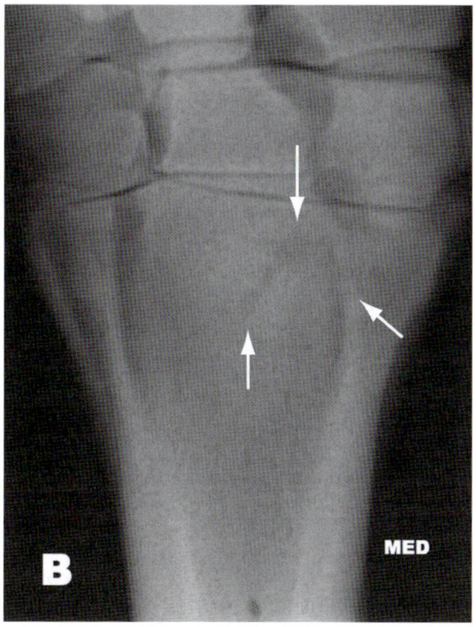

Figures 7.58a,b Nuclear scintigraphic image (A) and dorsopalmar radiographic projection (B) of the right proximal metacarpal region of a 3-year-old Standardbred. **Avulsion fracture of the origin of the suspensory ligament:** In the scintigraphic image, there is intense isotope uptake at the palmar margin of the third metacarpal bone (arrow). In the dorsopalmar radiographic projection, the fracture appears as an inverted V-shape (arrows) in the proximal medial metacarpus. Mild bone sclerosis is noted around the fracture; this makes the fracture easier to see and indicates chronicity. Avulsion fracture of the suspensory origin can also occur in the hind limb where the lesion is seen on the lateral aspect of the third metatarsus. Injury to the suspensory ligament is often present concurrently with the avulsion fracture. Ultrasound evaluation of the suspensory ligament is recommended for complete assessment.

Periostitis (Bony Reaction) at the Origin of the Suspensory Ligament

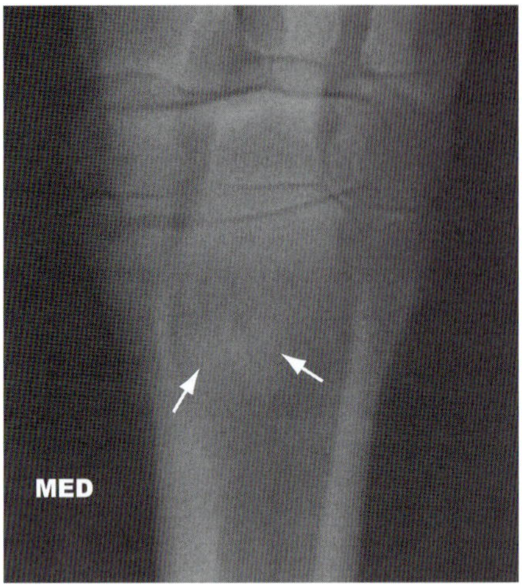

Figure 7.59 Dorsopalmar radiographic projection of the left proximal metacarpal region of a 2-year-old Standardbred. **Periostitis (bony reaction) at the origin of the suspensory ligament:** Rather than detach a piece of bone, the suspensory ligament may tear a piece away from its bony attachments. The result of this injury is a subperiosteal hematoma. Bony reaction (periostitis or enthesiophyte formation) then develops at the site of the hematoma. Radiographically, a localized area of increased opacity (sclerosis) is seen in the proximal medial metacarpus (arrows). This radiographic lesion will not be visible until approximately 2–3 weeks following the injury.

Splint Exostosis ("Splint") of the Second Metacarpal Bone

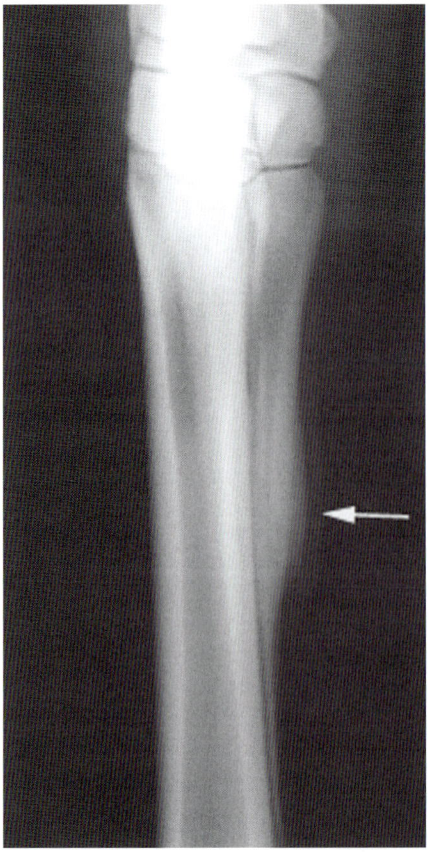

Figure 7.60 Dorsomedial-palmarolateral oblique radiographic projection of the left metacarpal region of a 4-year-old Thoroughbred. **Splint exostosis ("splint") of the 2nd metacarpal bone:** Interosseous ligaments are present between the 2nd and 4th metacarpal bones and the 3rd metacarpal bone. Strain on these ligaments leads to bony proliferation (periostitis). To horsemen, this lesion is a "splint." The bony proliferation is of variable size and is generally present in the proximal half of the bone. Splints occur most commonly between the 2nd and 3rd metacarpal bones. These radiographs show a very large splint arising from the 2nd metacarpal bone. The bony reaction is very smooth, and this is most likely an inactive splint and an incidental radiographic finding.

Fracture of the Fourth Metacarpal Bone with an Evidence of Osteomyelitis

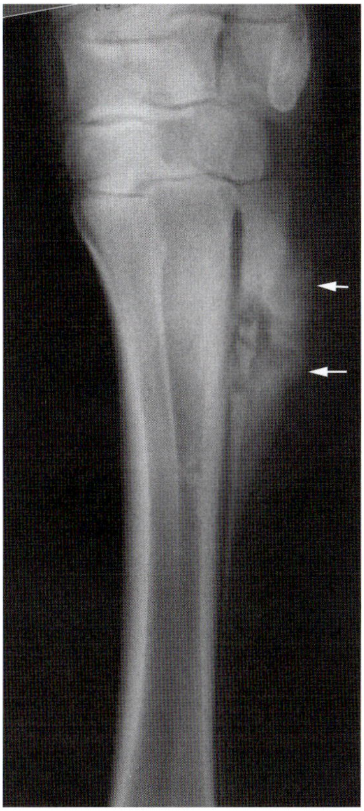

Figure 7.61 Dorsolateral-palmaromedial oblique radiographic projection of the right metacarpal region of a 1-year-old Thoroughbred. **Fracture of the 4th metacarpal bone with an evidence of osteomyelitis:** A fracture line is present in the proximal aspect of the 4th metacarpal bone. A large zone of lysis and excessive irregular periosteal response surrounds the metacarpal fracture (arrows). A fracture in this location is most likely the result of a traumatic injury. Penetration of the soft tissues with introduction of bacteria likely occurred at the time of the fracture. The fracture has been present for a long time, enough for osteomyelitis to develop.

The Tarsus and Metatarsus

Osteochondritis Dissecans (OCD)

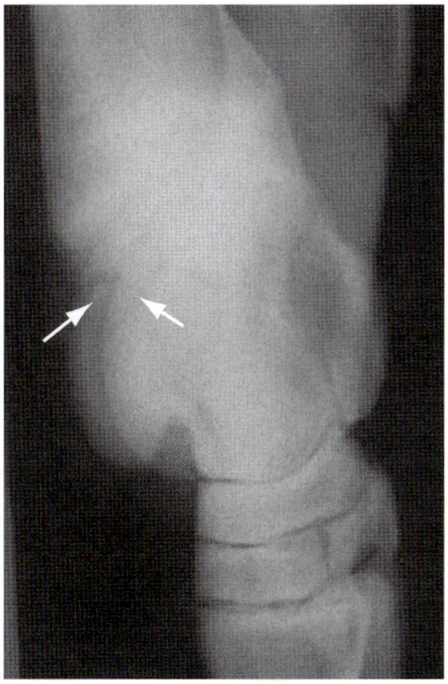

Figure 7.62 Dorsomedial-plantarolateral oblique radiographic projection of the left tarsus of a 2-year-old Standardbred. **Osteochondritis dissecans (OCD) of the distal intermediate ridge of the tibia:** There is an osseous fragment arising from the distal intermediate ridge of the tibia (arrows). The majority of OCD lesions in the tarsocrural joint occur in this location. The dorsomedial-plantarolateral oblique radiographic projection is the best view to see OCD lesions in this location. In this case the radiograph is only slightly obliqued from a lateral projection.

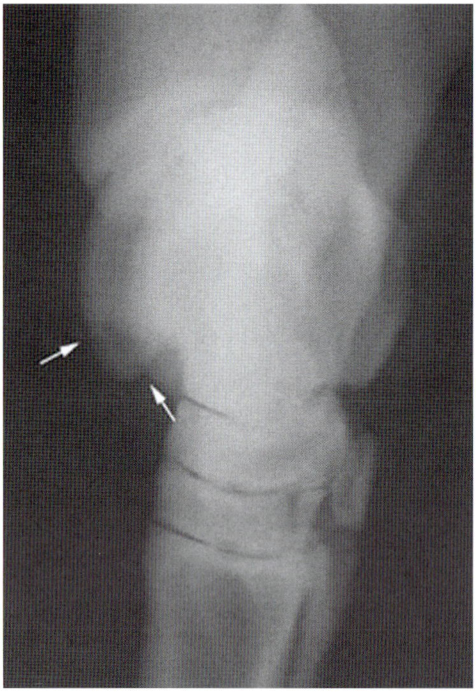

Figure 7.63 Dorsomedial-plantarolateral oblique radiographic projection of the right tarsus of a 3-year-old Standardbred. **Osteochondritis dissecans (OCD) of the lateral trochlear ridge of the talus:** A large area of lucency is present on the dorsal projection of the lateral trochlear ridge of the talus (arrows). This is the second most common location for OCD lesions although they occur much less frequently here than at the distal intermediate ridge of the tibia. The dorsomedial-plantarolateral oblique radiographic projection highlights the lateral trochlear ridge of the talus as well as the distal intermediate ridge of the tibia. This single radiographic projection will diagnose more than 90% of OCD lesions of the tarsocrural joint.

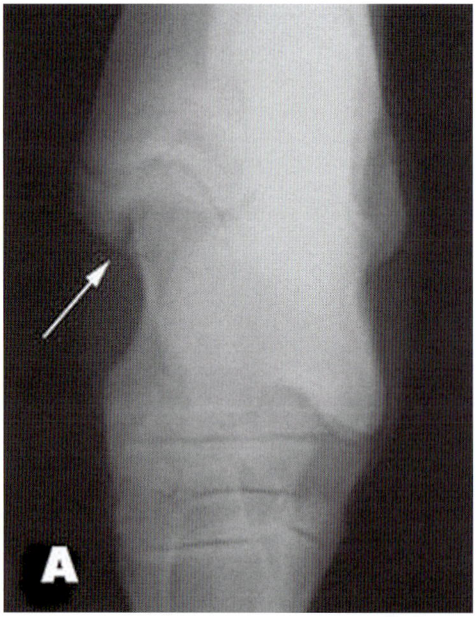

Figures 7.64a,b Dorsoplantar (A) and dorsolateral-plantaromedial oblique (B) radiographic projections of the right tarsus of a 3-year-old Standardbred. **Osteochondritis dissecans (OCD) of the medial malleolus of the tibia:** In the dorsoplantar view, a fissure line is visible separating an osseous fragment from the medial malleolus of the tibia (arrow). Superimposition of the talus in the dorsoplantar view makes evaluation of this area difficult. The dorsolateral-plantaromedial oblique radiographic projection better defines the medial malleolus of the talus and the osseous fragment is clearly seen (white arrow). Note that the oblique radiograph is only slightly oblique (~15 degrees) from dorsoplantar. This angle provides the best visualization of the medial malleolus.

Figures 7.64a,b *Continued*

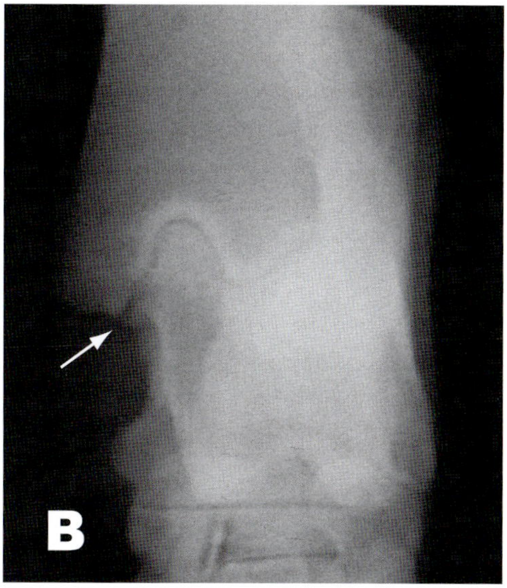

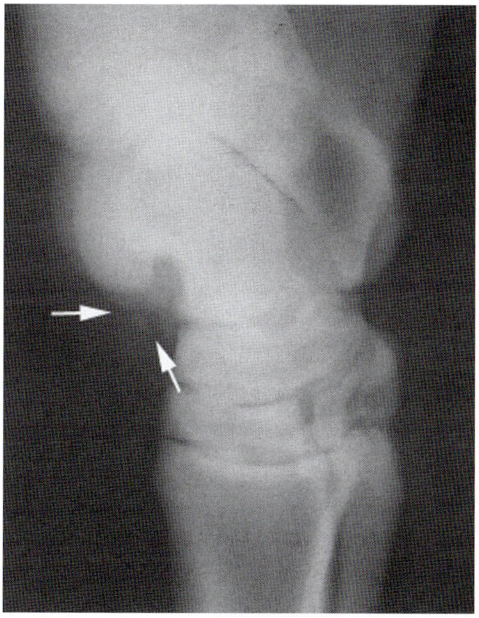

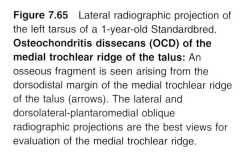

Figure 7.65 Lateral radiographic projection of the left tarsus of a 1-year-old Standardbred. **Osteochondritis dissecans (OCD) of the medial trochlear ridge of the talus:** An osseous fragment is seen arising from the dorsodistal margin of the medial trochlear ridge of the talus (arrows). The lateral and dorsolateral-plantaromedial oblique radiographic projections are the best views for evaluation of the medial trochlear ridge.

Osteoarthritis (Degenerative Joint Disease, "Spavin")

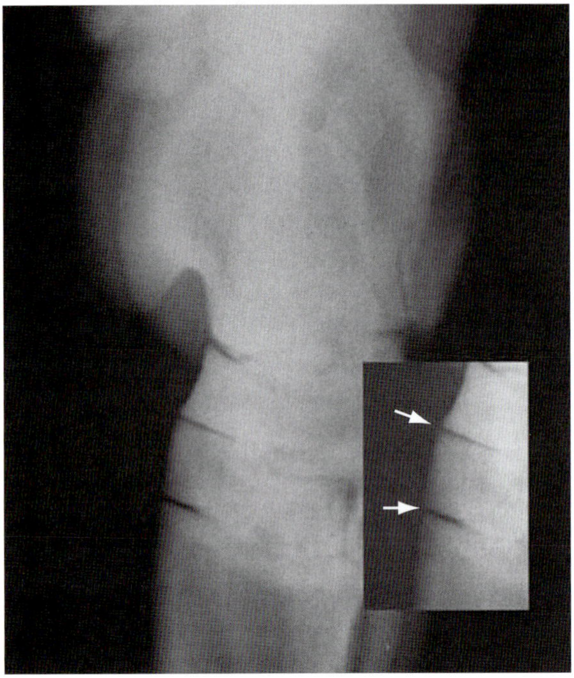

Figure 7.66 Dorsomedial-plantarolateral radiographic projection of the left tarsus of a 3-year-old Standardbred. **Mild osteoarthritis (synonym is degenerative joint disease, "spavin") of the distal intertarsal and tarsometatarsal joint:** Minor osteophyte formation is present on the dorsolateral margin of the distal intertarsal and tarsometatarsal joints (see arrows and inset). This creates an appearance of "lipping" or "spurring" of the joint margin. This degree of osteoarthritis is common in many athletic horses, even at a young age.

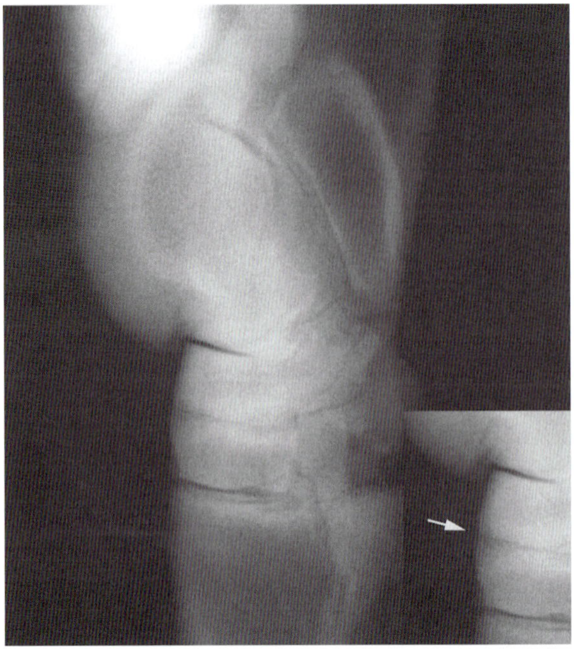

Figure 7.67 Lateral radiographic projection of the left tarsus of a 3-year-old Standardbred. **Moderate osteoarthritis of the distal intertarsal joint:** Osteophyte formation is present on the dorsal margin of the distal intertarsal joint. The dorsal distal intertarsal joint space is narrowed and lucency of the subchondral bone is seen at the dorsal margin of the joint (arrow and inset).

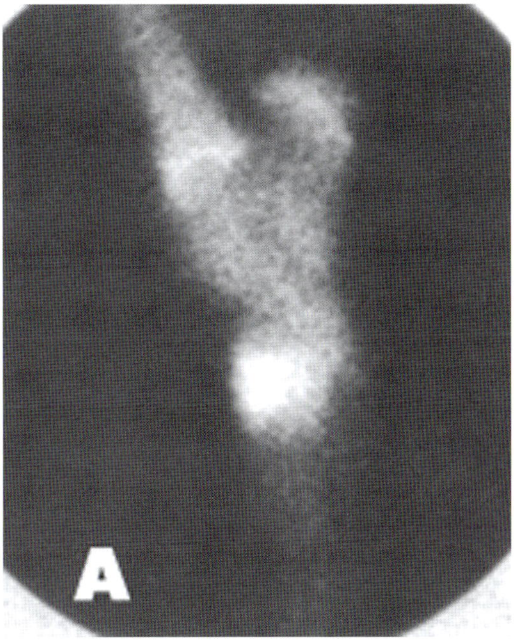

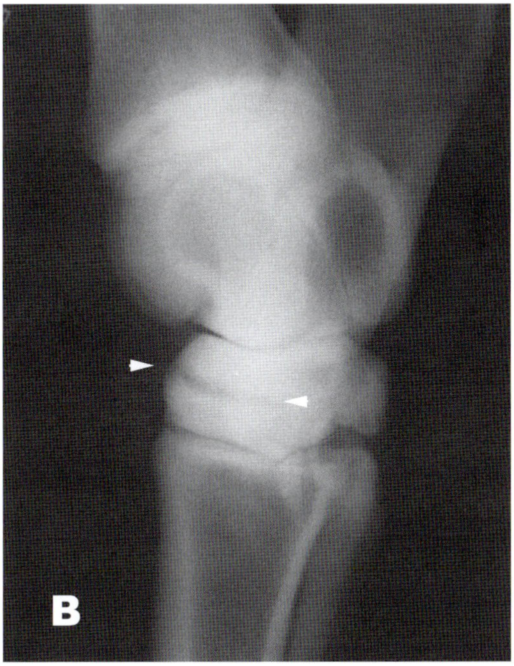

Figures 7.68a–c Nuclear scintigraphic image (A) and lateral radiographic projection of the left tarsus of a 10-year-old quarter horse (B) and dorsolateral-plantaromedial oblique radiographic projection (C) of the left tarsus of a 16-year-old Thoroughbred. **(A)Severe osteoarthritis of the distal intertarsal joint; (B)severe osteoarthritis of the proximal intertarsal joint, distal intertarsal joint, and tarsometatarsal joint:** In the scintigraphic image (A), there is intense isotope uptake (bright white area) on the dorsal margin of the distal intertarsal joint that extends into the joint space. In the radiograph of this horse (B), there is loss of the joint space and associated subchondral bone lysis in the same area as indicated by the scintigraphic study (arrowheads). The joint appears to be undergoing ankylosis. In (C) the distal intertarsal and tarsometatarsal joint spaces appear to be ankylosed. The dorsomedial margin of the proximal intertarsal joint space is visible but significant subchondral lysis is present. It is uncommon for osteoarthritis to affect the proximal intertarsal joint; those horses so affected are usually severely lame.

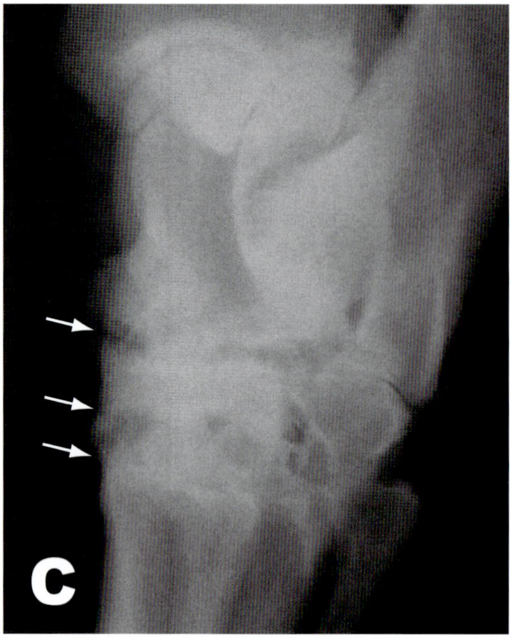

Figures 7.68a–c *Continued*

Fracture of the Talus

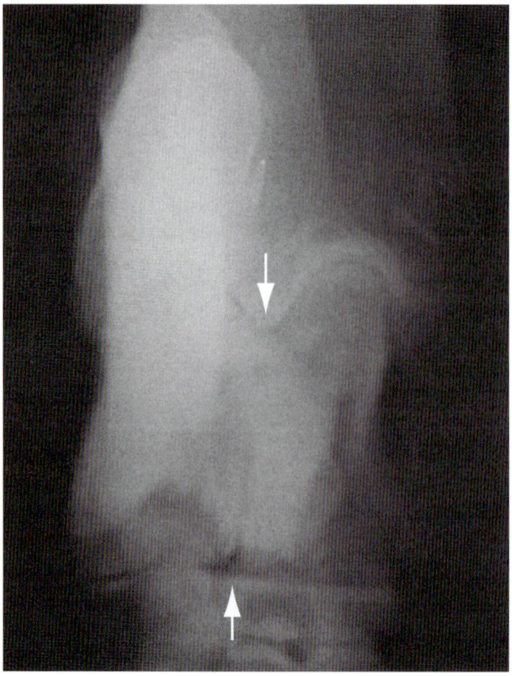

A

Figures 7.69a,b Dorsoplantar (A) and lateral (B) radiographic projection of the right tarsus of a 2-year-old quarter horse. **Comminuted fracture of the talus:** In the dorsoplantar view, a sagittal fracture is visible in the midbody of the talus (arrows). The fracture line extends from the tibiotarsal joint to the proximal intertarsal joint; this is by definition a slab fracture. In the lateral view, an additional fracture line is visible from the proximal to distal margins of the lateral trochlear ridge of the talus (black arrows). Multiple small bone fragments are visible dorsal to the talus and superimposed with the calcaneus (arrowheads). No fractures were visible in the calcaneus or in the bones of the distal tarsal rows.

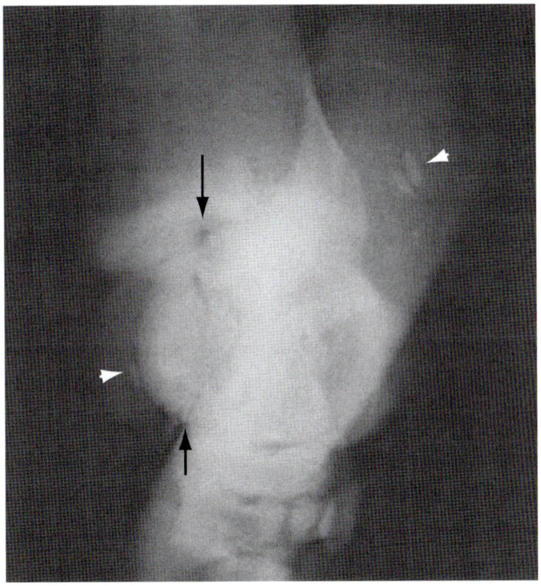

B

Figures 7.69a,b *Continued*

Sequestration of the Calcaneus

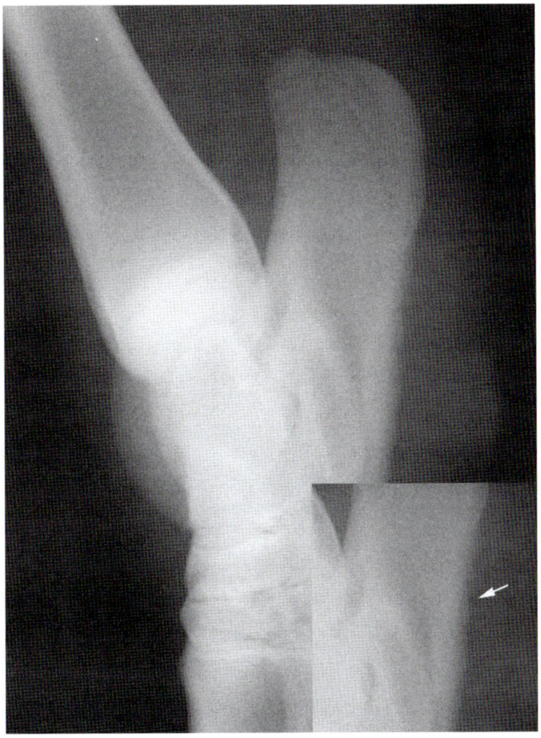

Figure 7.70 Lateral radiographic projection of the right tarsus of a 2-year-old quarter horse. **Sequestration of the calcaneus:** This lateral view is obtained with slight dorsolateral-plantaromedial obliquity to better define the plantarolateral aspect of the calcaneus. There is significant soft tissue swelling at the plantarolateral aspect of the limb. A small bone fragment (inset and arrow) is present on the margin of the calcaneus. This type of injury is not uncommon and is generally the result of a kick by another horse.

Fracture of the Fourth Metatarsal Bone

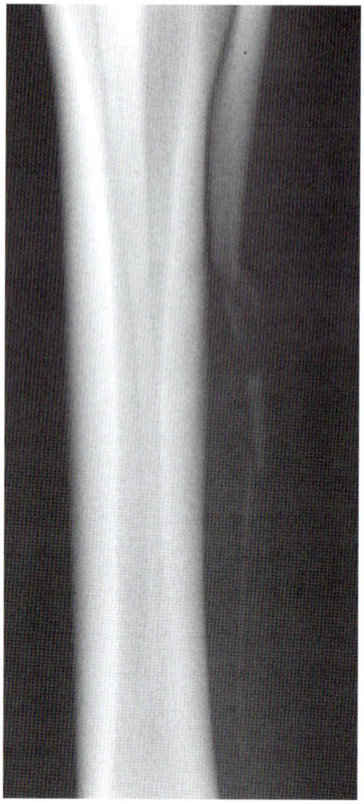

Figure 7.71 Dorsolateral-plantaromedial oblique radiographic projection of the left metatarsal region of a 6-year-old Thoroughbred. **Comminuted fracture of the 4th metatarsal bone:** The central portion of the 4th metatarsal bone is fractured; multiple fragments are present. Soft tissue swelling is present in the area. This type of fracture is most commonly the result of a kick by another horse and is most often seen in the 4th metatarsal bone.

Fracture and Osteomyelitis of the Fourth Metatarsal Bone

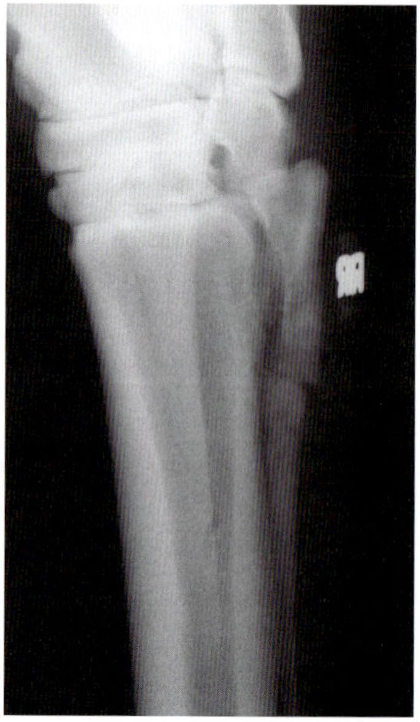

Figure 7.72 Dorsolateral-plantaromedial oblique radiographic projection of the right metatarsal region of a 1-year-old quarter horse. The lead marker indicates the location of a draining tract in the soft tissues. **Comminuted fracture of the 4th metatarsal bone with evidence of osteomyelitis:** Multiple fracture lines are present in the proximal aspect of the 4th metatarsal bone; some displacement of the fracture fragments is present. The fracture fragments are more lucent than the surrounding bone and there is irregular periosteal response on the margins of the affected portion of the metatarsal bone. The fracture has been present for several weeks and osteomyelitis has developed. Penetration of the soft tissues with introduction of bacteria likely occurs at the time of the fracture.

Figures 7.73a,b Lateral (A) and dorsoplantar (B) radiographic projections of the left metatarsal region of a 3-year-old Standardbred. The horse got his leg stuck in a gate approximately 4 weeks ago. **Sequestrum formation on the dorsal cortex of the 3rd metatarsal bone:** In the lateral view, a bone fragment, sequestrum, is seen arising from the dorsal cortex of the third metatarsus (arrows). The fragment is separated from the cortex by a lucent band; this band is the result of the accumulation of exudate with or without the presence of granulation tissue between the cortex and the bone fragment. In the dorsoplantar view, the lesion is seen "en face." The bone fragment is surrounded by a large zone of lucency and is clearly visible (black arrows). Sequestra occur following traumatic injury to the lower limbs that results in damage to the periosteal blood supply of the bone; penetration of the soft tissues is not necessary. Loss of periosteal blood supply to the bone causes the outer portion of the bone to die. The body mounts an inflammatory response against the necrotic bone fragment leading to the accumulation of inflammatory exudate and granulation tissue and thickening of the surrounding bone. These changes cause the characteristic radiographic changes seen here. Radiographic changes of sequestration are not visible for a minimum of 10–14 days following injury; 3–4 weeks is generally required for a distinct sequestrum to be visible.

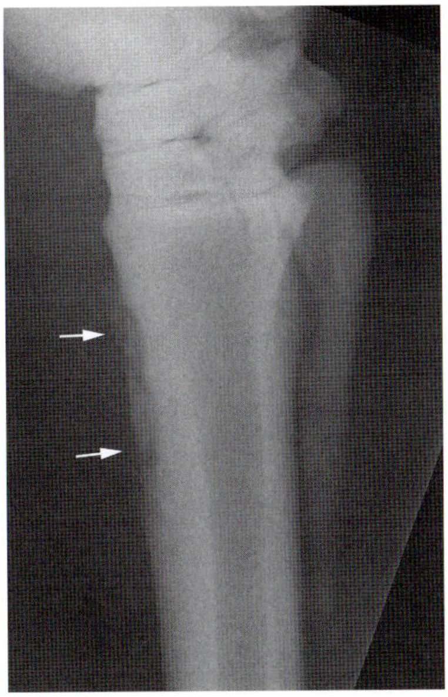

A

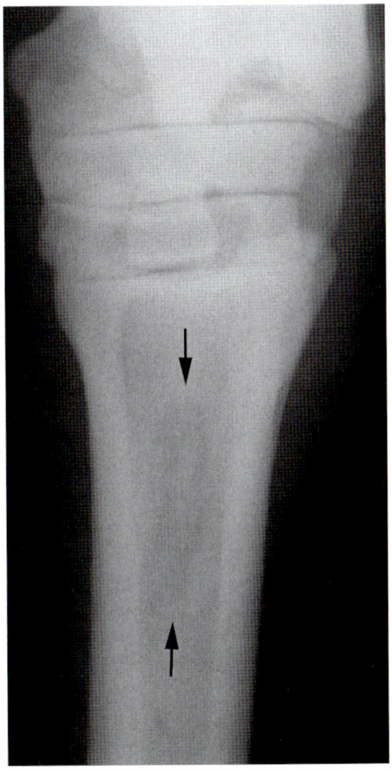

B

Subchondral Bone Cyst

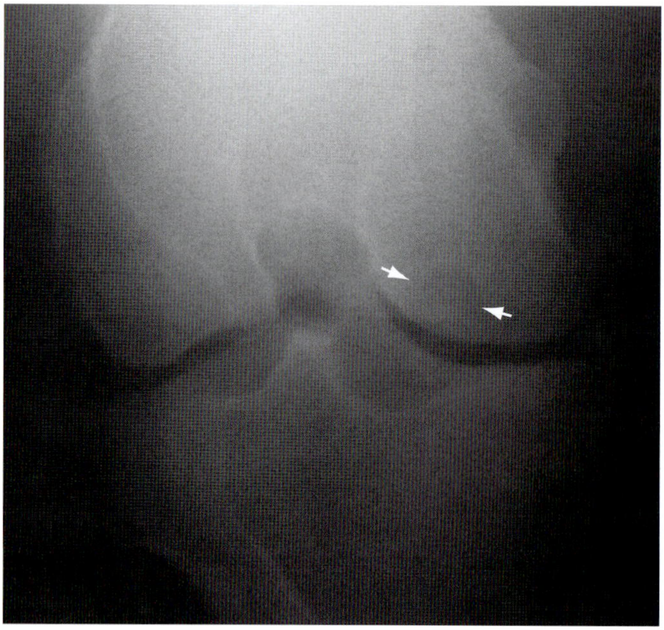

Figure 7.74 Caudocranial radiographic projection of the left stifle of a 3-year-old Standardbred. **Subchondral bone cyst of the medial condyle:** A large, well-defined lucency is present in the medial femoral condyle (arrows). This is a subchondral bone cyst (synonym is "osseous cystlike lesion"). This is a type of osteochondrosis lesion. These lesions are best seen in the caudocranial projection but may also be visible in the caudolateral-craniomedial oblique projection.

Osteochondritis Dissecans (OCD)

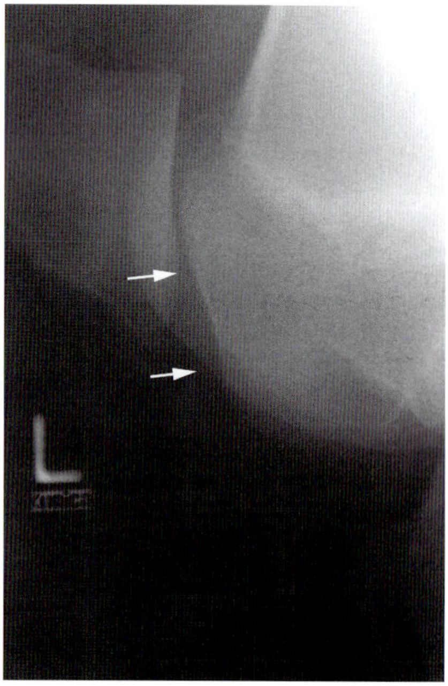

A

Figures 7.75a,b Lateral radiographic projections of the left (A) and right (B) stifles of a 1.5-year-old Standardbred. **Bilateral osteochondritis dissecans (OCD) of the lateral trochlear ridge:** In the left stifle, the lateral femoral trochlear ridge is flattened (arrows). In the right stifle, the lateral femoral trochlear ridge is flattened and irregular. An osseous fragment is seen cranial to the area of flattening. This is a cartilage flap that has ossified. These lesions represent two variants of osteochondritis dissecans (OCD) of the stifle joint. The caudocranial projection and caudolateral- craniomedial oblique projection highlight the femoral trochlear ridges and are necessary to diagnose this condition.

Figures 7.75a,b *Continued*

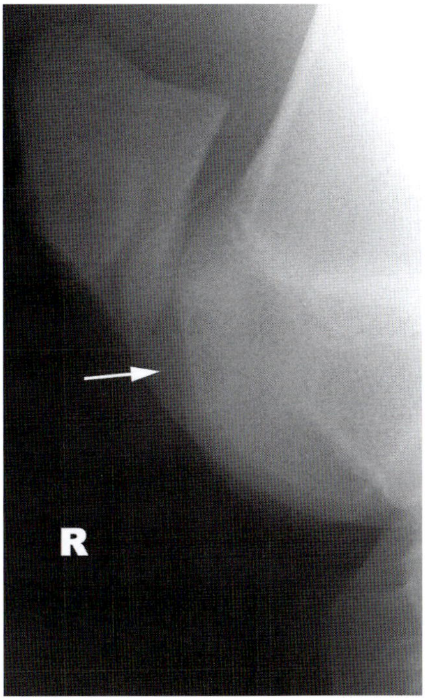

B

Osteoarthritis of the Stifle Joint

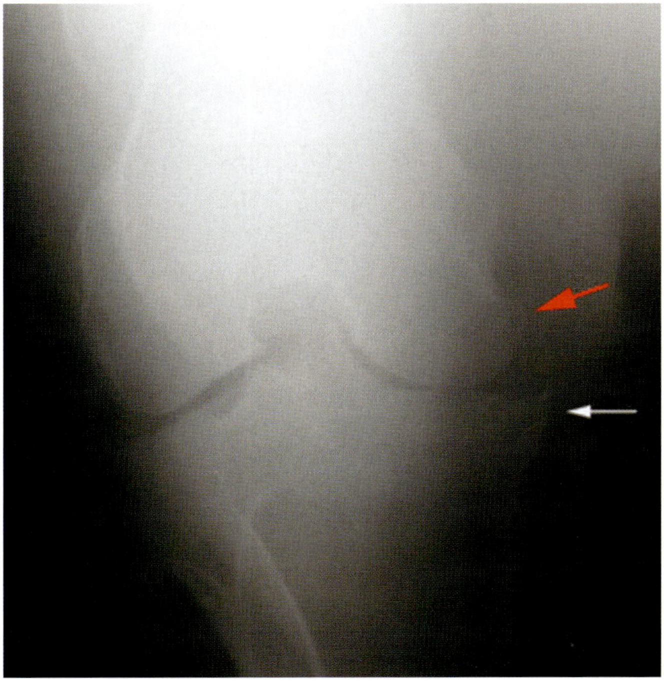

Figure 7.76 Caudocranial radiographic projection of the left stifle of a 13-year-old quarter horse. **Osteoarthritis of the stifle joint:** Osteophyte formation is present on the medial margin of the proximal tibial plateau and on the medial epicondyle of the femur (arrows). The medial femorotibial joint space is narrower than the lateral joint space; this may be an evidence for injury to the medial meniscus. However, this finding should be interpreted with caution as the apparent narrowing could be due to uneven weight-bearing in the standing patient. Osteoarthritis of the stifle is relatively uncommon. It is usually secondary osteoarthritis, the result of injury to the supporting structures of the joint, OCD, fracture, or sepsis. Radiographic changes of stifle osteoarthritis can be subtle and are best seen in the caudocranial radiographic projection.

Cranial Cruciate Ligament Injury

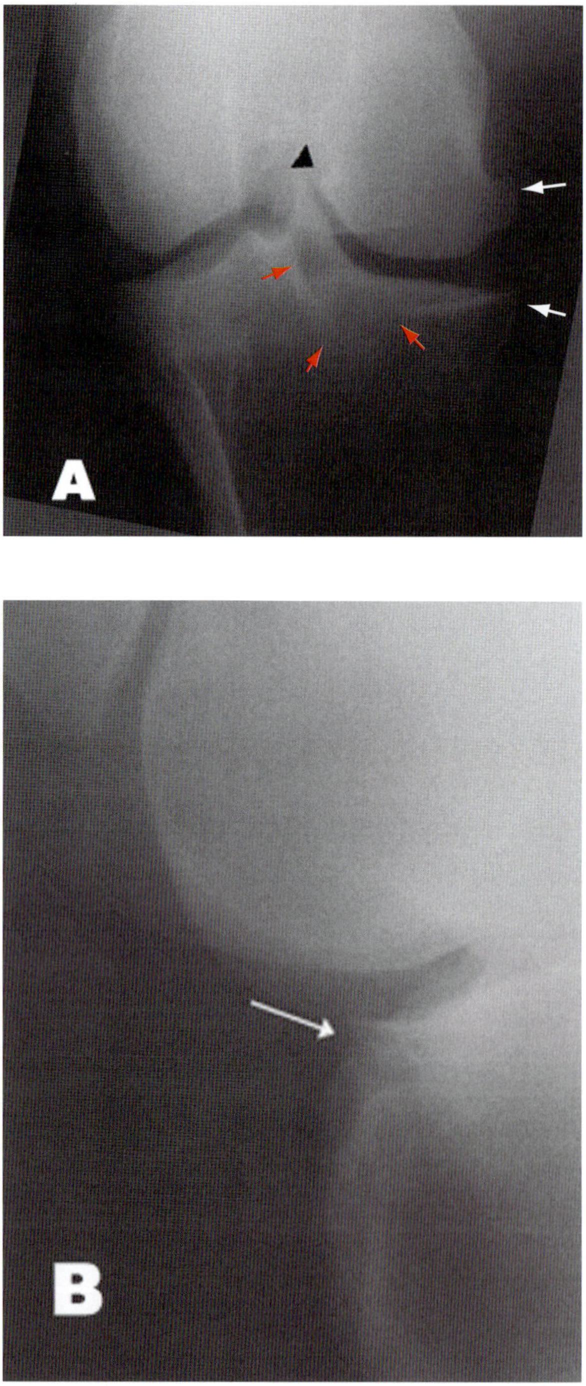

Figures 7.77a,b Caudocranial (A) and lateral (B) radiographic projections of the left stifle of a 6-year-old Standardbred. **Osteoarthritis of the stifle joint and chronic cranial cruciate ligament injury:** In the caudocranial radiographic projection, there is an osteophyte formation on the medial tibial plateau and medial epicondyle (white arrows) and on the axial margin of the medial femoral condyle (arrowhead). These changes are evidences of osteoarthritis. An ill-defined area of lucency with a sclerotic margin is visible distal to the medial tibial intercondylar eminence (red arrows). In the lateral radiographic projection, there is osteophyte formation on the tibial plateau (arrow) in the area of the intercondylar eminences. Osteoarthritis is present but is a nonspecific finding. The lucency ventral to the medial tibial intercondylar eminence and osteophyte formation cranial to the intercondylar eminences are radiographic changes seen as a result of injury to the cranial cruciate ligament. Acute injury to the cranial cruciate ligament does not cause radiographic changes. The radiographic changes characteristic of cruciate ligament injury are generally present by 3–4 weeks following injury.

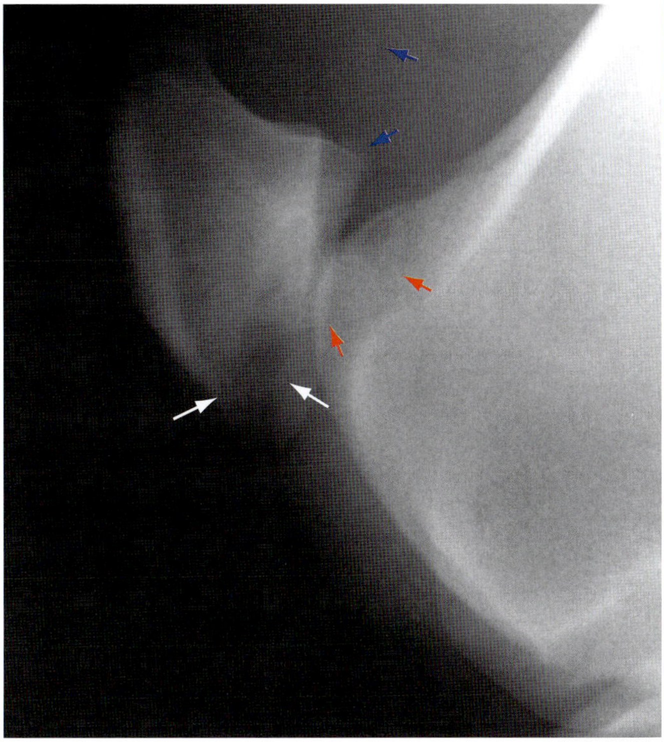

A

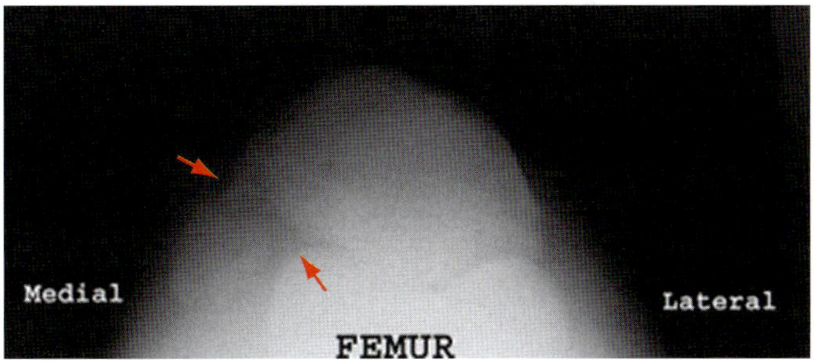

B

Figures 7.78a,b Lateromedial (A) and skyline (B) (cranioproximal-craniodistal oblique) radiographic projections of the stifle of a 12-year-old quarter horse. The horse had become lame after falling from an embankment 2 weeks earlier. **Chronic fracture of the patella:** In the lateral radiographic projection, careful evaluation of the patella reveals several abnormalities. A lucent area is present in the apex of the patella (white arrows) and a large bone fragment is superimposed with the patella and the femoral trochlear ridge (red arrows). Two smaller bone fragments are visible dorsal to the patella (blue arrows). The skyline projection provides the best visualization of the patella and is necessary to view where patellar fracture is suspected. In this case, a large fracture fragment is seen arising from the medial aspect of the patella. The fracture line is indistinct due to the chronicity of the fracture (red arrows).

Calcinosis Circumscripta (Tumoral Calcinosis)

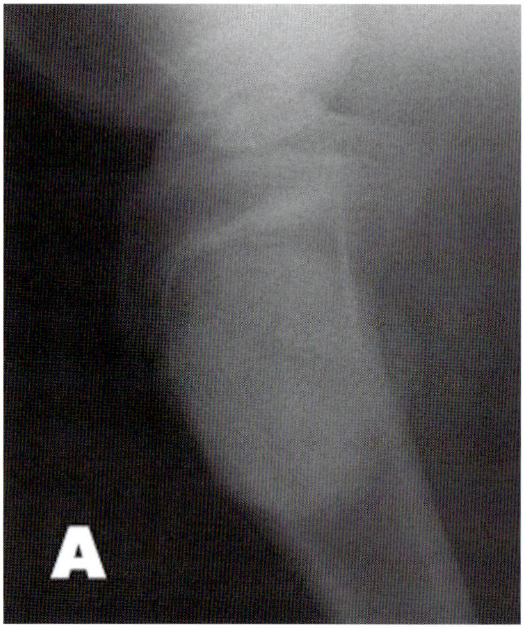

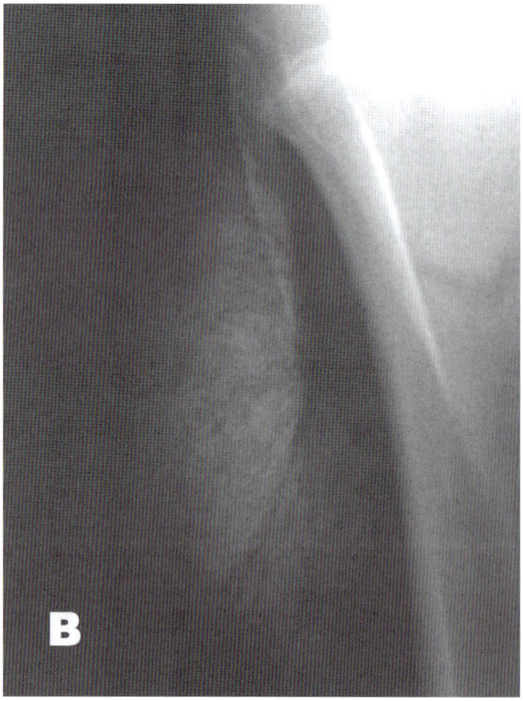

Figures 7.79a,b Lateral (A) and caudocranial (B) radiographic projections of the stifle of a 2-year-old Standardbred. **Calcinosis circumscripta (tumoral calcinosis):** There is large, well-circumscribed mass of stippled mineral opacity on the lateral aspect of the proximal tibia. The radiographic appearance of this lesion is characteristic of tumoral calcinosis (synonym is "calcinosis circumscripta"). The lesion is of unknown etiology and the result of deposition of calcium salts in the skin and subcutaneous tissues. Tumor calcinosis occurs mostly in young horses and the most common location is on the lateral surface of the stifle. Lesions are almost always bilateral. Horses with tumoral calcinosis are generally presented for cosmetic reasons; lesions rarely cause lameness.

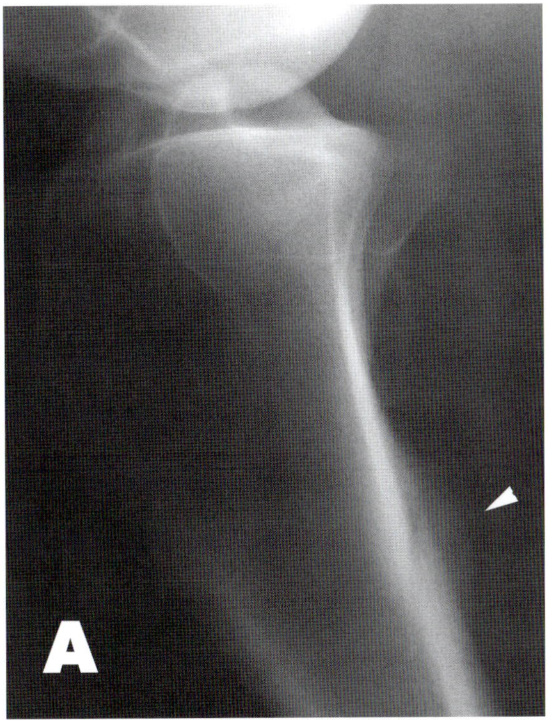

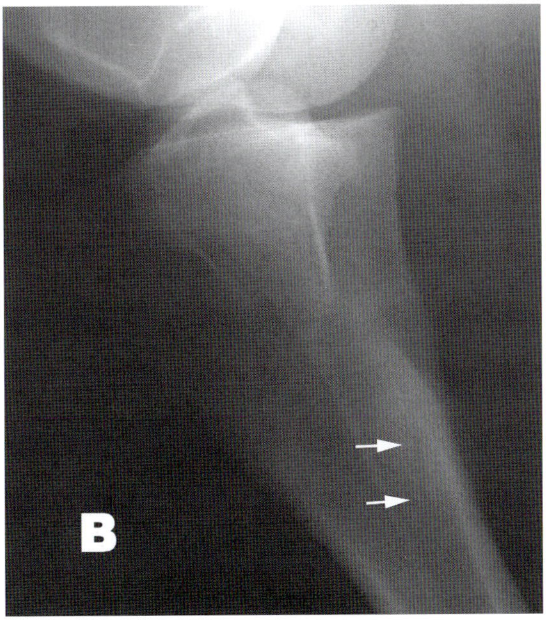

Figures 7.80a,b Lateromedial (A) and caudolateral-craniomedial oblique (B) radiographic projections of the right tibia of a 3-year-old Standardbred. **Tibial stress fracture:** In the lateral view, a smooth periosteal response is visible on the caudal aspect of the tibia (arrowhead). A lucent line is visible within the area of periosteal response; this appears to be the normal nutrient foramen. In the oblique radiographic projection, a linear lucency in an inverted V shape is present on the caudomedial margin of the tibia; this is the stress fracture (arrows). There is sclerosis of the bone surrounding the fracture and increasing its conspicuity. The lucent line in the proximal fibula is a normal separate center of ossification. Radiographic diagnosis of tibial stress fracture can be made in this patient due to the evidence for bone healing (periosteal response and bone sclerosis) that is present. In acute stress fractures, no radiographic changes are present. Nuclear scintigraphy (bone scan) is useful for diagnosis of an acute stress fracture.

Normal Cervical Spine

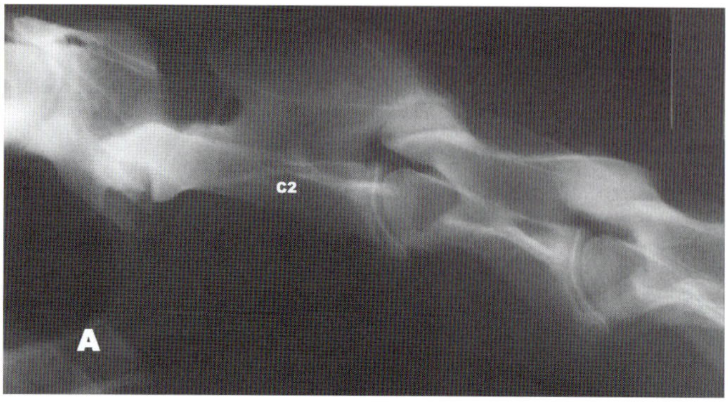

Figures 7.81a,b Lateral radiographic projections of the cervical spine in a 4-year-old Warmblood. **Normal cervical spine:** (A) is of the cranial portion of the cervical spine. The second cervical vertebra can be easily identified due to the presence of the large, distinctively shaped spinous process. (B) is of the caudal portion of the cervical spine. The 6th cervical vertebra is identified by the caudoventral extension of the transverse processes (arrows); the transverse processes of the 3rd, 4th, and 5th cervical vertebrae lack this extension. Note that the radiographic appearance of the 3rd, 4th, and 5th vertebrae is essentially identical. Accurate identification of these vertebrae relies on the presence of an identifiable anatomic landmark, either the 2nd or 6th cervical vertebra. * Contrast is visible in the subarachnoid space in (B). This figure is from a myelographic study.

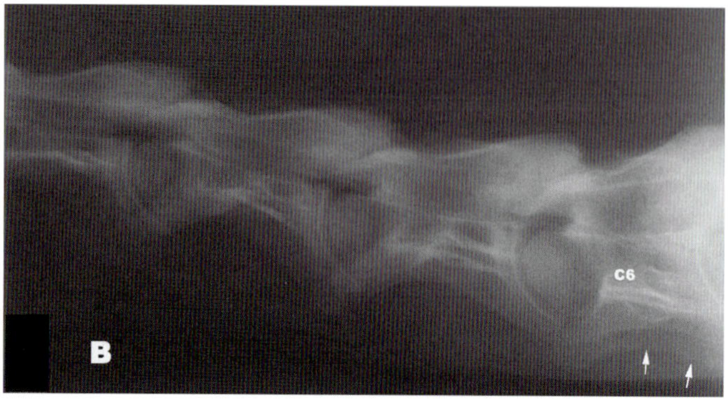

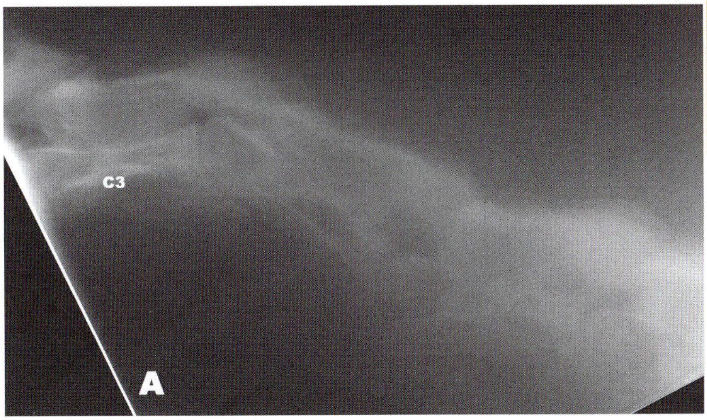

Figures 7.82a,b Lateral radiographic projections of the cranial cervical spine of a 2-year-old Standardbred. (A) is a survey film and (B) is from a myelographic study. **(A) Malalignment of the spinal canal at C 3-4; (B) compression of the spinal cord at C 3-4:** In the survey film (A), the spinal canal is malaligned at the C 3-4 level. The malalignment is static and did not change with a change in head position. Some bony proliferation is present at the articular facets. Prior fracture of the facets with malunion is suspected as the cause of these radiographic changes. Based on the appearance of the spinal canal, it is likely that compression of the spinal cord is present. However, myelography is required to confirm this supposition. In the myelogram (B), the ventral subarachnoid space is obliterated and the dorsal subarachnoid space is significantly narrowed (black lines). Decreased thickness of both subarachnoid spaces is the diagnostic criteria for spinal cord compression.

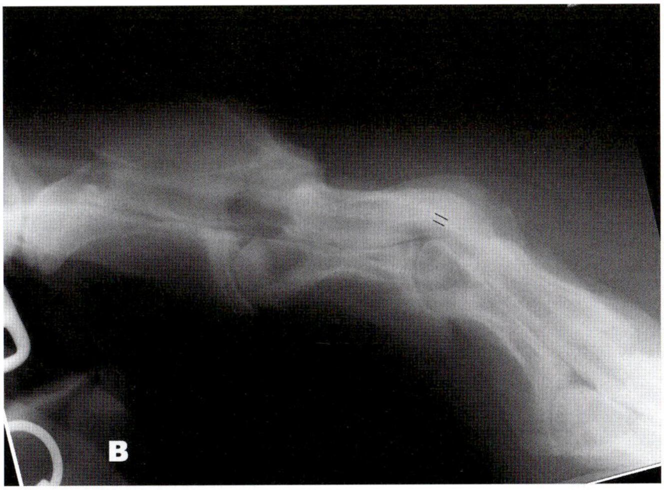

Articular Facet Reaction (Bone Proliferation)

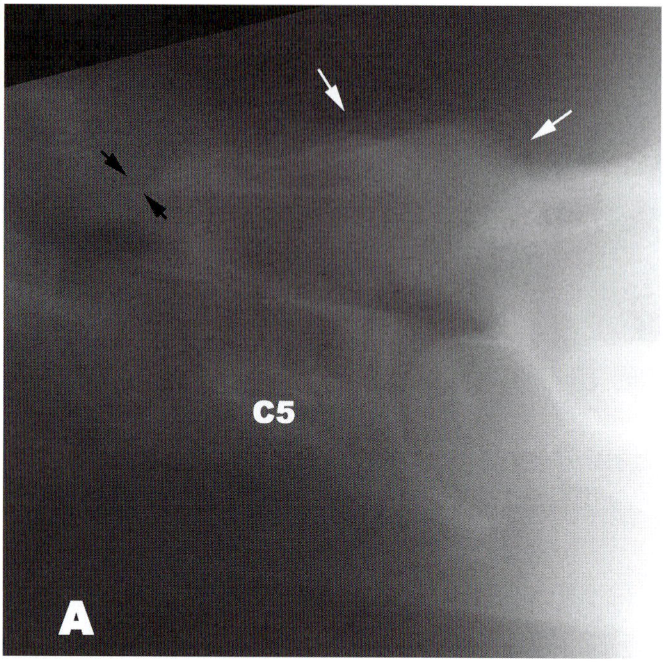

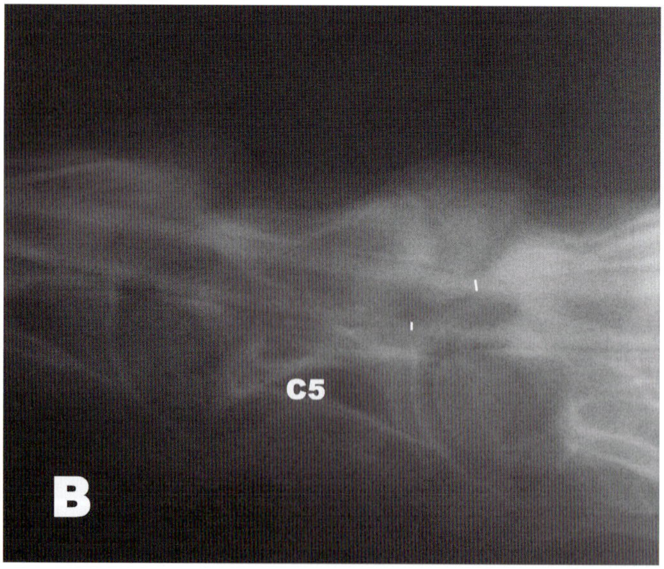

Figures 7.83a–c Lateral radiographic projections of the cranial cervical spine of a 2 year-old Standardbred. (A) a survey film and (B) and (C) are from a myelographic study. **(A) Proliferative bone at the articular facets of C 5-6; (B/C) Subtle compression of the spinal cord at C 5-6:** In (A), the articulation between the facets of the 5th and 6th cervical vertebrae (white arrows) is not as visible as the articulation at C 4-5 (black arrows). Smooth proliferative bone has caused increased prominence of the articulation. (B) is an extended view and (C) is a flexed view of the spine following the introduction of contrast into the subarachnoid space at the cisterna magna. Very subtle narrowing of the dorsal and ventral subarachnoid spaces is visible at the C 5-6 level (white lines). In this case, narrowing of the contrast columns is minimal and the lesion is considered mildly compressive. Possible causes for this abnormality include cervical vertebral malformation instability (CVMI, Wobbler's syndrome) or prior traumatic injury.

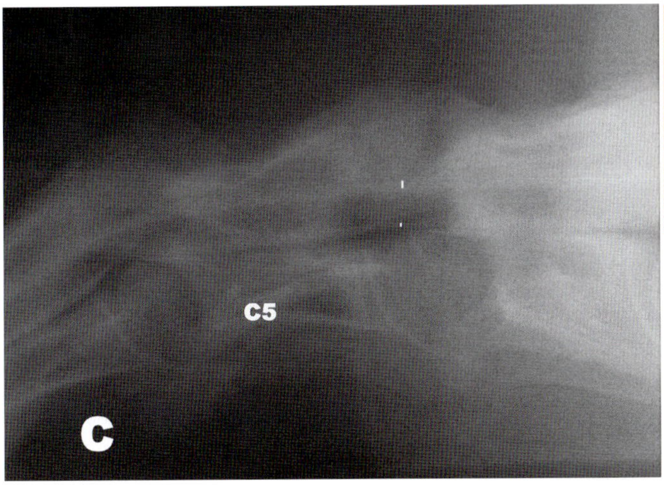

Figures 7.83a–c *Continued*

Cervical Vertebral Malformation Instability (Wobbler's Syndrome)

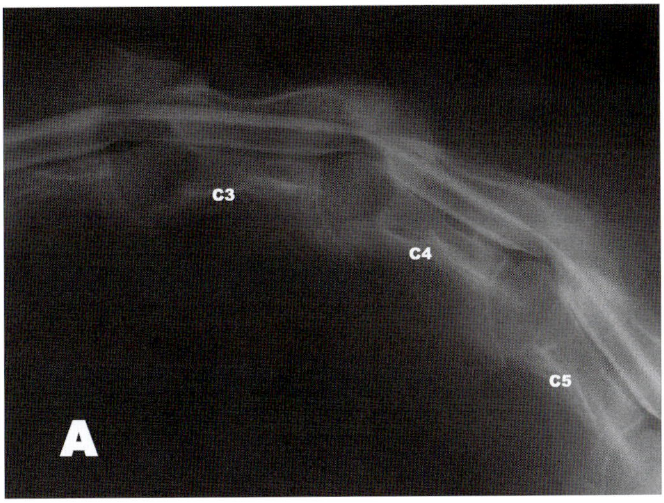

Figures 7.84a,b Lateral myelographic projections of the cervical spine of a 3-year-old Standardbred (A) and a 1 1/2-year-old Warmblood (B). **Compression of the spinal cord at C 3-4 and C 4-5; normal myelographic images:** In (A) there is narrowing of the dorsal and ventral subarachnoid contrast columns at C 3-4 and C 4-5. The narrowing is much more obvious at C 4-5. This view was obtained with the patient's neck in flexion; it is essential to obtain neutrally positioned, flexed, and extended views in the equine myelogram since many lesions are dynamic in nature and are not visible in neutral position views. The results of this myelogram are typical of those seen in patients with cervical vertebral malformation instability. (B) is included as an example of a normal myelographic study. With flexion of the neck, the ventral subarachnoid contrast columns are narrowed but the dorsal columns are slightly increased in width. This appearance of the contrast columns reflects redistribution of contrast within the subarachnoid space.

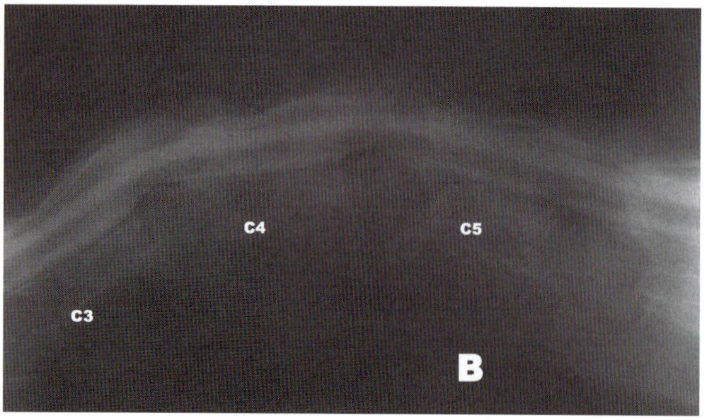

Figures 7.84a,b *Continued*

Osteomyelitis of the Third Cervical Vertebra

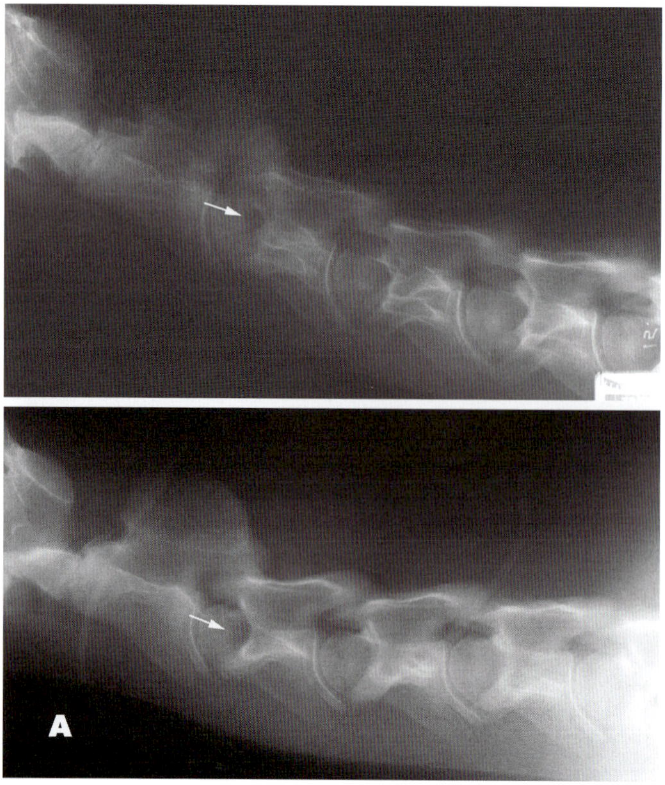

Figures 7.85a,b Lateral radiographic projections of the cervical spine of two 4-month-old Standardbred foals (A) and a lateral radiographic projection of the cervical spine of a 1-week-old Standardbred foal. **(A) Osteomyelitis of the third cervical vertebra. (B) Normal cervical spine:** In both films, in (A) a distinct lucency is present in the cranial aspect of the third cervical vertebra (arrows). The area of lucency is present in the vertebral body adjacent to the physis. The cranial vertebral physes appear to be closed but the caudal physes remain open. Hematogenous spread of bacterial infection is suspected as the cause of the osteomyelitis. The film in (B) is of a much younger foal and the cranial and caudal vertebral physes are very prominent. It does, however, provide a comparison for the normal appearance of the vertebral bodies.

Figures 7.85a,b *Continued*

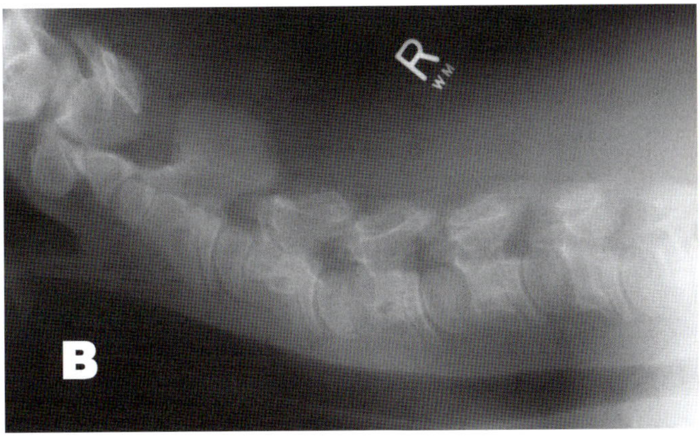

Figures 7.86a,b Lateral radiographic projections of the skull. **(A) Anatomy—conchofrontal sinuses; (B) anatomy—maxillary sinuses:** The paranasal sinuses are paired structures. The largest and most clinically important of these are the conchofrontal and maxillary sinuses. In **(A),** the red triangle outlines the frontal sinuses and white lines outline the dorsal conchal sinuses. These structures communicate to form the conchofrontal sinuses. The blue line is the infraorbital canal and the arrows indicate the ethmoid turbinates. In **(B),** the red lines show the rostral extent of the rostral maxillary sinuses; the blue arrowheads show the septum that separates the rostral and caudal maxillary sinuses.

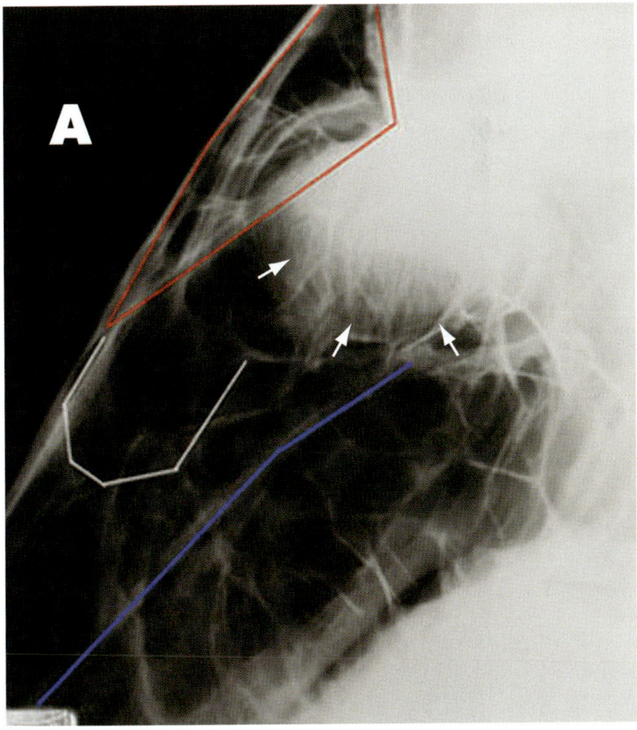

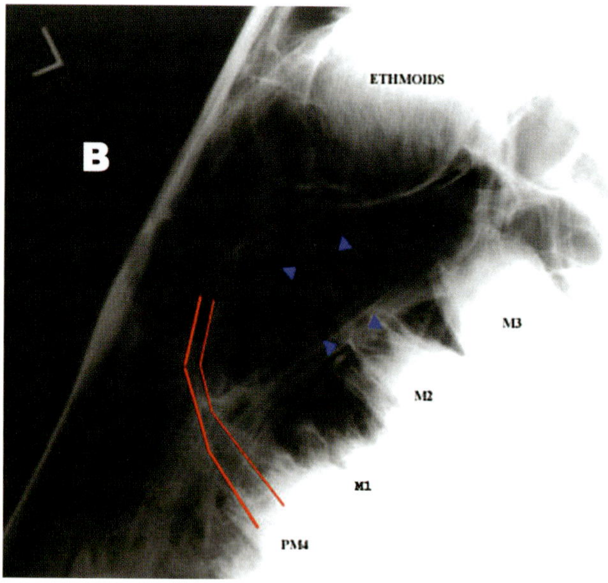

Figures 7.86a,b *Continued*

Sinusitis

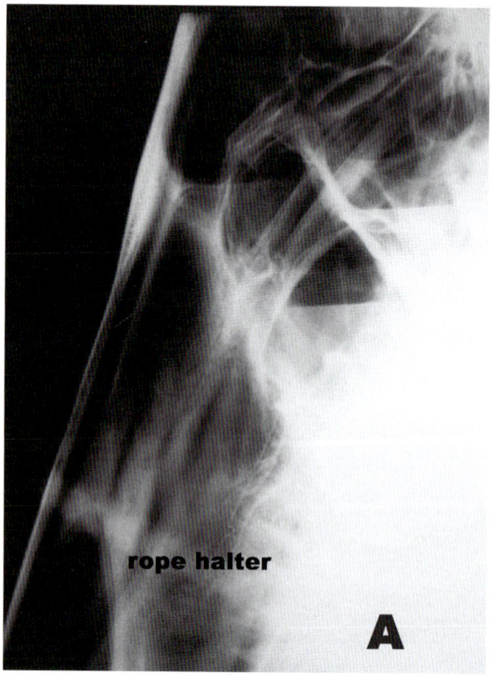

Figures 7.87a,b Unlabeled (A) and labeled (B) lateral radiographic projections of the skull. Fluid within the frontal, rostral maxillary, and caudal maxillary sinuses (sinusitis): The radiograph in (A) is unlabeled. In (B), lines have been placed to indicate the fluid-gas interface in each of the sinuses. Along with the clinical signs (foul-smelling unilateral nasal discharge), the presence of fluid-gas interface (fluid line) within the sinus on radiographs is usually an indication for sinusitis.

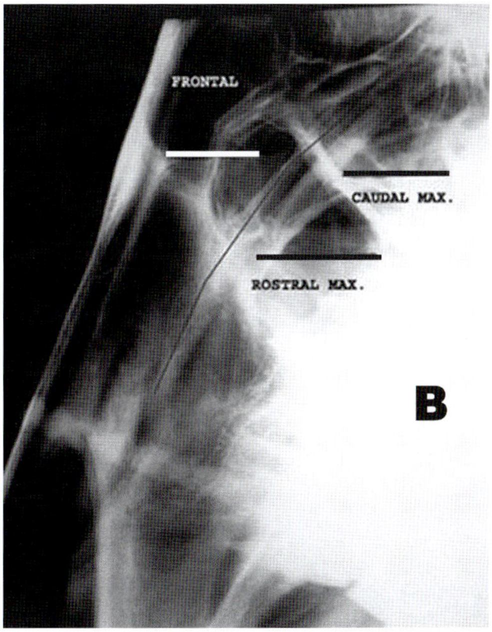

Figures 7.87a,b *Continued*

Sinus Cyst

Figures 7.88a,b Unlabeled (A) and labeled (B) lateral radiographic projections of the skull of a yearling Standardbred. **Sinus cyst:** There is increased fluid opacity throughout the region of the nasal cavity and paranasal sinuses (B—arrows). The rostral extent of the fluid opacity is rounded and well-defined and no fluid lines are visible. The absence of fluid lines suggests that the structure is a mass of some type. Differentials for this lesion include sinus cyst, abscess, or possibly a neoplastic process. In this young patient, a sinus cyst is considered most likely. With only a lateral view, it is not possible to determine if the fluid opacity is present within the sinuses or the nasal cavity or both. A ventrodorsal view of the skull would be needed to help determine the exact location of the structure. If it is not possible to obtain a ventrodorsal view of the skull, endoscopy could bc used to help determine if an involvement of the nasal cavity is present.

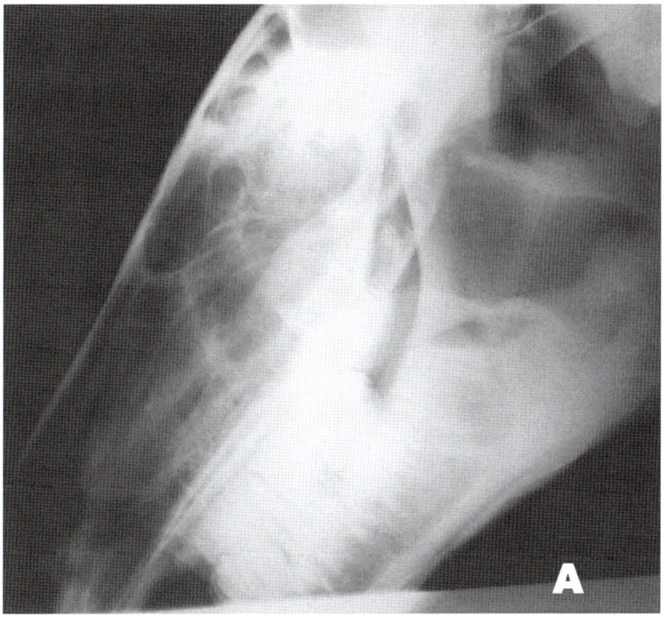

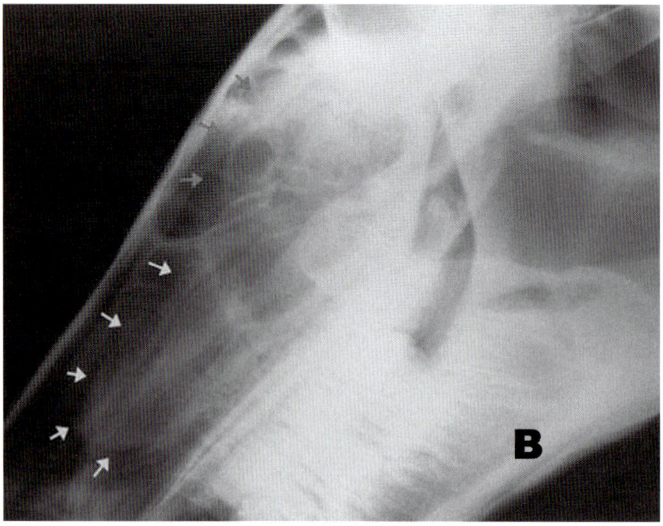

Figures 7.88a,b *Continued*

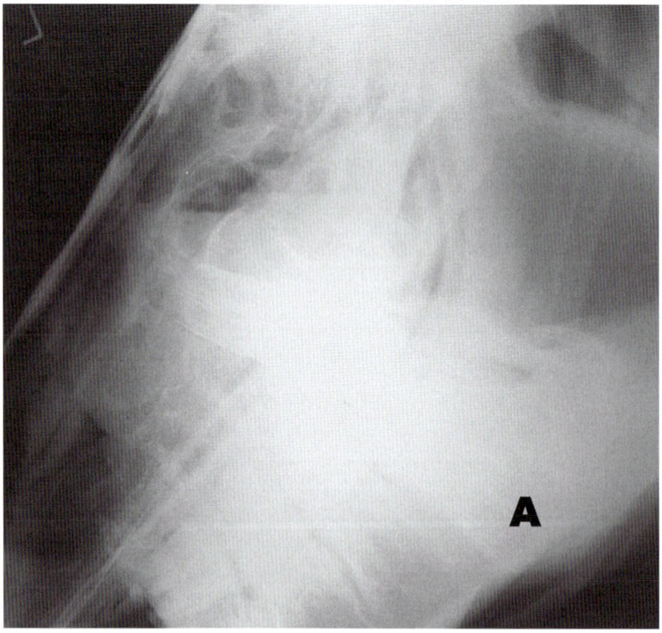

Figures 7.89a,b Unlabeled (A) and labeled (B) lateral radiographic projections of the skull of a yearling Percheron. **Sinus cyst and fluid within the rostral and caudal maxillary sinuses:** There is increased fluid opacity in the region of the maxillary sinus and nasal cavity. Fluid lines are visible in the rostral and caudal maxillary sinuses (arrows). The rostral extent of the fluid opacity is rounded and well defined (arrowheads). The rounded cranial margin of the structure suggests that a mass may be present. The fluid in the sinuses is likely present due to occlusion of the nasomaxillary opening. Differentials for this lesion include sinus cyst, abscess, or possibly a neoplastic process. In this young patient, a sinus cyst is considered most likely. With only a lateral view, it is not possible to determine if the fluid opacity is present within the sinuses or the nasal cavity or both. A ventrodorsal view of the skull would be needed to help determine the exact location of the structure. If it is not possible to obtain a ventrodorsal view of the skull, endoscopy could be used to help determine if involvement of the nasal cavity is present.

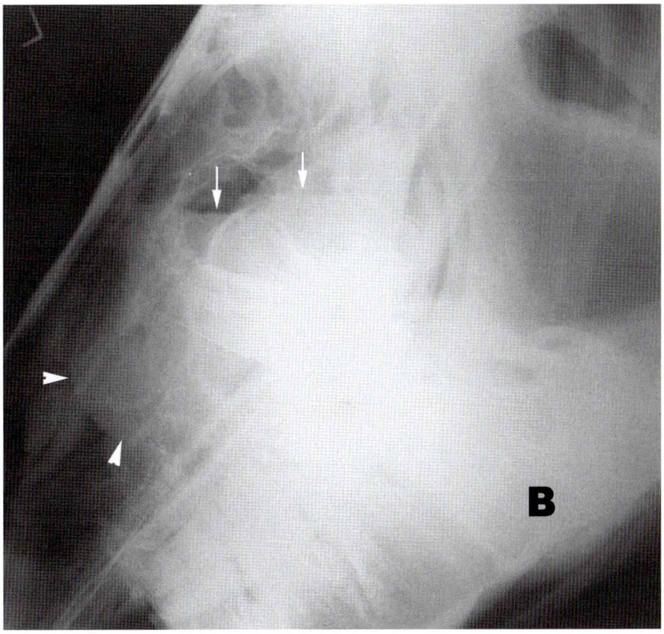

Figures 7.89a,b *Continued*

Ethmoid Hematoma

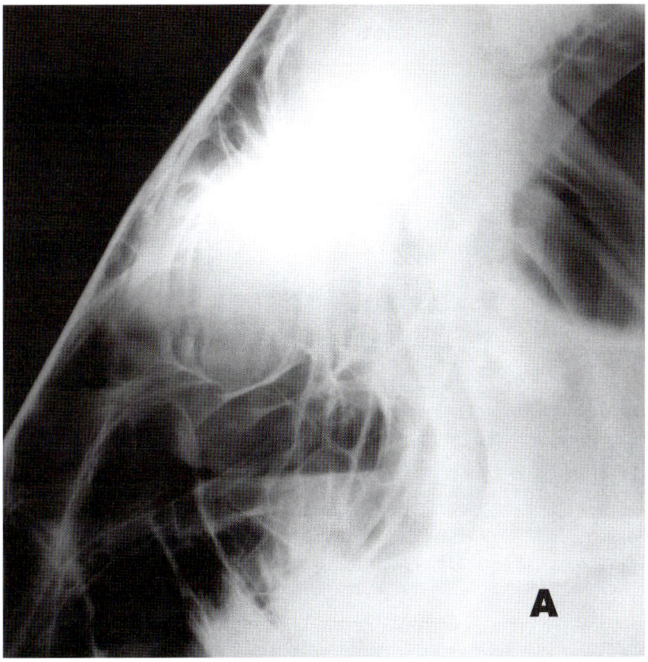

Figures 7.90a,b Unlabeled (A) and labeled (B) lateral radiographic projections of the skull. **Fluid within the caudal maxillary sinus and suspected ethmoid hematoma:** A round structure of soft tissue opacity is faintly visible projecting from the rostral extent of the ethmoid turbinates (arrowheads). This is suspected to be an ethmoid hematoma. A fluid line is visible within the caudal maxillary sinus (arrows). Fluid within the sinus may be secondary to extension of the hematoma into the sinus or to occlusion of the nasomaxillary opening by the hematoma. This diagnosis is best confirmed with endoscopy.

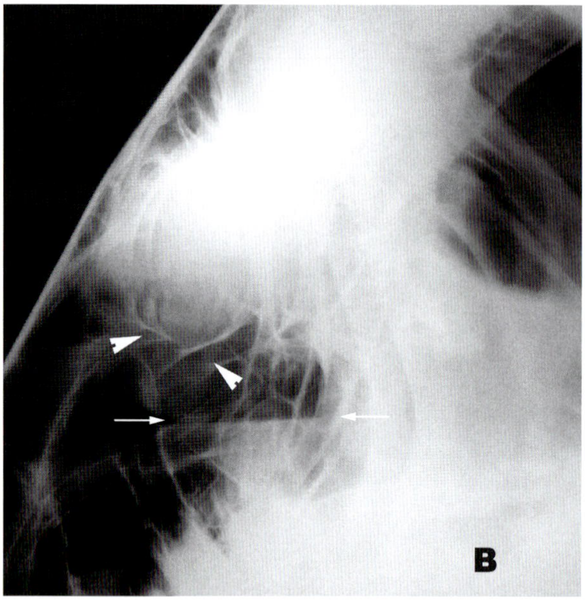

Figures 7.90a,b *Continued*

Normal Dental Structures

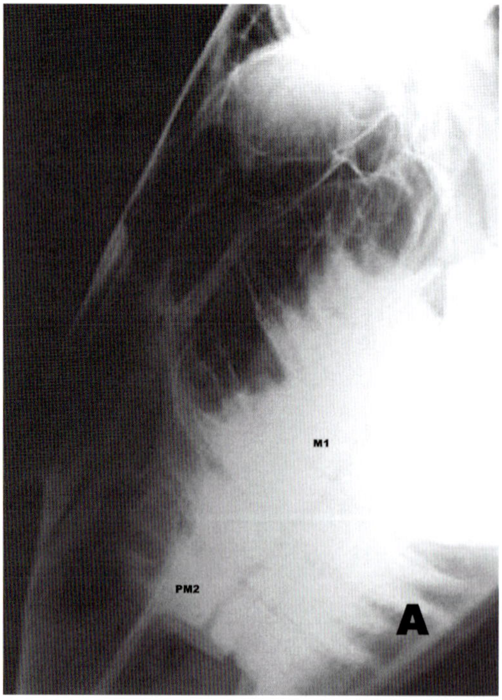

Figures 7.91a–c Lateral (A), right dorsolateral-left ventrolateral oblique (B), and ventrodorsal (C) radiographic projections of the skull. **Normal maxillary dental structures (aged horse):** The lateral view is needed to evaluate for the presence of fluid within the paranasal sinuses but provides limited evaluation of the maxillary dental structures. The left and right arcades are superimposed and the physical density of the enamel makes penetration of the teeth by the X-ray beam difficult. When evaluating the dental structures, oblique radiographic projections of the left and right arcades are taken. If disease is suspected on one side only, the second view will provide a comparison normal. The right dorsolateral-left ventrolateral oblique is obtained with the cassette on the right placed ventrally and the X-ray tube placed on the right dorsally; this highlights the right maxillary arcade. Ventrodorsal views are not often obtained due to difficulty in restraint and positioning. It is possible to obtain this view with the patient standing but requires heavy sedation and a compliant patient. In this view, note that the maxillary arcade is wider than the mandibular arcade and the radiographic pattern is created by differing opacity of dental enamel and cementum.

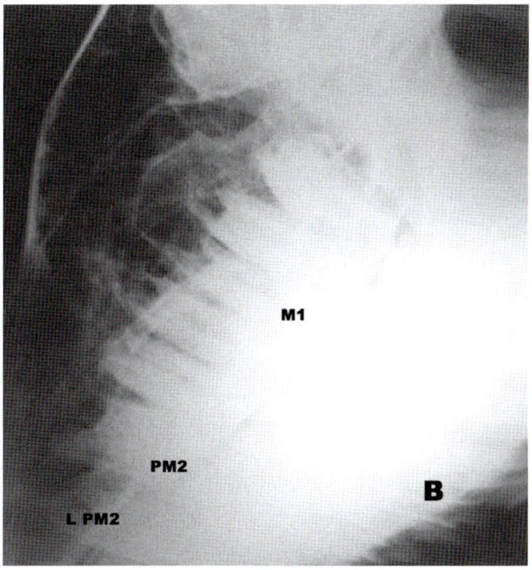

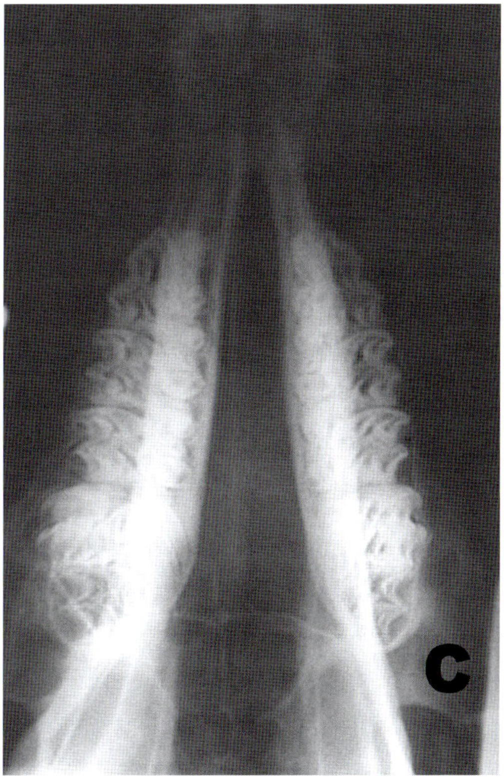

Figures 7.91a–c *Continued*

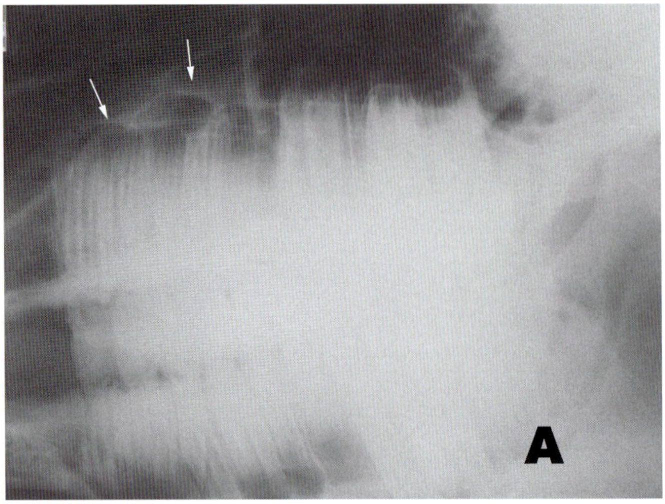

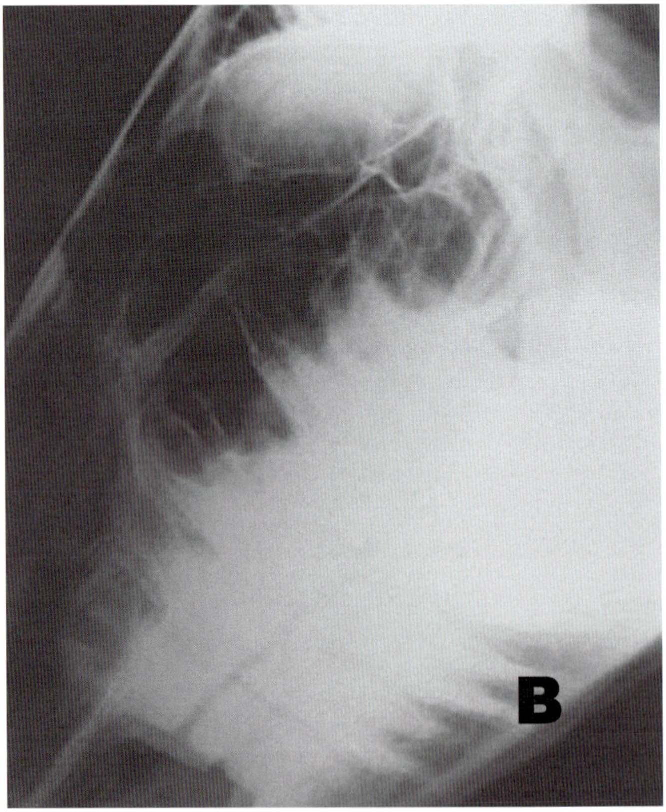

Figures 7.92a,b Oblique (A) and lateral (B) radiographic projections of the maxillary dental structures. **Normal maxillary dental structures in an immature horse; normal maxillary dental structures in a mature horse:** In the young horse (A), tooth roots have a round and lucent appearance (arrows); these are often described as tooth buds. This root appearance is normal for erupting maxillary and mandibular permanent teeth. Once the tooth is fully erupted and in wear, the tooth roots will lose this unusual appearance. This lateral radiograph (B) is from a much older horse. The tooth roots are clearly visible and very different from those present in the young horse. When the permanent teeth erupt, they are quite long and those that are present within the maxillary sinuses occupy the majority of the depth of the sinuses. As the horse ages, the teeth wear and continue to erupt and occupy less and less of the depth of the sinuses. In this case, little tooth root is visible in the sinuses indicating that this is an older horse, likely more than 10 years old.

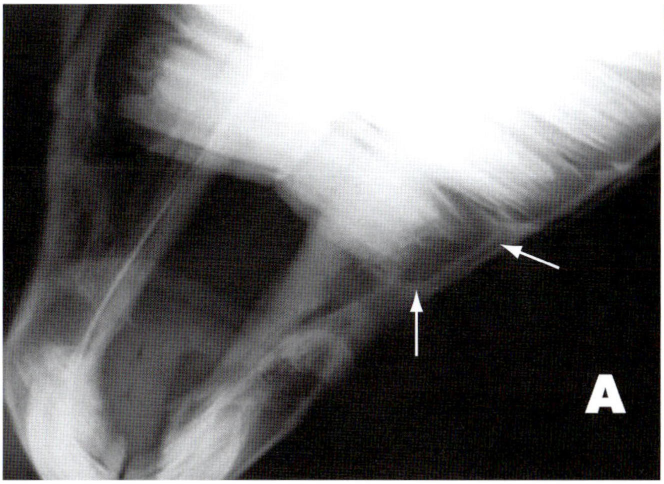

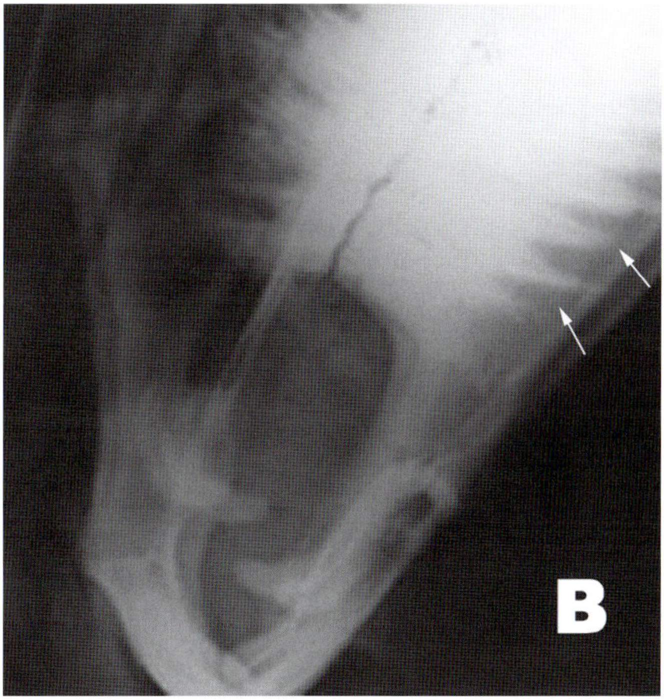

Figures 7.93a,b Lateral radiographic projections of the rostral mandibular dental structures. **(A) Normal mandibular dental structures in an immature horse; (B) normal mandibular dental structures in a mature horse:** In the young horse (A), tooth roots have a rounded and lucent appearance (arrows); these are often described as tooth buds. This root appearance is normal for erupting maxillary and mandibular permanent teeth. Once the tooth is fully erupted and in wear, the tooth roots will lose this unusual appearance. In the older horse (B), the tooth roots are clearly visible (arrows). This appearance of the roots is normal for teeth that are fully erupted and in wear. This horse has very prominent canine teeth likely indicating that it is a male.

Tooth Root Abscess

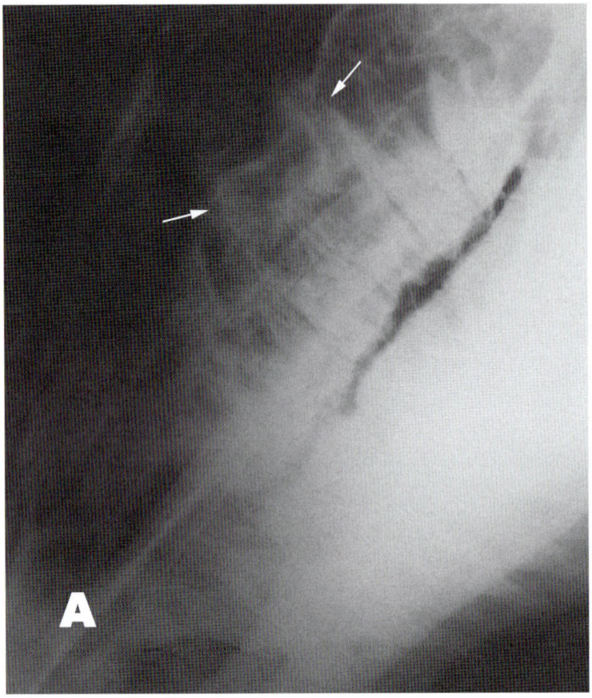

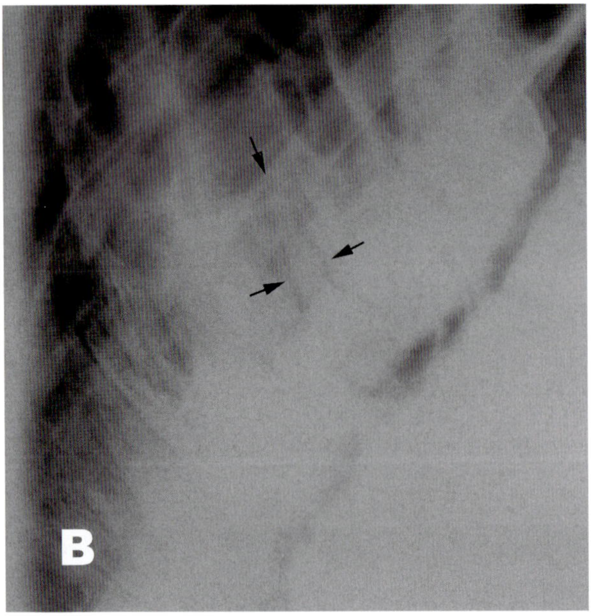

Figures 7.94a,b Lateral (A) and oblique (B) radiographic projections of the left maxillary dental arcade of a 10-year-old quarter horse. **Tooth root abscess of the left first maxillary molar:** Radiographic diagnosis of maxillary tooth root abscessation can be difficult. In many cases, the roots of the teeth are obscured by fluid within the sinus and the radiographic changes may be subtle. In this case, there is a large, relatively well-defined area of soft tissue opacity dorsal to the roots of the 4th premolar and 1st molar; this area is also the rostral extent of the rostral maxillary sinus. In the lateral view, a subtle band of lucency is seen surrounding the rostral root of the 1st molar (white arrows). In the oblique view, more obvious lucency is evident surrounding the caudal root of the 1st molar (black arrows). The lucent band has an irregular margin as does the surface of the tooth root. These changes are considered evidence of tooth root abscessation.

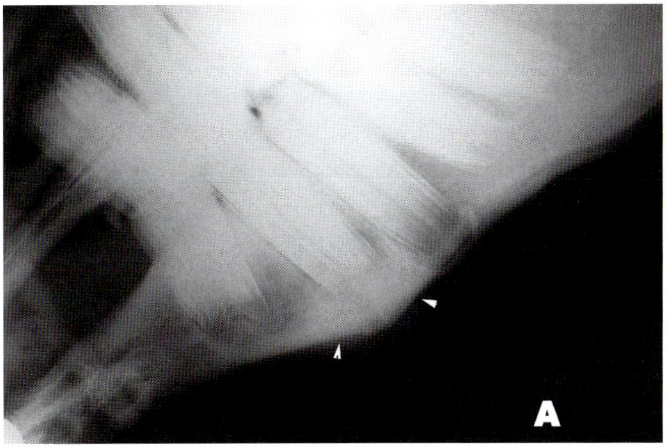

Figures 7.95a,b Lateral (A) and oblique (B) radiographic projections of the left mandibular dental arcade of a 3-year-old quarter horse. **Tooth root abscess of the left 3rd mandibular premolar:** Radiographic diagnosis of mandibular tooth root abscessation is easier than that of maxillary abscessation. These teeth are surrounded by bone, not within a sinus cavity, and reactive changes due to inflammation in the bone are visible. Clinical findings include prominent swelling in the region of the tooth root often with a central draining tract. In the lateral view, marked thickening of the ventral aspect of the mandible is evident (arrowheads). An ill-defined area of lucency is seen surrounding the root of the 3rd premolar and a lucent tract extends from the tooth root to the surface of the bone. The oblique view gives a better visualization of the lucency surrounding the root of the tooth (arrows). This area of lucency is less clearly defined and distinct than the normal tooth buds of the erupting teeth adjacent to it.

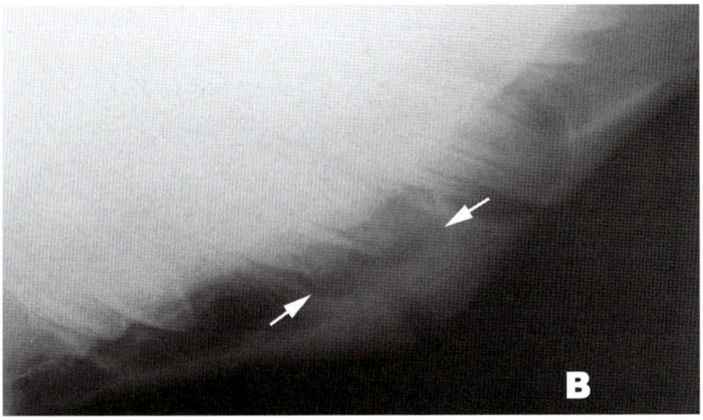

Anatomy of the Pharynx and Guttural Pouches (Auditory Diverticula)

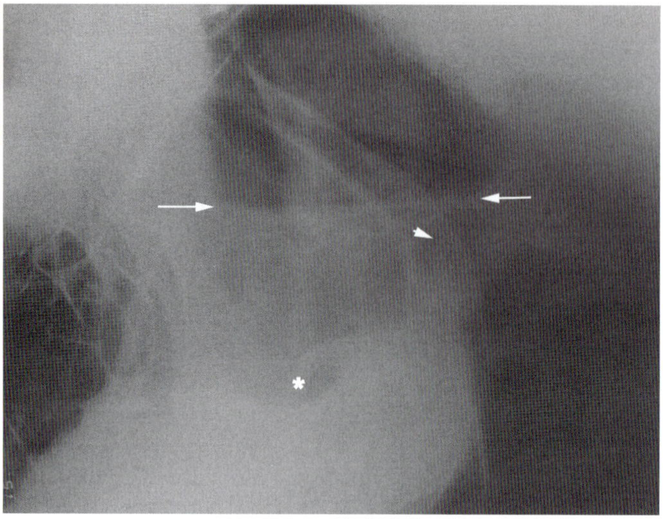

Figure 7.96 Lateral radiographic projection of the pharyngeal region. **Normal pharyngeal anatomy and guttural pouches (auditory diverticula):** The arrows indicate the thin tissue that is normally present between the guttural pouches dorsally and the pharyngeal cavity (pharynx) ventrally. Thickening of this tissue may be seen in animals with severe pharyngitis or enlargement of the retropharyngeal lymph nodes. Due to the presence of surrounding air, the structures of the larynx are well defined. The asterisk indicates the tip of the epiglottis; the linear soft tissue opacity ventral to the epiglottis is the soft palate. The ventral surface of the soft palate is rarely visible due to a normal lack of air in the oropharynx. The arrowhead is a portion of the arytenoid cartilages that projects into the pharyngeal cavity.

Guttural Pouches Empyema

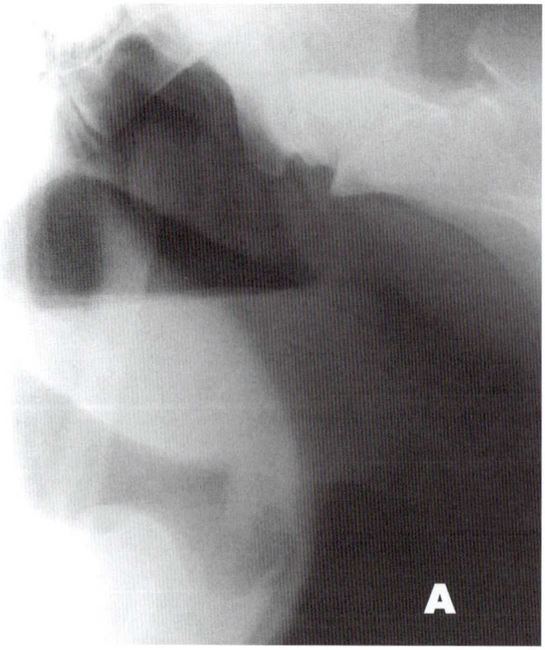

Figures 7.97a,b Unlabeled (A) and labeled (B) lateral radiographic projections of the pharyngeal region of a young Standardbred. **Fluid within the guttural pouches and pharyngeal compression:** The dorsal wall of the pharynx is ventrally deviated (arrows) and the arytenoid cartilage is shifted cranioventrally resulting in narrowing of the pharynx and laryngeal ostium. There is apparent thickening of the soft tissues between the air in the guttural pouches and the air in the pharynx. Two horizontally oriented gas-fluid interface lines are visible (arrowheads). This appearance is evidence of fluid within both guttural pouches. With this amount of fluid, it is not possible to determine if there is enlargement of the retropharyngeal lymph nodes or if chondroids are present.

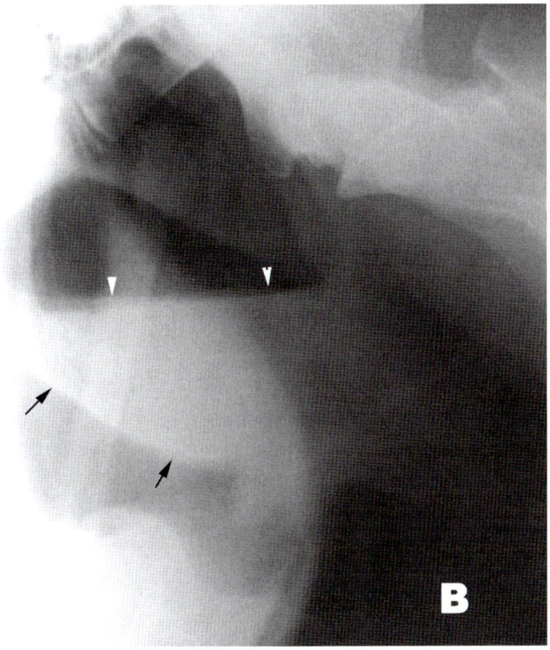

Figures 7.97a,b *Continued*

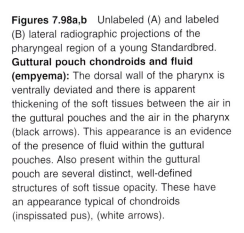

Figures 7.98a,b Unlabeled (A) and labeled (B) lateral radiographic projections of the pharyngeal region of a young Standardbred. **Guttural pouch chondroids and fluid (empyema):** The dorsal wall of the pharynx is ventrally deviated and there is apparent thickening of the soft tissues between the air in the guttural pouches and the air in the pharynx (black arrows). This appearance is an evidence of the presence of fluid within the guttural pouches. Also present within the guttural pouch are several distinct, well-defined structures of soft tissue opacity. These have an appearance typical of chondroids (inspissated pus), (white arrows).

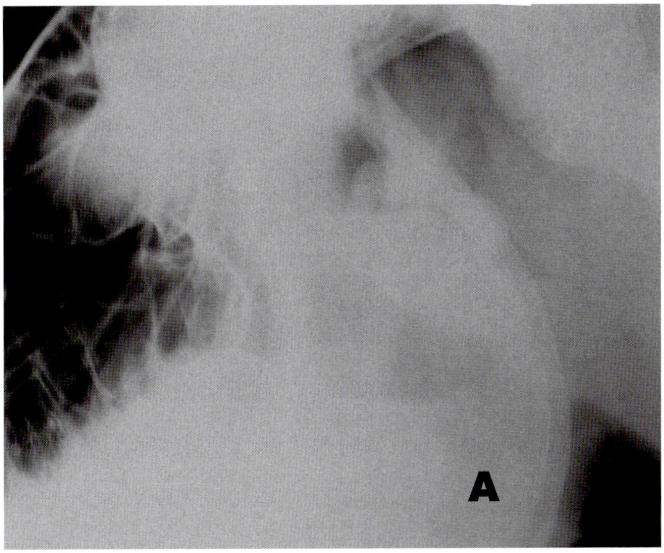

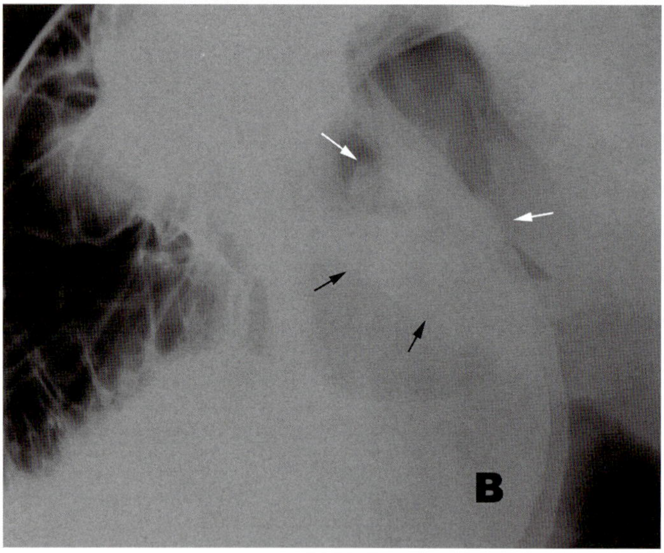

Figures 7.98a,b *Continued*

Normal Larynx and Aryepiglottic Fold Entrapment

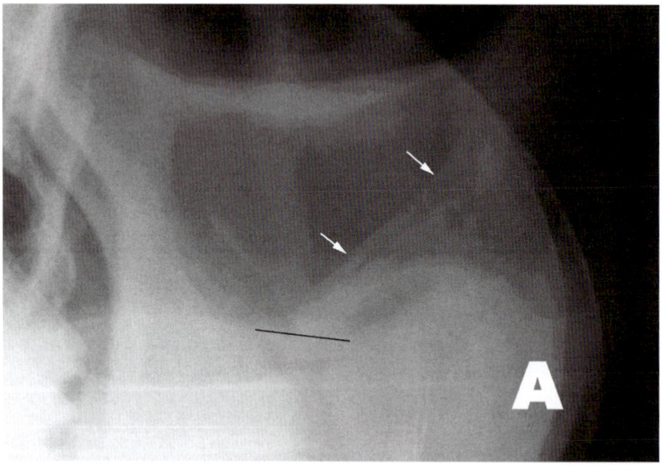

Figures 7.99a,b Lateral radiographic projections of the larynx. **(A) Normal larynx; (B) aryepiglottic fold entrapment:** In the normal larynx (A), the aryepiglottic folds are visible as two bands of tissue extending between each arytenoid cartilage and the base of the epiglottis (arrows). The tip of the epiglottis is visible dorsal to the soft palate (black line). Although aryepiglottic fold entrapment is usually diagnosed during an endoscopic examination, it may be diagnosed with a lateral radiographic projection of the pharynx. In (B), the body of the epiglottis is visible in a more dorsal location than normal and the tip of the epiglottis is no longer visible. The aryepiglottic folds are visible (arrows) and appear to "wrap around" the tip of the epiglottis. The soft palate is ventral to the epiglottis but in a more dorsal position than normal. The retracted position of the epiglottis may allow the soft palate to move dorsally and dorsal displacement of the soft palate may also occur.

Figures 7.99a,b *Continued*

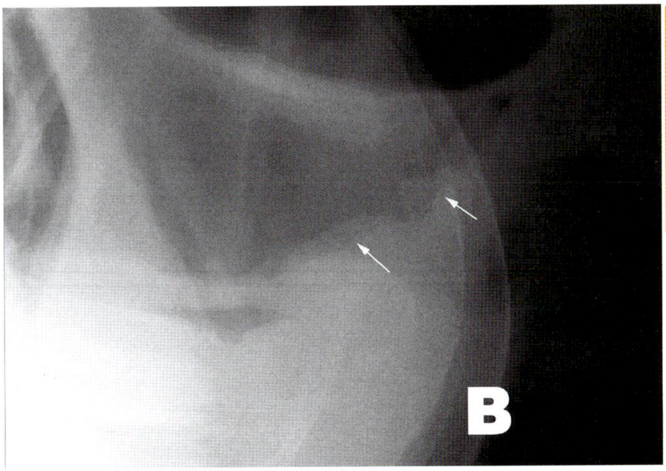

Fracture of the Sphenoid Bone and Guttural Pouch Hemorrhage

Figures 7.100a,b Unlabeled (A) and labeled (B) lateral radiographic projections of the pharyngeal region of a weanling Standardbred. **Fracture of the sphenoid bone and guttural pouch hemorrhage:** The guttural pouches are not visible as distinct air-filled structures. The dorsal wall of the pharynx is ventrally deviated (arrows) causing narrowing of the pharynx. An elongated bone fragment is visible caudal to the stylohyoid bones (white + signs). The bone fragment has avulsed from the sphenoid bone at its junction with the basilar portion of the occipital bone (black + signs). This injury occurs when horses fall backward and strike their heads. At the time of impact, the longus capitus muscle avulses from its attachment and hemorrhage occurs into the guttural pouches.

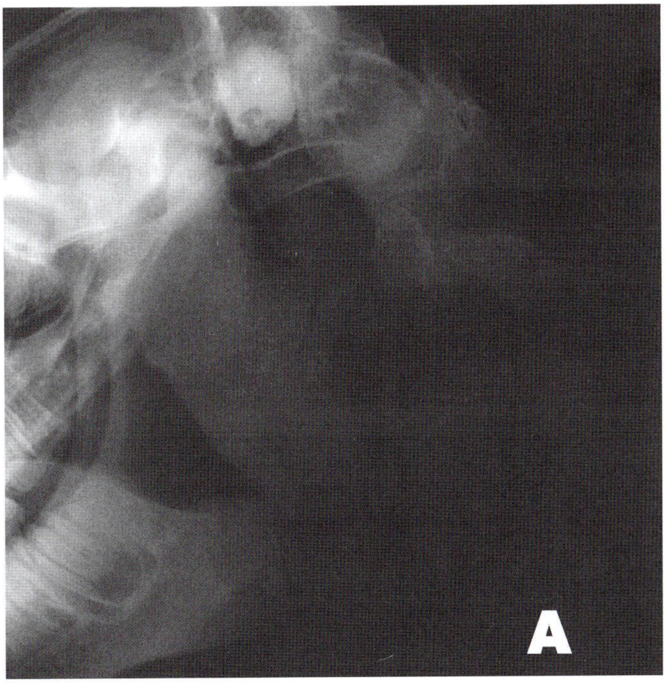

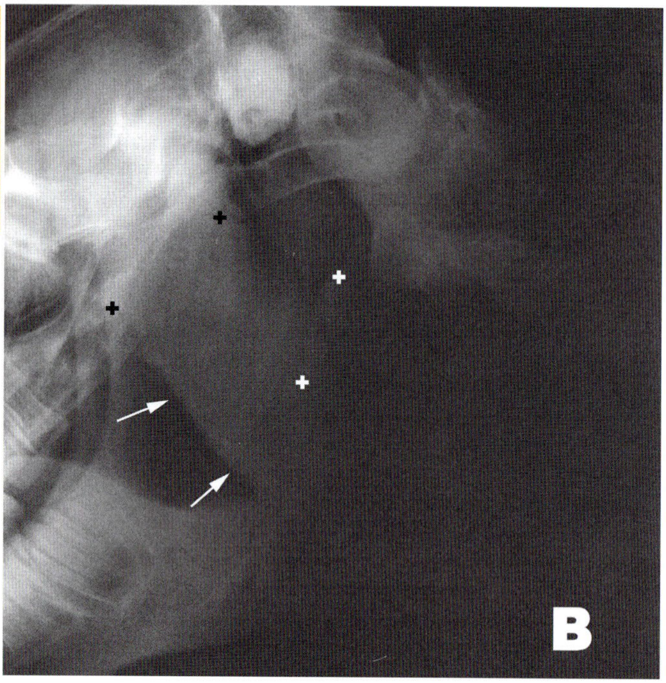

Figures 7.100a,b *Continued*

Dental Tumor of the Mandible

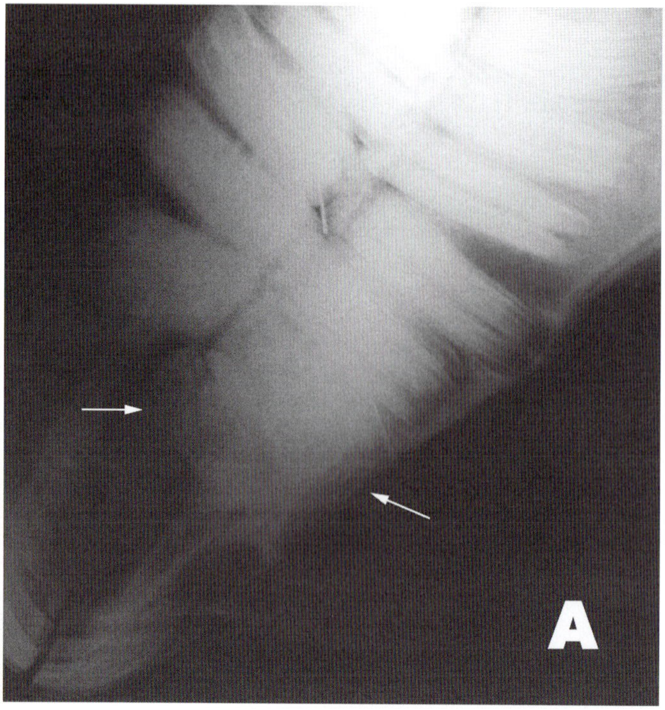

Figures 7.101a,b Lateral (A) and ventrodorsal (B) radiographic projections of the mandible of a 5-year-old Standardbred. **Dental tumor of the mandible:** A large expansile lesion is present on the left rostral mandibular ramus (arrows). In the lateral view, the dental structure immediately rostral to the 3rd premolar is thought to be the 2nd premolar. It appears to be impacting with the 3rd premolar, which is impeding its eruption. Focal areas of ill-defined opaque tissue within the expansile lesion resemble dental tissue. There is a large gap present between the 4th premolar and 1st molar; malalignment of these teeth may be due to compression by the abnormal 2nd premolar. The radiographic appearance of this structure is typical of a dental tumor (odontoma). These are most commonly seen in young horses and typically respond well to surgical resection. The metallic structure between the dental arcades is an artifact.

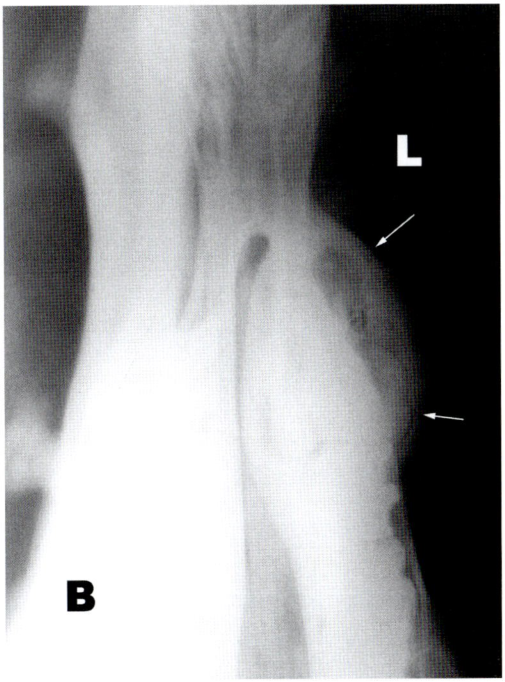

Figures 7.101a,b *Continued*

Mandibular Osteomyelitis

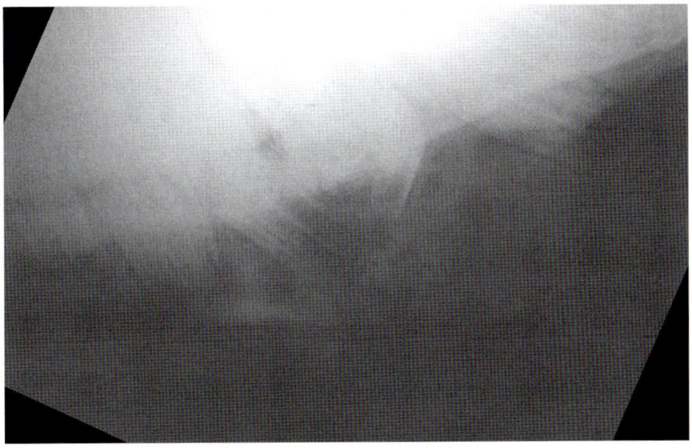

Figure 7.102 Oblique radiographic projection of the left ramus of the mandible of a 2-year-old Standardbred. **Mandibular osteomyelitis:** A mottled area of lucency is present in the ventral aspect of the left horizontal ramus of the mandible. The cortical bone appears thin and there is periosteal proliferation on the margin of the bone. The roots of the 4th premolar and 1st and 2nd molars are displaced due to the expansile nature of the mass. The root of the 1st molar is malformed. Differential diagnoses for this radiographic appearance include osteomyelitis, granulomatous disease, and neoplasia. This horse had a history of traumatic injury to the mandible as a foal and osteomyelitis was suspected. The diagnosis was confirmed by biopsy and culture of the abnormal tissue.

Recommended Reading

Butler JA, et al. Clinical radiology of the horse. Ames, IA: Blackwell Scientific Publications, 1993.
Moore JN, White NA. Current practice of equine surgery. New York: JB Lippincott Co., 1990.
Stashak TS. Adams' lameness in horses. 4th ed. Lea & Febiger. 1987.
Thrall DE. Textbook of diagnostic veterinary radiology. 4th ed. Philadelphia: WB Saunders, 2002.

8 Diseases of the Reproductive System

Reproductive System of the Male
- Cryptorchidism
- Hemosemen
- Neoplasia
- Kicking Injuries
- Testicular Hypoplasia
- Penile Paralysis and Amputation
- Scrotal Hernias
- Testicular Torsion and Hydrocele
- Smegma Accumulation "Beans" in the Fossa Glandis

Reproductive System of the Female
- Routine Diagnostics
  - Following the Estrous Cycle
  - Routine Monitoring of Early Pregnancy
  - Aging of the Fetus
  - Vaginal Examination
  - Clitoral Anatomy and Sampling the Clitoral Sinuses
- Neoplasia
  - Granulosa Cell Tumors
  - Other Tumors
- Infertility
  - The Transitional State
  - Pyometra
  - Transluminal Adhesions
  - Lymphatic Lacunae or Cyst (Endometrial Cysts)
  - Aneuploidy and Intersex
  - Poor Vulvar Conformation
  - Vulvar Injuries
  - Coital Exanthema
  - Cervical Tears
  - Periovarian Adhesions
  - Fetal Death Followed by Anestrus
  - Routine Culture and Cytology to Investigate Infertility
  - Endometrial Biopsy
- Dystocia
  - General Approaches and Forms of Dystocia
- Fetal Sexing
  - Early and Late Gestation Fetal Sexing
- Accidents During Advanced Gestation
  - Premature Placental Separation and Prolapse of the Bladder
  - Estimating the Time of Impending Foaling

Prematurity
Uterine Torsion
Ventral Edema in Late Gestation
Ventral Abdominal Rupture
Uterine Rupture
Hydrops Allantois
Foaling Injuries
Normal Contusion of the Vagina
Severe Vaginal Contusions and Pelvic Subluxation
Rectal Prolapse
Uterine Hemorrhage
Intra-abdominal Hemorrhage
Rectal, Vaginal, and Perineal Tears and Lacerations
Embryonic Death and Abortion
Early and Later Embryonic Death
Embryonic Death and Abortion due to Twinning
Fetal Death Followed by Mummification
Ascending Placentitis
Enlargement of the Mammary Gland Prior to Abortion
Stillbirth or Abortion Close to Term
Long Umbilical Cord as a Cause of Abortion
Yolk Sac Remnants on the Umbilical Cord
Retained Placenta
The Nature of Equine Placentation

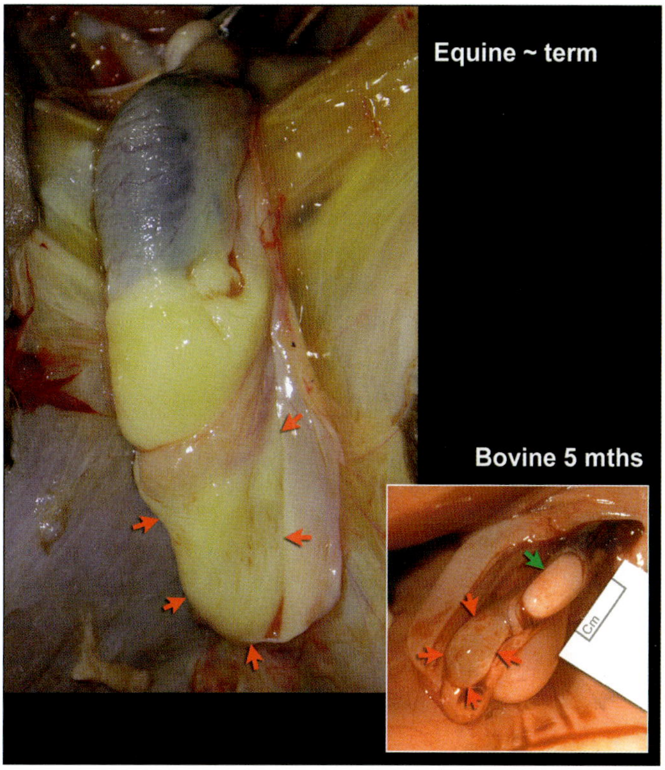

Figure 8.1 Testicular descent; species comparison: testicular descent in cattle (lower right) and horses (upper left). In bulls, the testicles descend into the scrotum by about the fifth month of gestation. By comparison, testicular descent is only complete in stallions close to the time that they are born. This comparative tardiness in testicular descent may be related to the relatively high incidence of cryptorchidism in stallions. In both of these illustrations, the gubernaculum has been indicated by red arrows. It is a large structure, which at some point in testicular descent is larger than the testicle itself. After testicular descent, the gubernaculum regresses to an insignificant ligament between the tail of the epididymis and the parietal vaginal tunic.

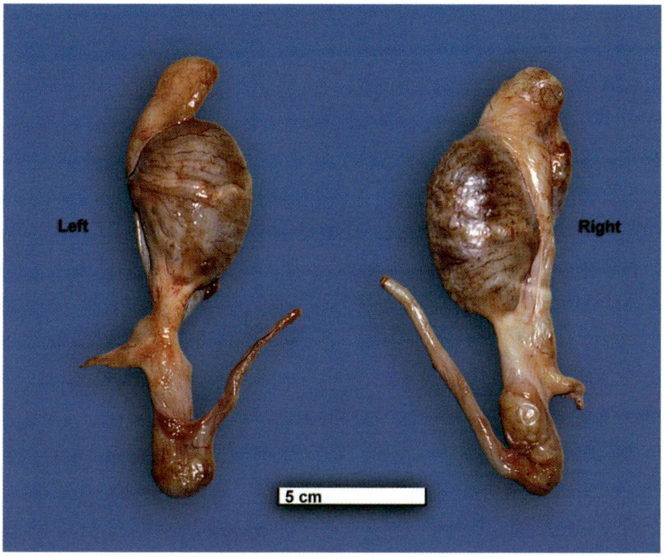

Figure 8.2 Bilateral cryptorchidism. Only about 10% of the cases of cryptorchidism in horses are bilateral. About 60% of all cryptorchid testicles are abdominal. These testicles were very soft and would have been difficult to palpate per rectum. They were removed from the abdomen of a 2-year-old Appaloosa stallion.

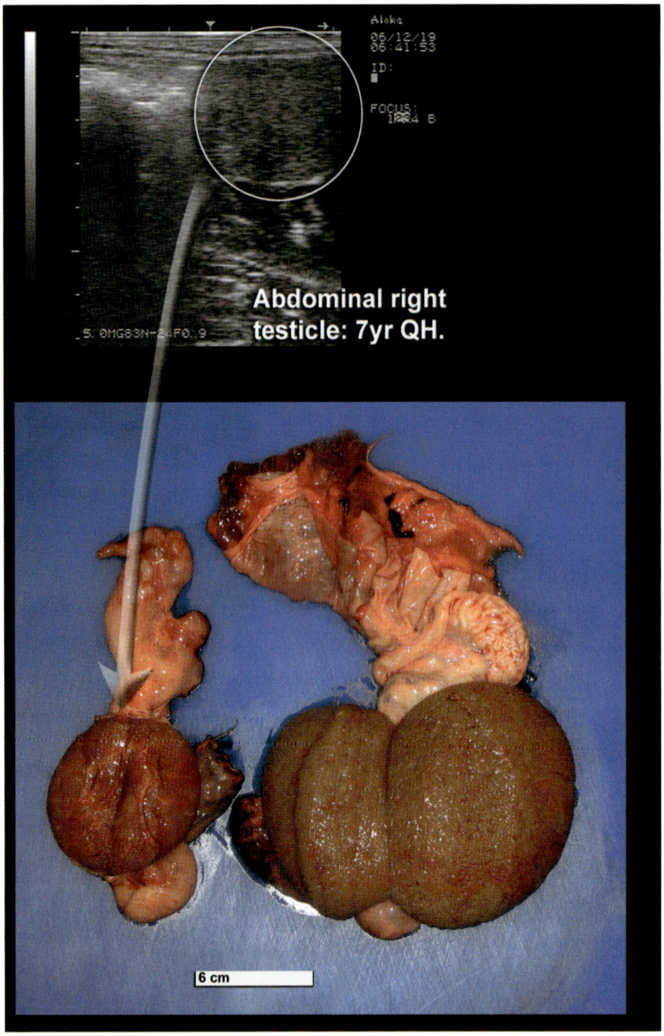

Figure 8.3 Cryptorchid testicle. The intra-abdominal testicles in this 7-year-old quarter horse stallion were not easy to palpate per rectum but the image was captured using a 5 MHz intrarectal transducer using almost random scanning in the area of the internal inguinal opening. As is often the case, these intra-abdominal testicles could not be seen by transabdominal scanning in the inguinal region. Although ultrasound images are best analyzed using video capture, this still image illustrates the testicular echo and its homogeneity fairly well. Note that the size of this testicle is considerably smaller than normal if one considers that the diameter of a transverse section of a normal testicle is about 5 to 6 cm. In this case, it is about 3.5 cm. Although spermatogenesis is suppressed completely in cryptorchid testicles, the function of the Leydig cells is only slightly compromised and steroidogenesis remains close to normal. This is why the hCG stimulation test (Cox test) and estrone sulphate tests are useful for diagnosing cryptorchidism.

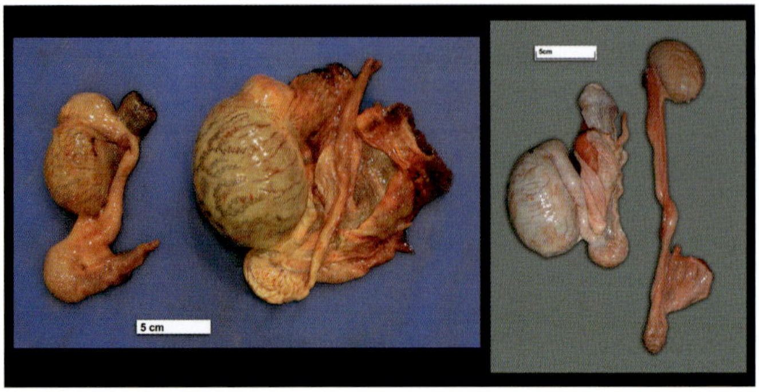

Figure 8.4 Comparison of normal and cryptorchid testicles. These are classic views of normal and cryptorchid testicles taken from the same animal in each image. The images show that there can be considerable variation in the distance between the tail of the epididymis and the testicle. In the left image, this distance is very short and it is likely that the testicle was seen by the surgeon when the tail of the epididymis was grasped during cryptorchidectomy. In the image on the right, the tail of the epididymis is a long distance away from the testicle. This may account for the fact that inexperienced surgeons sometimes remove the tail of the epididymis in the belief that this is an extremely hypoplastic, cryptorchid testicle; leaving the cryptorchid testicle in the abdomen. It is important to realize that this variation exists between stallions with cryptorchid testicles. It is logical to suggest that the distance between the testicles and the tail of the epididymis is at its longest when the cryptorchid testicle is retained entirely within the abdomen rather than within the inguinal canal. In the former case, the gubernaculum would be unable to draw the testicle into the scrotum but could move the tail of the epididymis well into the scrotum.

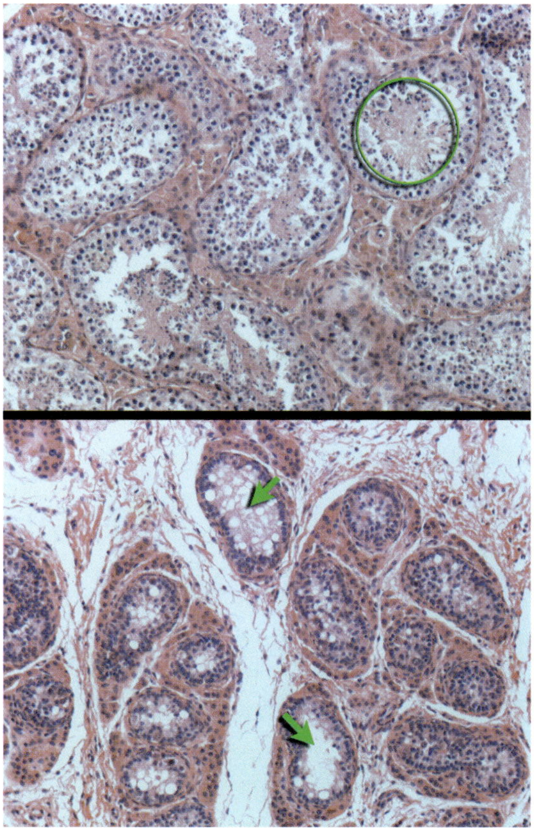

Figure 8.5 Disruption of spermatogenesis. Disruption of spermatogenesis mediated by high body temperature, in this case due to cryptorchidism. Spermatogenesis is disrupted by an increase in body temperature of only two to three degrees. Due to cooling by the pampiniform plexus, the temperature of arterial blood in the spermatic artery drops from approximately 39 °C to 34 °C within the scrotum. Even brief increases in systemic body temperature can disrupt spermatogenesis significantly. In the top image, spermatogenesis is proceeding normally. The area under the green ring shows spermiation (completion of spermatogenesis) occurring. By comparison, the lower image shows that the seminiferous tubules are empty (green arrows) except for spermatogonia and Sertoli cells. Just above the upper green arrow is a large population of Leydig cells that can be seen. These function comparatively normally, producing various androgens including testosterone.

Hemosemen

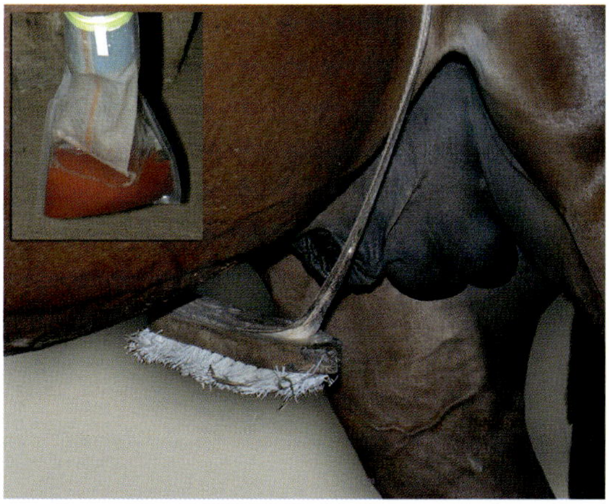

Figure 8.6 Trauma and hemosemen. This image shows a brush that has been placed under the abdomen of a stallion to stop masturbation. Stallions sometimes masturbate by slapping their penises up against the ventral abdomen, occasionally resulting in ejaculation. Despite the contention that this lowers the potential fertility of the stallion, objective studies have shown that masturbation has no significant effect on fertility. Unfortunately, masturbation brushes can traumatize the penis and have been associated with hemosemen as shown here.

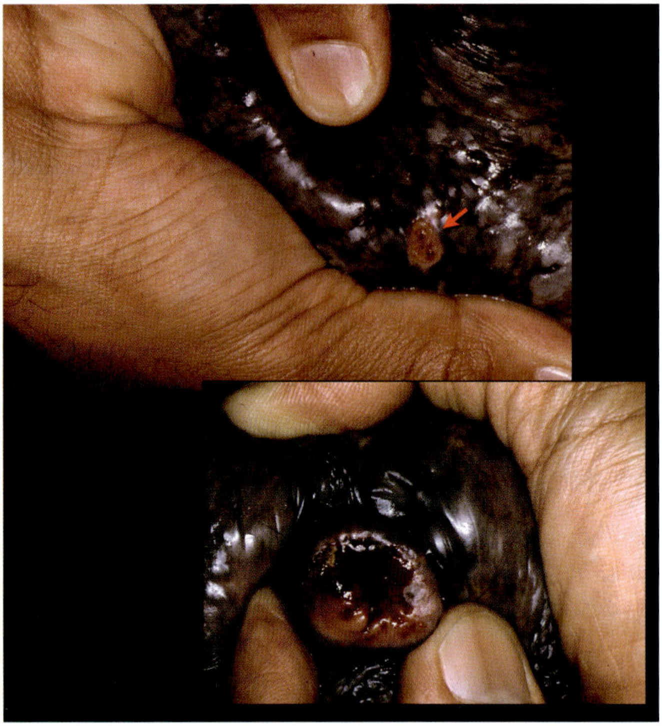

Figure 8.7 Habronemiasis. Habronemiasis on the penis of a quarter horse stallion. This is due to infestation by the fly-borne larvae of *Habronema muscae*, *H. microstoma*, and *Draschia megastoma*. The lesions these larvae cause are intensely pruritic and may occasionally cause hemosemen. Habronemiasis should be differentiated from squamous cell carcinoma by biopsy. A diagnosis is based on the presence of larvae in scrapings of the lesion. Oral ivermectin is an effective treatment for habronemiasis when two treatments are given one month apart. *Habronema* spp. lay their eggs in manure piles and their larvae are ingested by the larvae of the housefly (*Musca domestica*) or stable fly (*Stomoxys calcitrans*), which also develop in manure. The habronema larvae then emerge from adult houseflies or stable flies as they alight on horses. Fly control is therefore of great importance in the control of habronemiasis.

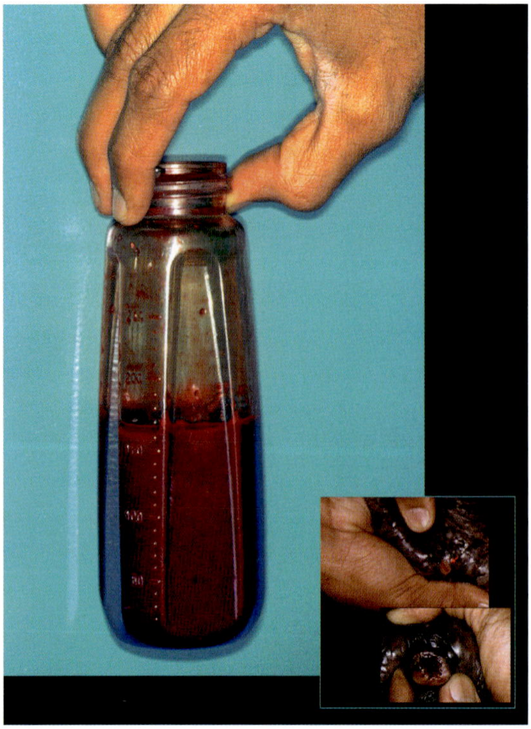

Figure 8.8 Hemosemen due to habronemiasis. This image shows semen that appears to be almost pure blood as a result of habronemiasis in a quarter horse stallion. In this case, as in most cases of hemosemen, hemorrhage was seen only during ejaculation. This is usually a transitory condition and resolves after appropriate treatment for habronemiasis. Most cases of hemosemen are not due to habronemiasis. In fact, the etiology often remains unknown and the ejaculate returns to normal with sexual rest alone. Despite some recommendations to the contrary, only a brief period of sexual rest is required in most cases—perhaps a week to 10 days. In that regard, it is important for veterinarians to realize that even severe hemosemen does not necessarily signal the end of the breeding season for a particular stallion. Although blood in the semen has been reported to decrease fertility, anecdotal reports suggest that some stallions maintain their fertility despite the regular presence of blood in their ejaculates.

Figure 8.9 Seminoma. An 18-year-old stallion with a seminoma in his left testicle. The stallion was presented because of remarkable enlargement (A) of his left testicle. Asymmetry due to the enlargement of this testicle was more evident in a lateral view than a caudal view. The appearance on ultrasound (B) of the seminoma (s) showed irregular masses of variable echodensity compared to normal (n) testicular parenchyma in the same testicle. A needle biopsy confirmed the diagnosis of a seminoma. Hemicastration of the affected testicle was done. The site of the needle biopsy (C) was obvious on the visceral surface of the tunica vaginalis of the testicle. On cut surface of the removed testicle (D), the seminoma was obvious, as were areas of avascular necrosis (orange arrows). The normal tissue (n) seen on ultrasound and the seminoma (s) are clearly visible here as well. This is the most common testicular tumor in stallions although Leydig cell and Sertoli cell tumors can occur. Seminoma should always be a differential diagnosis in older stallions with testicular asymmetry.

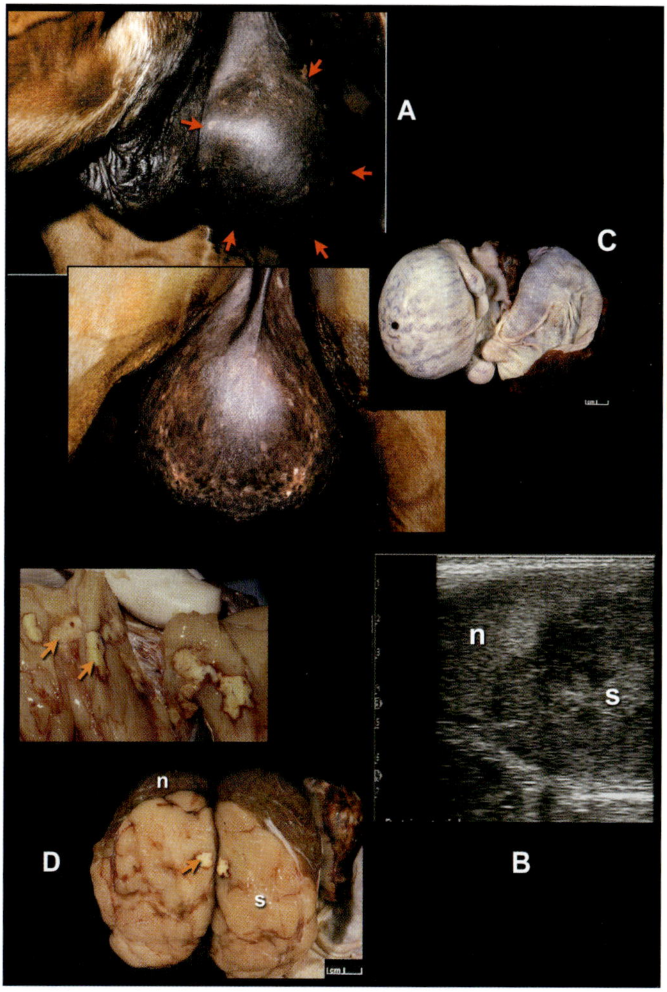

Figure 8.10 Precancerous lesions. Squamous cell carcinomas are common neoplasms on the penises of horses. Their etiology is unknown but it has been speculated that chronic irritation caused by accumulations of smegma in the prepuce may induce tumor formation. This is most likely in geldings where the frequency of spontaneous erections is low and, as a consequence, large amounts of moist, highly contaminated smegma accumulate in the prepuce. In both cases pictured here, the lesions were characterized as precancerous that could, in time, develop into squamous cell carcinomas. The penis at upper left was of an intact miniature stallion and the penis at lower right belonged to an aged gelding. The gelding was treated using cryotherapy.

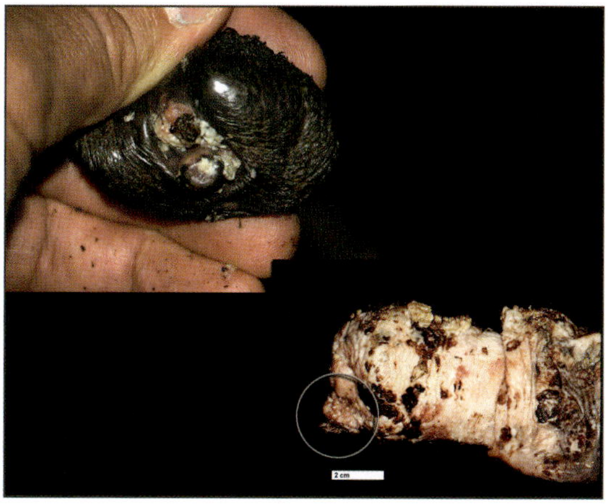

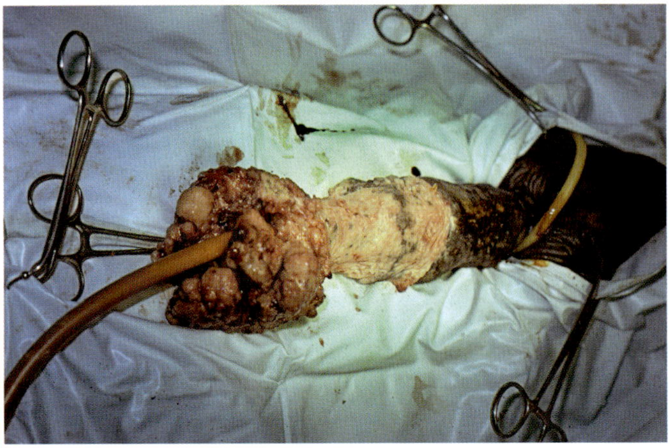

Figure 8.11 Squamous cell carcinoma. Squamous cell carcinoma is a common neoplasm of the equine penis. A large squamous cell carcinoma has developed on the glans of this stallion's penis. If cryosurgery and local excision are not successful, amputation of the penis (phallectomy), as shown here in this image, should be contemplated. A major consideration in phallectomy is hemostasis. Note the large rubber tube about to be used as a tourniquet on the right side of the operative field.

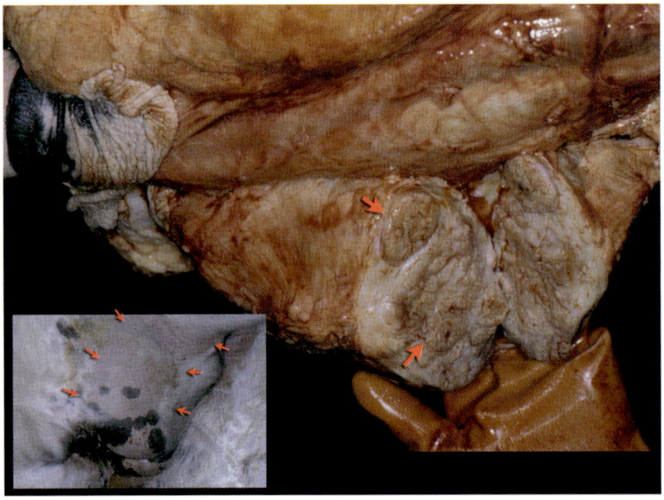

Figure 8.12 Lymphosarcoma. A lymphosarcoma, which developed between the legs of a gelding, ventral to and closely associated with the penis. This is an unusual tumor and an unusual site for its development in a horse. The enlargement was readily visible and palpable as shown in the inset at lower left. This animal was euthanized and the tumor was found to be well encapsulated and not locally invasive.

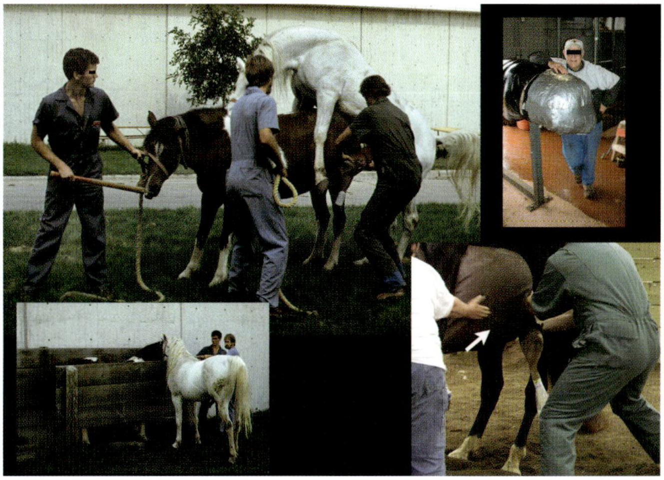

Figure 8.13 Safe semen collection. Both natural service and semen collection using a mare (a so-called mount mare or live mount) hold the potential for injury to a stallion. The illustrations that follow show that injuries to the penis are common and can be devastating. When natural service is practiced or if a live mount is to be used for semen collection, it is essential to tease the mare properly (nose-to-nose then nose-to-tail) to ascertain that she is in good standing heat before either of these procedures are attempted. The procedure for this is shown in the image at the lower left where a set of teasing stocks is being used to protect the stallion. The image at upper left shows how vulnerable the stallion's genitalia are during semen collection. At lower right a "phantom mare" or "dummy" is being used for collection. These structures are simple to build (upper right) and it is usually very easy to train a stallion to serve a phantom mare. This is much safer for the stallion than a live mount.

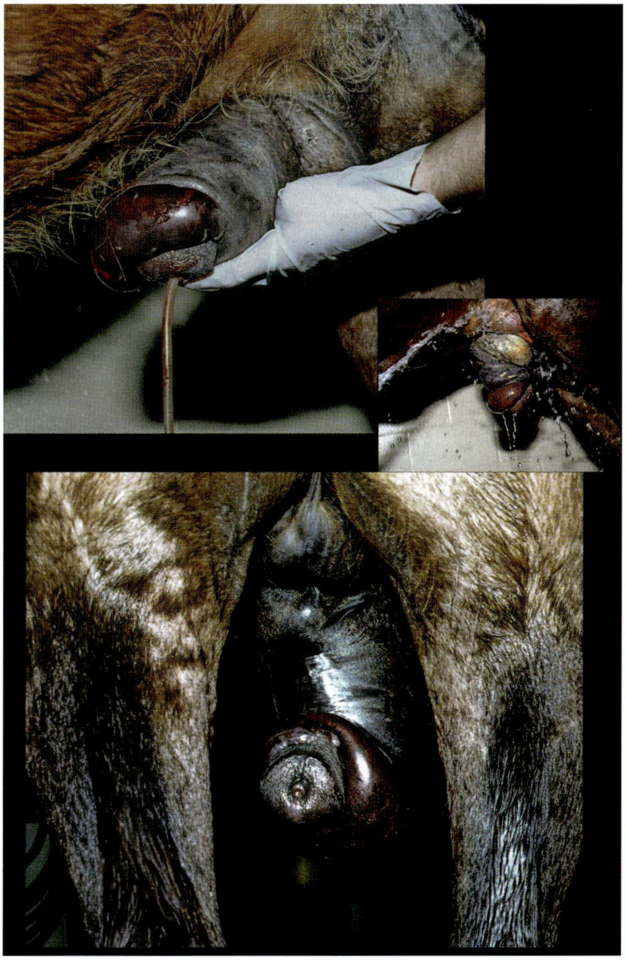

Figure 8.14 Typical kicking injury (penile hematoma). Damage to the penis of a stallion sustained by a kick from a mare during breeding. This is all too common and can be prevented by appropriate teasing and mare restraint or, preferably, the use of a phantom and artificial insemination (AI). On no account should inexperienced stallions be turned out into a group of mares to breed them; especially stallions that have been trained to serve a phantom or have bred mares in heat throughout their lives. Note how the penis has curved to face caudally. This is due to damage of a major venous plexus on the dorsal aspect of the penis, forming a hematoma that induces this curvature of the penis. This plexus is shown in the following image. A major priority in these cases is to catheterize the urethra to ensure normal urine flow. As the inset shows, hydrotherapy is an essential part of treatment as well. When injuries such as this occur, the stallion often cannot be used again for the rest of the breeding season. Also see fig. 8.16.

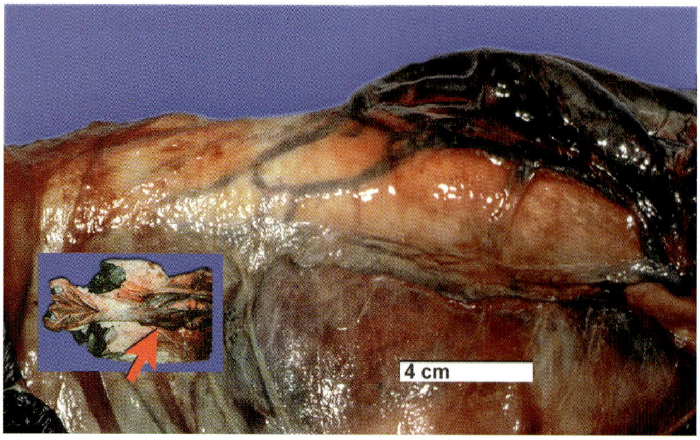

Figure 8.15 The dorsal venous plexus of the penis. An overview of the anatomy of a stallion's penis viewed from the lateral aspect and, in the inset, from the dorsal aspect. Of particular interest is the massive venous plexus that lies dorsal to the penis. As shown in the previous image, this plexus is often damaged when stallions are kicked on their penises during mounting.

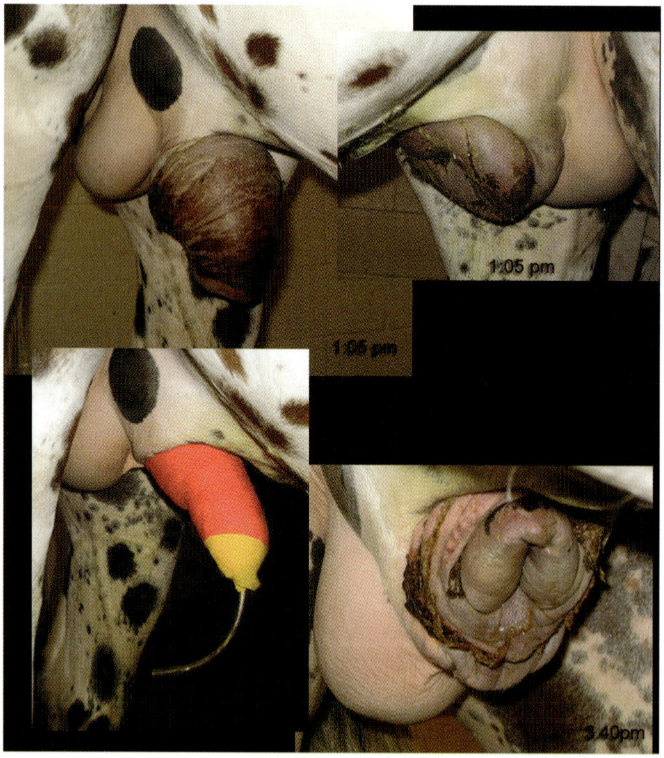

Figure 8.16 Penile injury and hematoma. These images show the penis and prepuce of a 3-year-old Appaloosa stallion. He stood in a pasture with a number of mares and was kicked while trying to serve one of them. The animal received tetanus prophylaxis, antibiotics, and pressure treatment on his penis. Note how the penis was wrapped with "Vet-wrap" after being catheterized. In this case, the wrap was only left in place for a period of approximately 3 hours. After removal of the wrap, the improvement was obvious. Examination of the scrotum using ultrasound suggested that there was very little effusion into the tunica vaginalis despite obvious subcutaneous edema in the scrotum. In general, treatment of kicking injuries to the penis includes: (1) catheterization of the urethra (as shown here) to ensure normal urine flow; (2) rebandaging of the penis every few hours with a gauze, nonstick dressing to decrease the size of the hematoma and any swelling due to edema; (3) suspension of the penis to prevent gravitational exacerbation of the swelling; (4) tetanus prophylaxis; (5) analgesia; (6) prophylactic antibiotics to prevent abscess formation in the hematoma.

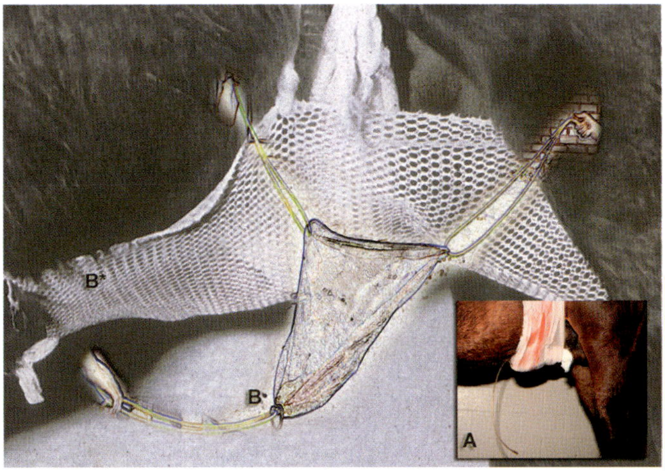

Figure 8.17 Suspensory choices for penile injuries. This composite image shows various options for penile suspension after kicking injuries. The main image shows a crude truss made from white netting, suspended using bandages. The superimposed image shows variation of that truss with two loops of surgical rubber tubing anterior and a single loop posterior. The single loop is passed up through the hind legs and joined to both of the anterior loops, which are passed up on either side of the abdomen. The inset shows how the same effect can be achieved with a simple belly bandage. Whichever system is used, it should allow for frequent bandage changes and access to the penis.

Testicular Hypoplasia

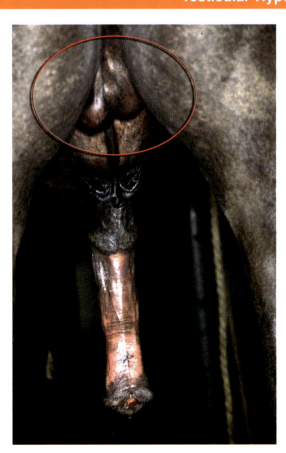

Figure 8.18 The average size of the equine scrotum (i.e., width when measured transversely) is about 10 cm, each testicle having a transverse diameter of about 5 cm. Although there is a considerable difference in the size of the testicles between breeds, one would not usually expect to encounter a scrotal width of less than 7 cm in any standard size breed. In this case, the scrotal width (see red ellipse) was marginally less than 7 cm. Despite this, the stallion had a normal libido and produced a normal ejaculate. Although stallions with small testicles produce fewer spermatozoa than those with large testicles and testicular size appears to be heritable, the importance of testicle size in a stallion breeding soundness evaluation is of little consequence in very prestigious stallions. Genetics outweigh fertility.

Penile Paralysis and Amputation

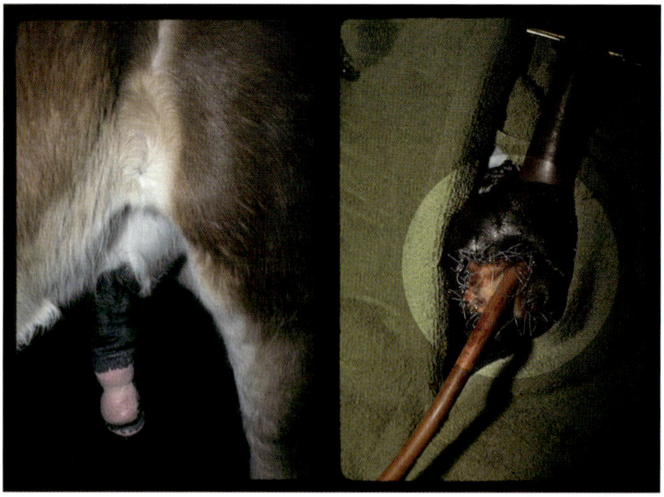

Figure 8.19 Penile "paralysis" or morbid engorgement of the penis. Although there is a classic association between the use of phenothiazine tranquilizers and penile paralysis in horses, most cases are actually associated with trauma. Other cases have an unknown etiology. Although the term priapism is sometimes used to describe this condition, it is probably inaccurate because priapism is persistent erection rather than one of passive engorgement. As shown in the image on the right side, phallectomy (penile amputation) was performed to prevent trauma in this stallion. Amputation is considered to be an extreme measure in such cases and not always necessary, especially if a special truss is made to support the penis. Affected stallions can even provide fertile ejaculates using pharmacological stimulation, usually with imipramine hydrochloride and xylazine.

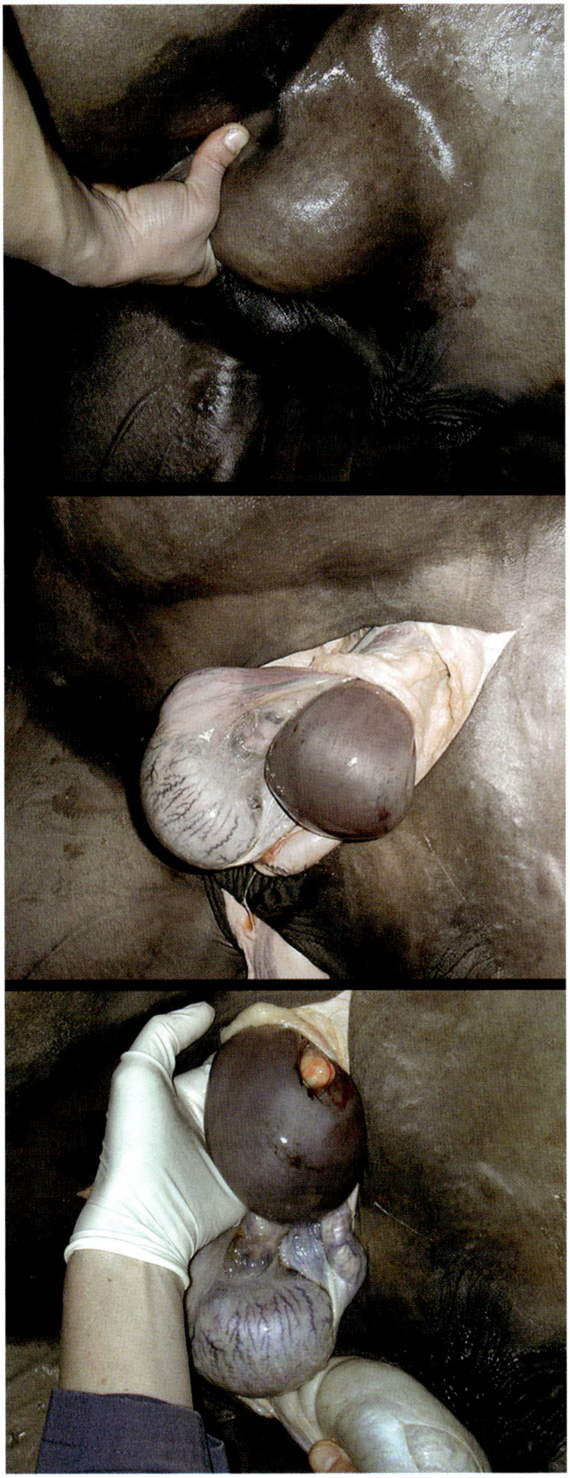

Figure 8.20 Scrotal hernia. Scrotal hernia of the small intestine in the right half of the scrotum in a stallion. This hernia was not obvious on casual observation or palpation but was easy to appreciate using transscrotal ultrasonography. The owner elected to have the horse euthanized and these images were taken shortly after euthanasia. The hernial ring was very tight, hardly permitting the insertion of a single finger, suggesting that loops of bowel can pass through very small inguinal openings. Occasionally these hernias are temporary and resolve spontaneously after a brief period of severe pain. In some cases, they can even be corrected via rectal palpation and traction. Ultimately, however, loops of bowel become trapped in the tunica vaginalis and surgery is usually necessary.

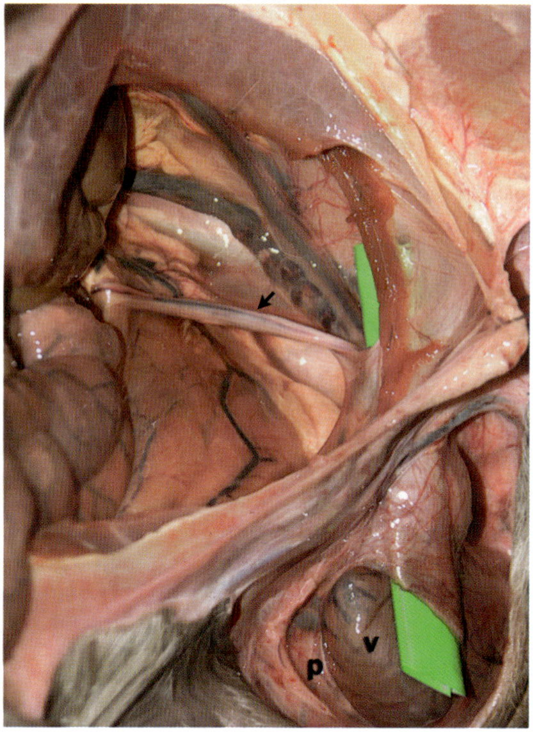

Figure 8.21 Anatomy of scrotal hernia. The left inguinal canal and vaginal cavity of a newborn male donkey viewed from a cranial-oblique aspect. A roll of green plastic, about 7 mm in diameter, has been placed in the inguinal canal, from the internal inguinal opening and into the tunica vaginalis, which has been opened. The visceral vaginal tunic (v) is part of the testicle while the parietal vaginal tunic (p) is the outer limit of the vaginal cavity. The ductus deferens is indicated by the black arrow emerging into the abdomen from the internal opening of the inguinal canal. When a scrotal hernia develops, the intestines usually occupy the same space as is occupied by the roll of green plastic in this illustration.

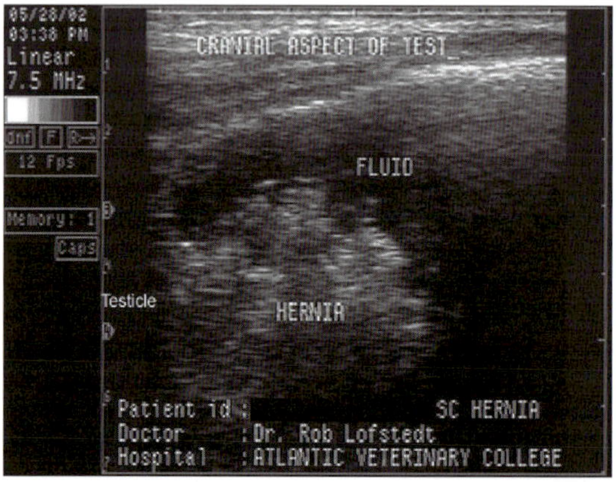

Figure 8.22 Ultrasonography of scrotal hernia. When intestines become entrapped within the vaginal cavity, edema and peritoneal fluid often accumulate around the herniated intestines. Together with the movement of intestinal contents, the contrast provided by this fluid facilitates a diagnosis of an intestinal hernia in the vaginal cavity.

Figure 8.23 Congenital scrotal hernia (diagnosis). A 30-day-old foal with a severe right-sided scrotal hernia. Although this initially appeared to be a left-sided hernia, it was later realized that the herniated intestines on the right side had displaced the left testicle and scrotum farther out than normal toward the left side. This created the impression of a left-sided hernia. This image shows how ultrasound was used to confirm the diagnosis of the hernia. (Image courtesy of Dr. N. Vos, Atlantic Veterinary College, UPEI)

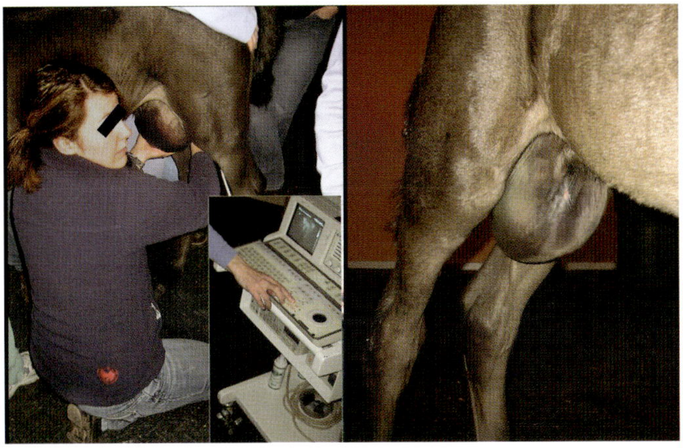

Figure 8.24 Congenital scrotal hernia (surgical treatment). The same foal shown in fig. 8.23. The head of the foal is at the top of the image. The abdominal opening seen here on the right side was made through an abdominal incision adjacent to the right scrotum, exposing these intestines. This was done in an attempt to reduce the hernia through an abdominal route beginning on what was believed to be the opposite side of the hernia. During the laparotomy, it was discovered that the hernia was actually on the same side as the abdominal incision; a section of the intestine entering the right inguinal opening. At that point, a herniorrhaphy was performed on the right side and the left testicle (green ring) was removed. The surgeon suggested that the testicle on the affected side should be removed as well, especially in view of potential physiological compromises after wound healing. The owner was warned of the possibility of propagating a heritable defect if the foal ever became fertile. However, at the insistence of the owner, the right testicle was left in situ. This image illustrates some of the potential pitfalls in the surgical correction of a scrotal hernia in a horse. (Image courtesy of Dr. N. Vos, Atlantic Veterinary College, UPEI)

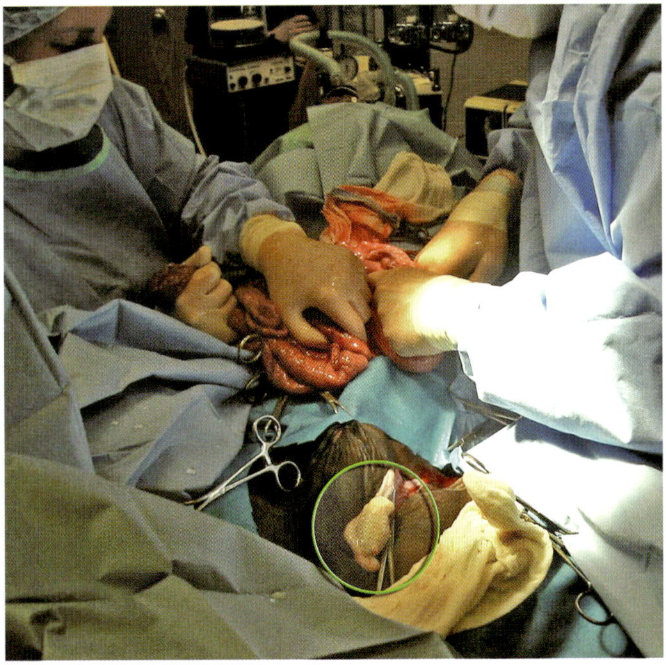

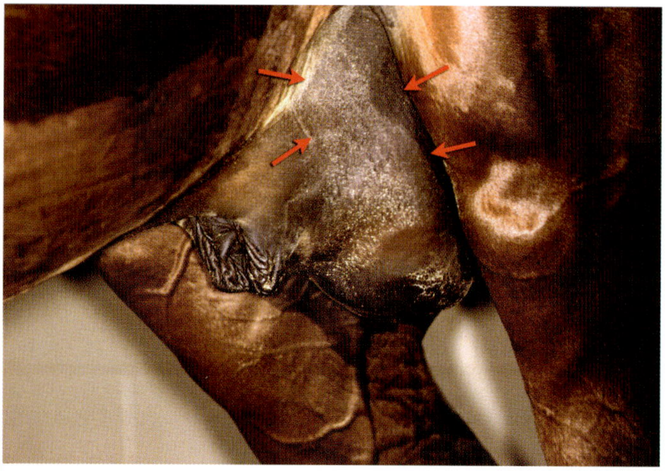

Figure 8.25 Scrotal hernia after castration. The scrotum of a stallion that herniated an intestinal loop into its scrotum 3 weeks after an open-type castration. The intestinal contents occupied the empty scrotum (red arrows). Fortunately the scrotal incision had healed sufficiently to prevent evisceration and, probably, death. Closed castration with double transfixing ligation of the inguinal canal will usually prevent this problem from occurring. When the inguinal canal is left open to the exterior, the risk of fatal evisceration always exists. Herniorrhaphy was performed on this stallion.

Testicular Torsion and Hydrocele

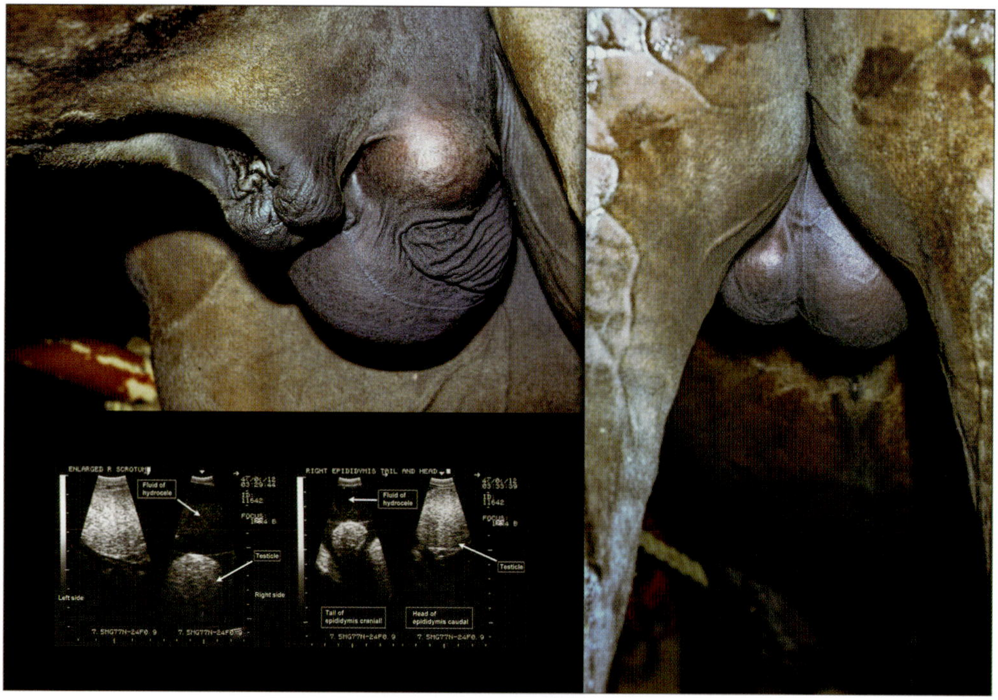

Figure 8.26 Testicular torsion with hydrocele. Caudal view of a 3-year-old Standardbred stallion presented for castration after discomfort during exercise. Examination revealed a right-sided hydrocele. Testicle torsion was suspected by palpation and ultrasonographic examination (inset) and confirmed during surgery. Bilateral castration was performed. It is not clear how testicular torsion develops in stallions because the mesorchium is usually a short ligament between the parietal and visceral vaginal tunics, along the entire dorsal aspect of the testicle. Therefore testicular torsion should, in theory, be almost impossible. However, it certainly occurs. Perhaps the mesorchium stretchs under some circumstances, such as hydrocele in this case, allowing the testicle to rotate horizontally on its dorsoventral, transverse axis. In this case, there was neither strangulation nor vascular embarrassment of the spermatic cord. Therefore, the discomfort this stallion experienced may have been unassociated with torsion of the testicle. In some cases, testicle torsion appears to be congenital and is innocuous, causing neither infertility nor vascular embarrassment.

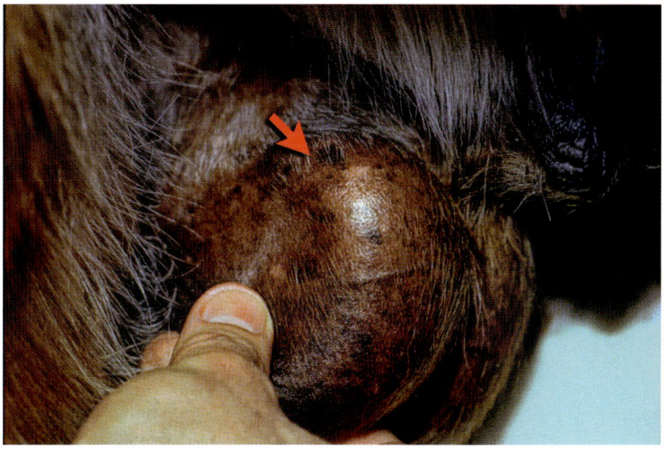

Figure 8.27 Congenital testicular torsion. A 4-year-old paint stallion with 180 degrees (estimated) torsion of the right testicle. A bulge caused by the tail of the epididymis is indicated by a red arrow. This was discovered during a routine breeding soundness evaluation. In this case, torsion was probably congenital because the stallion was fertile and did not experience any pain from the condition.

Smegma Accumulation "Beans" in the Fossa Glandis

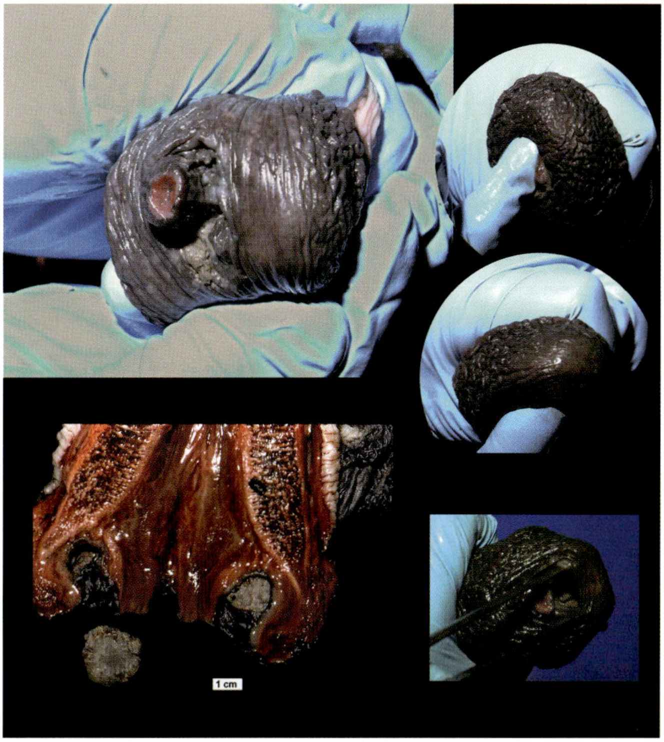

Figure 8.28 The fossa glandis (also called the urethral diverticulum; a somewhat misleading term) is a paired structure with a diverticulum dorsolateral on each side of the opening of the urethra. It is frequently the site of accumulations of concretions of smegma, colloquially called "beans." Beans are considered to be innocuous structures but may provide a substrate for bacterial multiplication because many stallions harbor potential pathogens such as *Klebsiella* and *Pseudomonas* spp. in these diverticulae. The fossa glandis is also a somewhat anaerobic environment and is therefore an ideal site for the maintenance and propagation of the bacteria *Taylorella equigenitalis*, the cause of contagious equine metritis (CEM). It is important to know the anatomy of the fossa glandis, the characteristics of beans, how to remove them (circular images), and where to insert culture instruments when screening stallions for CEM.

Routine Diagnostics

Following the Estrous Cycle

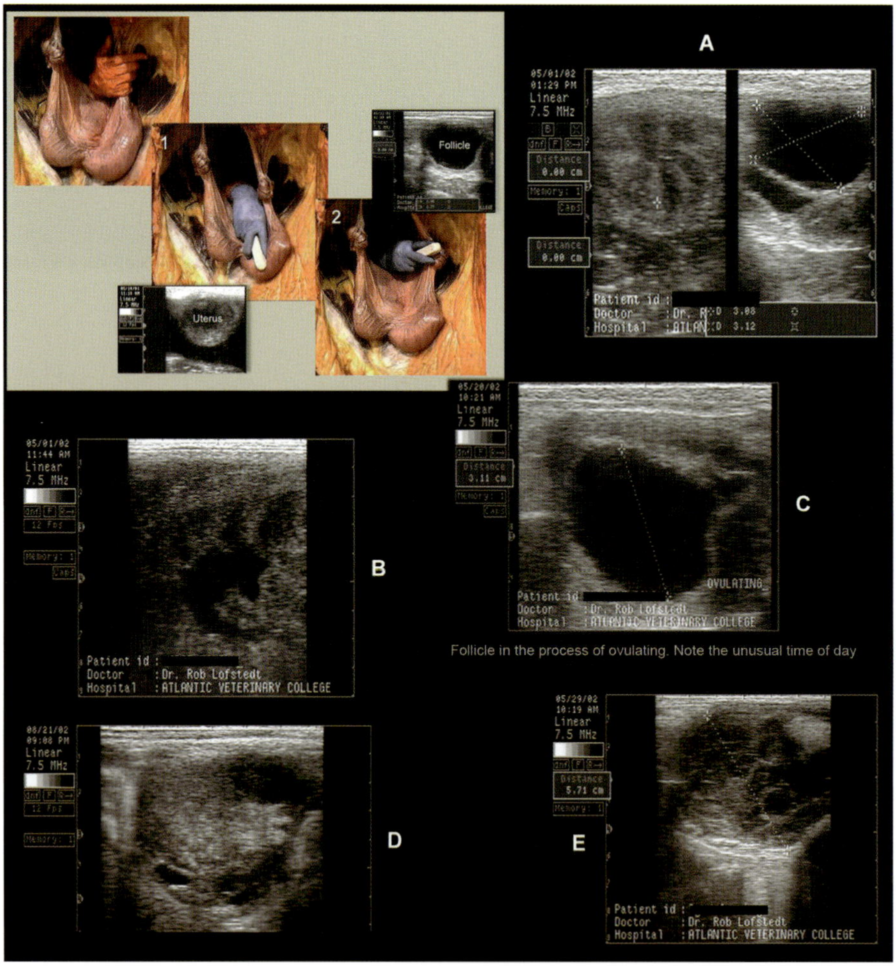

Figure 8.29 With the advent of ultrasonography, routine teasing has become far less essential than it once was for tracking the estrous cycle. An exception to this is in Thoroughbreds, where natural breeding is practiced exclusively and behavioral estrous is essential for breeding. At top left it can be seen that the uterus is palpated first, before ultrasonography is attempted. After establishing the dimensions and position of the tract, all the palpated structures are viewed on ultrasonography. In image **A**, a large preovulatory follicle appears on the right side of the split image, with obvious uterine edema on the cross section of the uterus on the left side. Collectively, these are excellent indications of impending ovulation and the need to inseminate the mare. If fluid is present in the uterine lumen as shown in image **B**, and is shown to be innocuous using cytology, oxytocin is usually administered until the fluid is expelled. In image **C**, a follicle is in the process of ovulating and insemination must have occurred already or within the next 18 hours, the expected life span of an oocyte after ovulation. This follicle is ovulating at 10 a.m., slightly unusual because most ovulations occur late in the evening through early morning. In image **D**, a corpus luteum (CL) has formed where the follicle once existed. The homogeneous echogenic appearance is typical of the majority of corporate lutea but considerable variation in the echodensity of the CL is possible. In image E, a hematoma has formed instead of a normal CL. It is usually diagnosed by its large size (almost 6 cm in this case) and it has nonhomogeneous echogenicity. Large hematomas are not very common and seem to have no endocrinological significance, usually disappearing within a few estrous cycles.

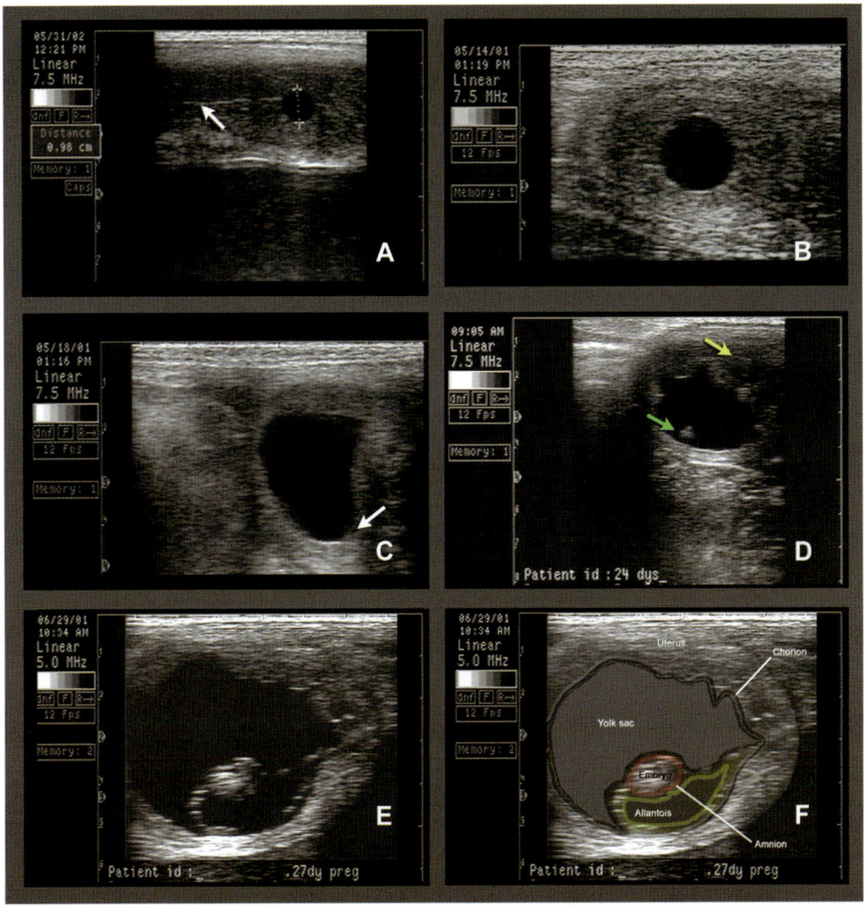

Figure 8.30 This sequence of images illustrates the author's philosophy in monitoring early pregnancies. Mare owners are encouraged to submit their mares for all of these steps in diagnosis. In this manner, twins can be managed properly, early embryonic death can be detected, and the normal development of the conceptus can be monitored. Image A shows a conceptus presumed to be about 14 days old. The precise age of an embryo is actually unknown in normal stud practice because mares are examined and inseminated at 2- to 3-day intervals. Therefore the precise time of ovulation is unknown. The embryonic vesicle migrates throughout the uterus until the embryo is about 16 days old. In this case, the echogenic line that characterizes the uterine body (arrow) shows that the embryo is just cranial to the cervix. Image B shows a conceptus that is approximately 16 days old. It has already become fixed in the uterine horn. The thick homogeneous "doughnut" that surrounds it is the tonic myometrium that characterizes early pregnancy in this species. The nonechogenic (black) center of the vesicle is almost entirely yolk sac. The embryo itself is not yet visible. Image C shows an approximately 19-day-old pregnancy. The sodium pump in the wall of the trophoblast is less active than earlier in gestation, therefore the osmotic pressure within the trophoblast is lower and the trophoblast loses some of its turgidity. This is normal and should not lead one to assume that embryonic death is about to occur. A small echogenic "blip" on the lower right extremity of this vesicle (arrow) is the embryo itself. In image **D**, the embryo (green arrow) has lifted away from the ventral portion of the trophoblast, about 23 to 24 days of age. The characteristic thickening of the uterine wall opposite the embryo (yellow arrow) is typical of this stage of pregnancy. In images **E** and **F**, a pregnancy is about 27 days old. The embryo itself is clearly visible and the embryonic membranes can be distinguished as well. These are clarified in image **F**. The heartbeat of the embryo clearly visible at this time, usually in the range of 120 to 160 bpm.

Aging of the Fetus

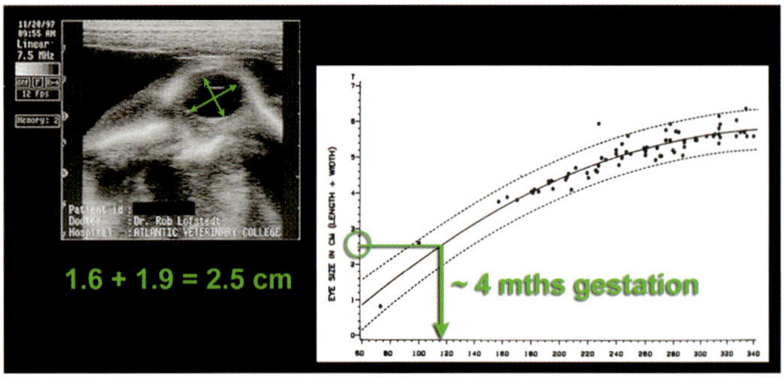

Figure 8.31 The fetal eye is seen here as a large anechogenic circle in the skull of the foal. Its size may be used to determine the approximate age of the fetus. Unfortunately, it is not a very sensitive indicator of age. Nevertheless, this author has found it to be valuable in practice. To estimate fetal age, the two largest diameters of the eye are measured and the sum of those results is plotted against a chart as shown. The diameters of the eye can be measured throughout gestation with the correct equipment.

Vaginal Examination

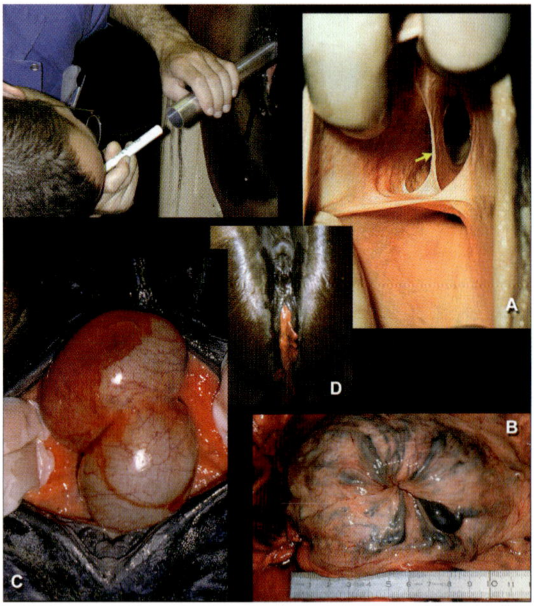

Figure 8.32 Congenital and acquired pathology of the vagina make it essential to perform routine prebreeding per-vagina examinations, especially when natural breeding is used. When artificial insemination is used, vaginal defects are usually discovered when a gloved hand is inserted into the vagina during insemination. In the case of Thoroughbreds, however, failure to recognize structures such as persistent hymens and remnants of the Mullerian system will result in breeding accidents. Such an accident is shown in image **D** where a persistent hymen was not noted before natural breeding. Although speculum examination (top left) can be used to diagnose many vaginal defects, a gloved-hand examination is even more rewarding, especially with cervical injuries, because of one's ability to palpate injuries when they are not obvious during speculum examinations. For completeness, both examinations should probably be done. Image **A** shows the vestibule of a mare with a persistent medial wall of the Mullerian system in the vagina (yellow arrow) and a normal, large external urethral orifice just ventral to it. Image **B** shows a mass of large varicose veins in the everted portion of the cranial vagina of an aged mare. This postmortem specimen shows how large these vessels can become, often causing hemorrhage that is visible at the vulvar lips. This often occurs during late gestation under the effect of high serum estrogen concentrations. In such cases, owners must be assured that this is not a sign of impending abortion. Image **C** shows an intact hymen, bulging through the vulvar lips in this mare. It is slightly twisted on its dorsoventral axis, with a remnant of the Mullerian system providing a central raphe to the structure. The author has seen a case of a complete hymen that became so stretched, presumably due to changes in intravaginal pressure, that it became extended and socklike, intermittently hanging from the vulvar lips or covering the cervix. Although complete hymens are unusual, partially persistent hymens are quite common.

Clitoral Anatomy and Sampling the Clitoral Sinuses

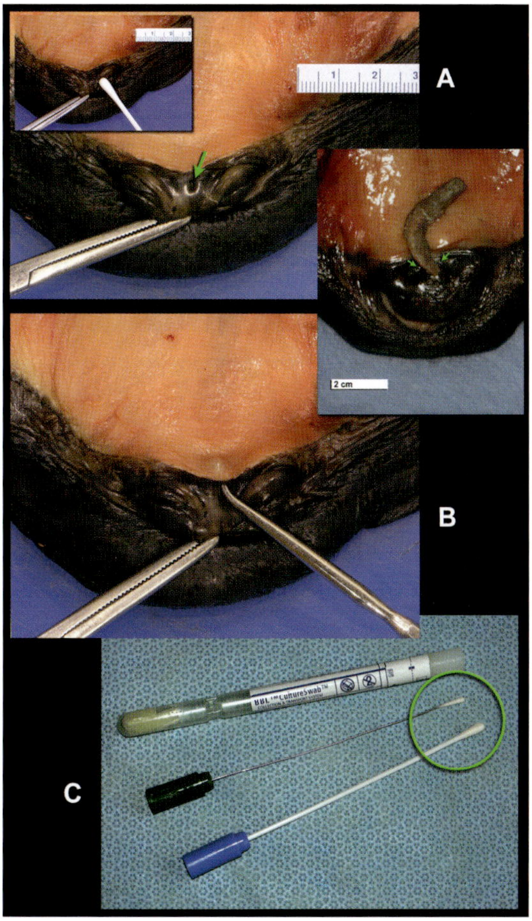

Figure 8.33 Clitoral sinuses are routinely cultured for the contagious equine metritis (CEM) organism, *Taylorella equigenitalis*, which is able to grow in this relatively anaerobic environment. Image A shows the location of one of the largest clitoral sinuses, usually the central sinus on the dorsal surface of the clitoris. Image B shows the approximate depth of the largest sinus, certainly deep enough for an anaerobic environment. The inset between images A and B shows that this central sinus can stretch and harbor large amounts of smegma. This mass of accumulated smegma is analogous to a "bean" found in one of the urethral diverticulae in a stallion. In this case, the smegma contents of the sinus have been cleaned out by squeezing the margins of the clitoris. The smegma itself probably provides an anaerobic environment for the growth of *T. equigenitalis*. Due to the small size of the clitoral sinuses, it is best to use small-diameter swabs to culture for CEM. A conventional swab with a blue cap is shown in image C next to a narrow bore swab that is ideal for sampling the clitoris. In the image at top left, it is apparent that a large swab cannot easily fit into a clitoral sinus.

Neoplasia

Granulosa Cell Tumors

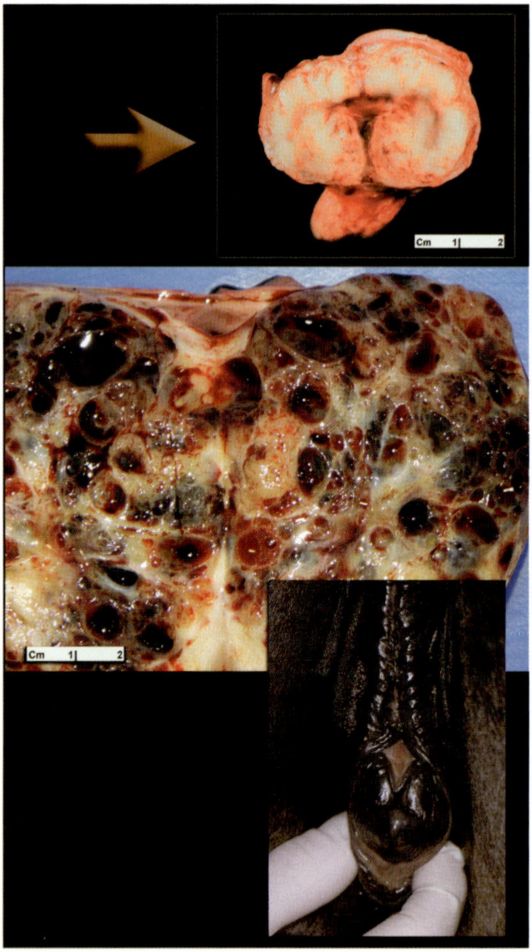

Figure 8.34 Typical granulosa cell tumor, top and middle images. Granulosa cell tumors (GCTs) such as this one are common forms of ovarian neoplasia in mares. Although they have been related to both male and female behavior in the affected animal, they are also a common cause of pathological anestrus. Granulosa cell tumors produce a multitude of sex steroids that may cause negative feedback and suppress hypothalamic-pituitary function. In fact, high serum concentrations of testosterone are sometimes diagnostic of these tumors, but GCTs sometimes produce very little testosterone. When they do produce testosterone, clitoral enlargement may be seen as shown in the inset at lower right. Although their steroid production is variable, GCTs almost invariably produce a complex polypeptide hormone called inhibin, which causes suppression of FSH production and, consequently, decreased ovarian activity. This is why follicle growth in the contralateral ovary is severely suppressed, a useful diagnostic feature of the condition. Sometimes ovarian suppression is chronic, persisting for prolonged periods of time even after the removal of the tumor. Owners should be warned of this possibility. The cut surface of a GCT usually has a honeycomb appearance as shown in this case, middle image. This is obvious on preoperative ultrasonography. As shown in fig. 8.35, however, they can also be solid or consist of only one or two major cystic cavities. Treatment consists of surgical removal using either a flank or ventral midline approach.

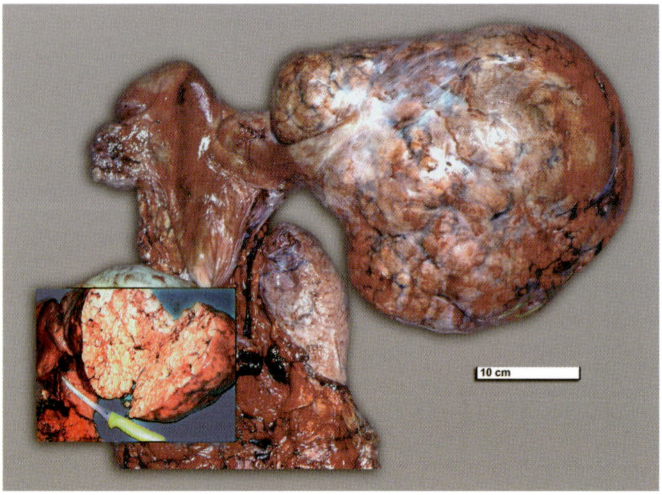

Figure 8.35 Solid granulosa cell tumor. A large granulosa cell tumor (GCT) that was solid on cut surface. Its cut surface is shown in the inset. This is an unusual appearance for a GCT because most of these tumors are cystic or polycystic in nature.

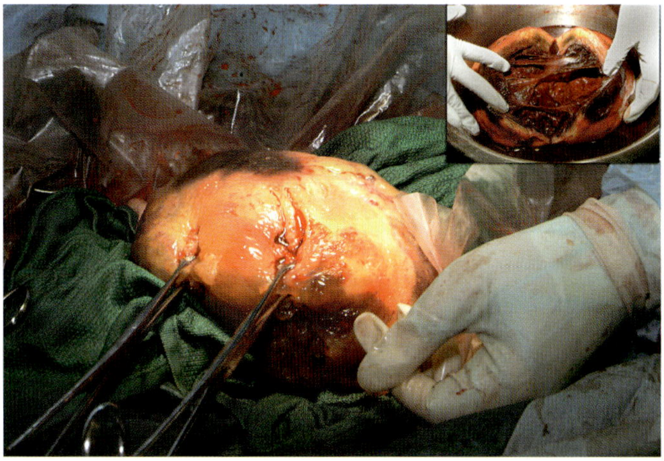

Figure 8.36 Monocystic granulosa cell tumor. An 8-year-old pony mare presented for surgical resection of a mass on her right ovary, which was discovered incidentally during a workup for mild colic. The mare had been observed mounting another mare on one occasion. On palpation, the mass was quite large (25 × 28 cm), ovoid, and very firm. Ultrasonographic examination revealed it to be fluid filled, consisting of one large cyst containing what appeared to be a network of fibrin strands, reminiscent of a postovulation hematoma. There were also two small follicles on the contralateral ovary, therefore a diagnosis of a GCT was uncertain. The tumor is pictured here during its removal. The inset shows its monocystic character and a network of connective tissue strands spanning the cyst. Preoperative serum fluid samples for progesterone, estradiol, and testosterone were within normal ranges for serum concentrations in mares. However, the serum inhibin concentration was approximately twice that of a normal mare, consistent with a diagnosis of a granulosa cell tumor. It is interesting that the inhibin concentration in the cyst itself was about a hundred times higher than the normal serum concentration of inhibin.

Other Tumors

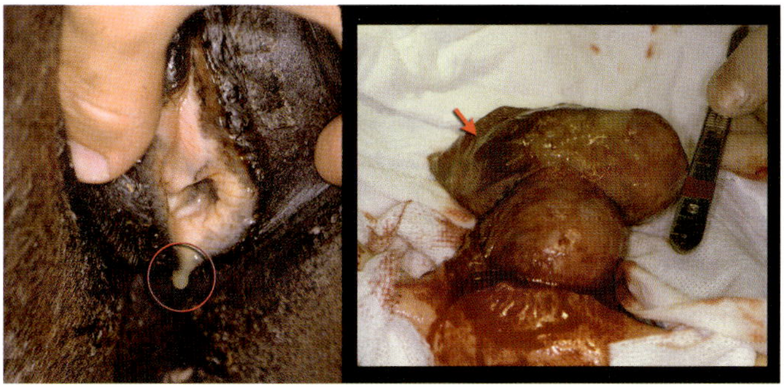

Figure 8.37 Leiomyosarcoma. Leiomyosarcoma is a very unusual tumor in mares. This tumor caused a chronic vulvar discharge in an aged Morgan mare (circle). It had outgrown its blood supply and was partially necrotic, the source of the discharge (arrow). The tumor was removed surgically and the mare conceived within two months.

8

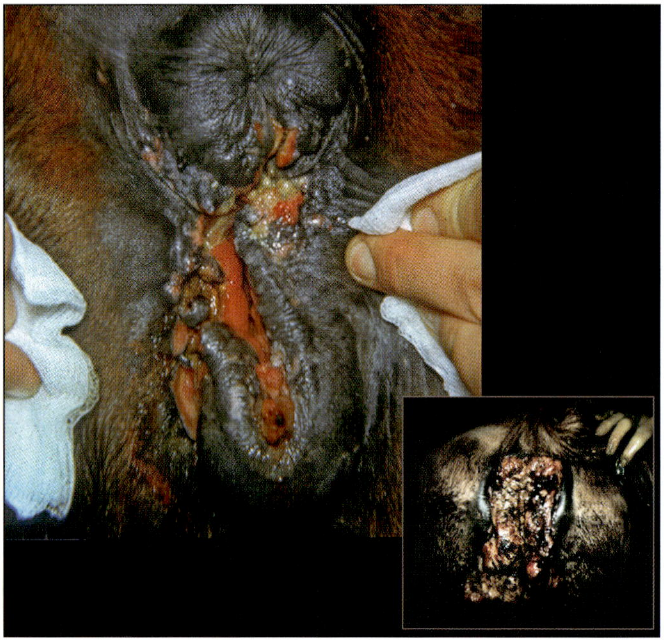

Figure 8.38 Squamous cell carcinoma. These old but unique images illustrate the severe destructive nature of locally invasive squamous cell carcinomas. These tumors do not usually metastasize and are most often treated using cryotherapy. (Image courtesy of the Department of Theriogenology, Iowa State University)

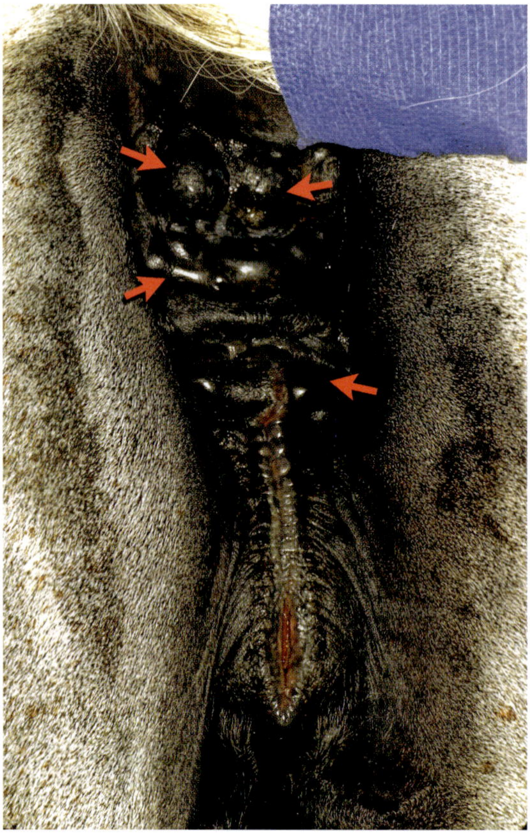

Figure 8.39 Melanoma. Focal melanomas (arrows) are not unusual, especially in gray horses; this one occurred in an Arab mare. Although melanomas are often regarded as potentially malignant, those that occur in the perineal region are usually benign and seldom invasive. As a result, they may not even be treated. Occasionally, local resection or cryotherapy is used.

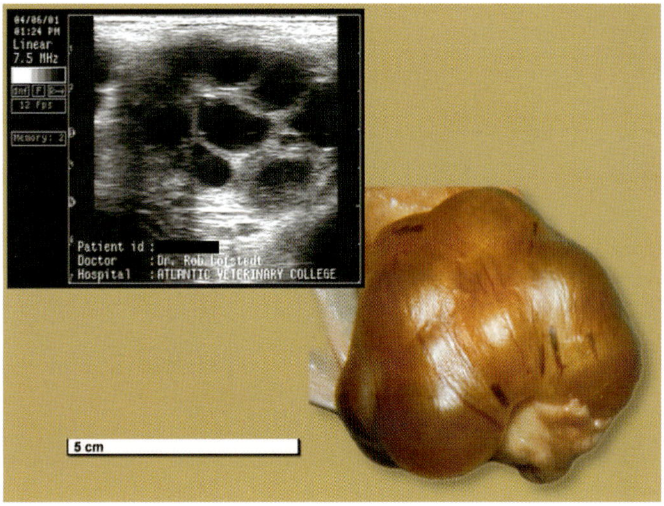

Figure 8.40 A transitional ovary from a mare. This appearance of both ovaries is typical of mares in the springtime when multiple medium-sized follicles predominate on the ultrasonographic image because a dominant, preovulatory follicle has not yet been "selected." This is well illustrated in the ultrasonographic image. Transition is a normal condition, an intermediate state between anestrus and normal estrous cycles. Although transitional mares are in estrus for prolonged periods of time, they are not cystic and do not require treatment. Therefore, this condition is not analogous to cystic ovarian disease in cattle. Mares in transition may be bred repeatedly because they will usually stand for the stallion but they will obviously not become pregnant until estrous cycles begin. Therefore, this is a common cause of "infertility." When such mares arrive at a stud farm, this author normally suggests that the owner take the mare home and return in about 2 weeks to see if the mare has started to ovulate. When these mares return to the stud farm, the presence of a CL visible on ultrasound confirms that they have begun to have estrous cycles. From a practical standpoint, there is nothing one can do to hasten the onset of ovulation in these mares. When owners become impatient at the lack of progress of such mares, a lighting program may be used the following year, at least 8–10 weeks before breeding is anticipated.

Pyometra

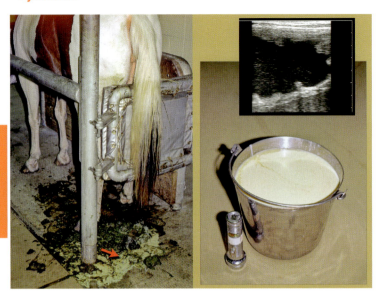

Figure 8.41 The general characteristics of pyometra. A mare with pyometra discharging pus from her vulva. Frequently this may be the only sign of disease as mares are not affected systemically. Pyometra in mares is unlike the condition in cows. It is not usually a postpartum phenomenon and does not invariably block estrous cycles as it does in cows. Pyometra is often an incidental finding in mares unless there is a purulent discharge as occurred here. It is usually due to infection with *Streptococcus zooepidemicus*. Also, affected mares (and cows) are not usually systemically ill like bitches; not even the hemogram is significantly affected. Contrary to what is occasionally stated, the cervix does not have to be abnormal for mares to develop pyometra. Although affected mares are treated with prostaglandin if a corpus luteum is present, the cornerstone of treatment involves physical drainage of the uterus. During treatment, the cervix is dilated manually and a sterile stomach tube or stallion catheter is inserted. Saline is admitted to the uterus to start a siphon and the pus is then drained. Volumes of pus are variable but can be large; this bucket was one of two drained from this mare. The uterus is flushed with saline after it has been drained and about 10 million IU of penicillin (Na or K) in 100 ml of saline were left in the uterus. Systemic antibiotics are not usually required. Unfortunately, the condition often reoccurs; some mares require physical drainage every 2 or 3 months. Hysterectomy is not a common form of treatment because of its surgical difficulty in mares. Although there is little evidence to support such a statement, it is thought that failure to drain pus on a regular basis may predispose mares to uterine rupture.

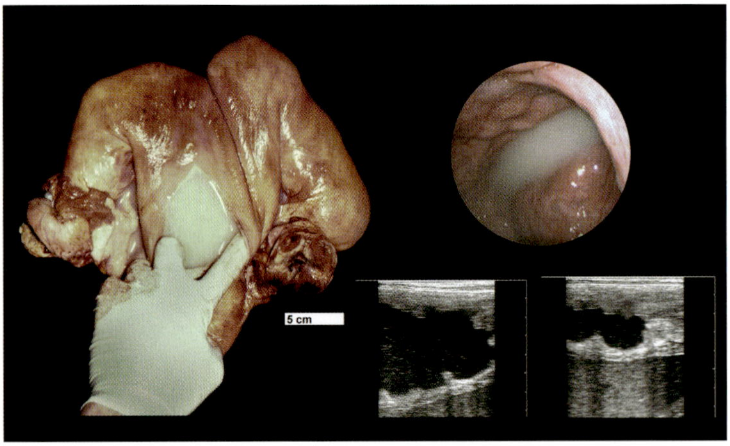

Figure 8.42 Endoscopy and ultrasonography of pyometra. This image shows the appearance of pyometra in the uterus of a mare at postmortem. In this case, the condition was supported by a progestogenic environment; two corpora lutea being visible on the right ovary. In such a case, the mare would have been treated with prostaglandins and physical drainage if she had not been euthanized. Pyometra may be characterized by a purulent discharge but often it is only discovered on routine ultrasonography. As seen in the insets, pus is often highly echogenic due to its cellular content. Occasionally, however, it can be remarkably nonechogenic. In such cases, cytology or endoscopy (as seen here) will confirm the diagnosis.

Transluminal Adhesions

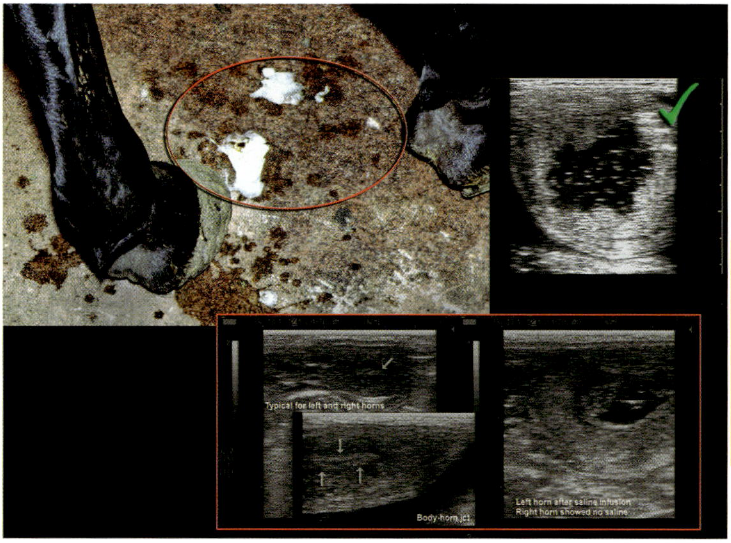

Figure 8.43 Purulent discharge seen on the floor (red ellipse) behind a mare. This mare discharged pus intermittently because of multiple draining abscesses that had formed in her vagina. These abscesses formed between transluminal adhesions caused by vaginal irritation. This followed prolonged intervention during dystocia and caused obliteration of the cervix. Unfortunately, this complication arising from the management of dystocia is not uncommon. To prevent transluminal adhesions of the vagina, a lubricating substance such as oil-based paste that is used to treat mastitis can be applied to the vaginal wall every 48 hours several times after relieving dystocia. This illustration also shows how the extent of transluminal adhesions can be evaluated using an infusion of saline. At the upper right corner, a green checkmark shows the normal appearance of saline in a uterus. Its echogenicity is due to microscopic bubbles of air normally found in saline. This makes saline an ideal contrast medium for the evaluation of the uterine and vaginal integrity using ultrasound. In the red rectangle, one can see how poorly an infusion of saline had distributed itself within the uterine lumen. That mare had severe transluminal adhesions throughout her uterus, probably as a result of a foaling injury.

Lymphatic Lacunae or Cyst (Endometrial Cysts)

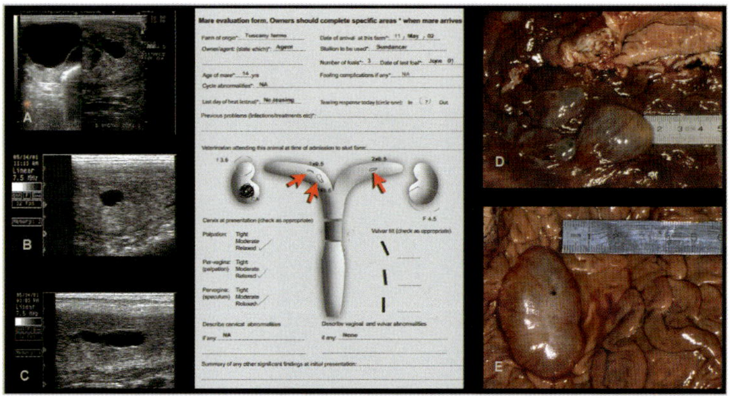

Figure 8.44 Appearance of lymphatic lacunae or cyst (endometrial cyst); lymphatic lacunae (lymphatic cysts) in the endometrium. These are easily confused with embryos at 12–16 days of gestation. All of the ultrasonographic images on the left are in fact cysts, although two of them resemble embryos that are adjacent to cysts. Unlike embryos, however, they are never mobile. To avoid confusion, lymphatic lacunae should be mapped during the first ultrasonographic examination of every breeding season. A diagram suitable for mapping of cysts is shown in the center of this image. The pathogenesis of lymphatic cysts is obscure but they are not always associated with endometrial fibrosis as is sometimes suggested. Instead, cysts appear to be a sort of lymphatic varicosity, occurring commonly in older mares. Endometrial cysts are not associated with infertility unless they prevent embryonic migration and thereby block the recognition of pregnancy. For that reason, endometrial cysts are sometimes ablated using laser surgery.

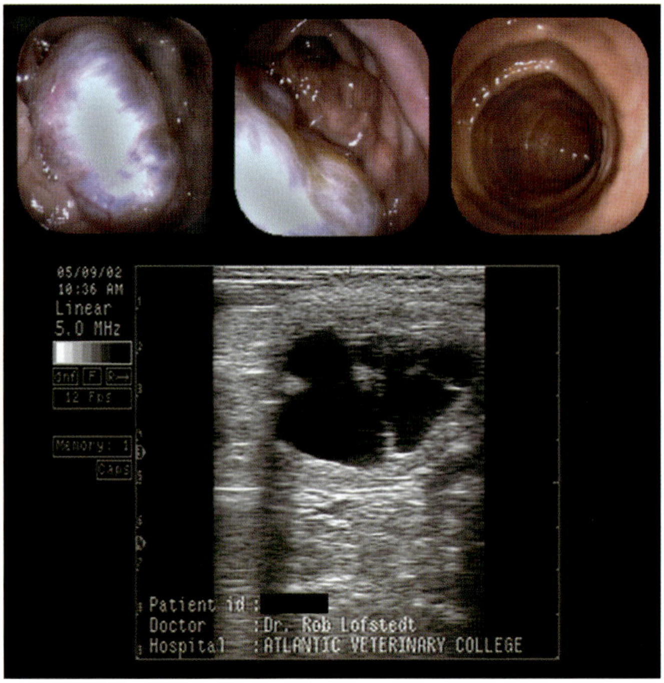

Figure 8.45 Endometrial cyst affecting the recognition of pregnancy. A 19-year-old mare with a long-standing endometrial cyst in her left uterine horn. This was a source of confusion for the referring practitioner because it resembled a 40-day pregnancy. It also appeared to be interfering with the migration of embryos in the uterus, resulting in infertility. The cyst is visible in this ultrasonographic image and two endoscopic views (with a normal section of the uterine horn on the extreme right). An endometrial biopsy was taken from this mare to prognosticate on her ability to maintain pregnancy and to justify laser treatment of the lymphatic lacuna. Apart from mild lympangectasis in one area of the biopsy, there was no obvious endometrial fibrosis. Therefore, the cyst was ablated using a CO_2 endoscopic laser. Unfortunately this mare was lost to follow-up. Therefore, her postoperative fertility is unknown.

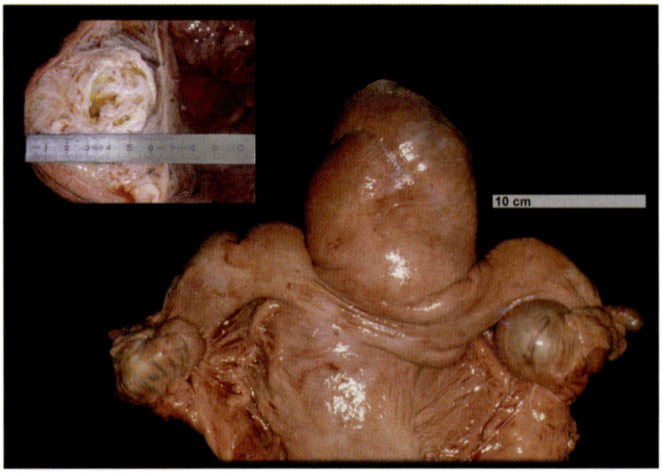

Figure 8.46 A large lymphatic cyst. This large structure was detected on transrectal palpation and resembled a leiomyoma on ultrasonographic examination. A tentative diagnosis of leiomyoma, or leiomyosarcoma, was made. On postmortem examination, however, this massive multilocular cyst was seen. In the absence of any neoplastic tissue on histopathology, it was presumed to be a large lymphatic cyst.

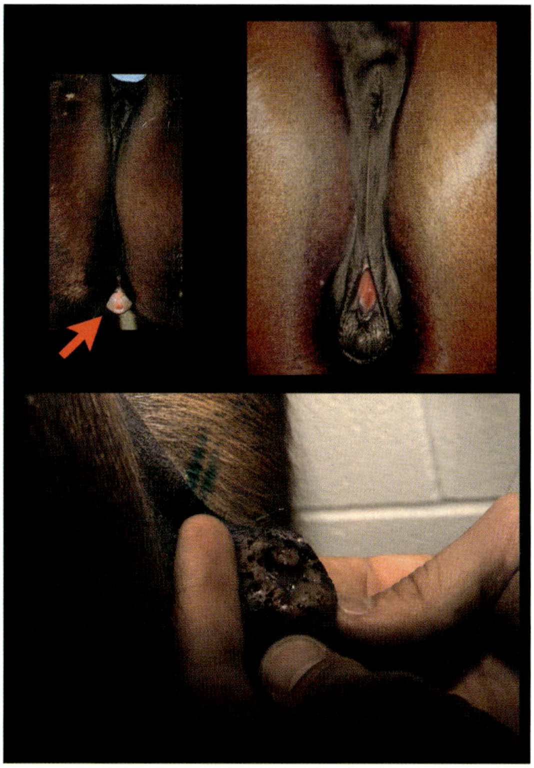

Figure 8.47 The intersex condition with abnormal genitalia is not rare in horses. In such cases, the external genitalia are sometimes bizarre (as seen here) but in others, the tract may appear to be almost normal. Animals with aneuploidy (any derangement of the chromosomal makeup) may have a wide range of karyotypes based on the absence, presence, or duplication of X and Y chromosomes and sometimes autosomes as well. These anomalies are often logically divorced from the gonadal sex of the animal. For example, intersex animals with XX karyotypes often have testicles. Instead, sex determination is made principally by the presence or absence of the SR-y gene. However, many other genetic factors are involved as well. The animals in these images are all male pseudohermaphrodites (a common form of intersex) where testicles are present but the external genitalia are ambiguous. None of them had a vagina. All showed predominantly male behavior and they had enlarged clitorises, resembling small glans penises. This resemblance is not surprising because the clitoris is the homolog of the glans penis in females. Turner's-like syndrome (XO) is not a case of intersex although these mares have aneuploidy. The external genitalia are normal in appearance. Although smaller than usual, their uteruses and ovaries are also normal in appearance. The primary source of pathology lies with ovarian function and absence of folliculogenesis. Aneuploidy should be excluded in all cases of mares that are not cycling during summertime. In many cases, owners will elect not to pursue either gonadectomy or karyotyping. Therefore, many cases of aneuploidy remain incompletely diagnosed, the cause unknown. Occasionally, intersex animals are used as teasers because male pseudohermaphrodites have testicles and can have good libido.

Poor Vulvar Conformation

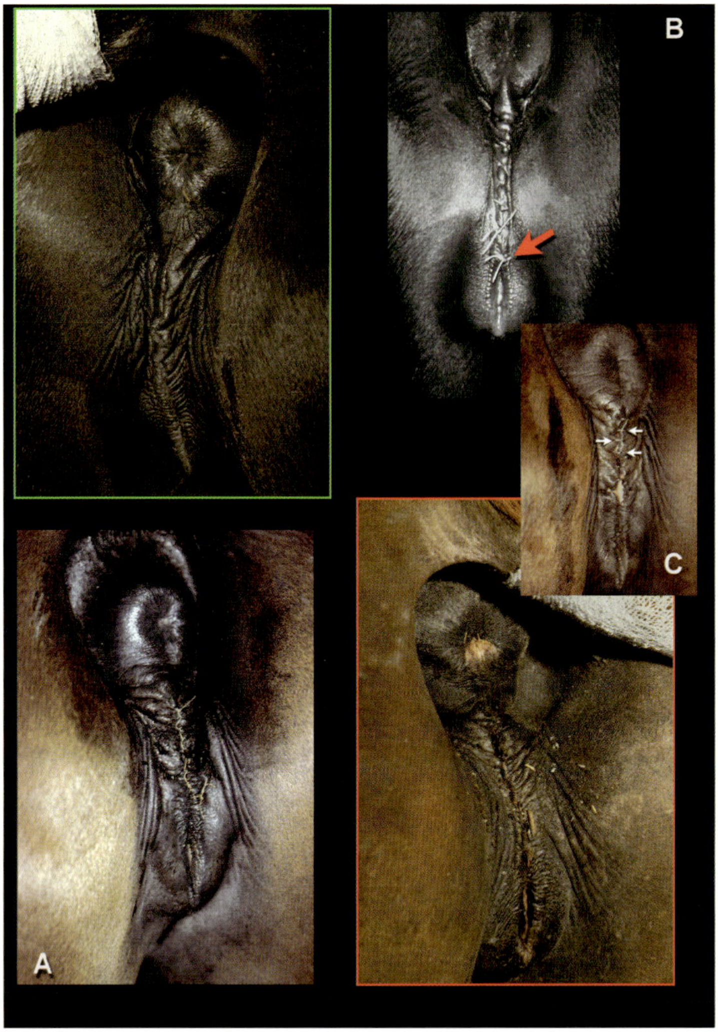

Figure 8.48 Vulvar conformation. A large field study showed that there was an association between vulva conformation and infertility. Essentially, it was shown that the vulvar lips should be as close to vertical as possible and should not tilt forward, increasing the amount of vestibule riding above the pelvic brim. For almost 30 years, mares with poor vulva conformation have been exposed to an operation that effectively corrects this problem. This is the so-called Caslick's operation where the dorsal two-thirds of the vulvar lips are surgically apposed. In all likelihood, this has selected for mares with poor conformation. The image contained within the green rectangle shows a mare with good vulvar conformation but the image contained within the red rectangle shows the opposite. In the second case, the vulvar slopes forward and the vulvar lips are not well apposed, allowing contaminated air from the perineum to be drawn into the vagina and uterus. This happens when abdominal pressure decreases during inhalation and is colloquially known as "wind sucking." This situation worsens with age because the perineum is pulled cranially and ventrally as the weight of the uterus increases and connective tissue attachments relax. In image A, the vulva lips have been opposed by debriding the dorsal two-thirds of the mucocutaneous junction and suturing the vulvar lips together using a continuous interlocking suture. In some cases, as shown in image B, a strengthening suture (colloquially known as a "breeding stitch" and indicated by a red arrow) is inserted in the most ventral part of the apposed lips. This strengthens the operative site for natural breeding. In such cases, care must be taken to prevent the suture from injuring the stallion's penis by guiding the penis under one's fingers during intromission. In our practice, 35 W metal staples (image C) are used to appose the vulvar lips temporarily, until the cervix closes during pregnancy.

Vulvar Injuries

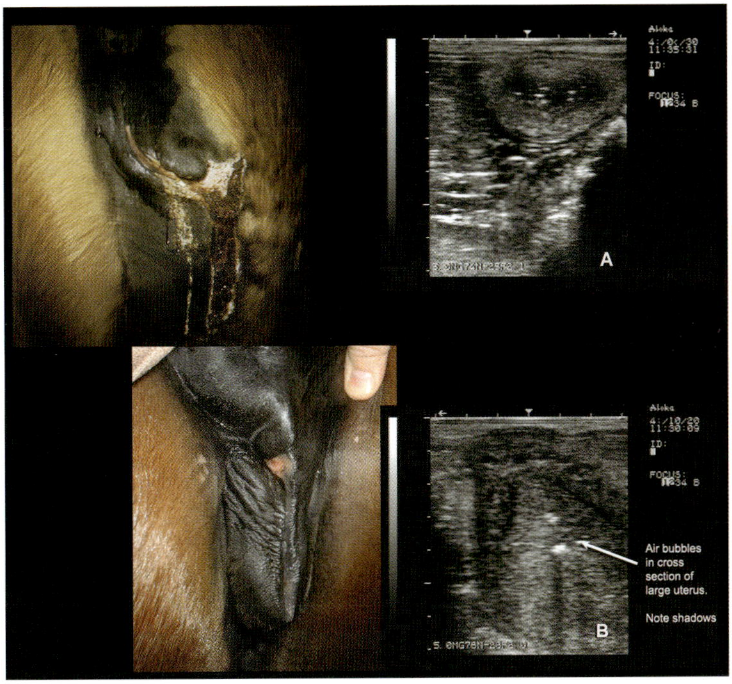

Figure 8.49 Injuries from foaling or other causes may result in mild to severe distortion of the vulvar lips after healing. This can be similar to congenital poor conformation and affected mares may become "wind suckers." In images A and B, bubbles of air can be seen in uterine cross sections using ultrasonography in a wind-sucking mare. The cause of the injury at upper left was never determined but it was not due to foaling. This contributed to wind sucking. In the image below that, mild distortion of the left vulva lip was a result of foaling, however, it did not result in wind sucking. When Caslick's operations are not reversed prior to foaling, similar injuries can occur.

Coital Exanthema

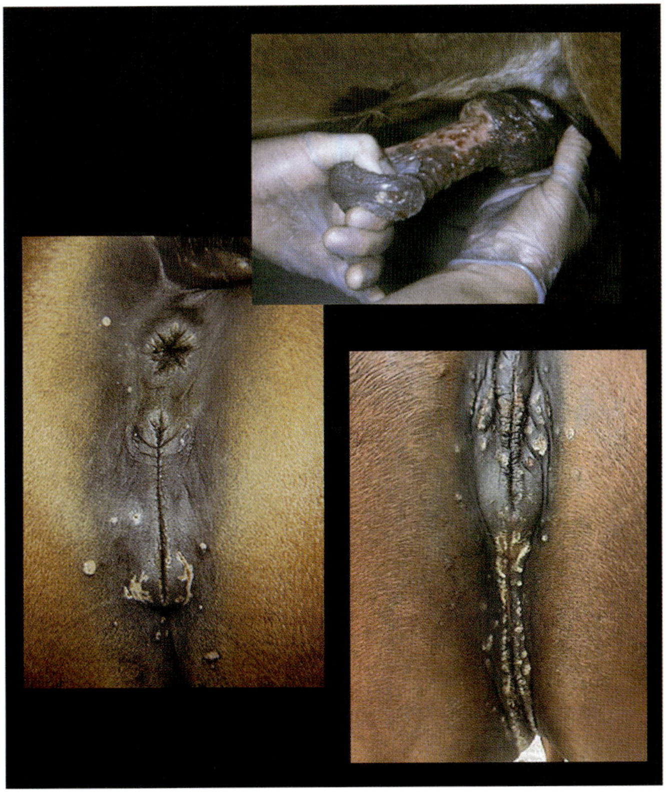

Figure 8.50 Coital exanthema ("spots") caused by equine herpes virus III (EHV III). This is a vesicular, then ulcerative venereal disease. It causes genital discomfort and reluctance to breed in both sexes. In that sense, it is a cause of infertility. As seen here, it can affect the area surrounding the genitalia as well as the genitalia themselves. The two main routes of infection are venereal and iatrogenic, in the acute phase when fresh lesions are present on the genitalia. To prevent transmission, affected animals should not be allowed to breed for at least 3 weeks after the lesions are first seen. Secondary infection may complicate the condition but lesions usually heal within 14 days. (The two lower images are courtesy of Dr. Charles T. Estill, College of Veterinary Medicine, Corvallis, Oregon)

Cervical Tears

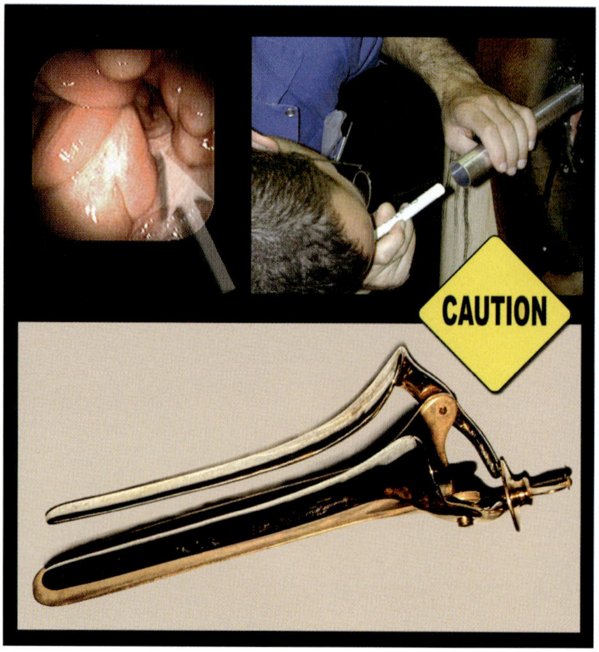

Figure 8.51 Cervical tears often arise as a result of foaling, especially in maiden mares. When the cervical integrity is sufficient to protect the uterine environment during pregnancy, cervical tears do not affect fertility. However, in many cases they do affect fertility; mares fail to conceive or conceive then experience early embryonic death. The mare with this cervical tear (top left) was presented after a failure to repair it surgically. This is not unusual because surgical repair of the cervix is difficult, and healing is usually compromised because of its relatively poor blood supply. The mare was infertile but her endometrial biopsy indicated that her uterus can maintain pregnancy. Therefore, a Shirodkar-like suture (a circumferential suture used for cervical closure in humans) was placed in the cervix and the mare was inseminated at two successive estrous periods, but failed to conceive. This illustration also emphasizes that speculum examination using either a Polanski or tubular speculum can fail to demonstrate cervical tears. This is especially the case during estrus when the cervix is relaxed. Gloved-hand examination is a more thorough method of examining the cervix.

8

Periovarian Adhesions

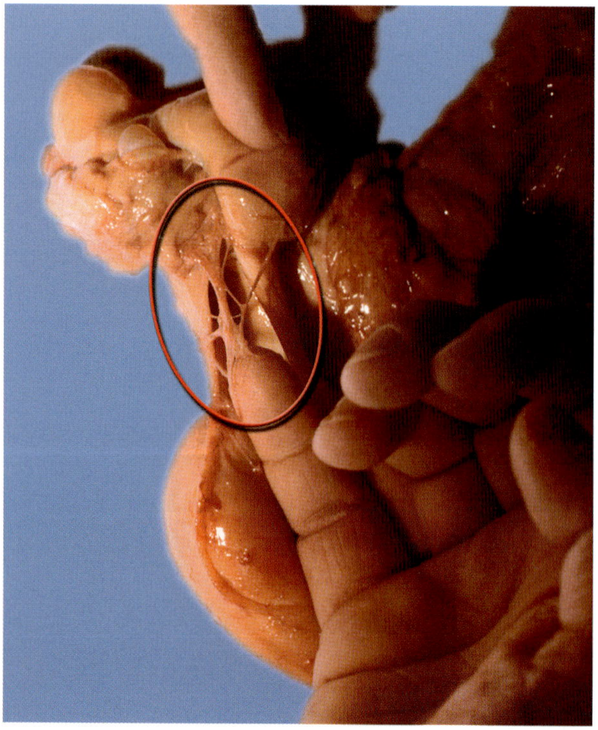

Figure 8.52 Periovarian adhesions are rare in mares. In this case, a finger has been placed under some adhesions between the ovary and the mesosalpinx. It is not known if this pathology causes infertility, however, it is possible. The rarity of periovarian adhesions in mares may be due to the one-way valve nature of the utero-ovarian junction. In postmortem specimens, a dye solution can be forced from the uterus into the fallopian tube quite easily in cattle but this is very difficult in mares.

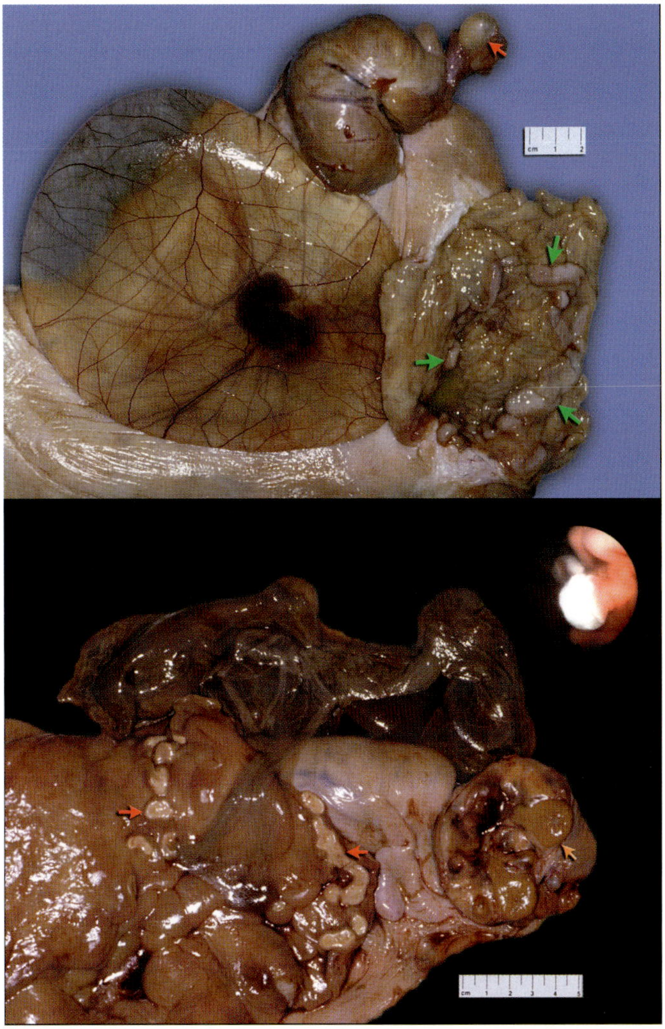

Figure 8.53 Endometrial cups, equine chorionic gonadotropin (eCG), and infertility. At about 28 to 35 days of gestation, cells from the embryo invade the endometrium forming endometrial cups. These structures are sources of equine chorionic gonadotropin (eCG) and are shown in the upper image of a healthy embryo. They are indicated by green arrows. If the embryo dies after the formation of endometrial cups, the endometrial cups persist as shown in the lower image indicated by red arrows. This embryo died at about 60 days of gestation, when large amounts of eCG were being produced. In the circular inset, endometrial cups are seen by endoscopy after the death of a fetus. Interestingly, endometrial cups are difficult to see using ultrasonography. Even after fetal death, the endometrial cups continue to produce eCG because their cells are supported by the endometrium. For an unknown reason, continued production of eCG in such cases causes anestrus or prevents the mare from having normal estrous cycles. This can persist for long periods of time, perhaps several months, eliminating the chances of breeding an affected mare again during that breeding season. Although it has been reported that endometrial cups can be destroyed using laser surgery, it is seldom performed in practice because of the expense of such equipment.

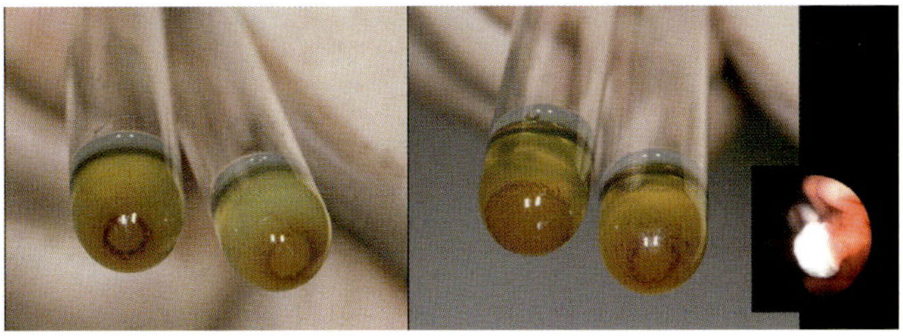

Figure 8.54 Fetal death and anestrus; the mare immunopregnancy (MIP) test. As shown elsewhere, endometrial cups often persist after fetal death, causing disruption of estrous cycles. Because endometrial cups are difficult to see using ultrasonography and many practitioners do not possess endoscopes, one must often rely on endocrinological tests to ascertain if endometrial cups are still present and are still producing eCG. Some laboratories offer quantitative assays for eCG but others still rely on the mare immunopregnancy (MIP) test, a qualitative assay for eCG. In this illustration, the set of tubes on the right-hand side have produced a positive test result because endometrial cups were present in this mare (see inset of endoscopic view). The image on the left shows a negative test result.

Routine Culture and Cytology to Investigate Infertility

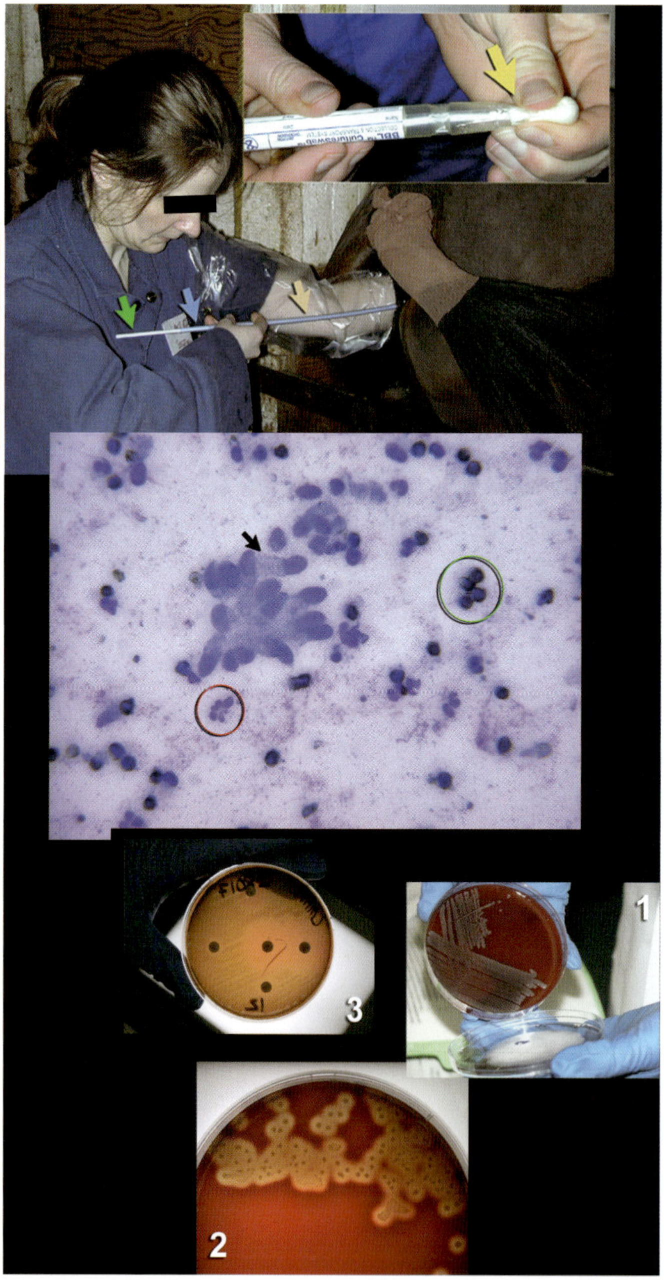

Figure 8.55 This illustration shows common diagnostic techniques that are employed in equine stud medicine. During routine breeding soundness evaluation or when fluid is seen in the uterus on ultrasonography, both culture and cytology are usually performed. The yellow arrow at top right shows how bacterial culture swab is transferred to a special transport medium immediately after culture. Common culturing instruments for mares do not contain transport media and are inclined to dry out before they can be plated for culture. The blue, green, and light orange arrows merely indicate the double-guarded nature of the culture instrument. The image at top left shows routine cytology. This is done with an extension on a cytology brush used for sampling the cervix in humans, providing excellent cytology specimens. Such a specimen is seen in the center of this collection of images. The black arrow shows normal epithelial cells from the endometrium; the length of their cytoplasm indicates that this mare was in estrus at the time of sampling. Some round cells (probably lymphocytes) are shown under the green ring. Their presence may indicate that the infection in this mare has become chronic although the neutrophils in this preparation (one lies under the red ring) indicate that there is an acute component to this infection as well. Signs of infection are not usually seen on cytology, and therefore the role of intrauterine fluid in infertility is questionable. In the three images at the bottom of this composite, both culture and sensitivity are demonstrated. Plate 1 shows a pure culture of coliforms. Plate number 2 shows beta hemolysis (alpha hemolysis is far less dramatic) caused by a culture of *Streptococcus zooepidemicus*, a common commensal and pathogen in mares. Plate 3 is an antibiogram, showing clear growth inhibition by two antibiotic discs and little inhibition by the others.

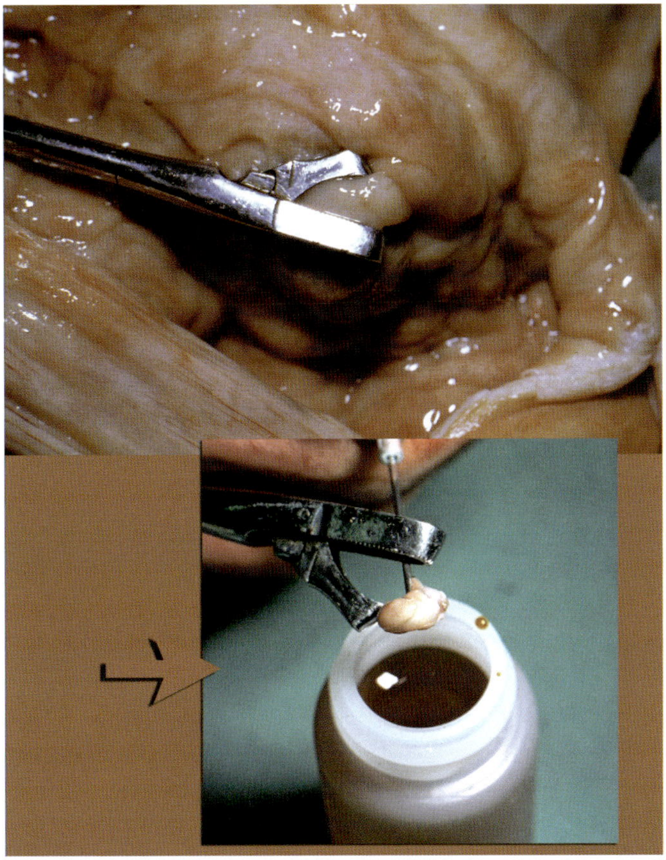

Figure 8.56 General comments. Endometrial biopsy is an important tool in diagnosing endometritis and other causes of infertility in mares. The jaws of the biopsy instrument are shown here on the dorsal endometrial surface where biopsies are normally taken. This is because the biopsy instrument is placed in the uterus and the dorsal endometrium is pushed down (per rectum) into the jaws of the punch. Sometimes this is referred to as a "guided" biopsy technique. It is far superior to a "blind" biopsy technique where the endometrial biopsy punch is inserted through the cervix and its jaws are closed in the hope of obtaining a satisfactory biopsy. When taking a biopsy, It is safer to feed the endometrium into the side of the jaws as shown here rather than into the front of the jaws. A large, deep, and penetrating biopsy can result in the latter case. This instrument is made by the Pilling Company, USA. The inset shows the biopsy itself being deposited into a container of Bouin's fluid, which is 80% picric acid and 20% formalin. This is a so-called hard fixative suitable for genital and embryonic tissue because the histological architecture is not destroyed when large amounts of water in these tissues are extracted during processing. However, the use of Bouin's fluid is by no means mandatory because ordinary formalin also provides satisfactory results.

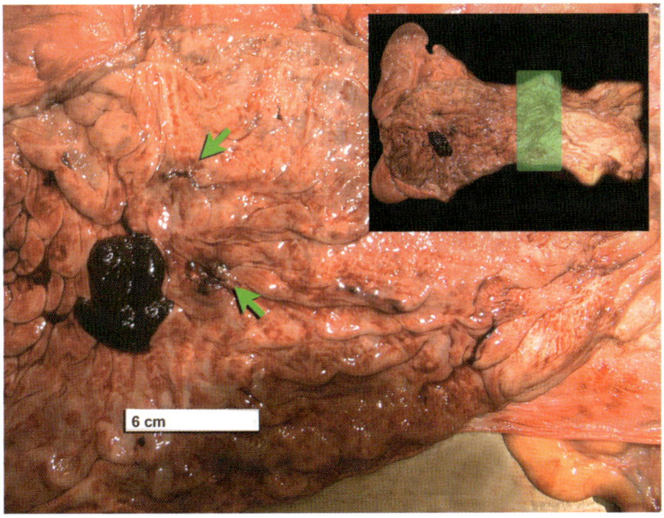

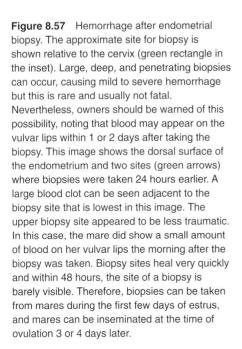

Figure 8.57 Hemorrhage after endometrial biopsy. The approximate site for biopsy is shown relative to the cervix (green rectangle in the inset). Large, deep, and penetrating biopsies can occur, causing mild to severe hemorrhage but this is rare and usually not fatal. Nevertheless, owners should be warned of this possibility, noting that blood may appear on the vulvar lips within 1 or 2 days after taking the biopsy. This image shows the dorsal surface of the endometrium and two sites (green arrows) where biopsies were taken 24 hours earlier. A large blood clot can be seen adjacent to the biopsy site that is lowest in this image. The upper biopsy site appeared to be less traumatic. In this case, the mare did show a small amount of blood on her vulvar lips the morning after the biopsy was taken. Biopsy sites heal very quickly and within 48 hours, the site of a biopsy is barely visible. Therefore, biopsies can be taken from mares during the first few days of estrus, and mares can be inseminated at the time of ovulation 3 or 4 days later.

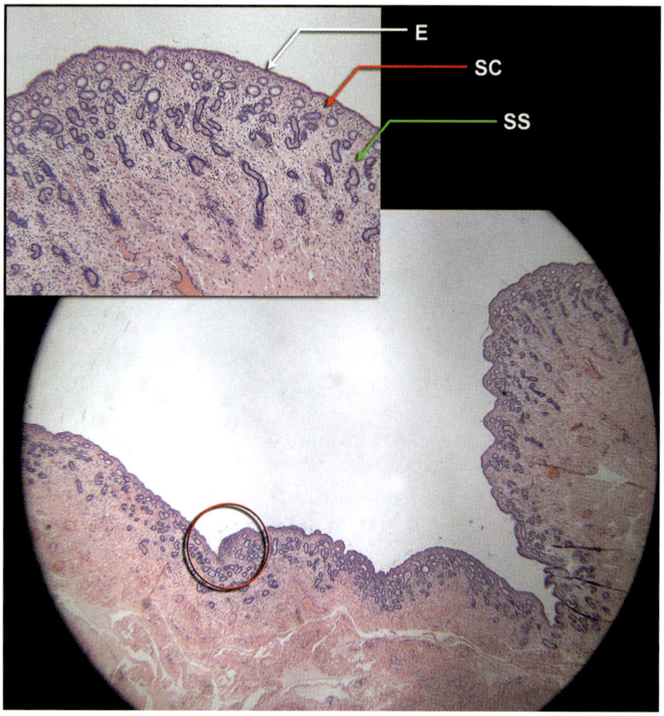

Figure 8.58 Examining an endometrial biopsy. This image shows the annotated anatomy of an endometrial biopsy. Endometrial biopsy is usually viewed at low power first. In this manner, a general impression of the biopsy is obtained and focal areas of cell infiltration, fibrosis, etc., can be appreciated. As an example, in the global view of a sample seen in the lower part of this composite, the focal area of cell infiltration under the red ring would have been missed if the biopsy had been examined immediately under high power. In the top rectangle, an area of endometrium is shown under higher power. E is the luminal epithelium; SC is the stratum compactum; and SS is the stratum spongiosum. Below those layers, toward the peritoneal surface, lie the inner circular and outer longitudinal layers of smooth muscle. In addition to cell infiltration, areas of periglandular fibrosis, evidence of estrous cycles, previous foaling, and stage of estrous cycle (estrous or diestrus) are also recorded.

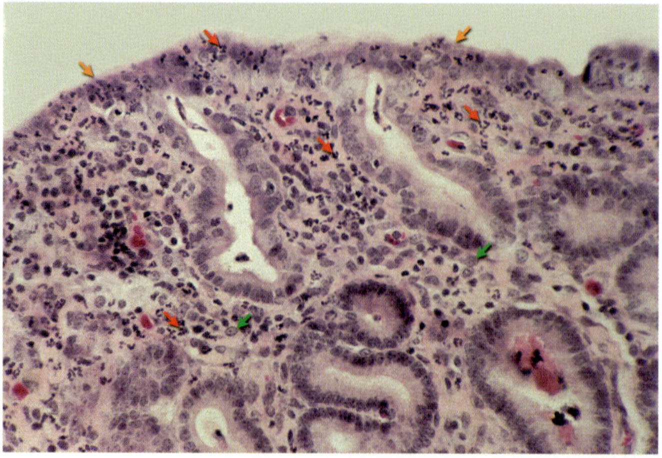

Figure 8.59 Severe suppurative endometritis. This is an image of severe suppurative endometritis. The red arrows show neutrophils, the predominant inflammatory cells in this histological section. The luminal epithelial cells indicated by the yellow arrows have been largely destroyed by the inflammatory process. The green arrows point to nuclei of normal connective tissue cells in the endometrium.

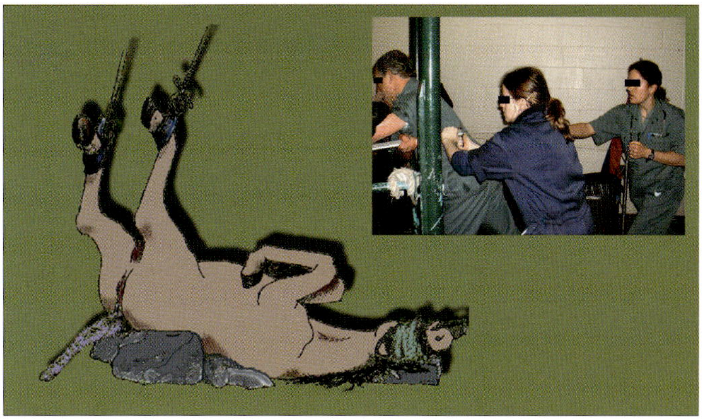

Figure 8.60 General comments. In most cases of the equine dystocia, the foal dies quickly or will be dead by the time the veterinarian arrives. This is because the equine placenta separates from the endometrium very rapidly during the birth process. The major image in this composite shows how a mare is hoisted up by her hind limbs after induction of general anesthesia. Although clenbuterol can be used as a tocolytic, general anesthesia provides excellent restraint as well as uterine relaxation. When the hind quarters are elevated, the foal also moves cranially providing space in the uterus for fetal mutation. In the event that mutation and traction are not successful within 10–15 minutes, the mare can be prepared for a cesarean section. Epidural anesthesia is slow and unpredictable in mares and therefore of limited value in cases of dystocia. However, it is used for fetotomy in standing restraint. Before fetotomy was performed in the mare at upper right, epidural anesthesia was used. When an epidural anesthetic fails in a mare, brief periods of relief from straining can be obtained by pulling out the tongue of the mare so that she is unable to close her glottis and strain.

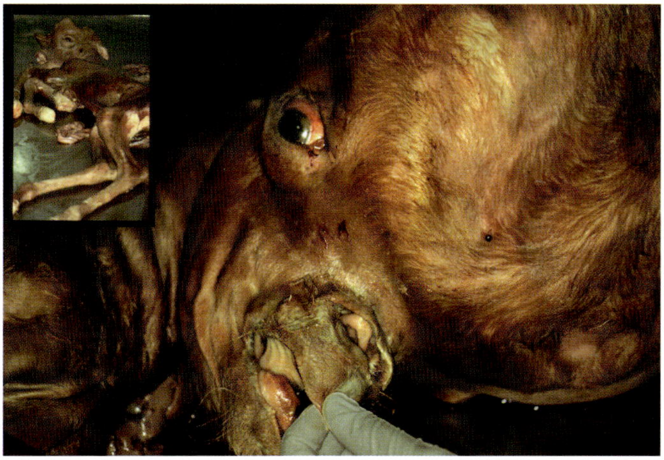

Figure 8.61 Hydrocephalus as a cause of dystocia. Hydrocephalus is not an unusual cause of dystocia due to fetal malformation. In such cases, it is likely that the bulbous shape of the head prevents normal distention of the cervix, resulting in dystocia. Occasionally, hydrocephalus can be reduced by puncturing the cranium within the uterus (see inset) thereby allowing delivery of the foal. In other cases, cesarean section is necessary.

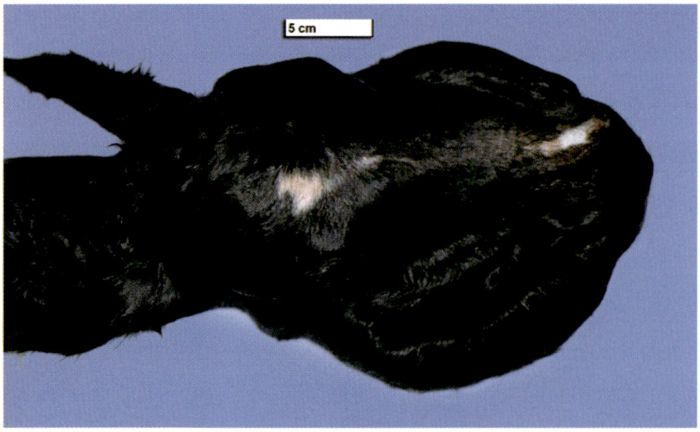

Figure 8.62 A salivary cyst as a cause of dystocia. This was a very unusual case of dystocia caused by a massive submandibular salivary cyst. Puncture and drainage of the cyst allowed delivery of the foal.

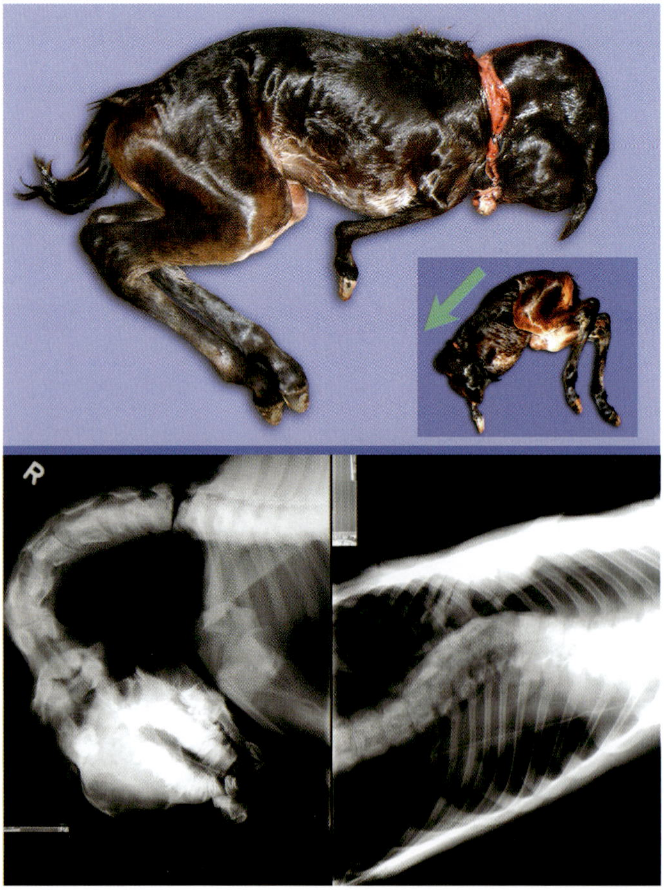

Figure 8.63 Severe skeletal malformation as a cause of dystocia. A pluriparous mare was referred for dystocia of several hours duration. An epidural was given and clenbuterol were administered IV. The foal was in anterior longitudinal presentation and dorso left-ilial position. There was an obvious wryneck. Wryneck is permanent ossification of the neck in a flexed posture—unique to the horse among domestic animals. The head was also deformed. Initially, one gained the impression that there was also bilateral shoulder flexion with both forelimbs retained. Using a fetotome, the head was removed uneventfully; but when an attempt was made to locate the forelimbs, they appeared to be absent. Because of the absence of the forelimbs, uterine tone and an inability to rotate the foal into a dorsosacral position, the foal was delivered by cesarean section. Her recovery was uneventful. Radiology showed that both the left and right scapulae were present but only the right forelimb was present. Also, the right forelimb was vestigial, about the thickness of a thumb, and it was also rotated on its longitudinal axis so that the hoof faced backward. There was severe scoliosis and the head of the left femur did not articulate with the acetabulum.

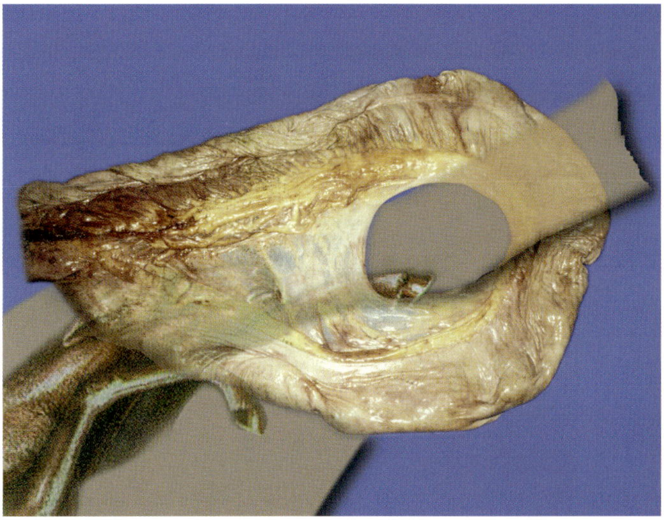

Figure 8.64 A mesenteric tear as a cause of dystocia. An extremely unusual case of dystocia in a Belgium draft mare. This mare was referred several hours after starting to foal. Attempts by the local veterinarians to deliver the foal were unsuccessful. On initial transrectal examination to ascertain the presence of uterine torsion, the foal was not palpable at all. However, the foal was clearly palpable during per vaginal examination. This led to some uncertainty and speculation about the cause of dystocia and the owners elected to euthanize the mare. On postmortem examination, a large rent was found in the mesentery. Evidently, this rent had healed completely some time before the mare had become pregnant. During early pregnancy, the uterus had passed through this hole in the mesentery. The foal had developed to term, within the uterus, on the other side of the mesentery. This explained why the foal could not be palpated per rectum yet was easily palpable per vagina. Essentially the hand of the operator passed down the vagina, through the hole in the mesentery, and into the uterus. Yet, the large bowel that lay over the uterus, disguised its presence and the presence of the fetus. The illustration provides a picture of the situation at the time of presentation. Here, the foal lies within the uterus and is unable to be born because it cannot pass through the cervix, constrained by the hole in the mesentery.

Fetal Sexing

Early and Late Gestation Fetal Sexing

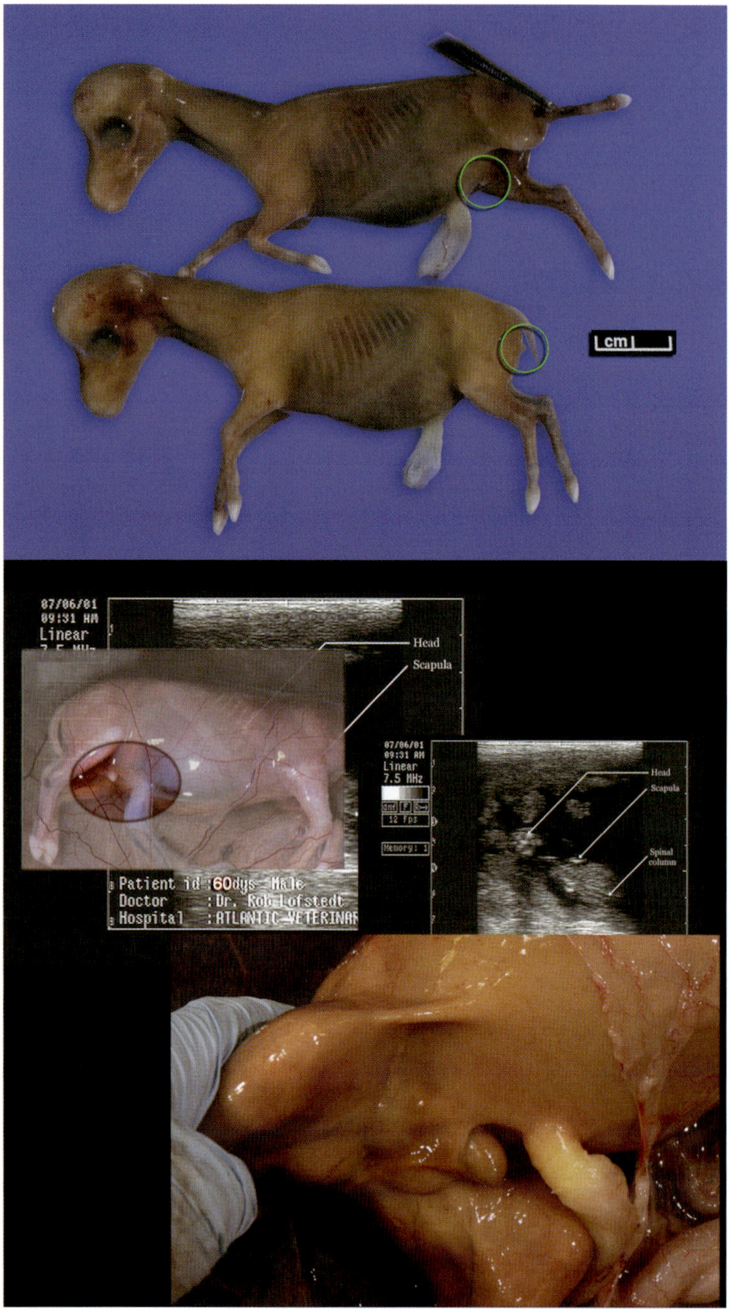

Figure 8.65a General comments. Equine fetal sex determination is possible early in gestation by transrectal ultrasonography. Between about 55 and 65 days of gestation, gender is based on the identification and location of the genital tubercle. In males, it is proximal to the umbilical cord and in females, it is just ventral to the tail. The genital tubercle in these 60-day-old twin fetuses, one male and one female, are indicated by green rings in the upper image. The genital tubercle in another male fetus about the same age is shown in the central image, together with its ultrasonographic image taken in utero. The optimal time for sexing embryos transabdominally is between 120 and 210 days for both sexes. In the 150-day-old male fetus at the bottom of this illustration, the scrotum and penis can be seen easily on ultrasonography, no longer a single genital tubercle. In females of the same age, the mammary gland with it two teats is used to identify its gender. This is shown elsewhere (fig. 8.65b).

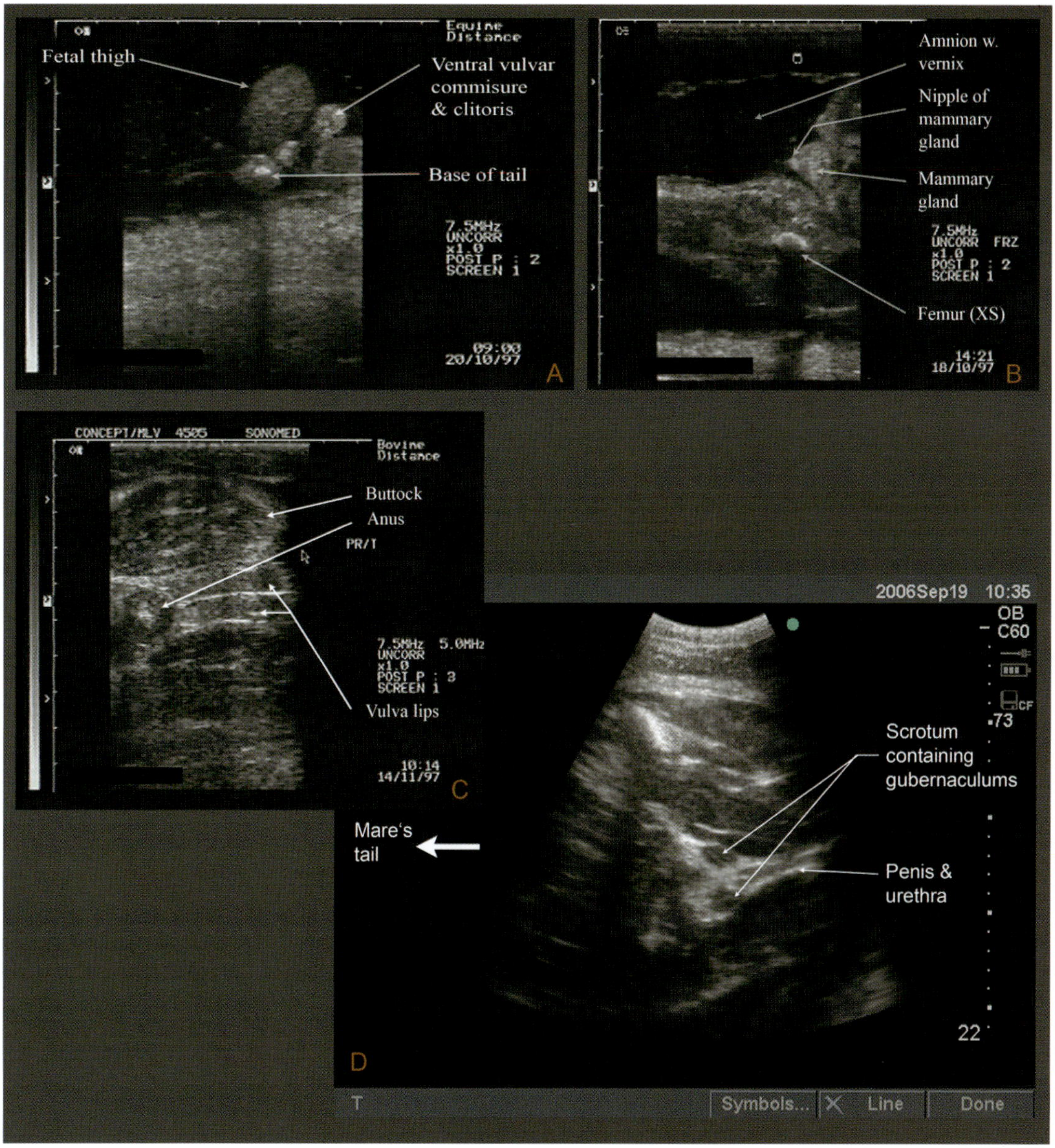

Figure 8.65b Fetal gender diagnosed during advanced gestation. (A) A transrectal scan at 123 days of pregnancy. The left side of the image is caudal in this mare. This is a female fetus in transverse/oblique presentation and dorsopubic position. The base of the tail is clearly visible with faint cross sections of some of the coccygeal vertebrae seen to the left of the tail base. Between the thighs is the anus and below that, the vulva and clitoris. (B) A transrectal scan at 133 days of a female fetus. The left side of the image faces the caudal aspect of the mare. The fetus is still in posterior presentation showing one-half of the mammary gland and its nipple. By 8 months of age, very few fetuses are in posterior presentation. This fetus has one extended hind limb with its femur showing in cross section. Vernix is clearly visible in the amnion but not the allantois. (C) A transrectal scan at 219 days of a female fetus in transverse presentation. The left side of the image faces the caudal aspect of the mare. The image shows the buttocks of the fetus, and between the buttocks, the anus and the vulvar lips. (D) A transabdominal scan of a male fetus in posterior presentation at 7 months of gestation. The left side of the image faces the caudal aspect of the mare. The thighs of the fetus, its scrotum, penis, and urethra are clearly visible. The scrotum does not yet contain the testicles but the gubernaculum is large and occupies most of the scrotum at this stage of gestation. Each anechogenic area within each side of the scrotum, also called the scrotal lodges, is a gubernaculum. (Images courtesy of Dr. Stefania Bucca, Hodgestown, Co Kildare, Ireland)

Accidents During Advanced Gestation

Premature Placental Separation and Prolapse of the Bladder

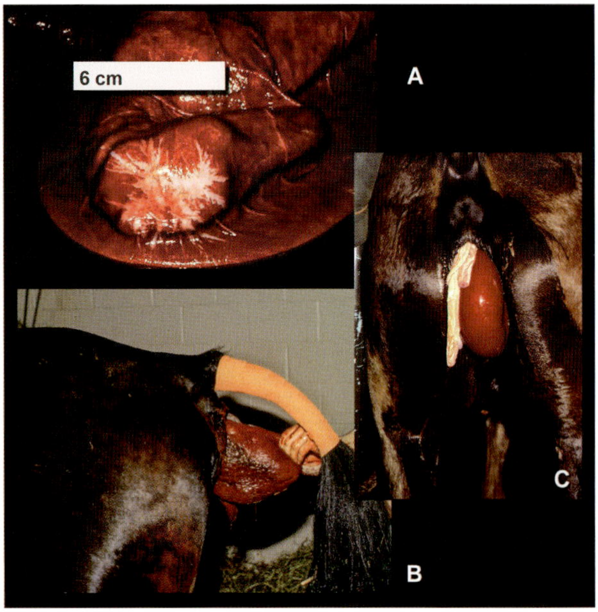

Figure 8.66 The chorioallantois is the bright red membrane seen at upper left (image A), covering the fetal placental head, revealing the cervical star. If this membrane appears at the vulvar lips during second stage labor (as seen in image B) the placenta is detaching prematurely. This is an obstetrical emergency. In such cases, the chorioallantois must be transected immediately and the foal delivered by forced traction. Additional effort may be required in neonatal resuscitation. Normally, the chorioallantois should rupture and remain adherent to the endometrium. The amnion, which is grayish and translucent, should appear at the vulvar lips. One should not confuse a prolapsed bladder with the chorioallantois. In the case pictured on the right side of this composite (image C), a Shire mare prolapsed her bladder before foaling. Clenbuterol was used to suppress foaling and epidural anesthesia was used to facilitate replacement of the bladder. Then, using conventional methods, a live foal was delivered. (Image at lower left is courtesy of Dr. Carole C. Miller, Athens Technical College, Athens, GA, and Dr. G. F. Richardson, AVC, UPEI.)

Estimating the Time of Impending Foaling

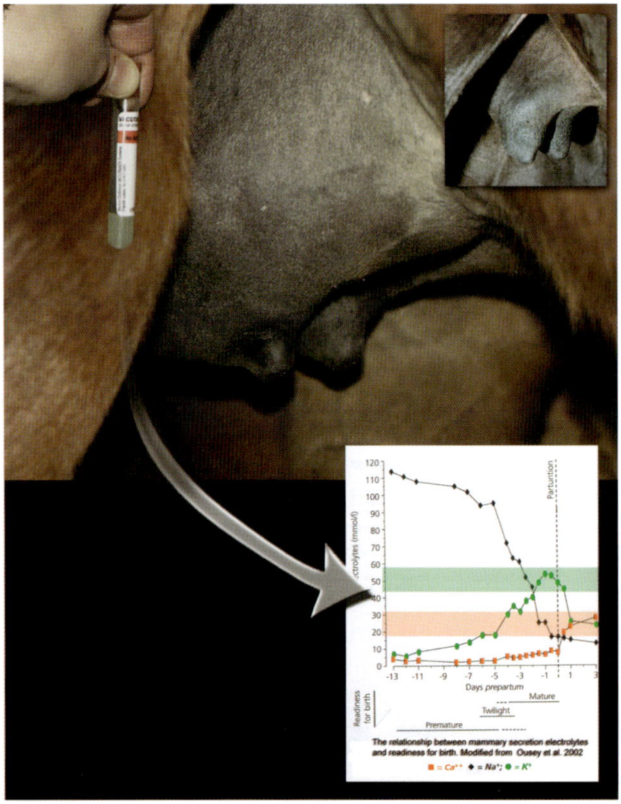

Figure 8.67 Estimating the time of foaling can be difficult. This is important during routine monitoring of foaling but absolutely critical when considering the induction of foaling. The first evidence that foaling is imminent is a sudden and remarkable increase in filling of the mammary gland. In this illustration, for example, there is a remarkable difference between the mammary gland in the inset, approximately 1 week before foaling, and the mammary gland in the main image, just 1 day prior to foaling. Changes in milk electrolytes must be measured as soon as the milk starts to become opaque because of an increase in content of kappa casein. Changes in milk electrolytes (calcium, sodium, and potassium) have also been well described; as shown in the graph, the combined results of milk electrolyte assays can be used to obtain a score for impending foaling. A table exists to simplify this process of "scoring" milk electrolytes. When a certain score is obtained, foaling is imminent and, when required, induction is usually safe.

Prematurity

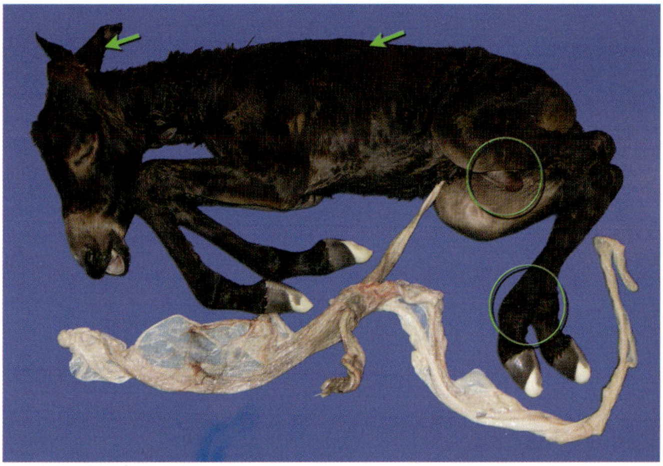

Figure 8.68 Jennys, or "jennets," have gestations that are somewhat longer than gestation in mares (perhaps a month longer on average) although the length of gestation is quite variable in both species. A monograph from the department of agriculture in Alberta (http://www1.agric.gov.ab.ca/$department/deptdocs.nsf/all/agdex598) suggests that gestation may even be as long as 14 months in donkeys. This donkey was born in a slightly immature state irrespective of its actual gestational age. If the gestational age can be shown to be significantly shorter than the mean for the species, the condition is correctly referred to as "prematurity." However, if the gestation length is consistent for that species yet the neonate still appears to be immature, the correct term for the condition is "dysmaturity." Signs of immaturity in this foal are indicated by arrows or circles and include its soft, floppy ears, a downy hair coat, and its flaccid joints in the distal extremities, allowing hyperextension at the fetlock joints. The testicles were still within the inguinal canal, the scrotum being filled predominantly by the gubernaculum. These statements are equally valid for both horses and donkeys.

Uterine Torsion

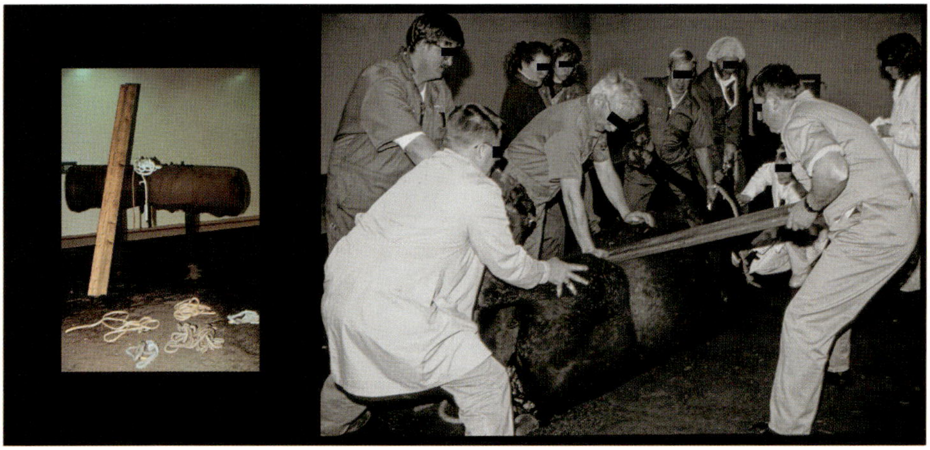

Figure 8.69 Uterine torsion is a problem that generally occurs in the last half of gestation in mares. It is essential to be aware of this because once uterine torsion has been relieved in a mare, no consideration is given to delivering the foal. It would usually be far too immature to survive. Uterine torsion should be suspected in any mare that is pregnant, in advanced gestation, and presented with colic. Torsion is usually easy to diagnose because the mesometrial ligament is pulled tightly to one side and the torsion is clearly palpable per rectum. The basic principle for nonsurgical correction of uterine torsion in mares is to introduce general anesthesia and to "roll the dam around her uterus" leaving her uterus behind. Essentially, therefore, one twists the animal around its own uterus. A plank such as that shown in both images can be used to stabilize the uterus while the mare is rotated on her longitudinal axis. When this method fails, one can resort to a laparotomy and surgical correction of the torsion. Occasionally, the foal dies as a result of blood vascular embarrassment and is aborted soon after the torsion is corrected. (Image courtesy of Dr. G. F. Richardson, AVC, UPEI)

Ventral Edema in Late Gestation

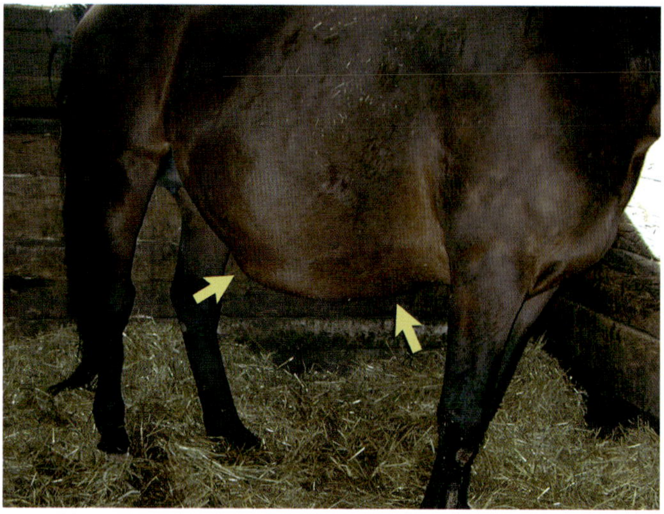

Figure 8.70 The plaque of ventral edema shown here (arrows) is typical of late gestation in mares. It is usually insignificant and pits on pressure but is not painful and the mare shows no discomfort at all. This makes this condition very different from impending rupture of the ventral abdominal structures, a condition illustrated in fig. 8.71.

Ventral Abdominal Rupture

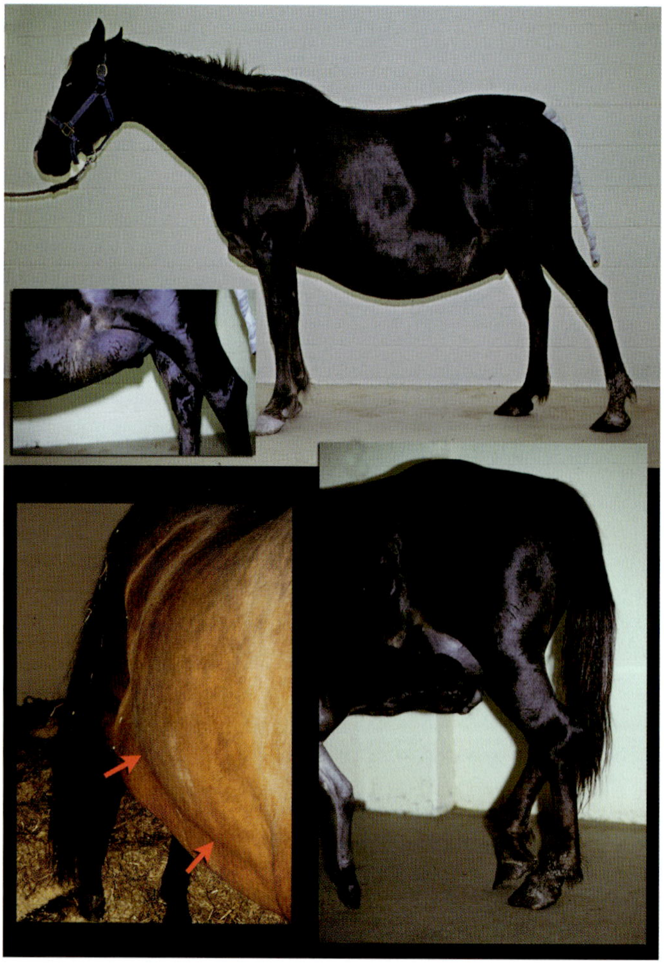

Figure 8.71 Impending rupture of ventral abdominal structures during late gestation. The massive ventral plaque of edema, usually more obvious than ventral edema of late gestation, and the painful gait of the mare are indicators of this condition. As shown in the inset of the dark mare, ventral edema can be so severe that the architecture of the mammary gland is largely obscured. It is also illustrated at lower left where the margin between the plaque of edema and the ventral abdomen is indicated by red arrows. The abdomen should be supported until foaling can be induced safely. After that, the ventral edema will usually subside enough to allow suckling (see lower right). Rupture may involve the prepubic tendon, rectus abdominus muscle, transverse abdominal muscles, or oblique abdominal muscles. It is seldom possible to tell which structure(s) is affected without a postmortem examination. It is not recommended to rebreed these mares as the condition will probably reoccur.

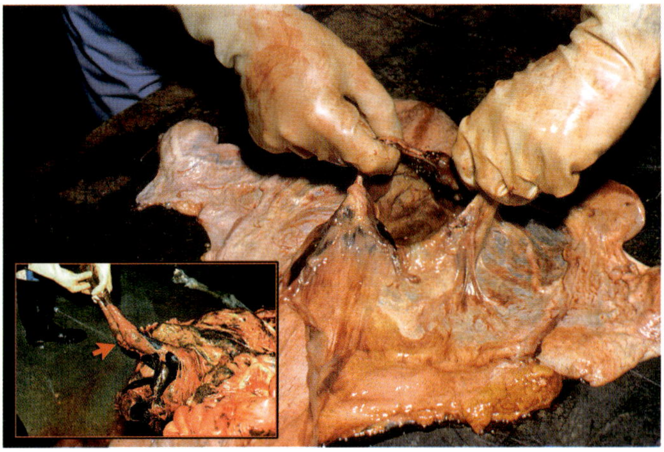

Figure 8.72 Uterine rupture occurred in this mare presumably as a result of uterine torsion. The mare was kept in a pasture so the symptoms of that condition would not have been noticed. Because of abdominal enlargement, however, the owner submitted this mare for a pregnancy diagnosis. A transrectal examination was performed and it was determined that a normal, nonpregnant uterus was present. The mare was in estrus at that time and was artificially inseminated. Within 48 hours, she had died from per acute peritonitis due to semen having escaped from the uterus into the peritoneal cavity. At postmortem, a dead fetus, close to maturity, was pulled from the abdomen of the mare (inset). As shown in the main image, a rupture site was discovered in the ventral portion of the uterus. It was from this hole that the foal had escaped into the peritoneal cavity. Amazingly, the rupture site had healed remarkably well, leaving only a small hole in the wall of the uterus. (Image courtesy of the Department of Theriogenology, Iowa State University, Ames)

Hydrops Allantois

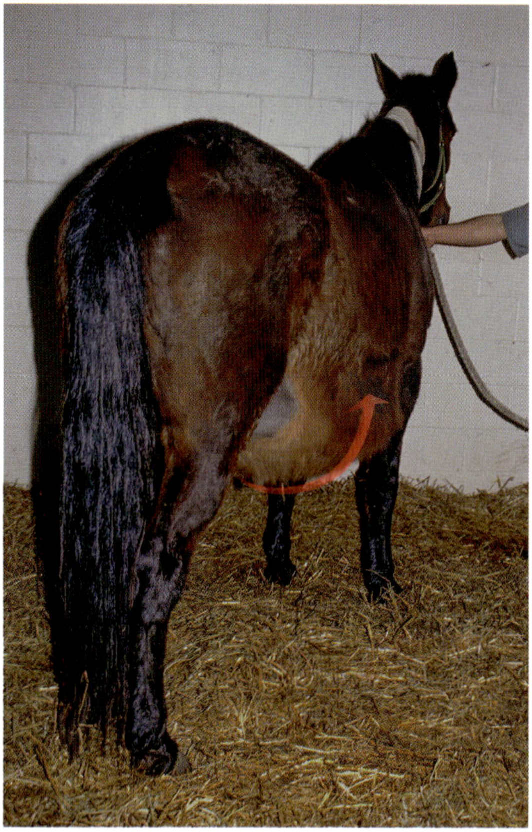

Figure 8.73 A 17-year-old Standardbred mare presented for signs of abdominal discomfort, anorexia, and a possible ventral abdominal rupture. This mare was due to foal approximately 2 weeks after the time of presentation. The referring veterinarian reported rapid abdominal enlargement over the 2-week period before presentation. The uterus was distended with fluid but a live fetus could be detected by ballottement per rectum. In a single day after admission, this mare gained 10 kg in weight, strongly suggesting some form of hydrops. The enlargement is indicated by a red arrow. This led to impending rupture of the ventral abdominal structures. In this case, however, the cause of the rupture was known. Because of serious discomfort, foaling was induced using oxytocin. Due to hypertrophy of the chorioallantois, it was transected and a small, live filly foal was delivered in posterior presentation. It was estimated that approximately 100 L of fluid had been released when the placenta was transected. The mare weighed 710 kg on admission and 570 kg immediately after foaling. The placental weight was 15 kg, approximately double its normal weight, and her foal weighed 30 kg. Therefore, the fluid content of the placenta was 90 kg or 90 L. The normal amount of allantoic fluid normally varies from 8 to 15 L and the amnionic fluid somewhat less. Shortly after foaling, the mare went into severe hypovolemic shock requiring aggressive fluid therapy. Due to continuing pain and severe damage of ventral abdominal structures that would preclude breeding, the mare was euthanized. Both hydrops allantois and hydrops amnion are rare in mares and little is known about either condition.

Normal Contusion of the Vagina

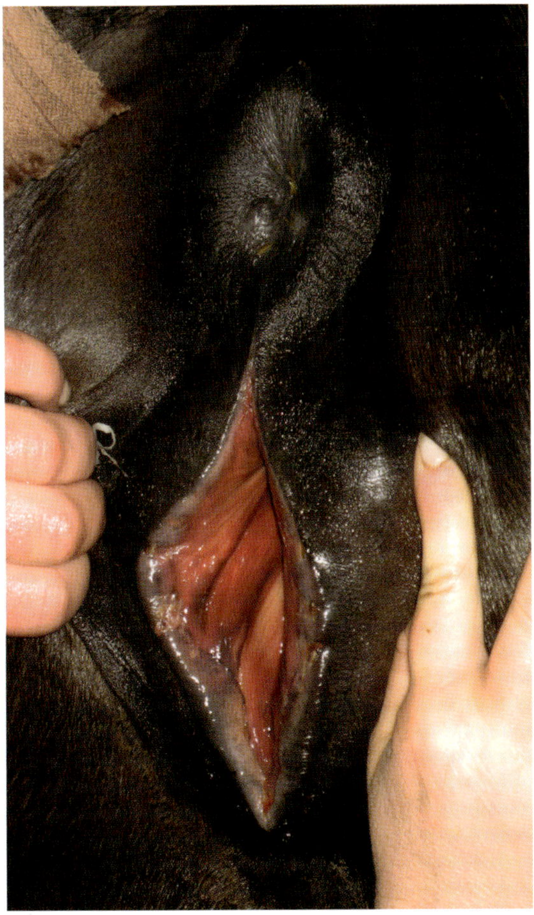

Figure 8.74 During normal foaling, there is always a degree of contusion of the vagina. This illustration shows contusion in the vestibule that is consistent with normal foaling. Optimally, one should perform a gloved-hand examination of the vagina after every foaling, in the event that serious vaginal damage has occurred.

Severe Vaginal Contusions and Pelvic Subluxation

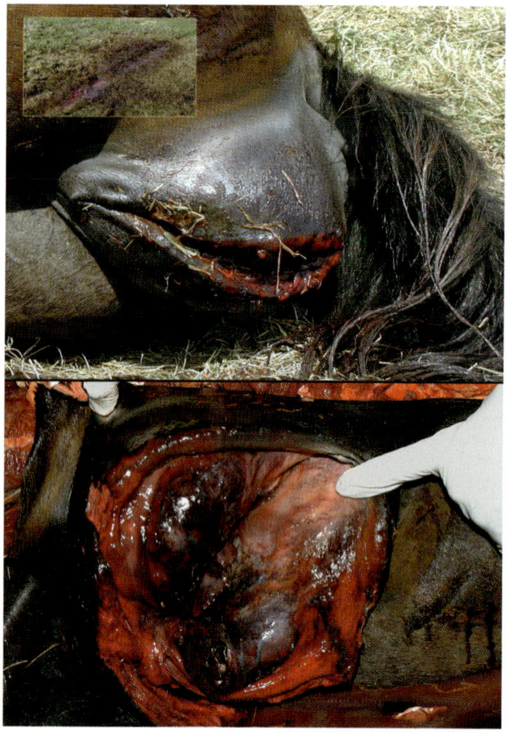

Figure 8.75 A 9-year-old Standardbred mare that had an assisted foaling. The mare appeared to be partially paralyzed in her hind quarters and was unable to rise. Hemorrhage from the vulvar lips was obvious, soaking the adjacent pasture (see inset). The owner elected to euthanize the mare. The lower image shows some of the postmortem findings: extensive muscular and fibrous tissue necrosis within the vaginal wall. There was also subluxation of the right sacroiliac joint. Severe coalescing vaginal and vulvar hematomas were also present.

Rectal Prolapse

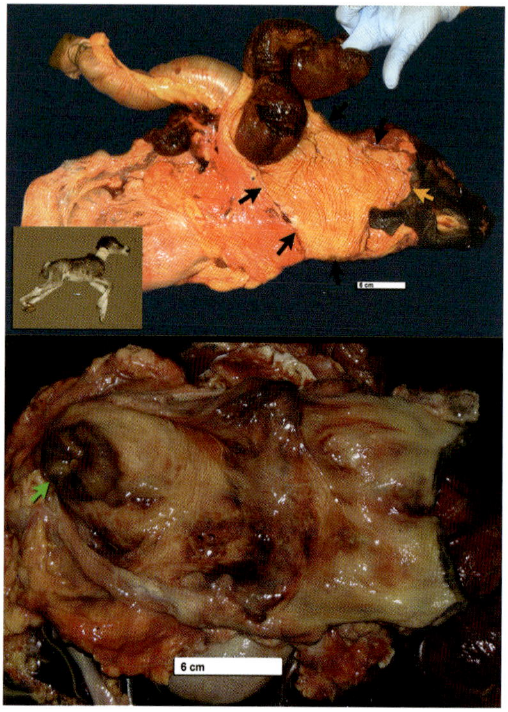

Figure 8.76 This pony mare foaled 48 hours earlier, producing a foal with arthrogryposis (inset) that lived for a short time after birth. Two hours after parturition, her rectum prolapsed and was reinserted by the attending veterinarian; a circumferential retention suture was placed in the anus. Forty-eight hours later, the mare began to show signs of shock and severe pain. She was euthanized. This image shows how the terminal part of the rectum intussuscepted causing circumferential strangulation and necrosis of the rectal wall. One presumes that this was a sequel to a painful birth (note the fetal hind limbs in the inset image), although the uterus and vagina, pictured in the lower image, showed no obvious signs of trauma.

Uterine Hemorrhage

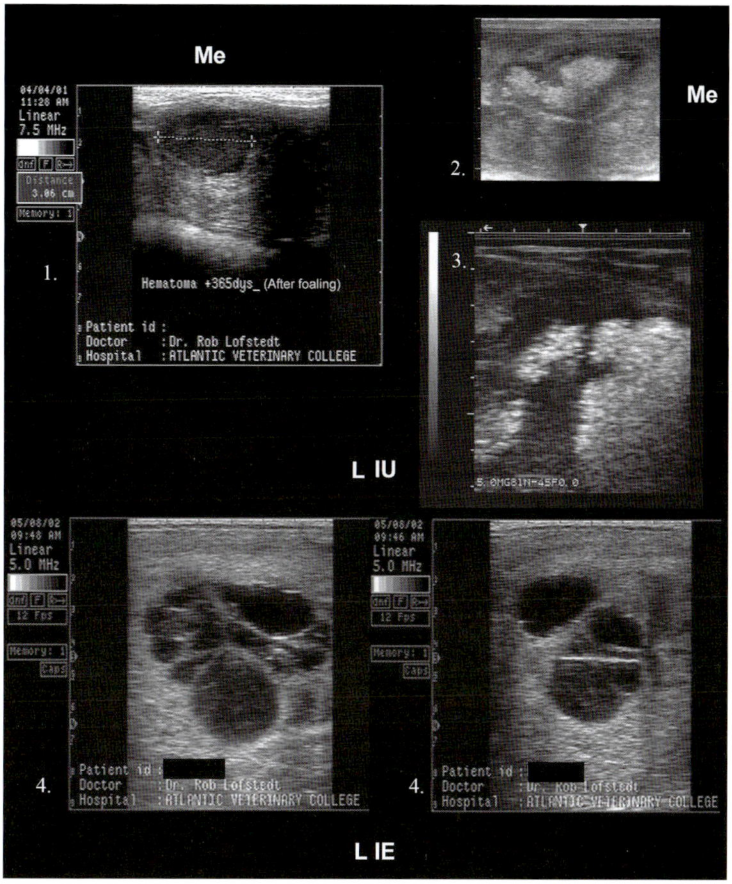

Figure 8.77 Ultrasonographic appearance of uterine hemorrhage. (1) A hematoma seen in the mesometrium at the time of foal heat breeding. This mare, like the majority of mares with postfoaling mesometrial hematomas, showed no symptoms at the time of foaling. The structure was clearly palpable per rectum. (2) A similar hematoma to that described above but more consolidated and echogenic. (3) Intraluminal hemorrhage in a mature mare was presented because of a foul-smelling vaginal discharge at 35 days postfoaling. The mare was systemically normal, but ultrasonography and a gloved-hand examination of the uterine contents revealed masses of clotted blood, shown here on ultrasound. This was presumed to be due to a severe partial thickness endometrial tear parturition. Uterine debris was removed carefully and the uterus was flushed with saline. Antibiotics and tetanus toxoid were administered. (4) Two images of an unusual intrauterine endometrial hemorrhage contained within a multilocular structure. Although this appears to be a multilocular endometrial cyst, its contents were not consistent with the nonechogenic fluid usually seen within cysts. However, this mare was known to have endometrial cysts before she conceived. Therefore, it is possible that this was a group of cysts that was traumatized during foaling, causing hemorrhage within the cysts.

Intra-abdominal Hemorrhage

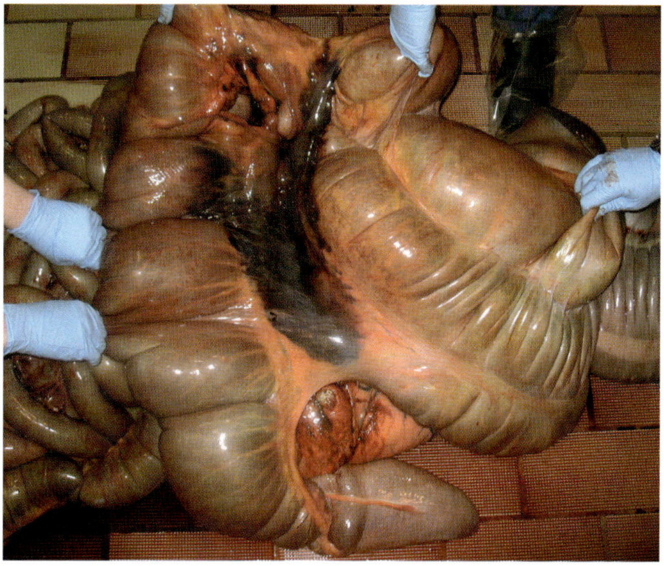

Figure 8.78 A mature Standardbred mare that died suddenly immediately after foaling. Her mucous membranes were extremely pale upon presentation, and postmortem examination revealed that she had suffered from an extensive intra-abdominal hemorrhage. This hemorrhage originated from one of the major vessels in the splenocolic ligament seen here. This accident was presumed to have been the result of verminous arteritis, rupturing as a result of hypertension during foaling.

Rectal, Vaginal, and Perineal Tears and Lacerations

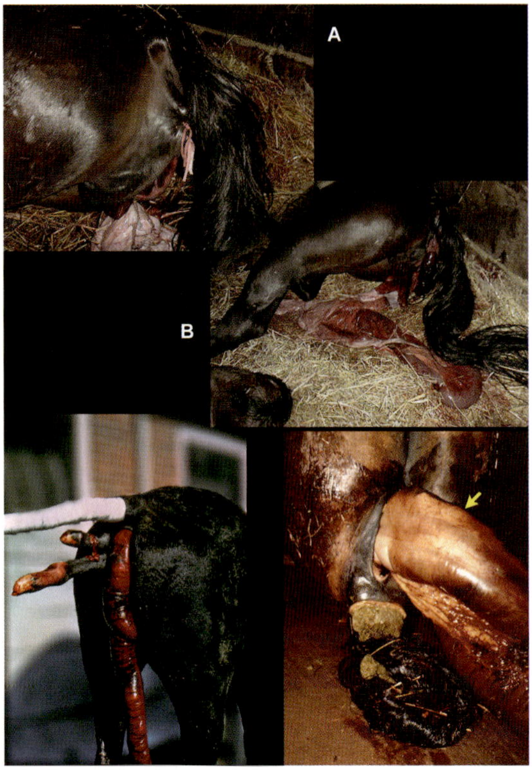

Figure 8.79 Injuries followed by evisceration. Foaling accidents are far more common in maiden mares than older mares. The two images at the top show a 6-year-old mare after her first foaling. Despite video surveillance, foaling occurred rapidly and was unattended. It was immediately followed by this evisceration. A temporary purse string suture was placed around the anus (A) by the attending veterinarian but when this was opened (B) intestines burst out of the anus. Both intestines and placenta are visible in the second image. It is believed that the rectum may have ruptured due to high abdominal pressure during foaling. It was unlikely that this was due to injury from the foal because the vagina was not damaged. Vaginal tears with fatal eviscerations are not rare but this case was remarkable because the evisceration occurred through a rectal tear, not a vaginal tear. As in most cases with eviscerations that occur during foaling, this mare was euthanized. The images at lower left and right show a more typical situation where the foal's feet have penetrated the cranial vagina, a part of the vagina that lies within the peritoneal cavity, allowing intestines to escape through the vagina. (Image at lower left is courtesy of the Department of Theriogenology, Iowa State University, Ames.)

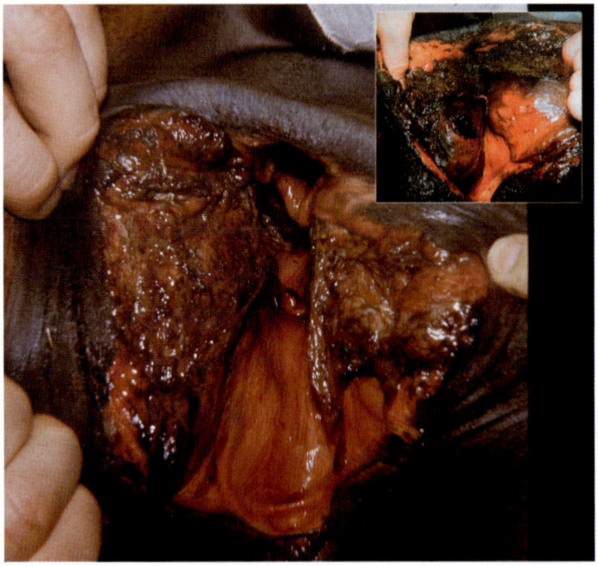

Figure 8.80 Third-degree perineal lacerations. Third-degree lacerations of the perineal body involve the rectal mucosa, vaginal mucosa, and the interposing muscle and connective tissue. They may take the form of fistulas or, more commonly, complete destruction of the perineal body as seen here. Usually there is little hemorrhage because of the blunt nature of the trauma. These injuries, which are most common in mares having their first foals, are seldom, if ever fatal. Immediately after the injury has occurred tetanus prophylaxis is recommended, however, the value of antibiotic treatment is debatable. One should resist the temptation to repair these injuries surgically until third intention healing has occurred. In practice, repair is usually attempted after weaning the foal because wound healing is complete and the dietary restrictions imposed on the mare, to decrease fecal production, do not retard the growth of the foal. Because of excellent uterine defense mechanisms in young mares, delaying surgical repair does not appear to have a detrimental effect on the future reproductive capacity of mares. (Images courtesy of the Department of Theriogenology, Iowa State University, Ames)

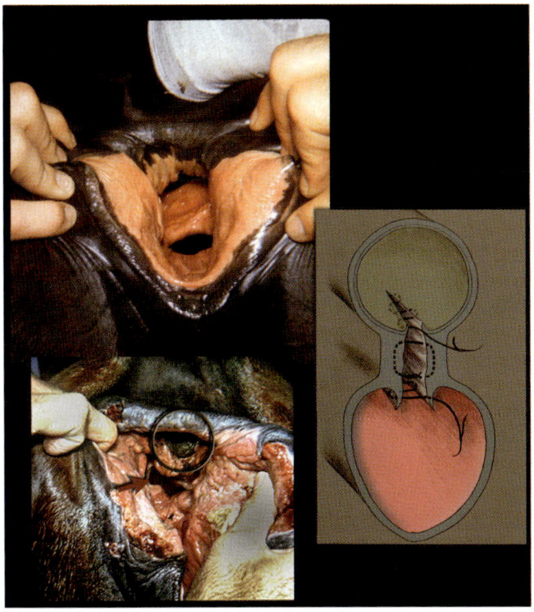

Figure 8.81 Surgical repair of third-degree perineal lacerations. As mentioned before (fig. 8.80), one should resist the temptation to repair these injuries surgically until third intention healing has occurred. This is because the wound margins are well defined and healthy by the time healing has occurred. The image at upper left shows how the perineum has been prepared for surgery. Although presurgical starvation is important to diminish the quantity of feces in the rectum, there is inevitably fecal material in the rectum, ringed in the lower image, at the time of surgery. This is prevented from entering the surgical field by placing a large cotton tampon in the rectum during surgery. There are several methods of repairing third-degree perineal lacerations, one of which is on the right side of this composite. (Images courtesy of the Department of Theriogenology, Iowa State University, Ames)

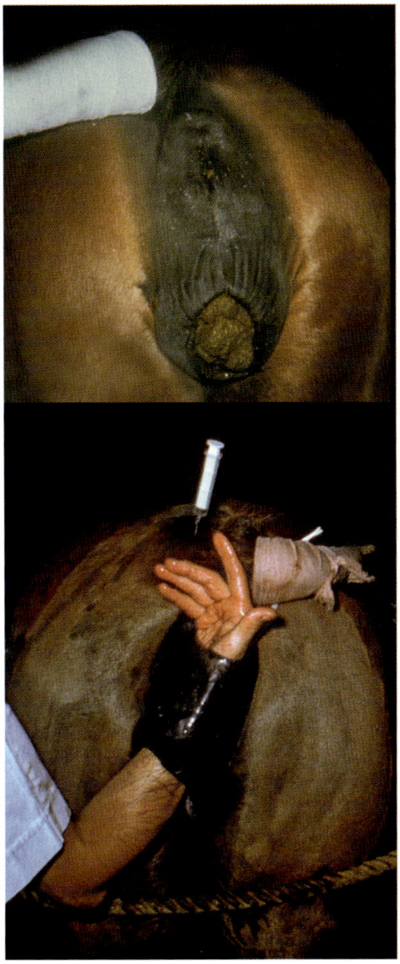

Figure 8.82 Rectovaginal fistula. Third degree lacerations of the perineal body involve the rectal mucosa, vaginal mucosa, and interposing connective tissue. Complete destruction of the perineal body is more common than perineal fistulas as seen here. In the top image, note that this mare is defecating through her vulvar lips. Third degree lacerations and perineal fistulas appear to be most common when foals are born in the foot-nape posture, but they may also occur when the foal's posture is normal. In cases of fistulas, the foal's forelimbs are thought to penetrate the dorsal vaginal mucosa and enter the rectum. After this, the foal probably slips back into the vagina and is born normally. In rare cases, foals may even be born through the anus. The surgical repair of fistulas is similar to that used for complete perineal destruction. (Images are courtesy of the Department of Theriogenology, Iowa State University, Ames)

Embryonic Death and Abortion

Early and Later Embryonic Death

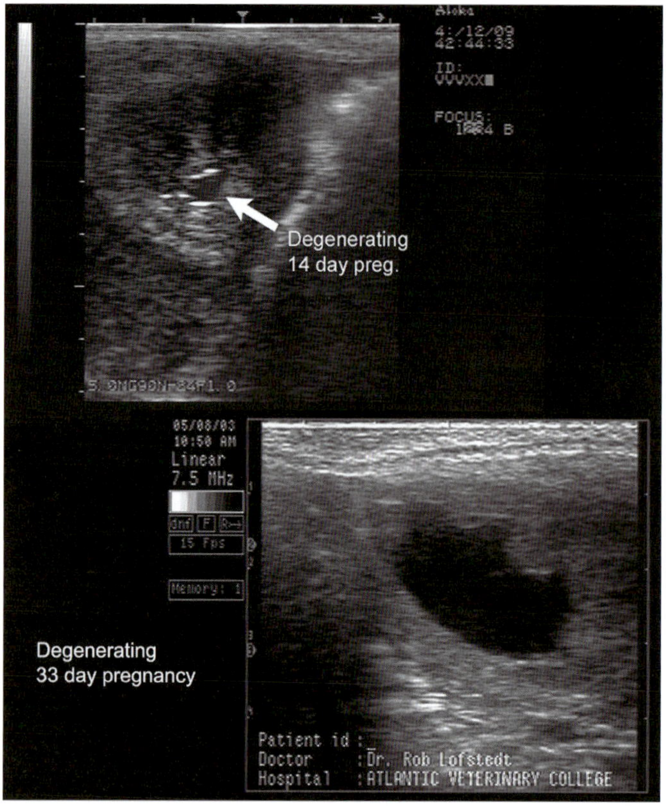

Figure 8.83 General characteristics of embryonic death. Early embryonic death is common in all animals. Some of this may be due to a hostile uterine environment but, undoubtedly, abnormal embryos, especially those with abnormal karyotypes, contribute largely to this phenomenon. The majority of embryos are lost even before they are detectable by ultrasonography. In this composite, the top image shows the hyperechogenic remnants of a degenerating 14-day-old embryo. The lower image shows a complete absence of the embryo, amnion, and allantois, which are normally typical features of this stage of pregnancy. The fetoplacental unit is also collapsing, a sign of impending death.

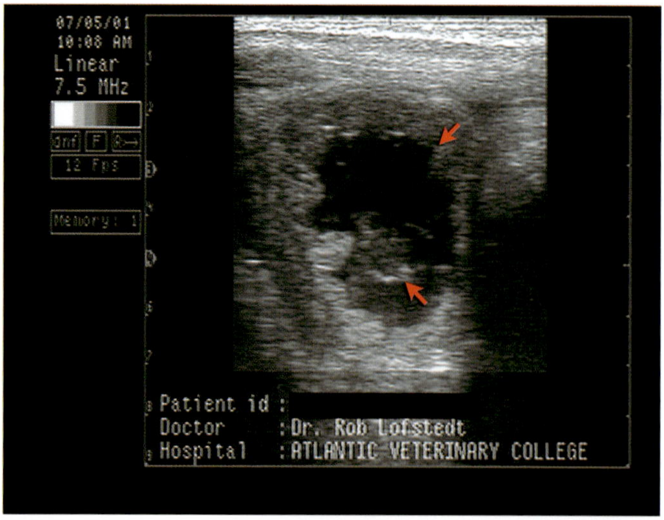

Figure 8.84 Embryonic death at about 55 days of gestation. This ultrasonographic image shows the fragmentation of fetal membranes and the collapse of a fetoplacental unit that typifies fetal death. The lower arrow shows the degenerating embryo and fetal membranes, the other shows the loss of tone in the placental unit. This is due to the collapse of the sodium pump within the fetal membranes with a consequent inability to retain water in the trophoblast. This was a 55-day pregnancy but on palpation resembled a 35–38-day pregnancy. Uterine tone was still present. Loss of pregnancy at this stage, 55 days onward, usually suggests endometrial incompetence as a result of endometrial fibrosis. This is because the yolk sac has been depleted by 55–60 days and the fetus becomes completely reliant on the endometrium for its sustenance. Abortion ensues. Endometrial biopsy is usually recommended before rebreeding is attempted.

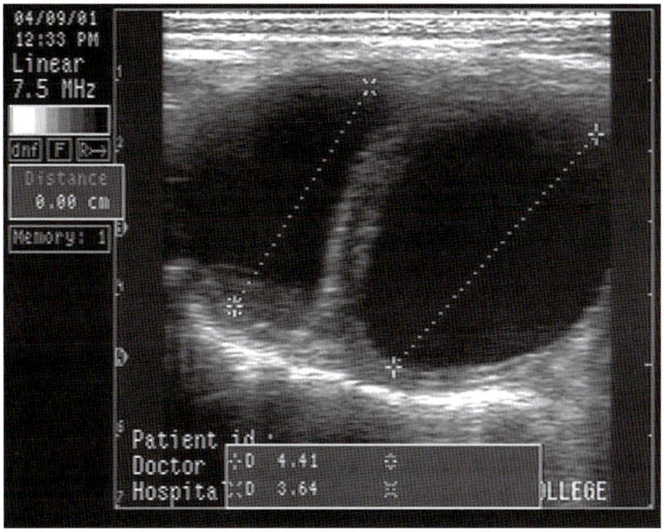

Figure 8.85 When there are two preovulatory follicles: twin preovulatory follicles seen on ultrasound. In the past it was recommended that mares should not be bred when twin follicles were present in the ovaries. This was based on the fact that twins are a common cause of abortion in mares. However, this would be considered poor management with the advent of ultrasound and our present philosophy on the management of twins. Indeed, if mares were not bred every time twin follicles were detected, perhaps 15%–20% of all breeding opportunities would be lost in most performance mares. This would be especially the case with the approach of the summer solstice when the twinning rate in mares is at its highest. Consequently, we always breed mares when twin follicles are present.

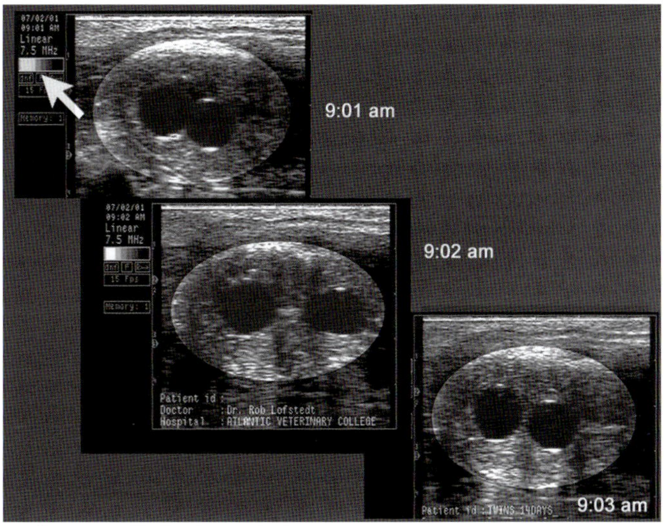

Figure 8.86 Tracking embryos during early pregnancy diagnosis. These ultrasonographic images show how quickly an embryo can migrate within the uterus before the time of fixation, which is about 16 days after ovulation. Because of myometrial contractions, embryos move together and apart and throughout the uterus during early gestation. This is thought to be important in the recognition of pregnancy. In practical terms, it is very important for the veterinarian to examine every part of the uterine horns and body before excluding the possibility of twins. Sometimes one of the twins may be present in a uterine horn while its cotwin is found in the uterine body, just cranial to the cervix. It is quite easy to miss a cotwin in the uterine body unless care is taken to ensure that the uterine epithelium is visible as a thin echogenic line on the entire length of the uterine body. An illustration of this echogenic line can be seen in image A in fig. 8.30 under the heading "Routine Monitoring of Early Pregnancy."

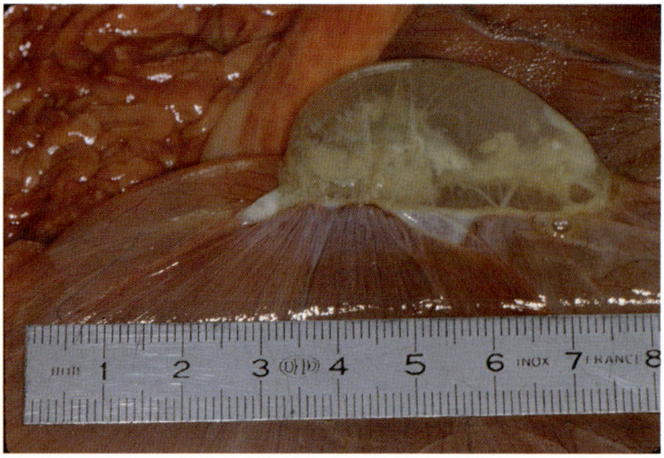

Figure 8.87 The fate of crushed cotwin embryos. A degenerating embryo seen on the chorion of its cotwin 21 days after it had been crushed by transrectal palpation. In general, little attention is paid to the cotwin that is crushed because the embryo and its fluids disappear almost instantly on ultrasonographic examination after a crush has been performed. This slide demonstrates that a crushed embryo may persist for some time alongside its normal cotwin.

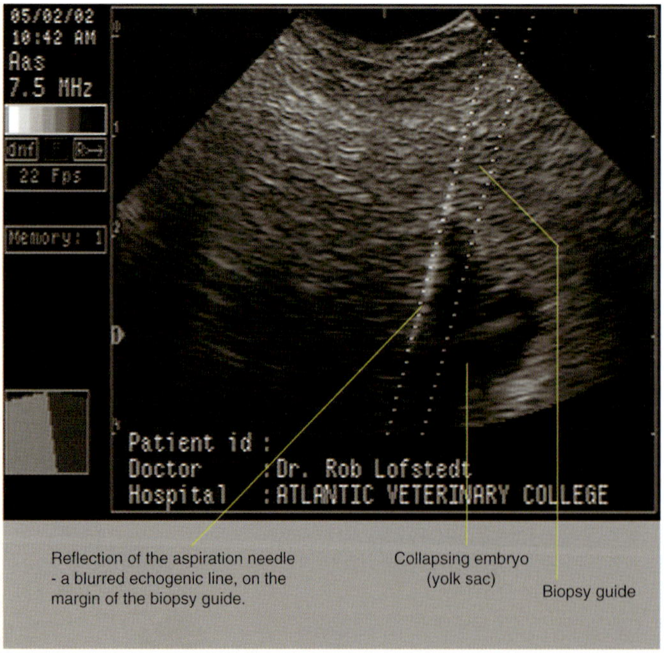

Figure 8.88 Twin reduction using transvaginal ultrasound guided aspiration. The mare in this case conceived twins at foal heat, an unusual phenomenon. At 15 days, the uterus was still enlarged enough to make routine crushing of one cotwin very difficult. At 17 days, the twins had fixed close to one another within the uterus and one was reduced by US guided per vagina aspiration as shown in this image. Serum progesterone concentrations should be monitored in the event that either crushing or aspiration have released enough prostaglandin to cause luteolysis and terminate the pregnancy. The progestogen altrenogest (Regumate) is given during this monitoring period in the event that luteolysis may have occurred. Fortunately, it is possible to measure endogenous progesterone concentrations while altrenogest is being given because altrenogest does not cross-react with most progesterone assays. If luteolysis occurs, pregnancy is maintained using altrenogest until the accessory corpora lutea are formed at about 35 to 40 days of gestation.

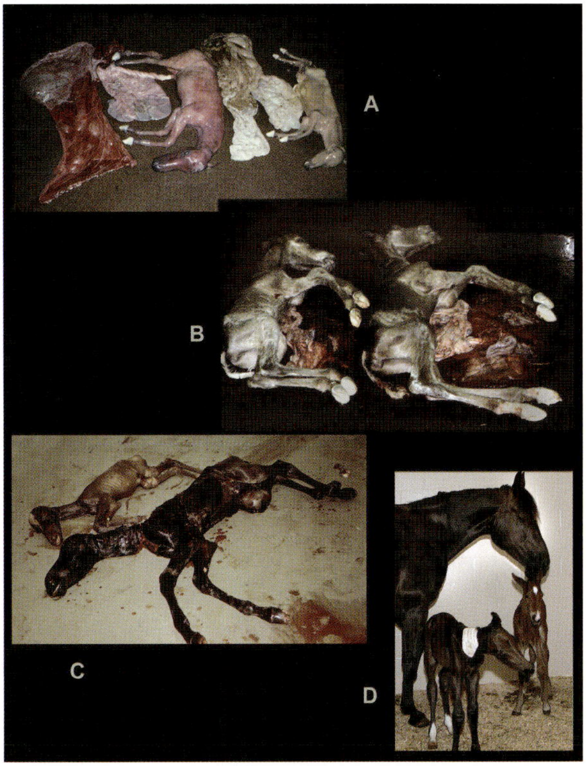

Figure 8.89 Consequences of poor twin management. This amalgam of images clearly demonstrates the devastating results of inappropriate management of twin pregnancies. Although many cotwin pregnancies are lost during early gestation, others progress into the last few months of pregnancy and are then aborted. Images A and B show typical twin abortions that occurred during the last trimester. One of the twins is almost inevitably significantly smaller than its cotwin. Interestingly, it is not always the larger of the twins that will survive if the pregnancy progresses to term. It has been speculated that this may be because the smaller twin has been under more stress than its cotwin, accelerating fetal maturation. Image C shows that twin pregnancies will sometimes cause dystocia during abortion or when they are born at term. In this case, the larger of the cotwins had a wryneck, which prevented foaling and required fetotomy. Image D shows the unusual state of a completed twin pregnancy. However, this is usually no cause for celebration because of the intensive care required by the twins and the high death rate in one or both of them.

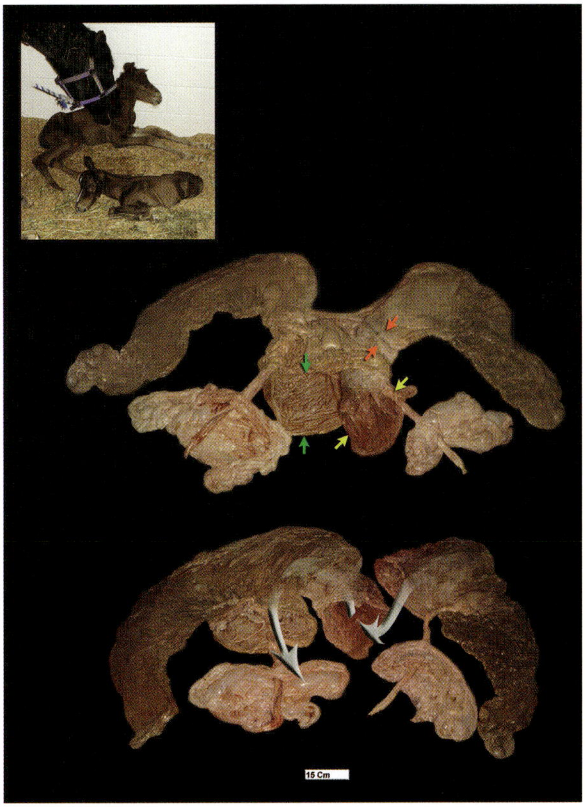

Figure 8.90 Variations in placentation in twin pregnancies. There is still some uncertainty as to how and why twin pregnancies usually result in abortion. Sharing of the available endometrial area is certainly a significant effect, but immunological rejection of one cotwin by another may also be important. This image shows one of numerous permutations of how twin placentas can be joined within the uterus and how the placental area can be shared. In this case, the red arrows indicate the start of an area of apposition between the two chorionic surfaces. In these placentas, there appeared to be little, if any, tissue reaction between the two conceptuses despite the intimacy of placental apposition. Approximately 40% of the chorionic surface from the smaller cotwin was invaginated into the placenta of the larger twin. The green arrows show the chorioallantois of the larger twin where it ruptured at the cervical star; the site of rupture necessary for the birth of the larger foal within its amnion (left amnion). The chorioallantois (yellow arrows) containing the smaller foal was also born through this rupture. This situation provided an obstetrical challenge during the assisted delivery of the foals. The lower image shows the path that had to be taken by the smaller foal to be born; through the placenta of the larger foal. Often, placentas of twin foals will lie side by side within the uterus and the foals will be born in a more conventional fashion.

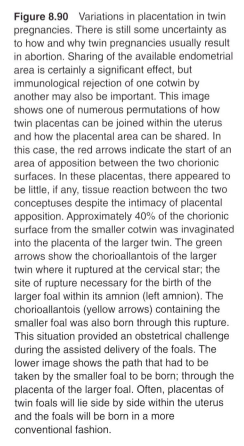

Fetal Death Followed by Mummification

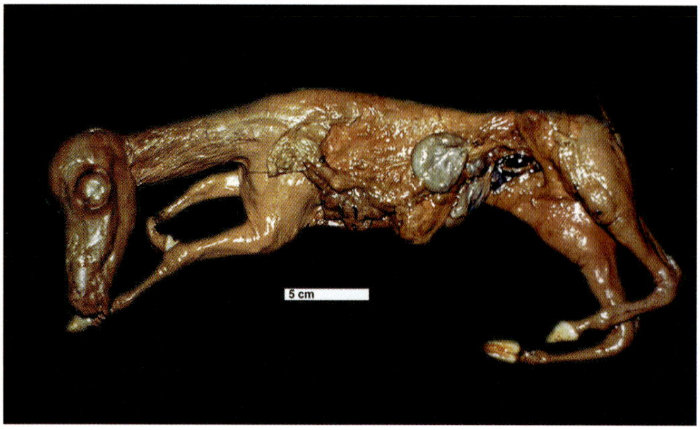

Figure 8.91a Equine mummies are rare and little is known of their pathogenesis. This image shows mummification of a single conceptus estimated to be about 120 days of age at the time of its death. It was not known if the mare pregnant with this fetus had any luteal tissue in her ovaries. However, it was presumed that luteal tissue would have to have been present to maintain this pregnancy. In the absence of luteal tissue, a single mummified conceptus is theoretically unlikely because a placenta is required to maintain pregnancy after 100 days of gestation.

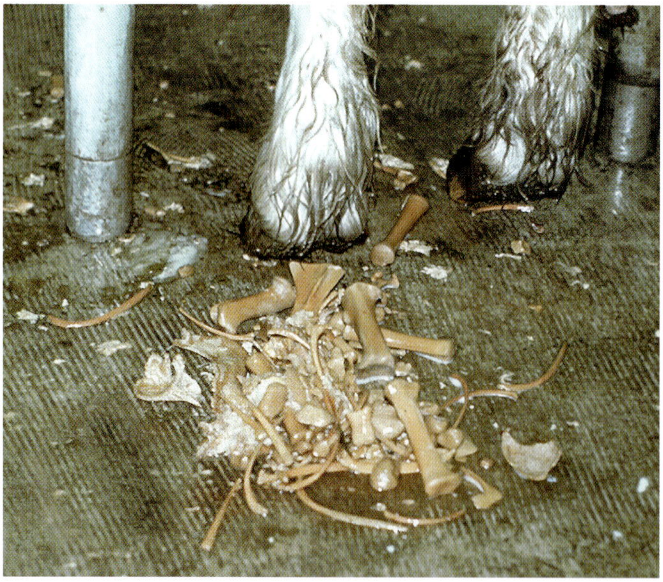

Figure 8.91b Maceration of an advanced age fetus in a mare. The fetus was discovered during transrectal examination after a complaint of prolonged gestation. As in cases of pyometra in mares, this mare showed no systemic signs of disease. Treatment included tranquilization followed by slow, manual dilation of the cervix, over a period of approximately 20 minutes. When the cervix was dilated enough to admit a hand, the bones and debris were extracted and the uterus flushed with saline and antibiotics. Oxytocin treatment could follow flushing if required.

Ascending Placentitis

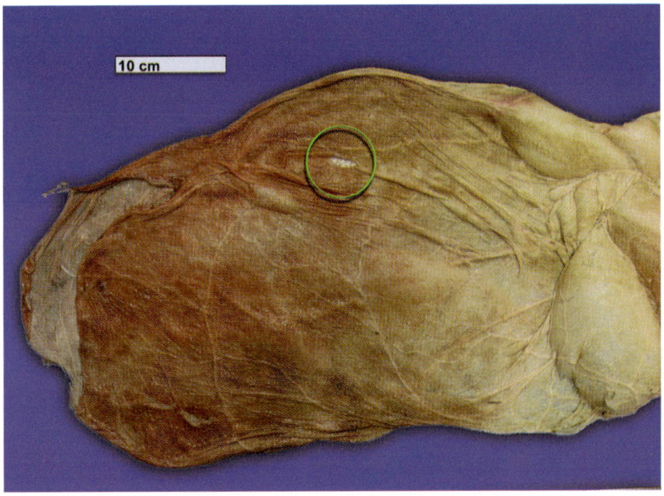

Figure 8.92 Although ascending placentitis is a common cause of abortion in mares, one should be cautious not to assume that there is placentitis based on the presence of hyperemia of the chorion in the vicinity of the cervical star. Although this image appears to illustrate a case of ascending placentitis from the cervix, this placenta was indeed, normal. A biopsy taken at the site indicated showed a complete absence of inflammation. The origin of this hyperemia was unknown.

Enlargement of the Mammary Gland Prior to Abortion

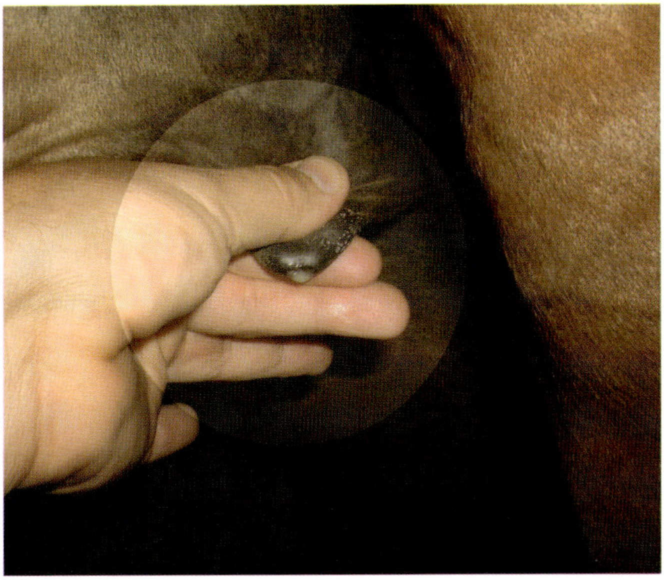

Figure 8.93 The first sign of impending abortion in a mare is premature enlargement of the mammary gland and production of milk. Abortion may follow within several days or several weeks. Occasionally, normal mares may begin to produce milk for several days, or longer, before foaling. Without electrolyte measurements of the milk and ultrasonographic examinations of the placenta and the fetus, it is difficult to tell the difference between these mares and those that are aborting toward the end of gestation. Contrary to the assumption of many horse owners, a hemorrhagic discharge from the vulva is not a harbinger of abortion in mares.

Stillbirth or Abortion Close to Term

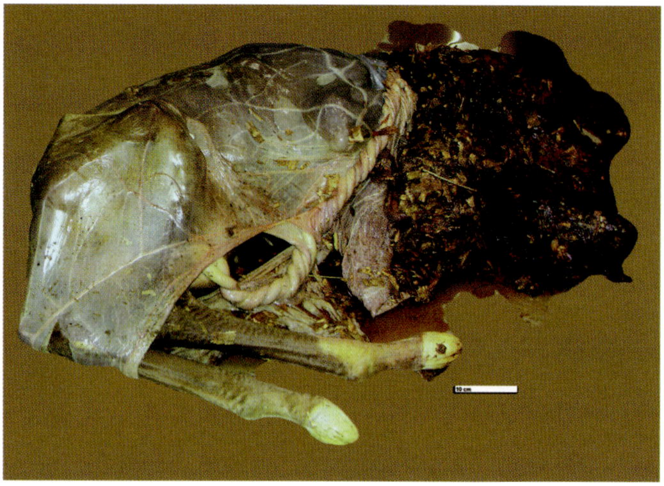

Figure 8.94 This image shows a Warmblood foal that was stillborn or aborted close to term. It was found wrapped within its amnion as shown here. Although definitive diagnosis of the cause of abortion was never made, it is possible that this foal was aborted as a result of vascular embarrassment in the umbilical cord, the cord being excessively twisted. This is discussed elsewhere. It is also possible that the foal suffocated within its amnion during the foaling in following images. This is possible in horses because the amnion is separated from the chorion completely by the presence of the allantois. A similar situation exists in carnivores.

Long Umbilical Cord as a Cause of Abortion

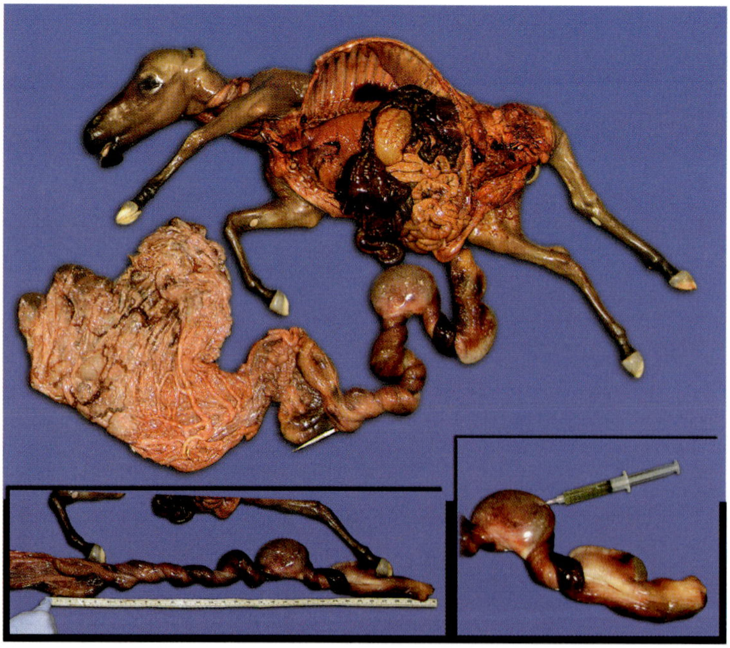

Figure 8.95 General characteristics of long umbilical cord. Since problems of twinning and equine herpes virus infections have been largely controlled, abnormalities associated with the umbilical cord are recognized as a common cause of abortion. Opinions vary as to how long a cord must be to be considered pathological. Those with a total length of more than 80 cm, intra- and extra-amnionic, are considered suspicious, while those over 100 cm in length are a probable cause of abortion. However, one should be careful with this categorization since normal foals are sometimes born with cord lengths within this range. The reason for the correlation between cord length and abortion is poorly understood but it may be related to disturbances of blood flow within the placenta, especially when there are more than five or six twists in the umbilical cord. In this 6-month fetus, abortion was probably due to the long and excessively twisted umbilical cord. In addition, the cord showed bullous dilations of the urachus, which are also considered abnormal. The insets show the measurement of the intra-amnionic cord and the bullous dilation of the urachus mentioned above. As expected, this dilation was filled with urine. In the main image, a pair of forceps has been inserted into the external orifice of the urachus, where urine drains into the allantois. The extra amnionic cord had been ripped off at this point with its vascular fragments visible on either side of the forceps.

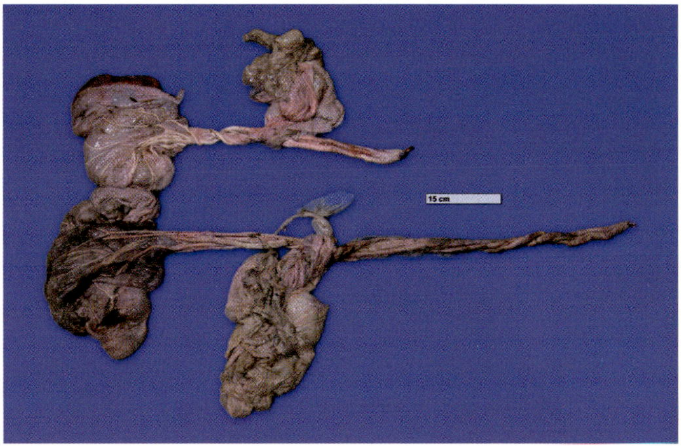

Figure 8.96 Variation in the normal length of umbilicus cords. As mentioned before (fig. 8.95), there is considerable variation in the lengths of normal umbilical cords. Because abnormalities associated with the umbilical cord are now the most common diagnosis, caution must be exercised when implicating the length of the umbilicus cord as a cause of abortion. This image shows placentas with total umbilical cord lengths of 55 and 91 cm; both are from normal Standardbred foals at term.

Yolk Sac Remnants on the Umbilical Cord

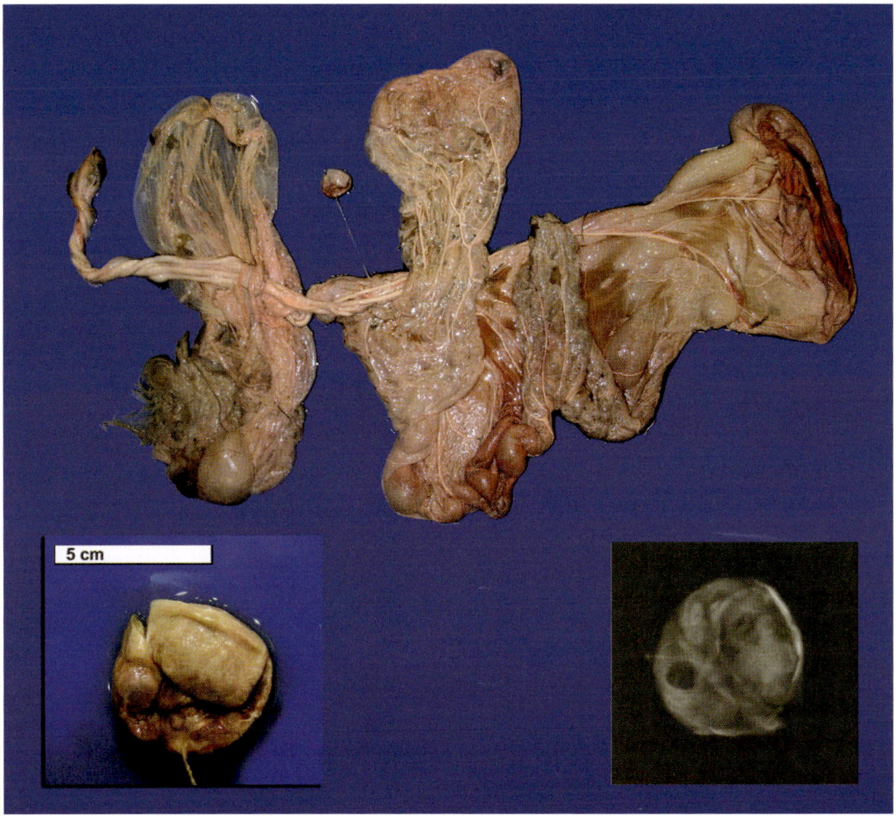

Figure 8.97 Occasionally, remnants of the yolk sac attached to the extra amnionic portion of the umbilical cord might be found. This is because the extra amnionic portion of the cord is formed when its contents (the yolk sac) are depleted by about 50 or 60 days of gestation. At that time, the sides of the yolk sac come together to form the extra amnionic cord. Sometimes these remnants are even calcified. In this case, a yolk sac remnant was attached to the cord by a thin strand of connective tissue. As shown in the radiograph at lower right, the remnant was highly calcified. These structures are not considered to be abnormal.

Retained Placenta

The Nature of Equine Placentation

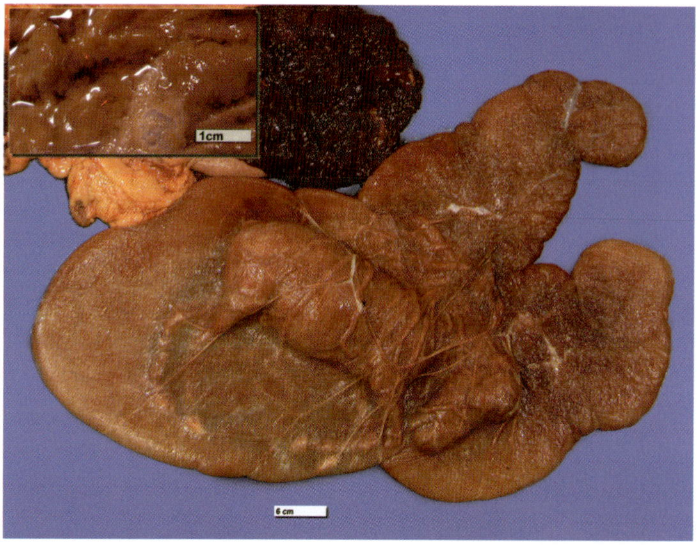

Figure 8.98 Practical anatomy. This image shows typical diffuse placentation of horses. The fetus in this image is about 2 months old and its placenta detached very easily from the endometrium in this fresh specimen. However, as shown in the inset, a close-up image of the placenta at term, microcotyledons shown by the red arrows eventually form an intimate attachment to the endometrium. These microcotyledons are similar in structure to those of cattle and form a tight bond to the endometrium by about 6 or 7 months of gestation. Surprisingly, detachment after foaling is usually very rapid despite the intimacy of its placentation.

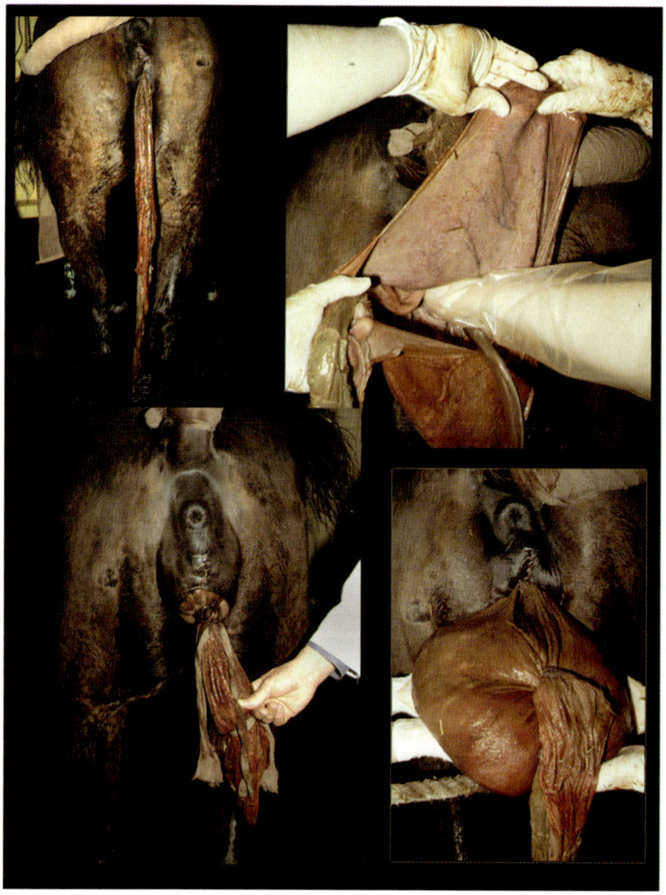

Figure 8.99 Treatment of retained placenta. The incidence of retained placenta in mares has been reported to lie between 2% and 10% of all foalings. Retained placenta in mares is a potentially life-threatening disease. If the placenta is still present 3 hours after foaling, it should be considered retained. It is unlikely that uterine atony does not contribute to retained placentas, because the vast majority of retained placentas are expelled after one or more injections of oxytocin. Intravascular injections of collagenase have been shown to be valuable in mares with retained placentas, but this treatment has not been widely used. An alternative is to inflate the chorioallantois with saline to loosen its attachment to the endometrium and, presumably, to stimulate myometrial contraction as well. This is colloquially known as the "Burns technique." This collection of images shows the typical appearance of a retained placenta and the application of the Burns technique in a mare. About 10 liters of saline are infused slowly and the tube is left in place in the standing mare. If the placenta has not been expelled within about 30 minutes, the tube should be removed and the fluid allowed to drain. Additional care should also be used including tetanus prophylaxis, antibiotics, nonsteroidal anti-inflammatory drugs, and vasodilators to prevent laminitis. Manual extraction of the placenta remains a contentious subject. In other parts of the world, it is more common to remove placentas manually than it is in North America.

Recommended Reading

Amann RP. Physiology and endocrinology. In McKinnon AO, Voss J, eds., Equine reproduction. Lea and Febiger, 1993.

Arthur CH. Veterinary reproduction and obstetrics. 4th ed. London: Balliere Tindall, 41–42, 1975.

Bucca S. Equine fetal gender determination from mid- to advanced-gestation by ultrasound. Theriogenology. 64:568–71, 2005.

Bucca S, Fogarty U, Collins A, Small V. Assessment of feto-placental well-being from the gestation to term: transrectal and transabdominal ultrasonographic features. Theriogenology. 64:542–57, 2005.

Haffner JC, Fecteau KA, Held JP, Eiler H. Equine retained placenta: technique for and tolerance to umbilical artery injections of collagenase. Theriogenology. 49:711–16, 1998.

McKinnon AO, Squires EL, Pickett BW. (No title) Eq Reprod Ultrason. Bulletin #4. Fort Collins: Colorado State University animal reproduction laboratory, 31–40, 1988.

Pascoe RR. Observations on the length and angle of declination of the vulva and its relation to fertility in mares. J Reprod Fert Suppl. 27:299–305, 1979.

Renaudin CD, Gillis CL, Tarantal AF. Transabdominal combined with transrectal ultrasonographic determination of equine fetal gender during midgestation. AAEP Proceedings. 43:252–55, 1997.

Thompson DL, Pickett BW, Squires EL, Amann RP. Testicular measurements and reproductive characteristics in stallions. J Reprod Fert Suppl. 27:13–17, 1979.

Vandeplassche M, Spincemaille J, Bouters R. Aetiology, pathogenesis and treatment of retained placenta in the mare. Equine Vet J. 3:144–47, 1971.

Whitwell, KE. Placental pathology: Morphological studies on the normal singleton foal at term. Res Vet Sci. 19:44–55, 1975.

9 Diseases of the Endocrine System

Pituitary Disease
- Pituitary Pars Intermedia Dysfunction (PPID) (Equine Cushing's Disease)

Diseases of Glucose Metabolism
- Insulin Resistance

Diseases of the Thyroid Gland
- Thyroid Adenoma
- Goiter in Newborn Foals (Neonatal Hypothyroidism)

Vitamin D/Parathyroid Hormone/Calcitonin
- Vitamin D toxicity
- Hyperparathyroidism
- Primary Hyperparathyroidism
- Secondary Hyperparathyroidism (Nutritional Hyperparathyroidism, Bran Disease, Osteodystrophia Fibrosa)

Adrenal Gland
- Adrenal Tumor: Adenoma
- Adrenal Tumor: Pheochromocytoma

Pituitary Pars Intermedia Dysfunction (PPID) (Equine Cushing's Disease)

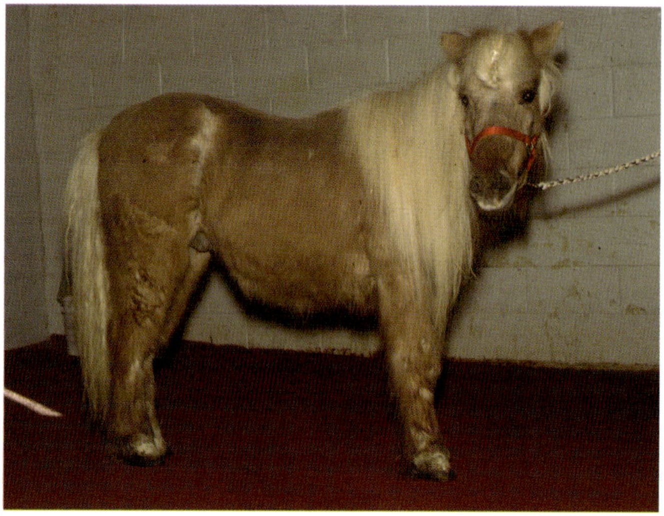

Figure 9.1 Pony with classic clinical signs of pituitary pars intermedia dysfunction (PPID), also known as equine Cushing's disease. Note the long, wavy hair coat or hirsutism. Also evident is poor muscle tone, a pendulous abdomen, hyperhydrosis, and rings on the hoof indicative of previous episodes of laminitis.

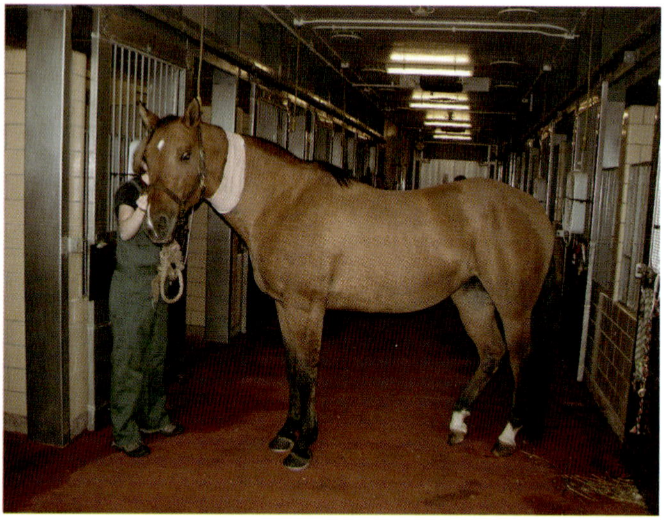

Figure 9.2 PPID in a horse with few other clinical signs associated with the disease. It presented for laminitis that occurred with no known inciting cause. If one looks closely, one can see long guard hairs on the legs, but there is no hirsutism per se. PPID should be suspected in any middle-aged horse with laminitis, even in the absence of other clinical signs.

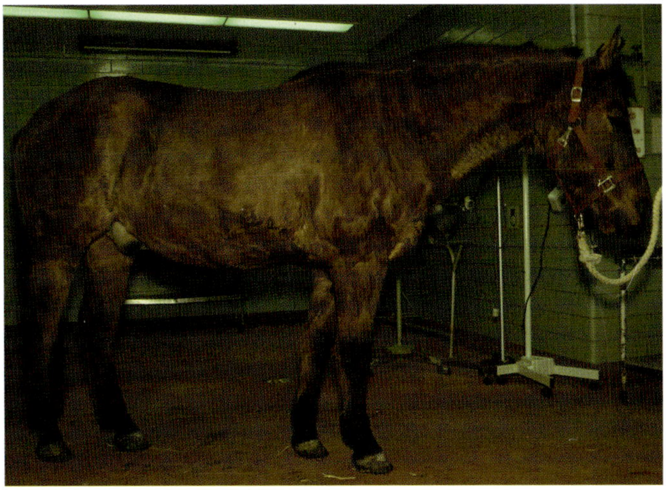

Figure 9.3 PPID with the beginning of the classical clinical signs. This includes a longer hair coat and loss of muscle tone.

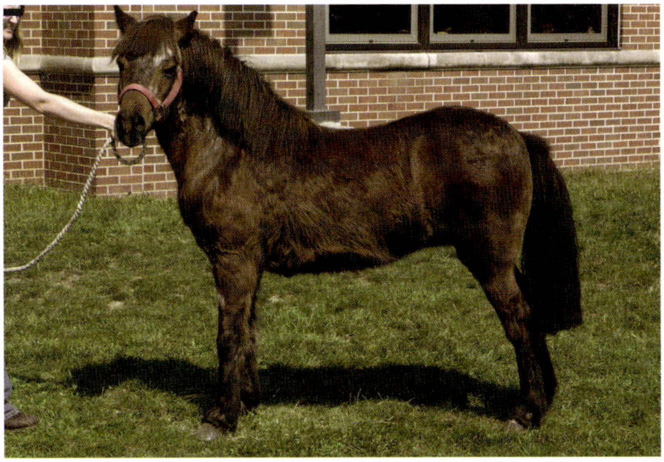

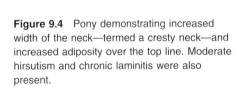

Figure 9.4 Pony demonstrating increased width of the neck—termed a cresty neck—and increased adiposity over the top line. Moderate hirsutism and chronic laminitis were also present.

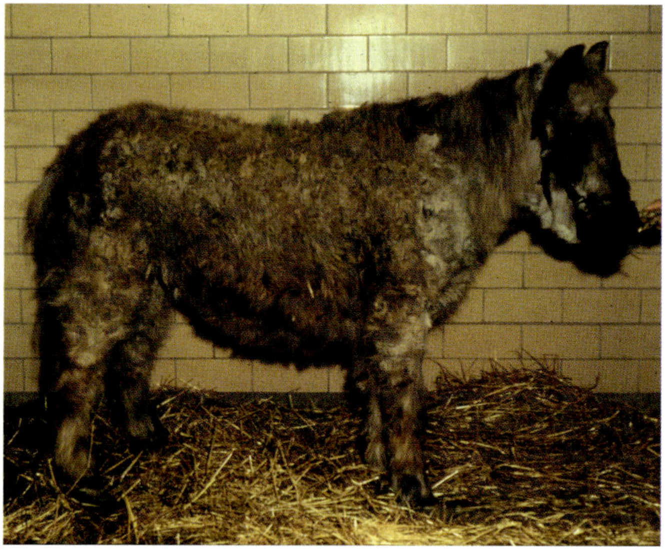

Figure 9.5 Pony with advanced signs of PPID including extremely long hair coat, hyperhydrosis, and laminitis.

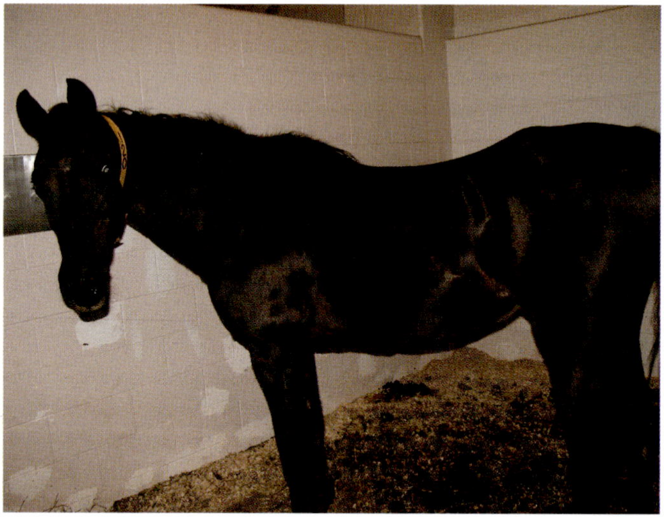

Figure 9.6 Horse with PPID exhibiting the overall lack of muscle tone and poor top line conformation characteristic of the disease.

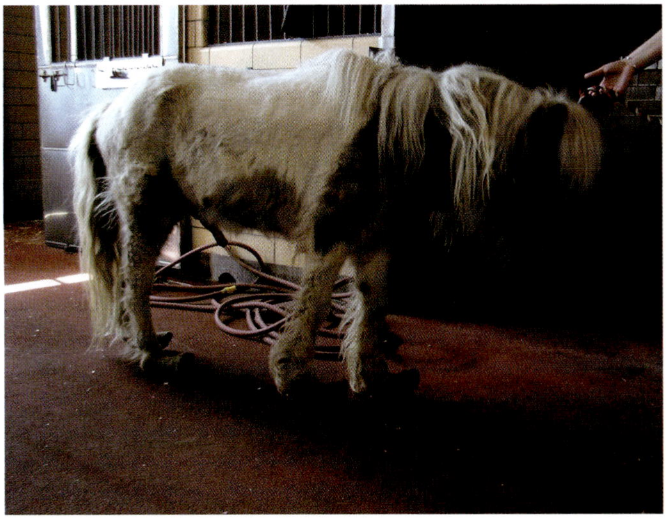

Figure 9.7 Pony with severe chronic laminitis. Laminitis is a common complication of PPID.

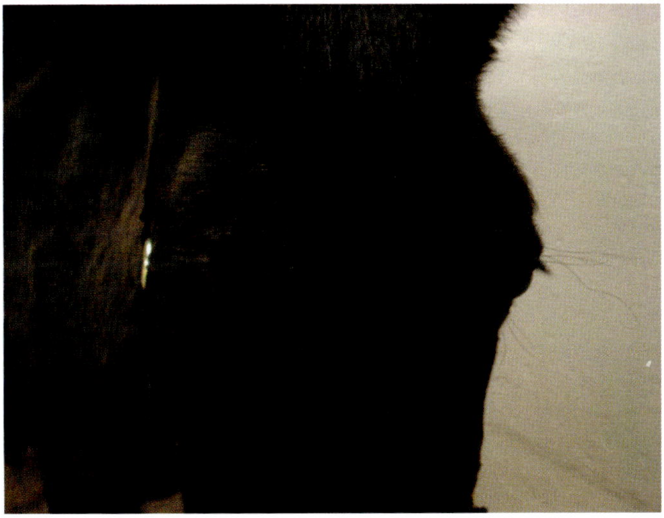

Figure 9.8 Bulging of the supraorbital fossa in a horse with PPID.

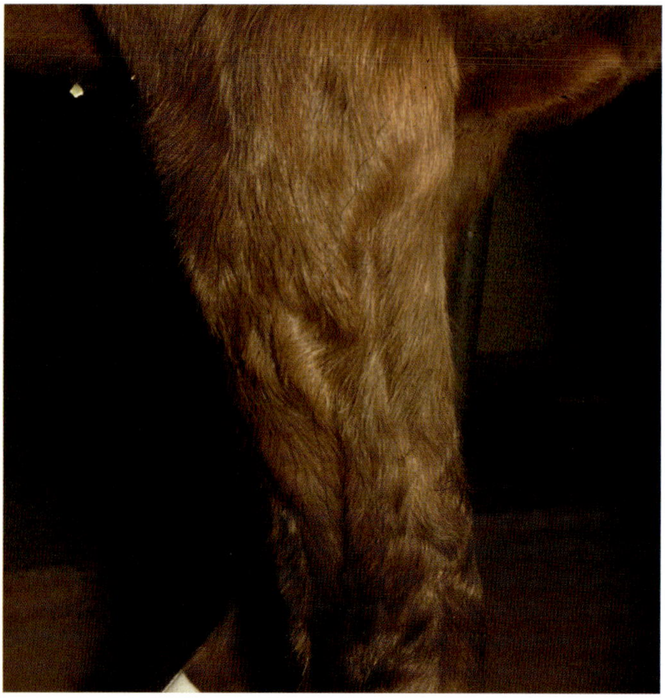

Figure 9.9 Hirsutism of the leg. Hirsutism often begins on the legs, under the chin, and on the ventral abdomen in horses with PPID.

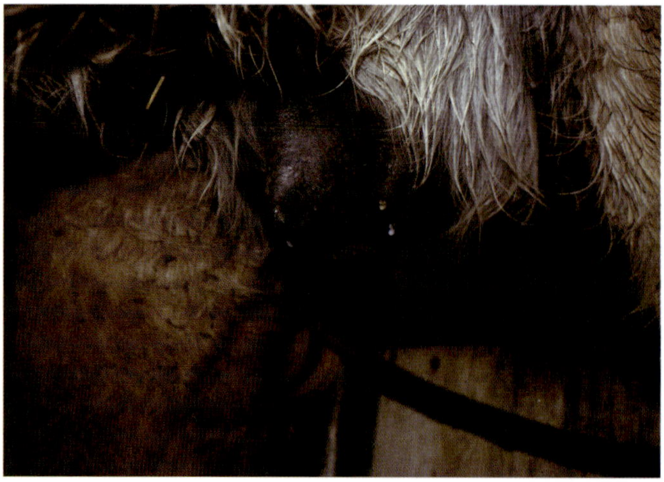

Figure 9.10 Inappropriate lactation in a horse with PPID. Loss of inhibitory dopaminergic tone from the hypothalamus may result in increased prolactin levels and the initiation of lactation.

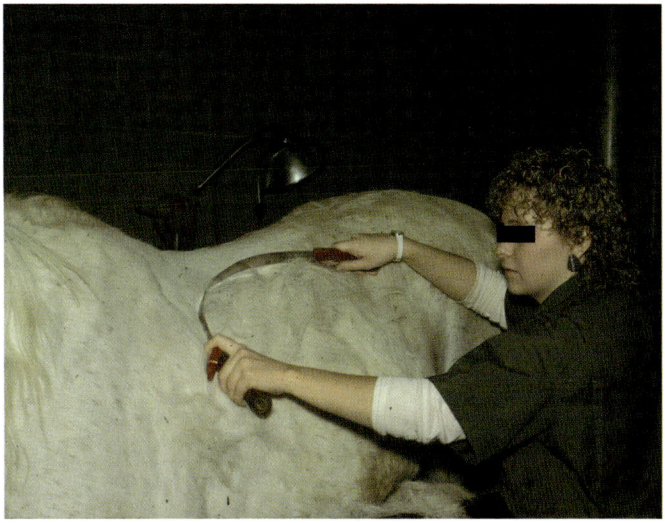

Figure 9.11 Horse with PPID that is responding to oral pergolide therapy by shedding out her excessive hair coat. Pergolide administration may result in a complete remission of all clinical signs for a period of time.

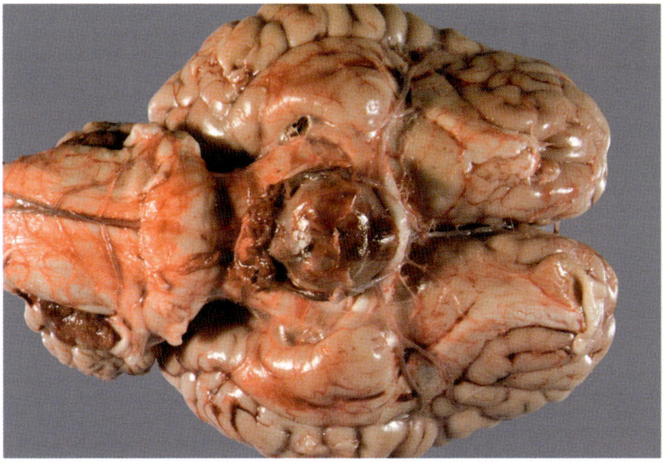

Figure 9.12 Postmortem photograph of a brain and extremely enlarged pituitary gland in a horse with PPID.

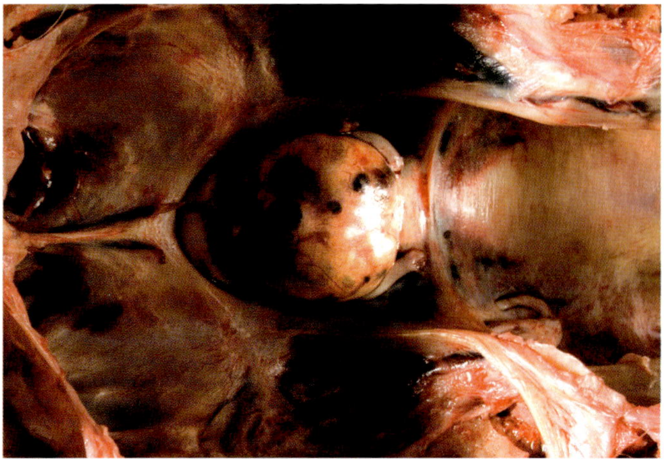

Figure 9.13 Postmortem photograph of an enlarged pituitary gland in situ on the bottom of the cranial vault.

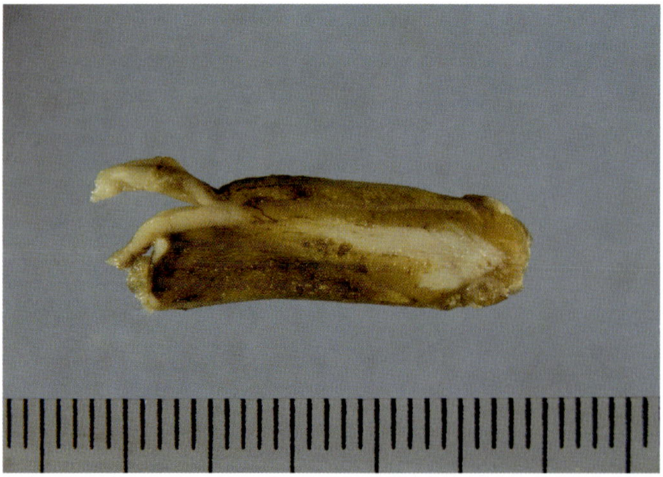

Figure 9.14 Pituitary gland cut lengthwise. One can see a small degree of thickening in the pars intermedia. This pituitary gland was classified as normal for an aged horse, or grade II.

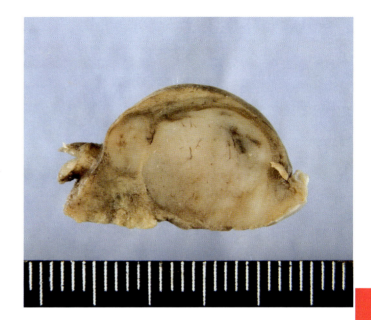

Figure 9.15 Pituitary gland cut lengthwise. A large pars intermedia adenoma can be visualized. It is distorting and compressing the normal pituitary tissue.

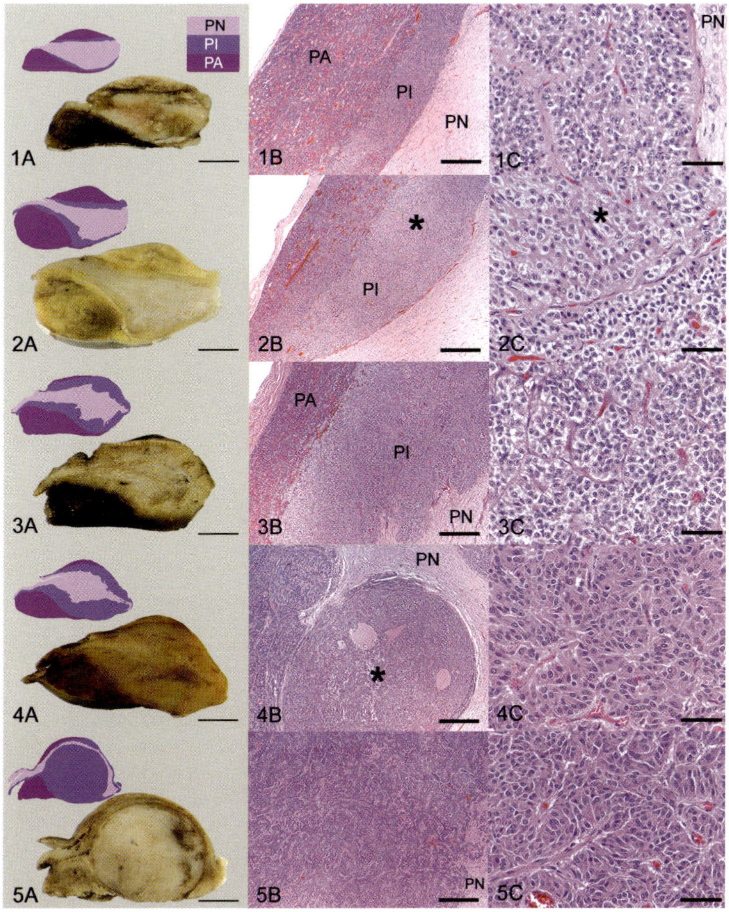

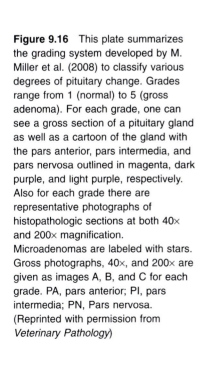

Figure 9.16 This plate summarizes the grading system developed by M. Miller et al. (2008) to classify various degrees of pituitary change. Grades range from 1 (normal) to 5 (gross adenoma). For each grade, one can see a gross section of a pituitary gland as well as a cartoon of the gland with the pars anterior, pars intermedia, and pars nervosa outlined in magenta, dark purple, and light purple, respectively. Also for each grade there are representative photographs of histopathologic sections at both 40× and 200× magnification. Microadenomas are labeled with stars. Gross photographs, 40×, and 200× are given as images A, B, and C for each grade. PA, pars anterior; PI, pars intermedia; PN, Pars nervosa. (Reprinted with permission from *Veterinary Pathology*)

Insulin Resistance

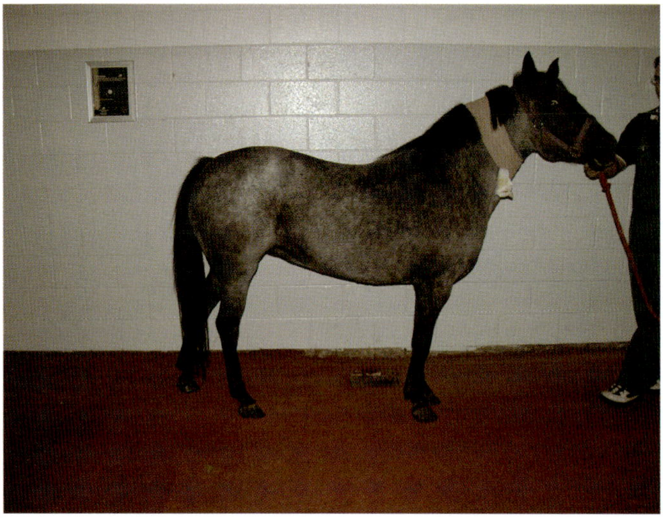

Figure 9.17 Typical phenotype of a horse with insulin resistance. Note high condition score, increased adiposity over the topline and neck resulting in a classic "cresty" appearance. Characterized by increased blood insulin concentrations and a poor ability to handle carbohydrates. Insulin resistance is often referred to as equine metabolic syndrome. At one time, this condition was termed hypothyroidism, although most often thyroid function is normal.

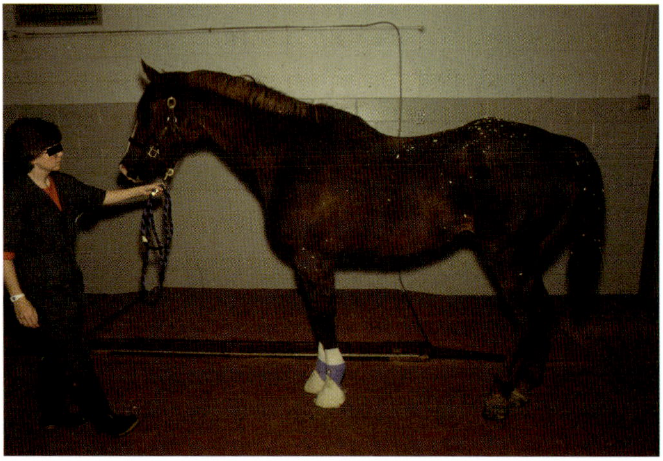

Figure 9.18 Insulin resistance in a horse that has a normal to low condition score. Despite this, there is a cresty neck and abnormal topline. This horse also suffers from laminitis, an extremely common complication of insulin resistance.

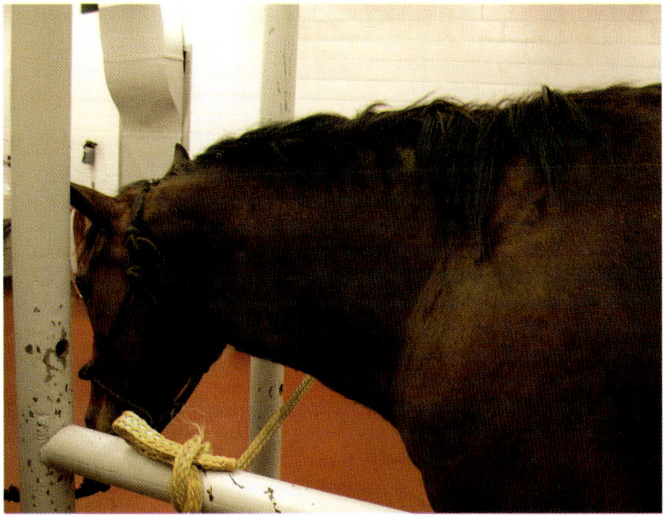

Figure 9.19 Close-up of the neck of a horse suffering from insulin resistance. Note overall thickness that is disproportionate to the horse's overall condition.

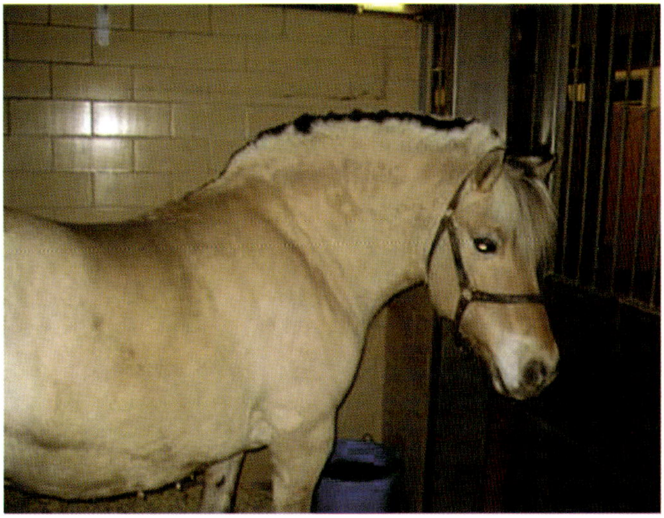

Figure 9.20 A Norwegian Fjord pony exhibiting the cresty neck that is typical for the breed. The pony had documented insulin resistance, an extremely common condition in breeds of horses and ponies with this phenotype. Perhaps insulin resistance provided a competitive advantage to horses kept in harsh environments, and is thus common in breeds developed in areas of the globe that commonly experience severe conditions.

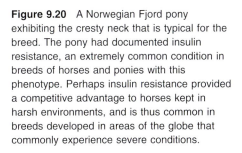

Thyroid Adenoma

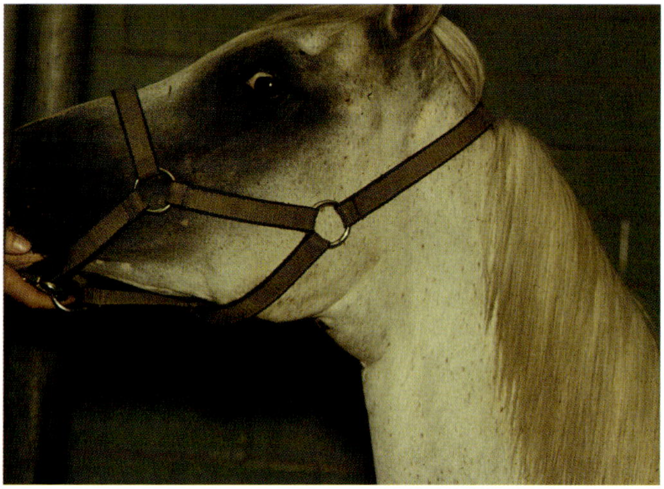

Figure 9.21 Enlarged thyroid gland in a 16-year-old horse with thyroid adenoma. Enlargement is clearly visible from a distance.

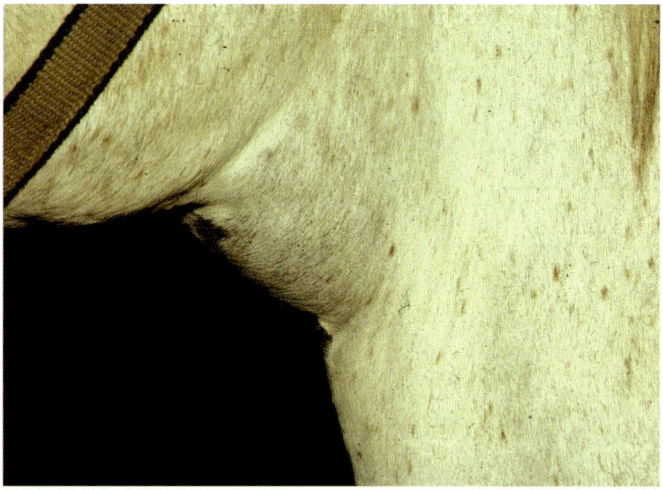

Figure 9.22 Close-up of enlarged thyroid gland. Note how the gland alters the neck line.

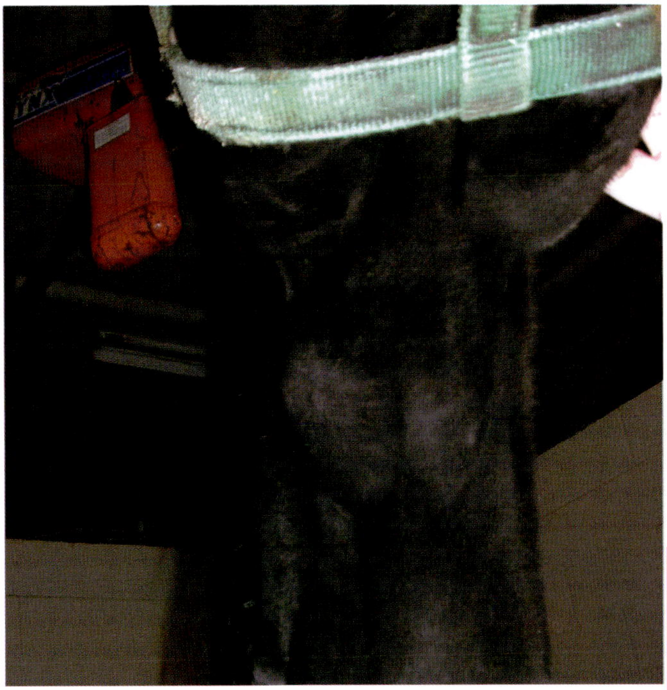

Figure 9.23 Unilateral enlargement of the thyroid gland due to thyroid adenoma. Sometimes the thyroid gland cannot be appreciated visually until hair is clipped, but could be palpated easily.

9

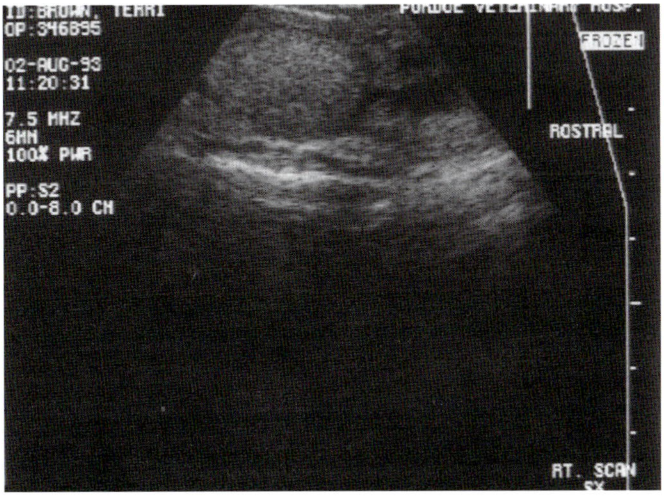

Figure 9.24 Ultrasound image of thyroid adenoma. Note oval, homogenous mass of similar echo texture within the gland.

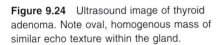

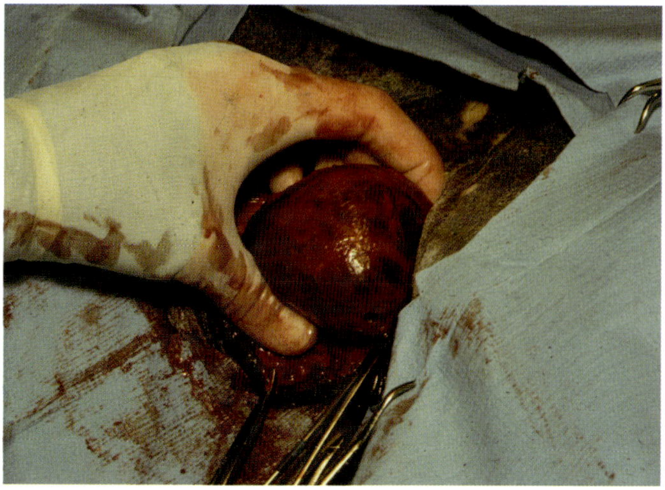

Figure 9.25 Surgical removal of a thyroid adenoma. In most instances the tumor is benign and well circumscribed, making its removal relatively easy.

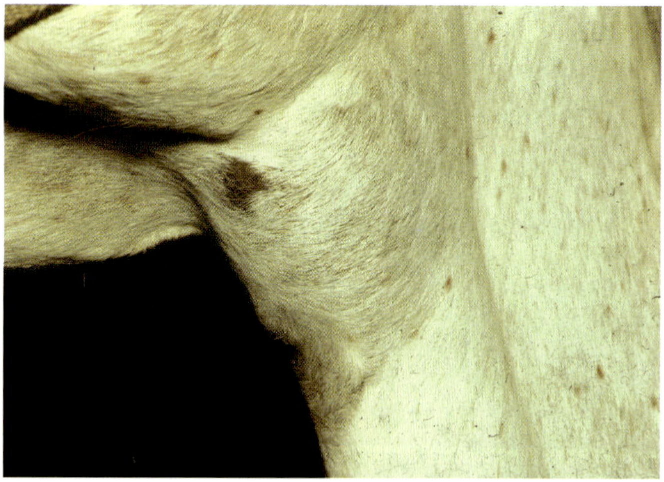

Figure 9.26 Postoperative picture of horse in fig. 9.21 after removal of thyroid adenoma.

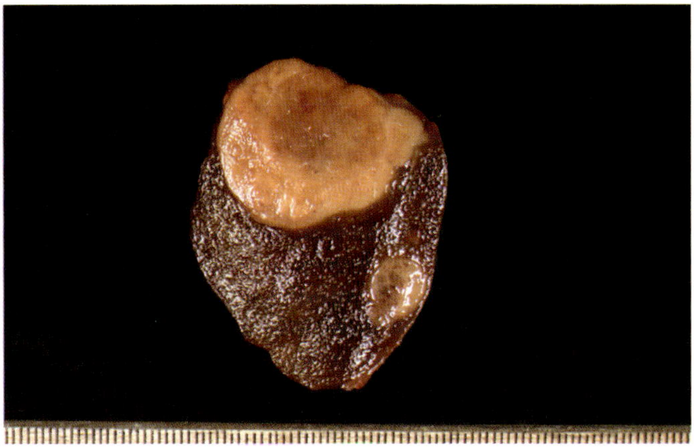

Figure 9.27 Thyroid gland containing two adenomas after surgical removal. Gland has been cut lengthwise.

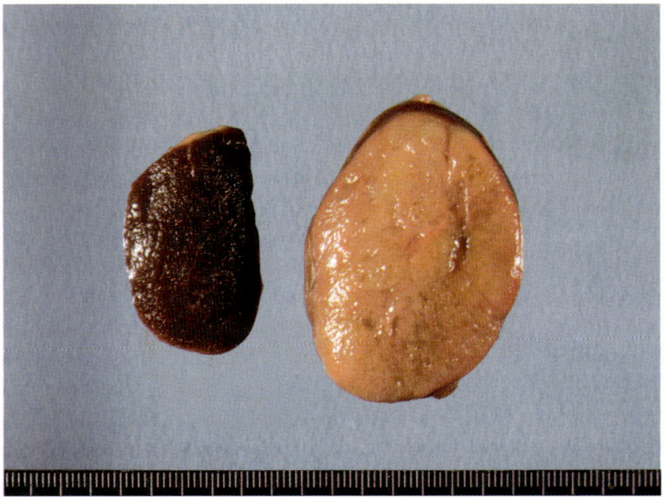

Figure 9.28 Left and right lobes of thyroid gland removed at postmortem. The right gland has been replaced by a homogenous tumor that was found to be a C-cell tumor via immunohistochemical staining.

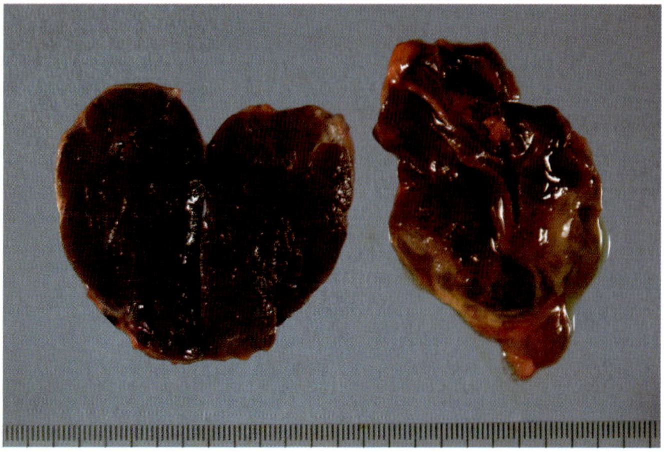

Figure 9.29 Brachial cysts attached to the thyroid gland found as incidental finding on postmortem examination. Such cysts are usually asymptomatic.

Goiter in Newborn Foals (Neonatal Hypothyroidism)

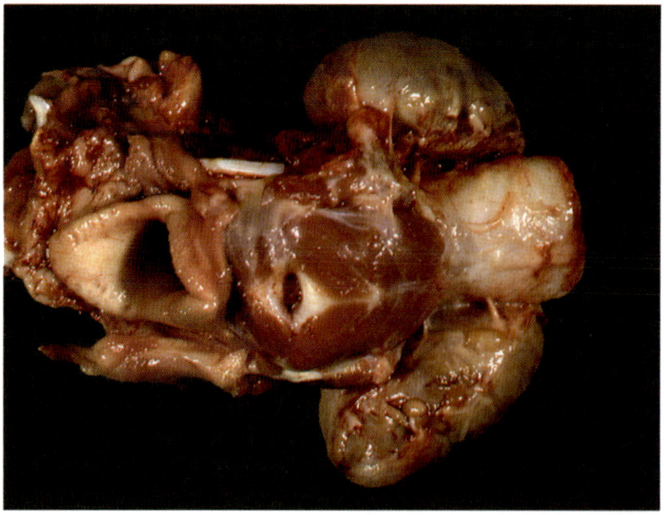

Figure 9.30 Congenital goiter from a newborn foal. Congenital goiter in foals is associated with increased iodine intake or the ingestion of goitrogenic plants or substances in pregnant mares. See also Chapter 12, Diseases of the Neonates.

Vitamin D Toxicity

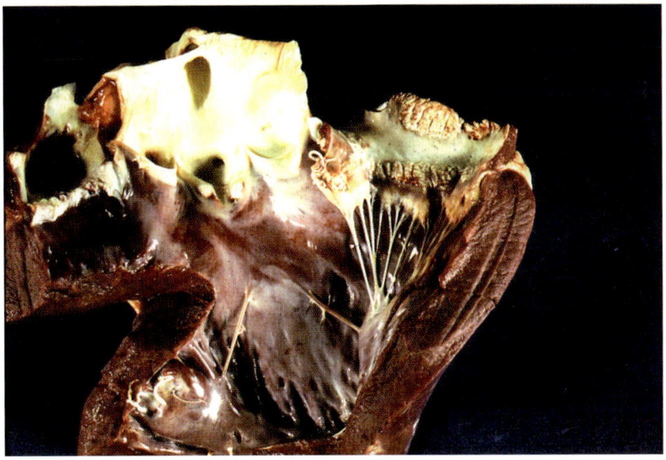

Figure 9.31 Calcification of heart valves in horse that was fed diet that had been incorrectly supplemented resulting in toxic levels of vitamin D. High levels of vitamin D result in increased blood calcium and phosphorus levels that precipitate causing calcification of large arteries and other tissues.

Hyperparathyroidism

Primary Hyperparathyroidism

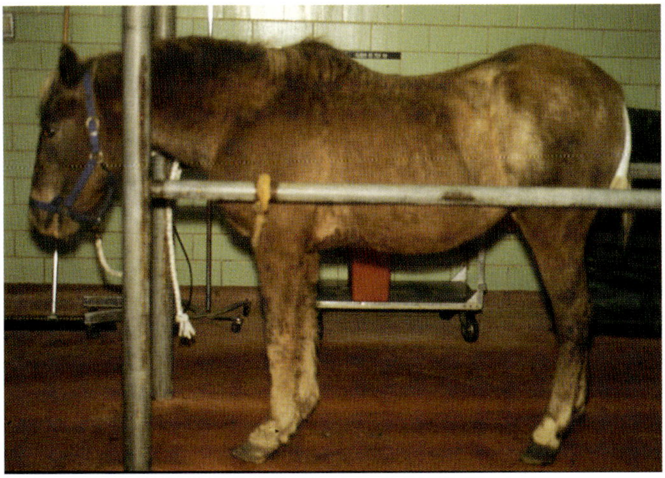

Figure 9.32 Side view of horse with primary hyperparathyroidism resulting in fibrous osteodystrophy of the skull (big head). Note how skull is disproportionately large when compared to the body.

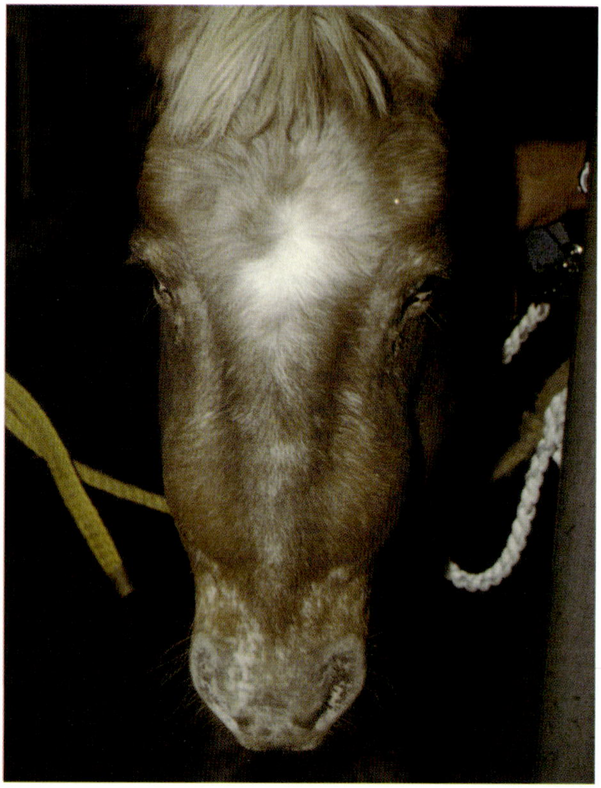

Figure 9.33 Close-up of horse with primary hyperparathyroidism revealing increased bone growth in the skull.

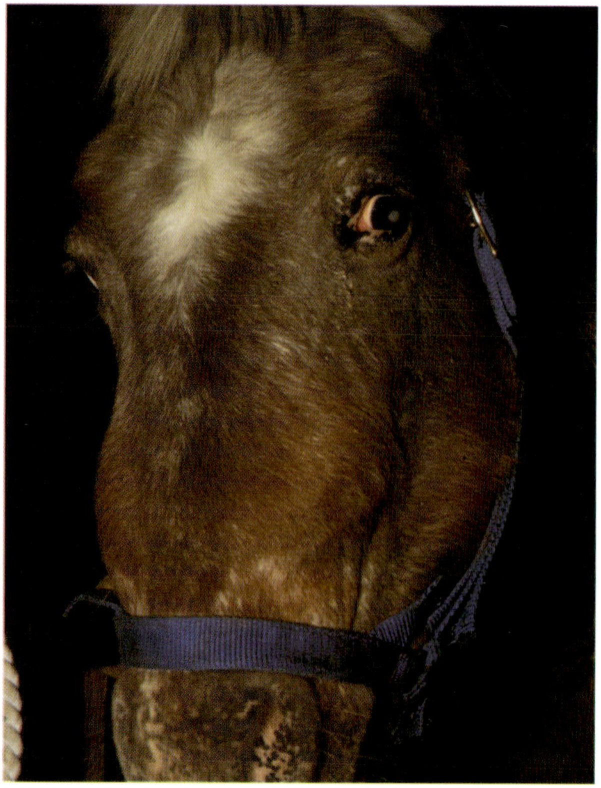

Figure 9.34 Primary hyperparathyroidism is caused by a PTH secreting tumor. Other forms of hyperparathyroidism may also result in fibrous osteodystrophy as illustrated in this photograph.

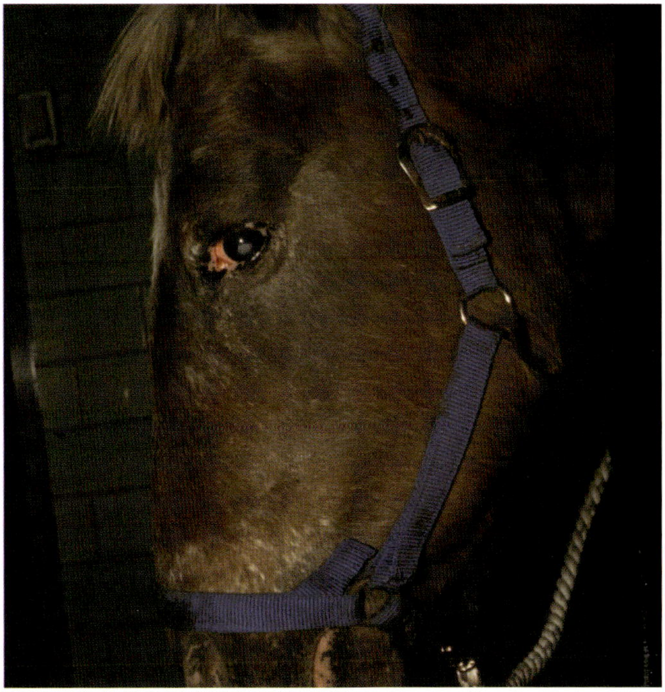

Figure 9.35 Side view of skull of horse with primary hyperparathyroidism.

Secondary Hyperparathyroidism (Nutritional Hyperparathyroidism, Bran Disease, Osteodystrophia Fibrosa)

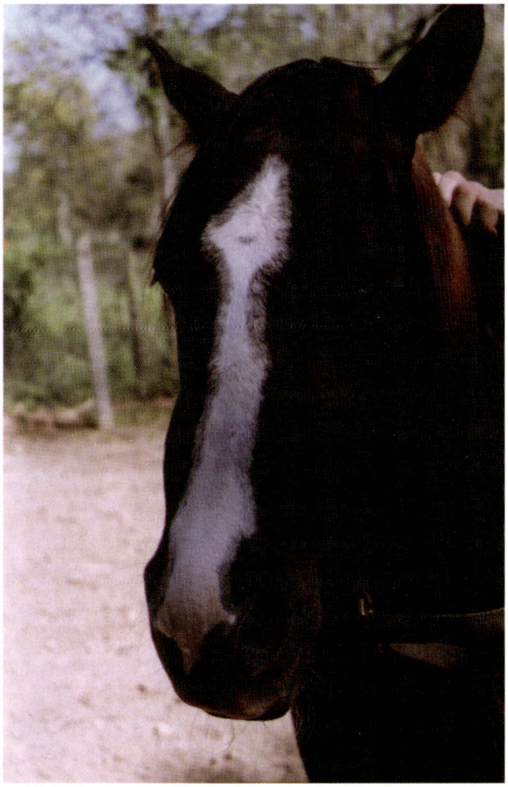

Figure 9.36 Photograph of a horse's head with distorted facial bones due to replacement with fibrous connective tissue. This photo is classical for secondary nutritional hyperparathyroidism. In this horse, clinical signs included slow mastication and a vague alternating leg lameness. The condition was diagnosed based on clinical signs and confirmed by high urinary fractional excretion of phosphorus. The condition is caused by absolute or relative calcium deficiency caused by excessive dietary phosphorus (Ca:P < 1). The horse in this picture was being fed grass hay and oats.

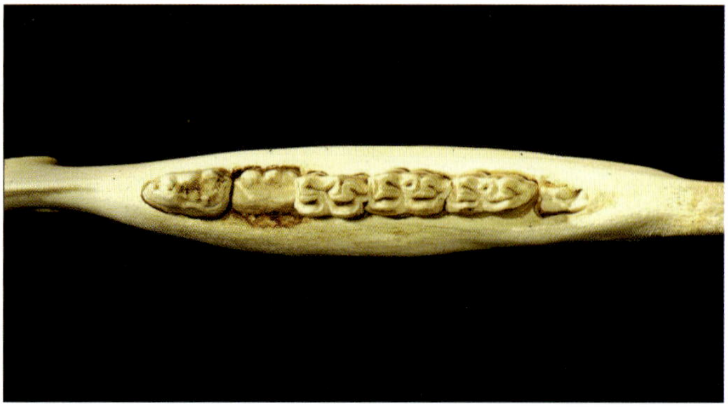

Figure 9.37 Postmortem photograph of one side of the mandible from a horse diagnosed with nutritional secondary hyperparathyroidism. Note the thickened and distorted mandible. (Courtesy of Dr. P. Fretz, WCVM, University of Saskatchewan)

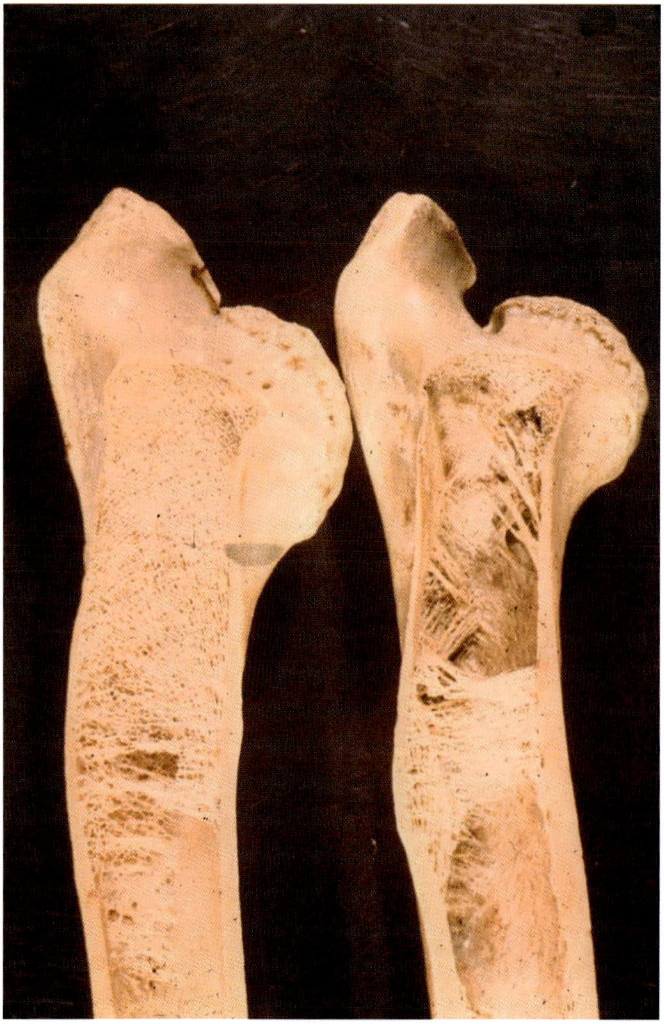

Figure 9.38 Sagittal section of a long bone from a horse with nutritional secondary hyperparathyroidism. (Courtesy of Dr. P. Fretz, WCVM, University of Saskatchewan)

Adrenal Tumor: Adenoma

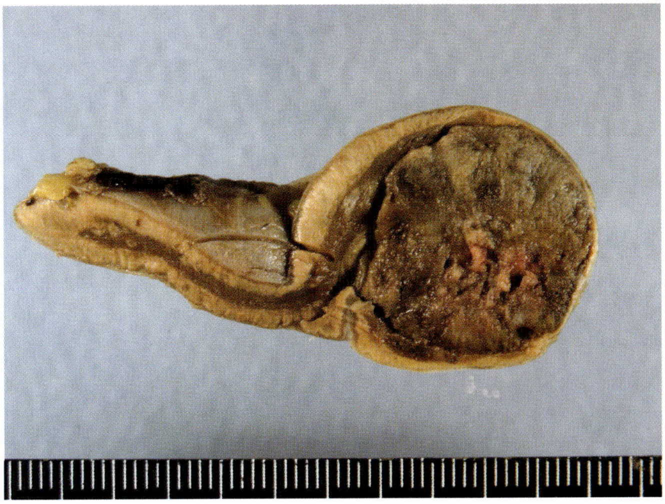

Figure 9.39 Adenoma of adrenal gland found in a horse with clinical signs of PPID.

Adrenal Tumor: Pheochromocytoma

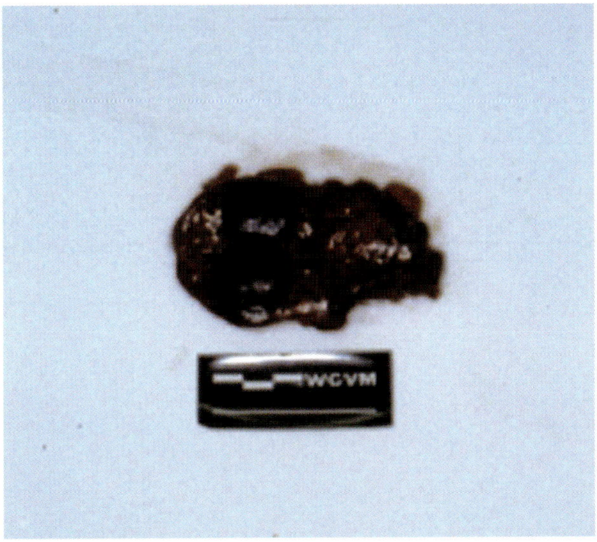

Figure 9.40 Postmortem photograph of a pheochromocytoma in the adrenal medulla of a horse. Pheochromocytoma is generally a nonfunctional tumor that is found incidentally on postmortem examination. However, a few can be functional and cause excessive sweating, apprehension, recurrent colic, increased heart rate, dilated pupils, and hyperglycemia. Diagnosis can be made by measuring blood and urinary catecholamines, which would be elevated.

Recommended Reading

Bailey SR, Baershon-Butcher JL, Ramsom KJ, Elliott J, Menzies-Gow NJ. Hypertension and insulin resistance in a mixed-breed population of ponies predisposed to laminitis. Am J Vet Res. 69:122–29, 2008.

Donaldson MT, LaMonte BH, Morresey P, Smith G, Beech J. Treatment with pergolide or cyproheptadine of pituitary pars Intermedia dysfunction (equine Cushing's disease). JACVIM. 16:742–46, 2002.

Donaldson MT, McDonnell SM, Schanbacher BJ, Lamb SV, McFarlane D, Beech J. Variation in plasma adrenocorticotropic hormone concentration and dexamethasone suppression test results with season, age, and sex in healthy ponies and horses. JACVIM. 19:217–22, 2005.

Frank N, Andrews FM, Sommardahl CS, Eiler H, Rohrbach BW, Donnell RL. Evaluation of the combined dexamethasone suppression/ thyrotropin-releasing hormone stimulation test for detection of pars intermedia pituitary adenomas in horses. J Vet Intern Med. 20:987–93, 2006.

Gold JR, Divers TJ, Barton MH, Lamb SV, Place NJ, Mohammed HO, Bain FT. Plasma adrenocorticotropin, cortisol, and adrenocorticotropin/cortisol ratios in septic and normal-term foals. J Vet Intern Med. 21:791–96, 2007.

Hudson NP, Church DB, Trevena J, Nielsen IL, Major D, Hodgson DR. Primary hypoparathyroidism in two horses. Aust Vet J. 77:504–8, 1999.

McFarlane D, Cribb AE. Systemic and pituitary pars intermedia antioxidant capacity associated with pars intermedia oxidative stress and dysfunction in horses. Am J Vet Res. 66:2065–72, 2005.

Messer NT, Johnson PJ, eds. Endocrinology. In the veterinary clinics of North America: equine practice. 18, 2002

Miller MA, Pardo ID, Jackson LP, Moore GE, Sojka JE. Correlation of pituitary histomorphometry with adrenocorticotrophic hormone response to domperidone administration in the diagnosis of equine pituitary pars intermedia dysfunction. Vet Pathol. 45:26–38, 2008.

10 Diseases of the Eye

Corneal Disorders
- Corneal Laceration
- Granuloma and Periocular Calcification
- Melting Corneal Ulcer
- Keratopathy
- Keratomycosis
- Perforated Corneal Ulcer
- Corneal Abscess
- Indolent Corneal Ulcer

Glaucoma
- Congenital Glaucoma
- Primary (Idiopathic) Glaucoma
- Secondary Glaucoma

Lenticular Disorders
- Immature Cataract
- Mature Cataract
- Hypermature Cataract
- Subluxated Lens
- Lens Rupture
- Uveal Disorders

Uveal Disorders
- Uveitis
- Uveitis and Intravitreous Hemorrhage
- Idiopathic Immune Mediated Keratouveitis
- Equine Recurrent Uveitis
- Leptospirosis and Acute Uveitis
- Chronic Uveitis
- Chronic Uveitis and Keratitis
- Iridal Prolapse
- Choroid Detachment
- Iridal Cysts
- Corpora Nigra Laceration
- Blue to White Irides
- Uveal Cyst
- Intrascleral Prosthesis

Ocular Tumors
- Bulbar Squamous Cell Carcinoma
- Third Eyelid Squamous Cell Carcinoma
- Spindle Cell Sarcoma
- Sarcoid
- Granuloma vs Neoplasm

Fundic Anomalies
- Normal Fundus
- Optic Nerve Degeneration
- Retinal Degeneration
- Peripapillary Butterfly Lesion
- Thin Retina

Corneal Laceration

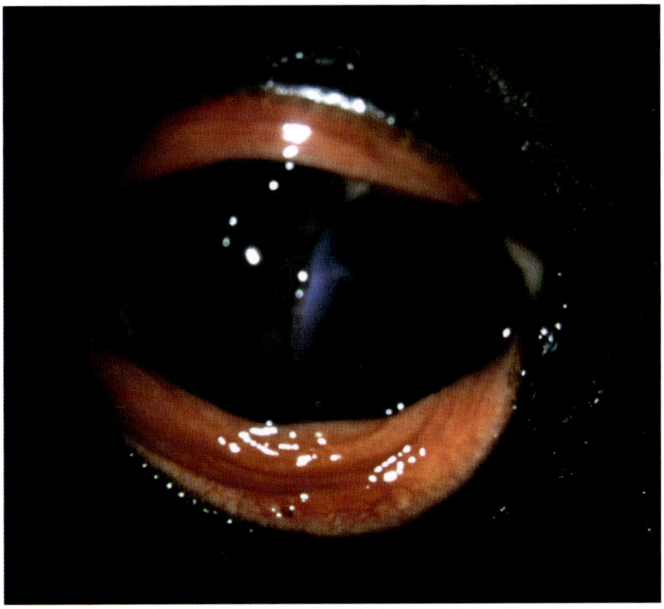

Figure 10.1 Corneal laceration. A full thickness corneal laceration with iridal prolapse has developed acutely after blunt ocular trauma due to a kick to the right facial area. Blunt ocular trauma such as this can result in severe intraocular trauma that often induces avulsion and lacerations of the retina, uvea, and lens. Ocular ultrasonography is advisable before repairing such lacerations surgically to assess the intraocular tissues. The lens was ruptured and expulsed and the retina and choroid, lacerated, and detached, so the eye was enucleated.

Granuloma and Periocular Calcification

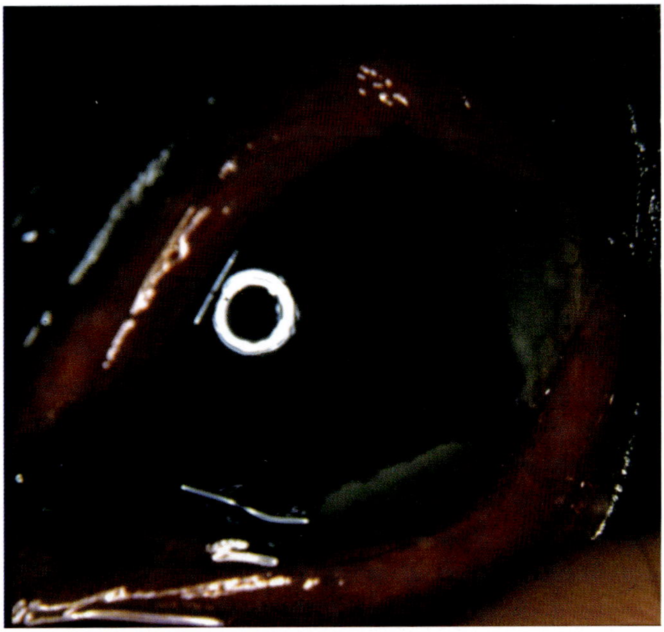

Figure 10.2 Granuloma and periocular calcification. Note the conjunctivitis and chemosis (conjunctival edema), miosis, and white corneal plaques in this Thoroughbred yearling filly. The plaques were gritty in texture when scraped. Cytological examination of the plaque material revealed many eosinophils. Periocular calcification and granulomas are occasionally associated with onchocerca and other migrating round worm infestations in the periocular region of horses. These lesions were debrided and then treated with topical steroidal anti-inflammatory medications.

Melting Corneal Ulcer

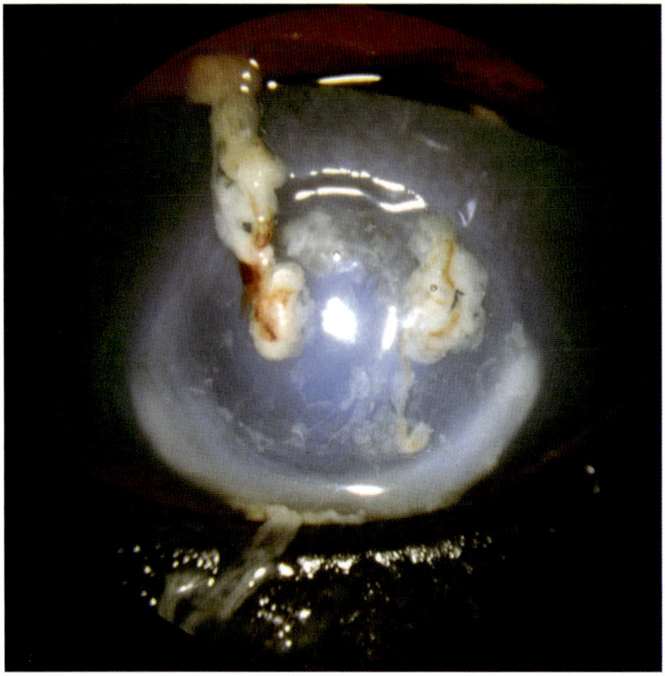

Figure 10.3 Melting corneal ulcer. A large deep melting corneal ulcer is present. Note the purulent ocular discharge and the crater that is present centrally. Collagenolysis develops in infected corneal ulcers in horses as collagenolytic enzymes are released from neutrophils, bacteria, and fungi. Most large collagenolytic corneal ulcers like this are treated surgically and are repaired with a conjunctival pedicle flap and appropriate antimicrobial and nonsteroidal anti-inflammatory medications.

Keratopathy

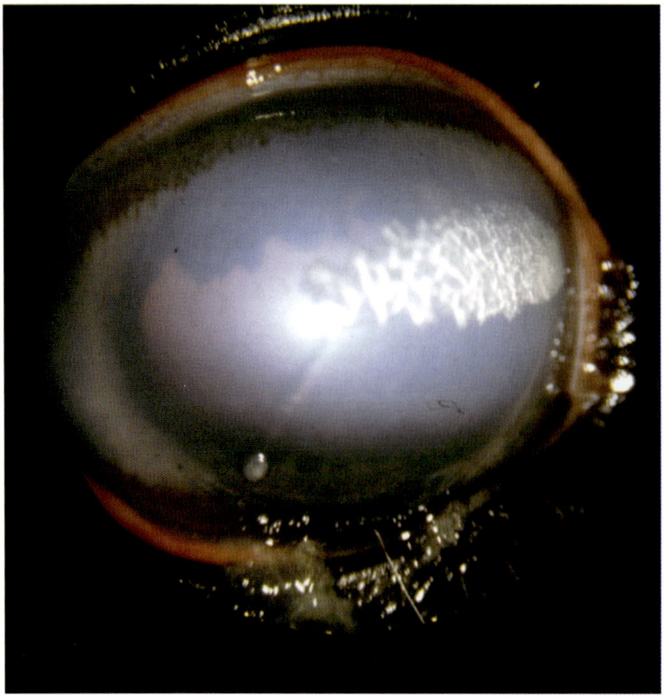

Figure 10.4 Keratopathy. This aged mare has a band keratopathy. Note the diffuse corneal blue haze (corneal edema), and the oval paracentral white stromal opacities typical of mineral or lipid infiltrate. Keratopathies such as this are best categorized as corneal degeneration. They usually develop due to mineralization or lipid infiltration around the keratocytes in the corneal stroma. Medical and surgical treatments are usually not effective or required for this chronic degenerative condition.

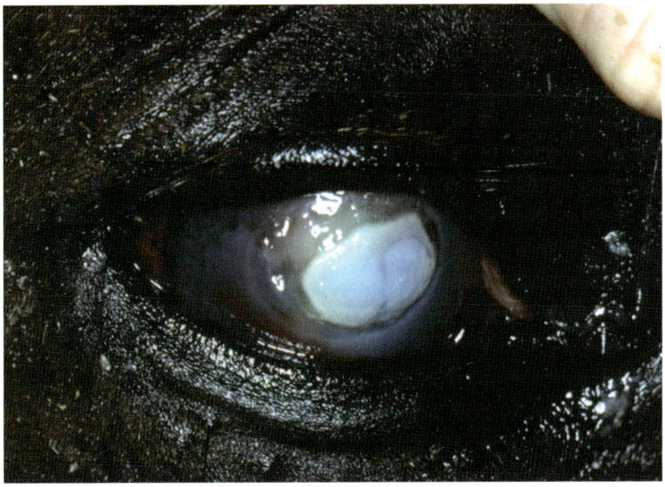

Figure 10.5 Keratomycosis. This is a complex corneal ulcer with a cake frosting–like plaque, cavitations due to collagenolysis, and vascular growth. These clinical manifestations are consistent with a clinical diagnosis of keratomycosis. Fungal organisms were documented with cytology, culture, and biopsy. Fungal keratitis was treated successfully with keratectomy, conjunctival pedicle flap, and topical antifungal, parasympatholytic, and antibiotic medications.

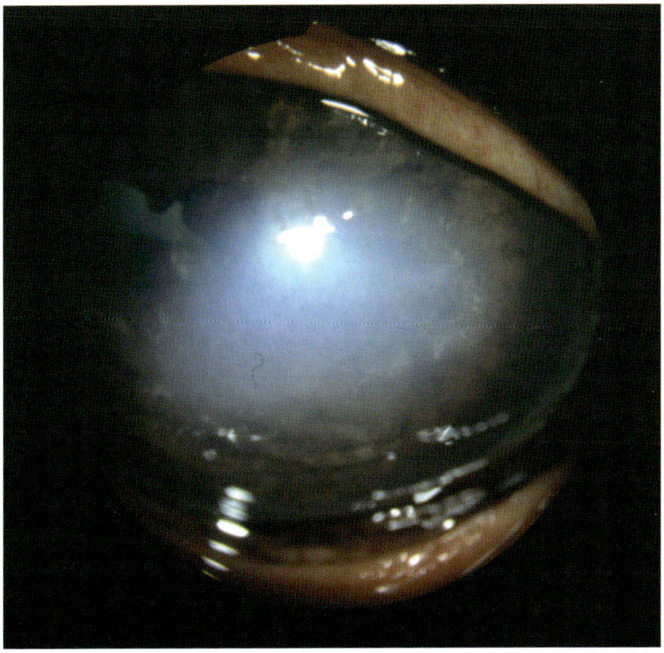

Figure 10.6 Keratomycosis. This is a large corneal ulcer with multiple satellite lesions (white opacities). These manifestations are consistent in appearance with some forms of keratomycosis, and septic corneal ulcers. The preferred diagnostic approach includes cytologic examination, fungal and aerobic and anaerobic bacterial cultures, and, if possible, corneal biopsy for histological examination. Keratomycosis was confirmed and treated with a keratectomy and conjunctival pedicle flap and appropriate topical medical ocular therapies.

Perforated Corneal Ulcer

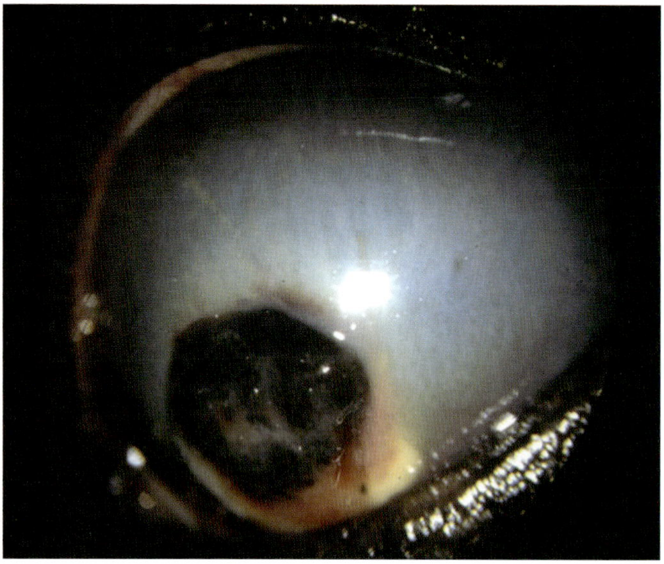

Figure 10.7 Perforated corneal ulcer. Note the iridal prolapse through a perforated deep corneal ulcer in this adult Standardbred gelding. The focal yellow opacity dorsally is consistent in appearance with a stromal abscess. The most likely cause of this prolapse was a perforated collagenolytic corneal ulcer that developed over the stromal abscess. The preferred therapy is surgical repair of the corneal defect, iridal prolapse replacement, and appropriate medical management (topical ocular antibiotic, parasympatholytic, and nonsteroidal and systemic nonsteroidal anti-inflammatory medications).

Corneal Abscess

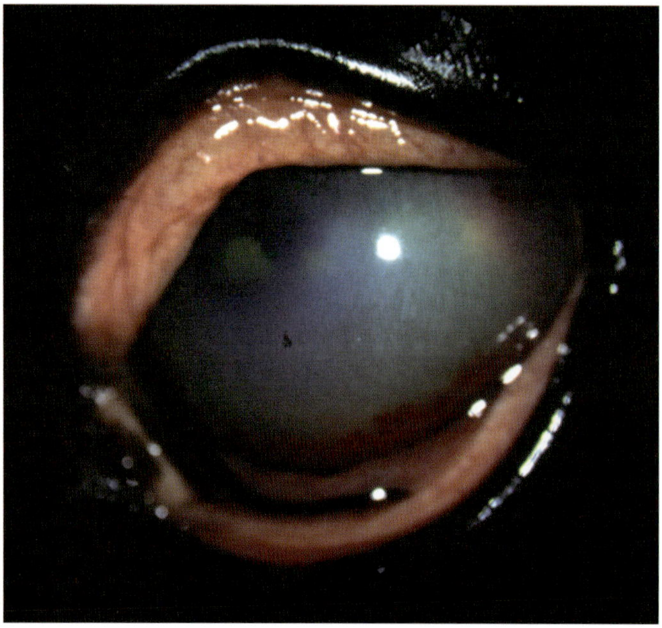

Figure 10.8 Corneal abscess. Conjunctivitis, chemosis, corneal vascularization and abscess, and miosis are present in the eye of this 3-year-old Thoroughbred gelding. Corneal abscesses can be septic or sterile, and may develop secondary to penetrating corneal stromal foreign bodies. They can be treated medically with long-term topical antibiotics and nonsteroidal anti-inflammatory medications, or surgically with a keratectomy, conjunctival pedicle flap, and appropriate adjunctive topical medical ocular therapies.

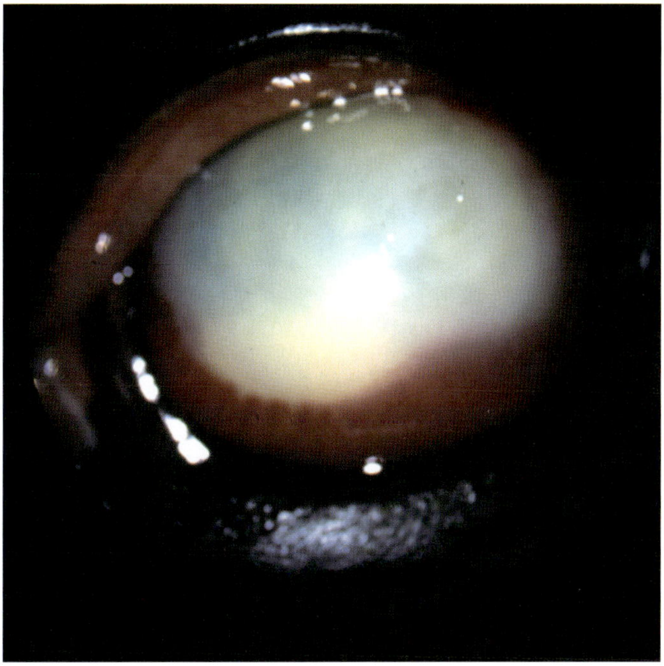

Figure 10.9 Corneal abscess. A nonulcerative corneal abscess extends across most of this cornea. A mixed bacterial and fungal keratitis was confirmed by keratectomy and laboratory culture. The eye was treated effectively with surgical keratectomy, conjunctival pedicle flap, appropriate topical antibiotics, topical nonsteroidal and systemic nonsteroidal anti-inflammatory medications.

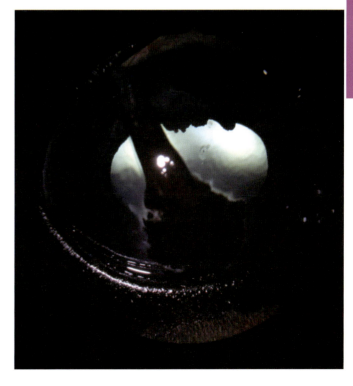

Figure 10.10 Corneal abscess treatment. A healed conjunctival corneal pedicle flap is present on this eye. This flap was sutured to a previous keratectomy site where an abscess was removed. The connecting stalk was severed under topical anesthesia to reduce the size of corneal opacity.

Indolent Corneal Ulcer

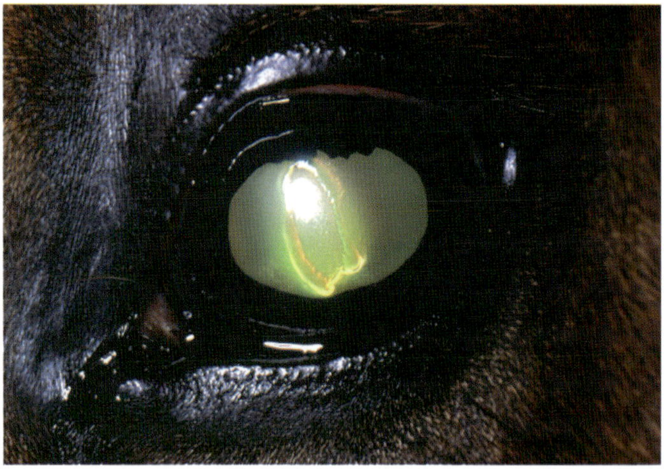

a

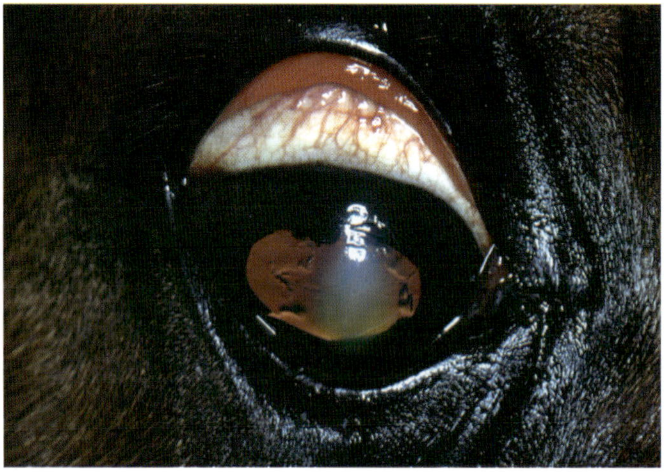

b

Figures 10.11a,b Indolent corneal ulcer. A chronic superficial nonhealing (indolent) corneal ulcer in a horse. Note the fluorescein stain migrates underneath the epithelial flaps, image A. The treatment of choice is a superficial keratectomy and striate keratotomy. These procedures were completed under sedation and topical anaesthesia and the cornea was photographed in B. Superficial keratectomy and striate keratotomy will convert most indolent corneal ulcers into simple ulcers, which are treatable with topical antibiotics with or without topical parasympatholytic, and nonsteroidal anti-inflammatory medications. This ulcer, although it had been present for many months, healed promptly within 10 days and all medications were discontinued.

Congenital Glaucoma

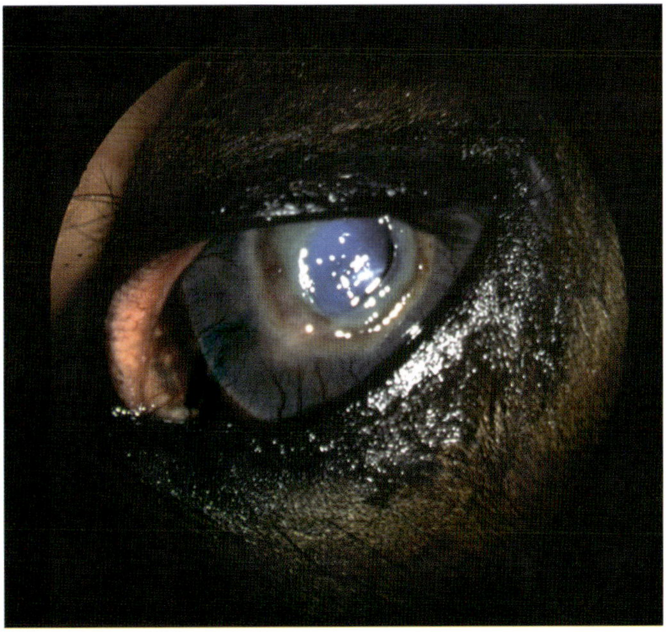

Figure 10.12 Congenital glaucoma. This is a buphthalmic globe in a 7-day-old Arabian filly. This filly was born with bilateral buphthalmos, microphakia, and uveal hypoplasia. The lenses were so small that it could not be identified until the eyes were examined histologically. The corneas were ulcerated and vascularized at birth, and this coupled with buphthalmos at birth. These findings confirm the diagnosis of bilateral congenital glaucoma. The filly was blind and the owner requested euthanasia. Congenital glaucoma develops secondary to an anterior segment dysgenesis, which includes multiple unilateral or bilateral anomalies including, most commonly, microphakia, uveal and filtration angle hypoplasia, and corneal anomalies.

Primary (Idiopathic) Glaucoma

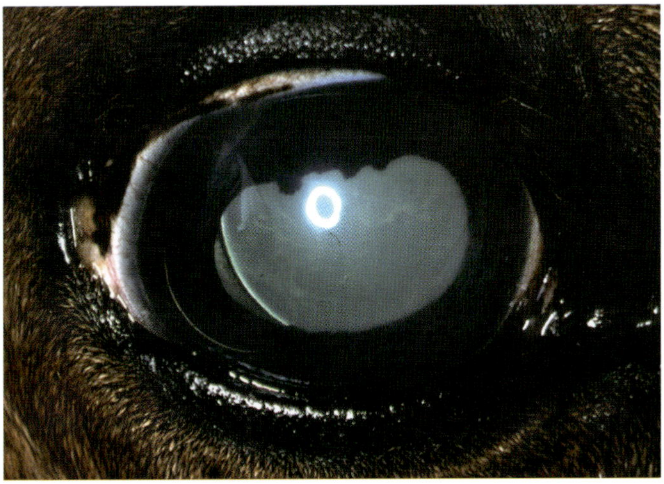

Figure 10.13 Primary (idiopathic) glaucoma. Corneal striae (breaks in Descemet's membrane), an aphakic crescent, and mild buphthalmia are present in this quarter horse. The intraocular pressure was 70 mmHg and the menace reflex was present in this eye. The presenting complaint was corneal opacity. No other ocular abnormalities were present and this supports the diagnosis of primary (idiopathic) glaucoma. Topical therapy with a carbonic anhydrase inhibitor was completed and the response was poor. The eye was treated with transcleral cytophotocoagulation and the intraocular pressure returned to normal reference ranges.

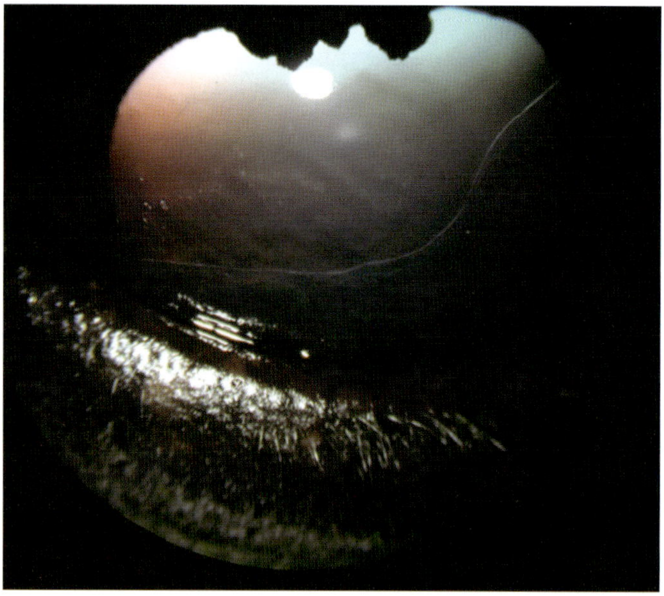

Figure 10.14 Glaucoma vs ocular trauma. Corneal striae (breaks in Descemet's membrane) are occasionally seen in horses in the absence of elevations of intraocular pressure, buphthalmia (rule out with ultrasonography of both eyes), or other intraocular abnormalities, as seen in this eye. In these cases, ocular trauma is assumed to be the etiology, not glaucoma.

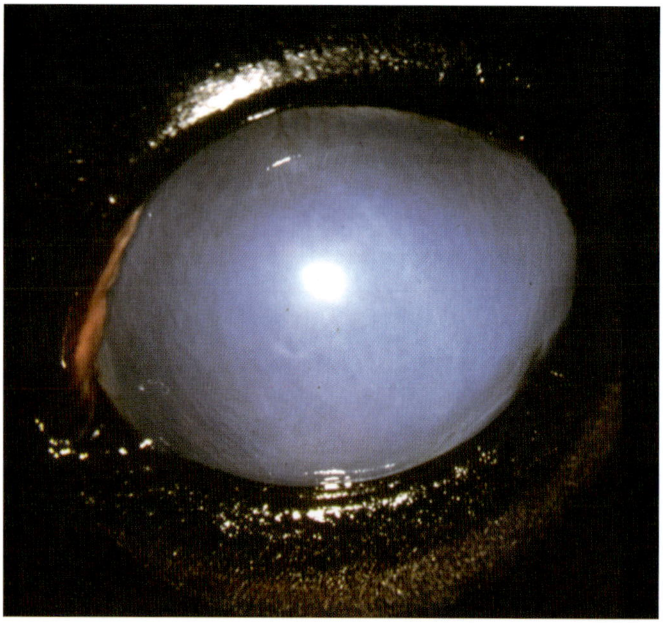

Figure 10.15 Primary (idiopathic) glaucoma. The intraocular pressure estimated with an applanation tonometer was 65 mmHg and confirmed the diagnosis of glaucoma. There was not evidence of other ocular diseases based on the biomicroscopic and indirect ophthalmoscopic and ultrasonographic examinations. The clinical diagnosis was idiopathic (primary) glaucoma and the eye was treated unsuccessfully topically with varied antiglaucoma medications for several weeks before it was enucleated. Light microscopic examination of the globe confirmed the diagnosis of idiopathic glaucoma.

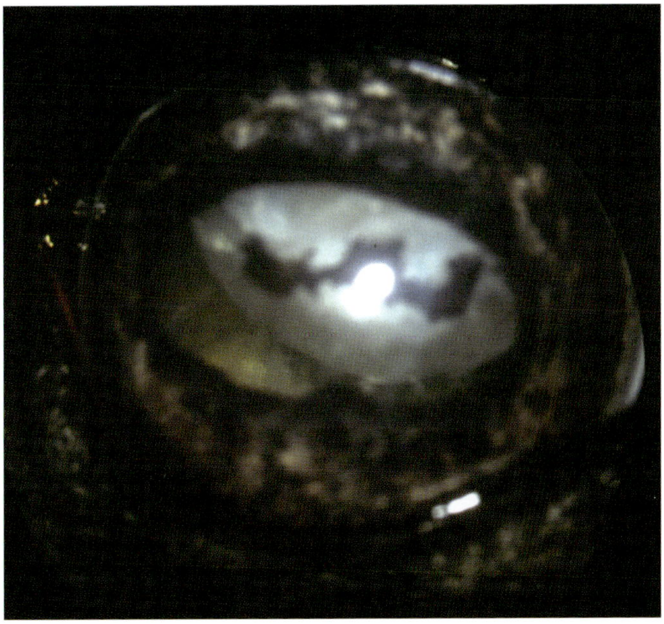

Figure 10.16 Secondary glaucoma. Note the aphakic crescent, cataract, and posterior synechiae in this ageing polo pony. The intraocular pressure was 55 mmHg and the diagnoses included traumatic uveitis, cataract, lens subluxation, and secondary glaucoma. The prognosis for return of vision in an eye such as this is poor. This globe was eviscerated and an intrascleral implant was completed.

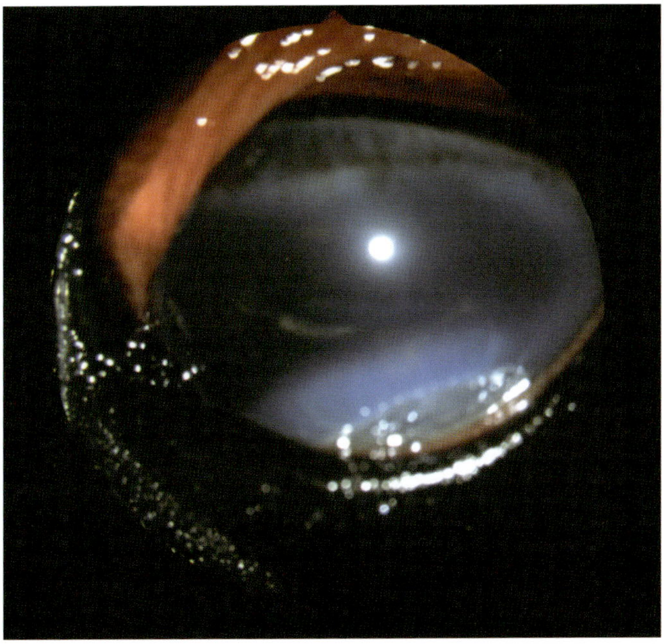

Figure 10.17 Secondary glaucoma. Note the peripheral corneal edema, miosis, and corneal stromal vascularization in this middle-aged horse. The intraocular pressure was 55 mmHg and the anterior chamber was shallow and posterior pupillary synechiae and peripheral anterior synechiae were present. Vitreous degeneration and aqueous and vitreous flare were present bilaterally and confirm the diagnosis of bilateral uveitis and secondary glaucoma. The prognosis for retention of a comfortable and sighted eye was poor. This eye was treated with transcleral laser cytophotocoagulation and topical carbonic anhydrase inhibitor medication, and the recurrent uveitis was treated with systemic nonsteroidal anti-inflammatory medications.

Immature Cataract

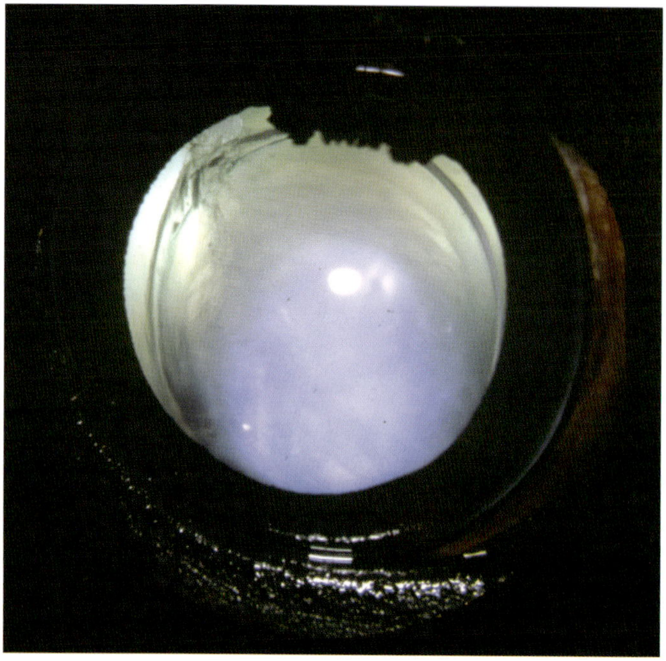

Figure 10.18 Immature cataract. An immature cataract in a yearling Arabian filly. Note the clear cortical rim of the lens, and the dense nuclear cataract. The recommended treatment for cataract in young horses is phacoemulsification, and when lens implants are available, synthetic lens implantation. This filly was affected bilaterally; both lenses were successfully removed by phacoemulsification, and aphakic vision was restored.

Mature Cataract

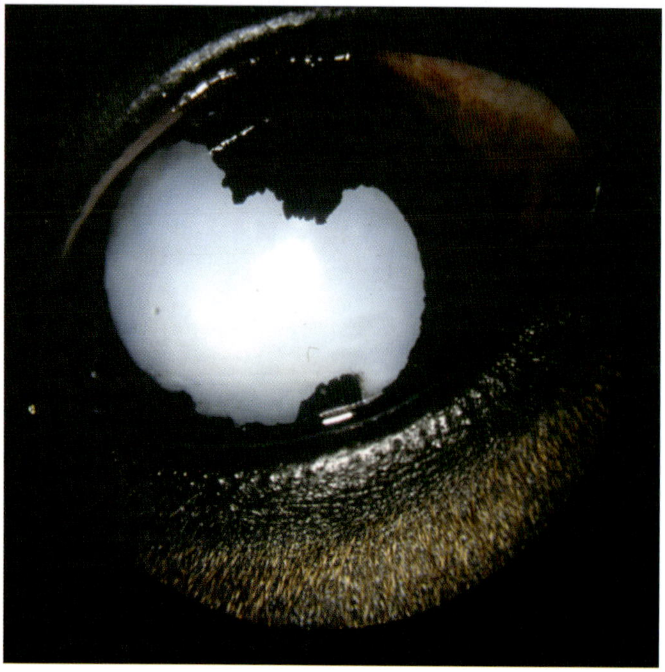

Figure 10.19 Mature cataract. A mature cataract is present in the eye of this young Arabian colt. Note the lack of tapetal reflex and the white leucocoria (white pupil). To restore vision, this lens should be removed and, when available, a lens implant should be placed within the lens capsule.

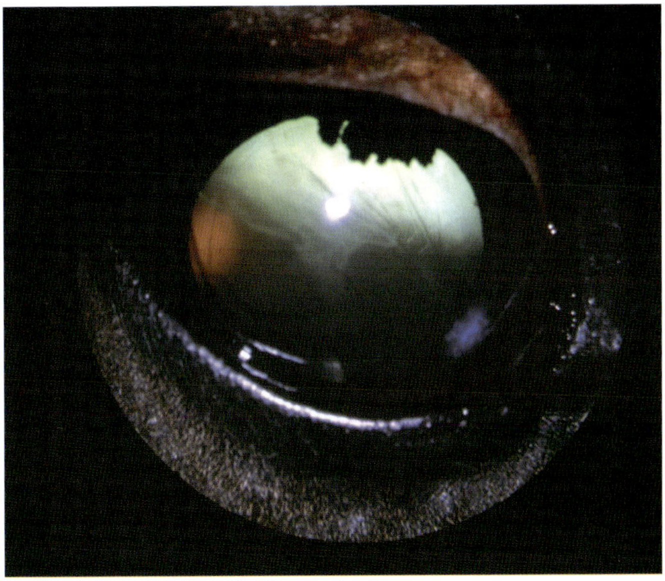

Figure 10.20 Treatment of cataract. The same eye of the horse in fig. 10.19, one month after phacoemulsification. Note the aphakia (i.e., the optic disc is visible at a distance through the pupillary aperture). The small pupillary opacities are folds in the remaining anterior and posterior lens capsules.

Hypermature Cataract

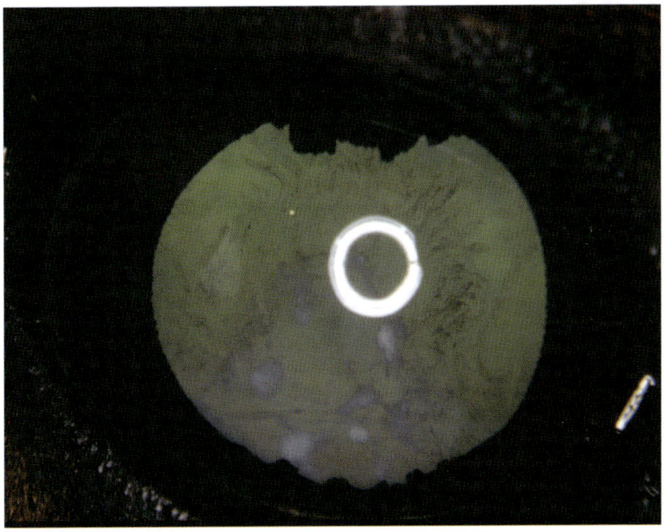

Figure 10.21 Hypermature cataract. This is a hypermature cataract in a young quarter horse. Note the green tapetal reflex is still present. There are multiple white lenticular opacities (incipient cataracts) present as well. The menace reflex was present and biomicroscopic examination confirmed the loss of most lens cortex. The anterior and posterior lens capsules were apposed in several areas, indicating a complete resorption of the lens in these areas. The dark brown iris is hyperpigmented, which commonly develops secondary to sustained uveitis that was likely induced by the ongoing cataract resorption in this young horse. Topical anti-inflammatory medications are indicated daily to suppress this lens-induced uveitis. Surgical removal of this lens is not warranted as the horse is regaining vision as the cataract continues to be absorbed.

Subluxated Lens

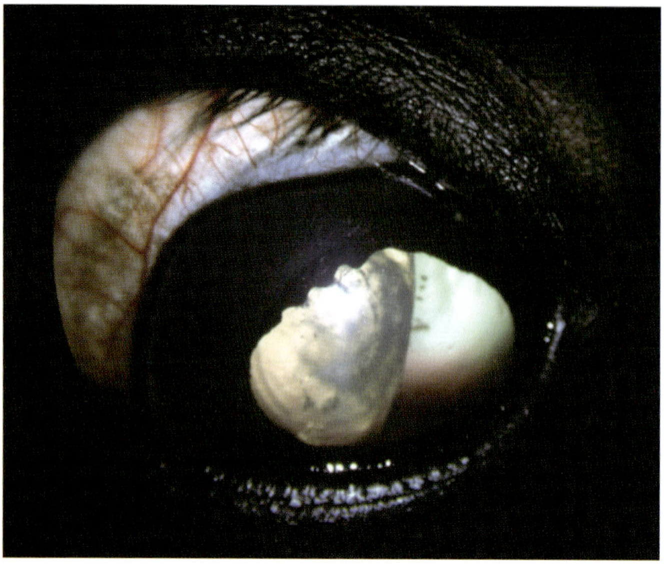

Figure 10.22 Subluxated lens. Note the aphakic crescent, subluxated lens with cataract, in this middle-aged polo pony, who has sustained ocular trauma for many years. This globe had an intraocular pressure within normal range. Ultrasonographic examination confirmed that the cornea to optic nerve depth was similar to the normal contralateral eye. The diagnoses were traumatic immature cataract, subluxated lens, and uveitis. The prognosis for retaining a visual healthy globe in this pony is poor. Treatment options include topical anti-inflammatory medications and intracapsular lens extraction. If the eye becomes blind and inflammation is not controllable, then an enucleation or an evisceration and intrascleral prosthesis implant are warranted.

Lens Rupture

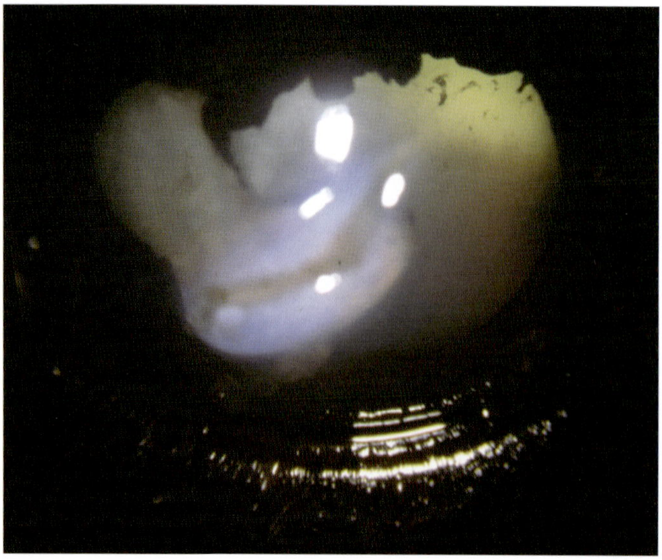

Figure 10.23 Lens rupture. Note the acute corneal and anterior lens capsule perforations in this Thoroughbred gelding. The lens cortex is streaming out of the perforated lens capsule into the corneal perforation. This confirms the diagnosis of acute phacoclastic (lens rupture) uveitis. The only vision retaining therapeutic option is phacoemulsification to remove the ruptured lens. Cornea requires surgical repair and then appropriate medical management to control the uveitis.

Figure 10.24 Lens rupture. This is an inflamed eye of an adult Percheron mare who had sustained a penetrating corneal injury 1 month previous to presentation. The corneal perforation healed and a marked aqueous flare was noted biomicroscopically. Note the salmon pink material (lens cortex debris) within the anterior chamber and covering the pupil. Biomicroscopic examination confirmed the diagnosis of phacoclastic (lens rupture) uveitis. The treatment of choice for this condition is lens removal by phacoemulsification, enucleation, or evisceration with intrascleral prosthesis placement depending on the chronicity and extent of the uveitis and the financial resources of the owner. This eye was enucleated and light microscopic examination confirmed the diagnosis of phacoclastic uveitis.

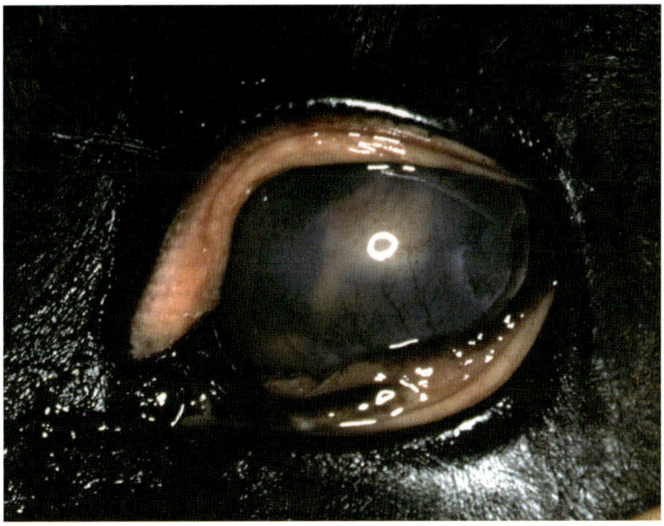

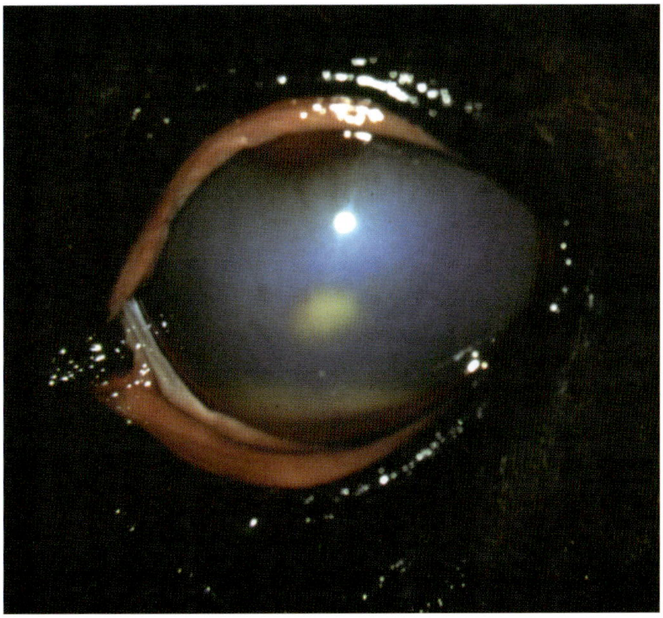

Figure 10.25 Uveitis. Corneal edema, dorsal corneal stromal vascularization, hypopyon, and yellow exudates that extend over the miotic pupil are present in the eye of this adult mare. The clinical diagnosis of phacoclastic uveitis was based on the low intraocular pressure and biomicroscopic identification of aqueous flare and a full thickness corneal scar, and lens rupture. The prognosis for saving a visual globe is poor and the eye was enucleated. Light microscopic examination confirmed fungal endophthalmitis and phacoclastic uveitis.

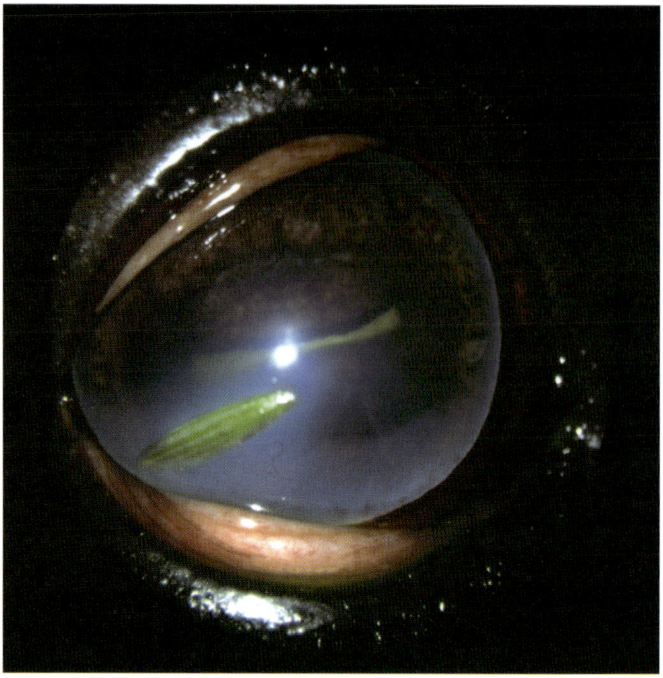

Figure 10.26 Uveitis. Note the corneal foreign body, miosis, and subtle ventral hypopyon. The clinical diagnoses are corneal foreign body and ulceration, and secondary anterior uveitis. The recommended therapies include removal of the grass hull, which was completed under sedation and topical anesthesia. The eye was treated topically with antibiotics and parasympatholytic and nonsteroidal anti-inflammatory medications until the ulcer and uveitis resolved in approximately 10 days.

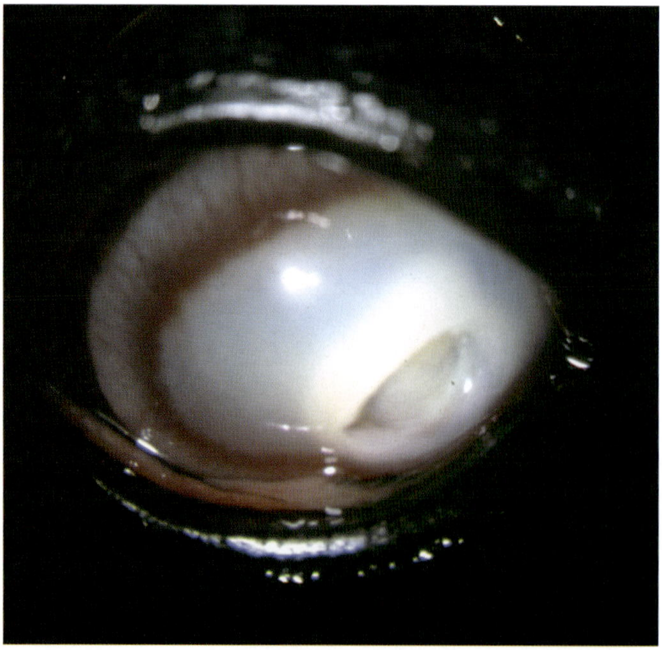

Figure 10.27 Uveitis. This is a perforated corneal abscess with septic endophthalmitis, and phthisis bulbi (shrunken globe). This eye was promptly enucleated as septic endophthalmitis. Although uncommon in the horse, septic endophthalmitis can result in septic meningitis because the infective organisms may invade the optic nerve, which is surrounded by cerebrospinal fluid and is covered by meninges. This horse was treated with systemic antibiotics (penicillin) for approximately 1 week postenucleation, and recovered without complication.

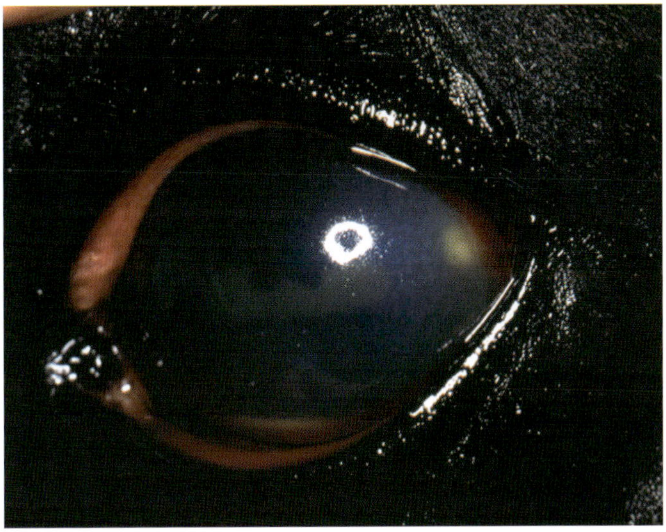

Figure 10.28 Uveitis. A corneal stromal abscess and secondary anterior uveitis are present in this 2-year-old quarter horse mare. Severe anterior uveitis that is accompanied by hypopyon as seen in this case can develop secondary to corneal diseases such as corneal abscesses or septic corneal ulcers.

Uveitis and Intravitreous Hemorrhage

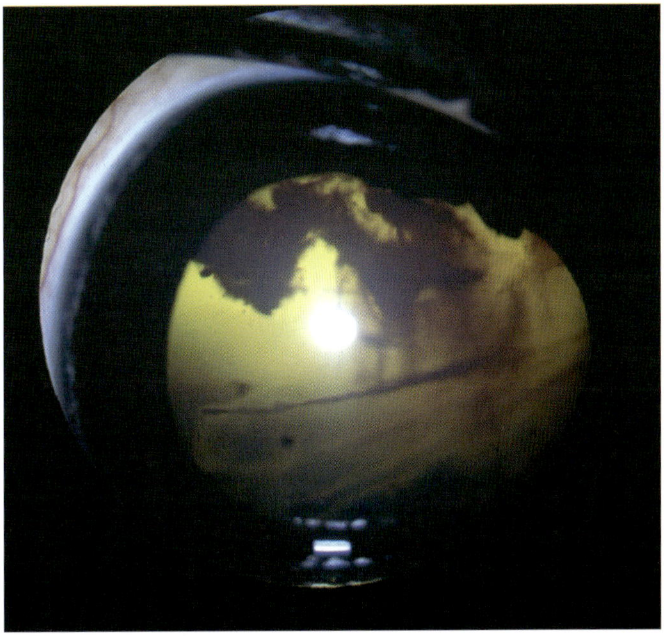

Figure 10.29 Uveitis and intravitreous hemorrhage. Intravitreous hemorrhage is diagnostic of uveitis and there are many potential etiologies, including penetrating or blunt trauma, coagulopathies, intraocular neoplasia, equine recurrent uveitis, etc. A thorough physical, ocular examination and several laboratory tests (coagulation panels, ultrasonography, etc.) are usually required to establish an etiologic diagnosis.

Idiopathic Immune Mediated Keratouveitis

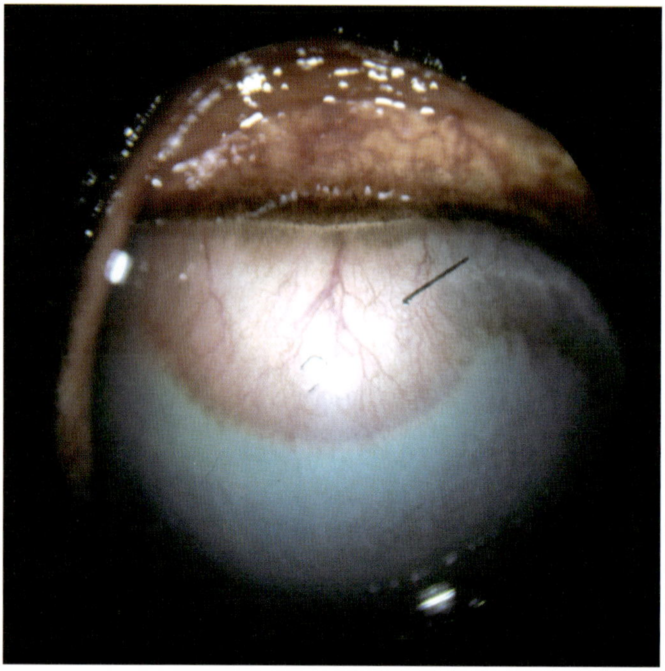

Figure 10.30 Idiopathic immune mediated keratouveitis. Note the vascularized limbal-based mass and marked corneal edema in this quarter horse. The uveitis in this eye was unrelenting and associated with keratitis. The tentative diagnosis was idiopathic immune-mediated keratouveitis. The keratouveitis eventually responded to systemic and topical nonsteroidal anti-inflammatory and steroid medications every 6 hours.

Equine Recurrent Uveitis

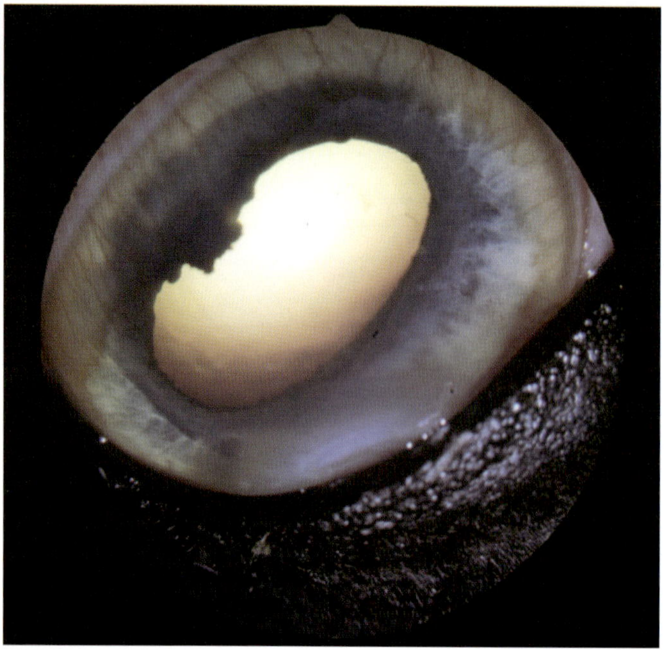

Figure 10.31 Equine recurrent uveitis. Note the corneal stromal vascularization, a subtle miosis, and a yellow discoloration to the aqueous and vitreous in this Appaloosa mare that has been diagnosed with equine recurrent uveitis. The intraocular pressures were consistently low and eventually the uveitis progressed and the mare became blind despite topical and systemic anti-inflammatory therapy. Secondary glaucoma and lens luxations are common sequelae to this bilateral progressive uveitis. The Appaloosa breed is predisposed to this condition.

Leptospirosis and Acute Uveitis

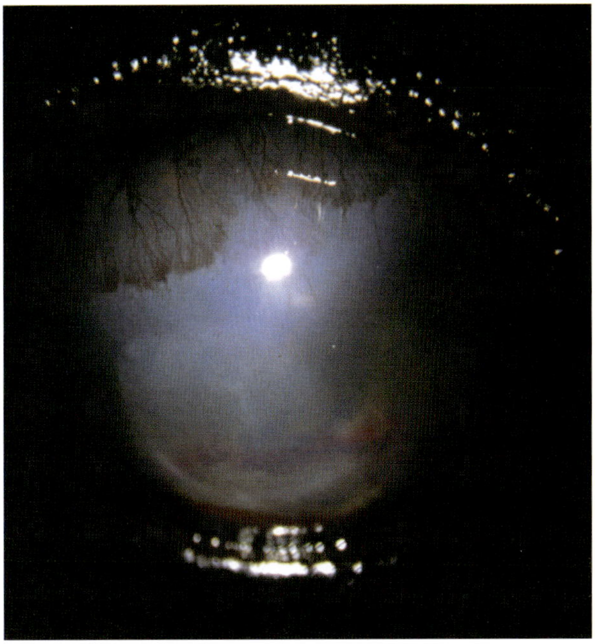

Figure 10.32 Leptospirosis and acute uveitis. Acute uveitis is present in this eye based on the blood clots, corneal vascularization, miosis, and swollen pale iris. These findings confirm the diagnosis. The contralateral eye was affected similarly. This 2-year-old Thoroughbred stallion was hyperthermic and anorexic. A complete blood count revealed neutrophilia. Systemic leptospirosis and uveitis were diagnosed based on positive urine culture and serum titers.

Chronic Uveitis

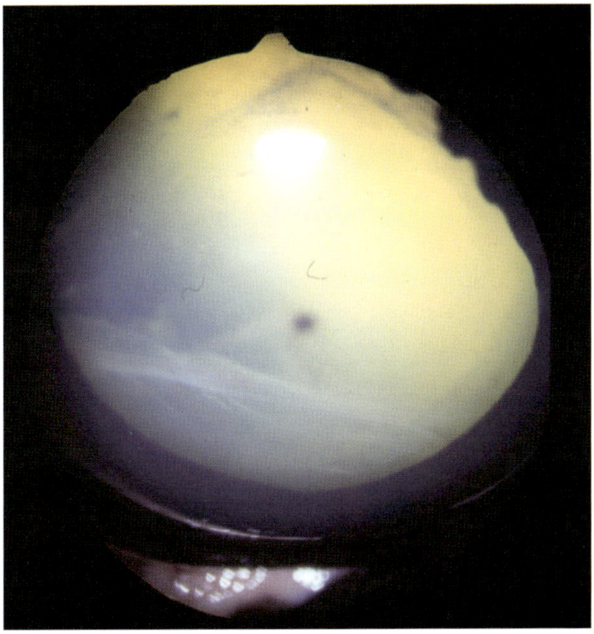

Figure 10.33 Chronic uveitis. Vitreous floaters, collagen clumping, vascularization, and focal pigment dispersion into the vitreous are synonymous with chronic uveitis and can all be seen in this photo. This Appaloosa had been diagnosed with immune-mediated equine recurrent uveitis 3 years previously and had been receiving topical and systemic nonsteroidal anti-inflammatory therapy during the recurrent bouts of uveitis. The prognosis is poor for this progressive condition. Surgical vitrectomy and slow release cyclosporine implants are perhaps the only viable treatment options for progressive bilateral equine recurrent uveitis.

Chronic Uveitis and Keratitis

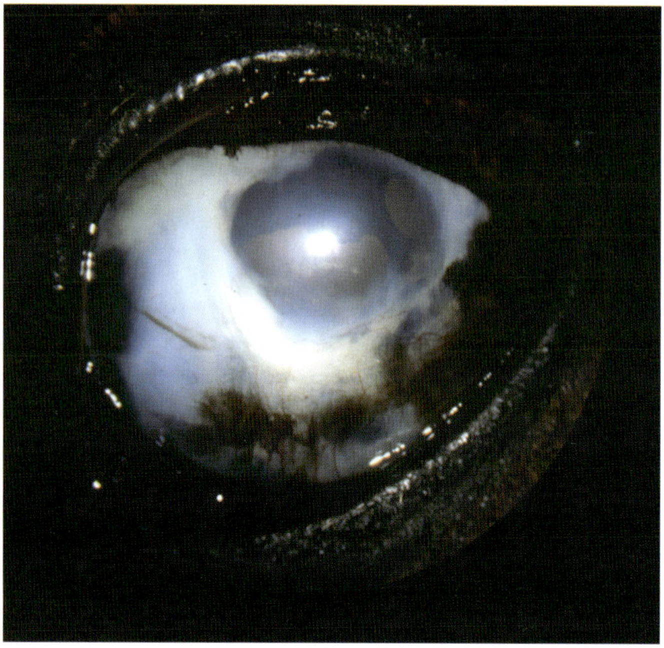

Figure 10.34 Chronic uveitis and keratitis. Note the corneal pigmentation, scarring, and anterior and posterior synechiae in this aging saddle horse gelding. These clinical signs are characteristic of chronic keratitis and uveitis. The intraocular pressure was within normal range and there was no evidence of an active uveitis. The contralateral eye had no abnormalities.

Iridal Prolapse

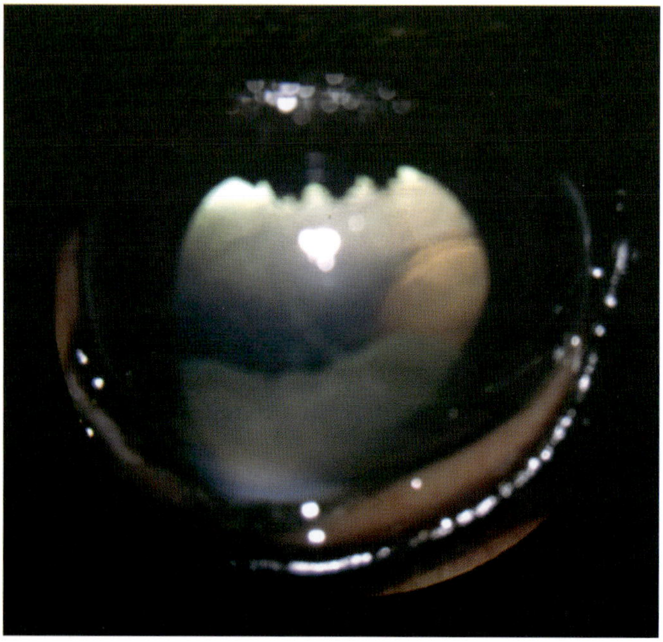

Figure 10.35 Iridal prolapse. There is yellow-tan colored fibrin within the anterior chamber of the eye of a young filly. Note how it streams ventrally and exits through a ventral corneal perforation, where there is a small iridal prolapse. The diagnosis is corneal perforation, iridal prolapse, and secondary anterior uveitis. The treatment of choice is surgical repair of the cornea, which was successfully performed in this horse. The eye was also treated with topical parasympatholytic, antibiotic, and nonsteroidal anti-inflammatory medications until the cornea had healed and the uveitis had abated.

Choroid Detachment

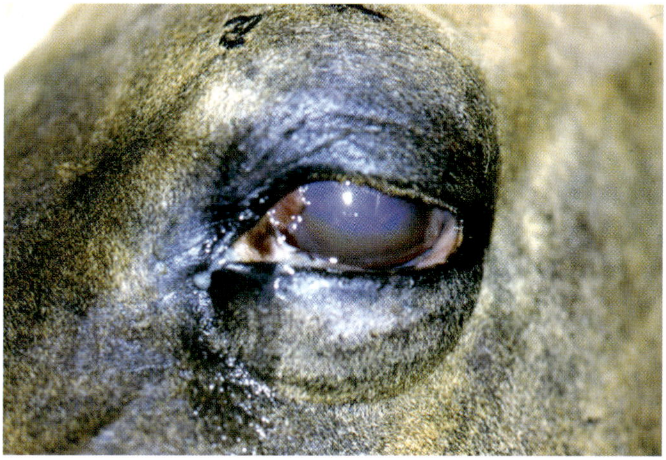

Figure 10.36 Choroid detachment. Note the swollen periocular tissues, eyelid hemorrhage, hyphema, and corneal edema, which are common accompaniments to blunt ocular trauma that occurred in this horse. The prognosis for vision is poor as the intraocular tissues are often severely traumatized at the time of injury. An ultrasonographic examination is warranted to assess the retina, lens, and uvea before advising therapy. Ruptured lens, avulsed retinas, and detached choroid are common accompaniments. If they are present, the eye may be eviscerated and have an intrascleral prosthesis placed. Alternatively, the eye may be enucleated as these complications will often lead to phthisis bulbi.

Iridal Cysts

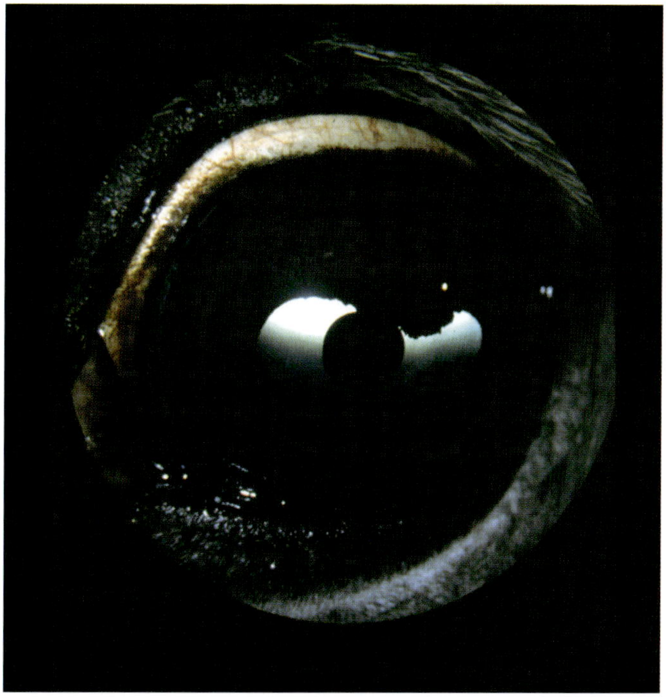

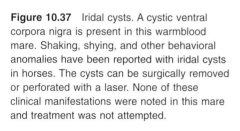

Figure 10.37 Iridal cysts. A cystic ventral corpora nigra is present in this warmblood mare. Shaking, shying, and other behavioral anomalies have been reported with iridal cysts in horses. The cysts can be surgically removed or perforated with a laser. None of these clinical manifestations were noted in this mare and treatment was not attempted.

Corpora Nigra Laceration

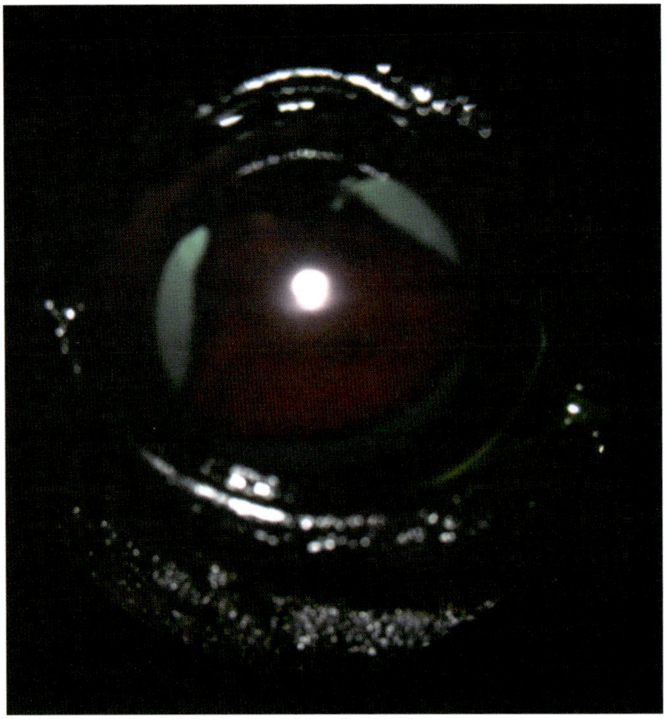

Figure 10.38 Corpora nigra laceration. A large anterior chamber blood clot is present that originated from a lacerated corpora nigra secondary to ocular trauma. The diagnosis was traumatic anterior uveitis and the eye was treated topically with mydriatics and corticosteroids until the clot dissolved and the uveitis was controlled. Further ocular complications were not observed.

Blue to White Irides

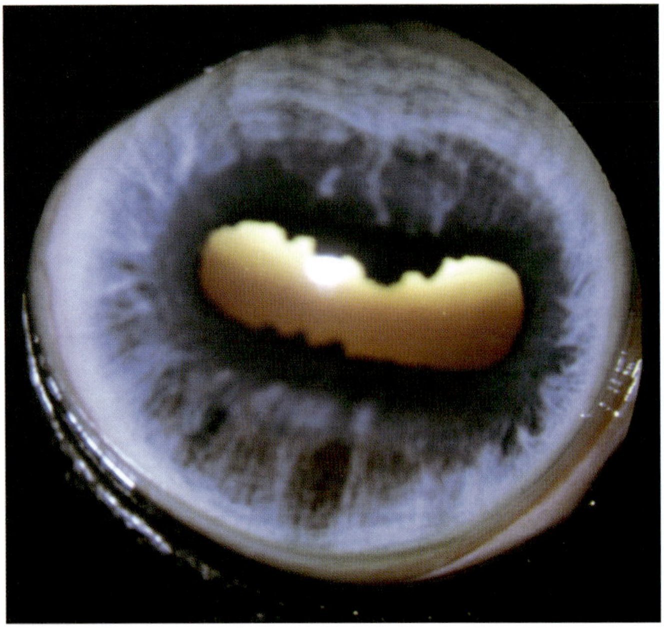

Figure 10.39 Blue to white irides. Blue to white irides are common in color dilute horses. The uvea is hypoplastic and thin in these animals. Note that the posterior iris epithelium is visible through the ventral iridal stroma in this horse. This is a normal eye.

Uveal Cyst

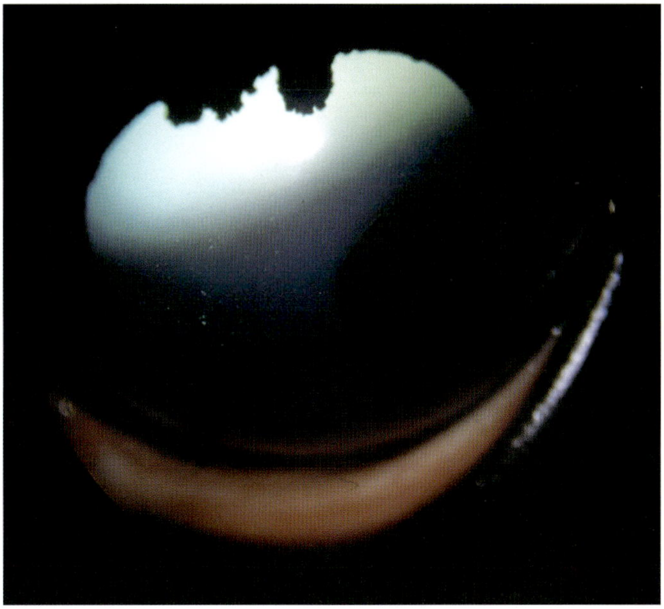

Figure 10.40 Uveal cyst. A uveal cyst has floated into the anterior chamber of this warmblood gelding. Uveal cysts are usually idiopathic in horses and they originate from the iridal or ciliary epithelium. They break free and float forward into the anterior chamber. Treatment is usually not required. However, if the horse develops clinical signs such as head-shaking or shying, the cyst can be perforated by a laser and left to settle in the anterior chamber. It also can be surgically aspirated.

Intrascleral Prosthesis

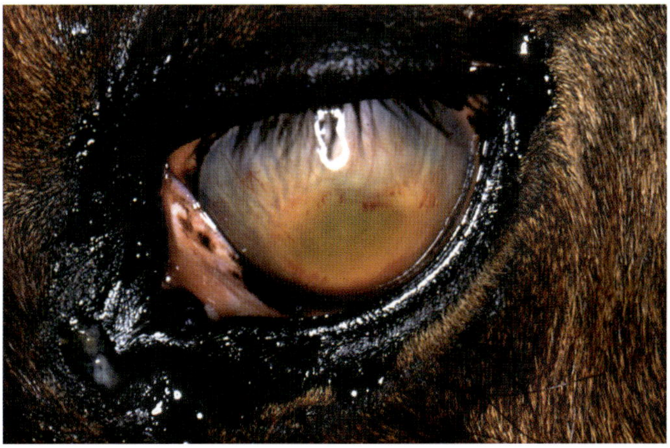

Figure 10.41 Intrascleral prosthesis. This eye is 3 weeks postintrascleral prosthesis surgery. This eye was blind and the glaucoma was not responsive to topical medical management. The cornea is vascularized and scarring around the intraocular implant. All medications have been discontinued. The cornea will continue to remodel and scar and will turn grey in color in a few weeks.

Bulbar Squamous Cell Carcinoma

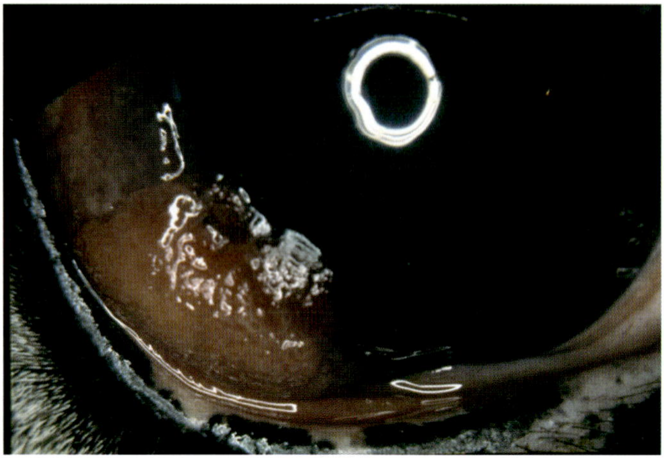

Figure 10.42 Bulbar squamous cell carcinoma. This is a classic appearance of bulbar squamous cell carcinoma, which has invaded the temporal cornea from the limbal conjunctiva in this 10-year-old paint mare. The prognosis for curing this neoplasia is excellent provided that clean surgical margins are established. Map biopsies of the perimeter of the conjunctiva and an accurate keratectomy with the aid of an operating microscope are essential. Adjunctive therapies are commonly employed including cryotherapy.

Third Eyelid Squamous Cell Carcinoma

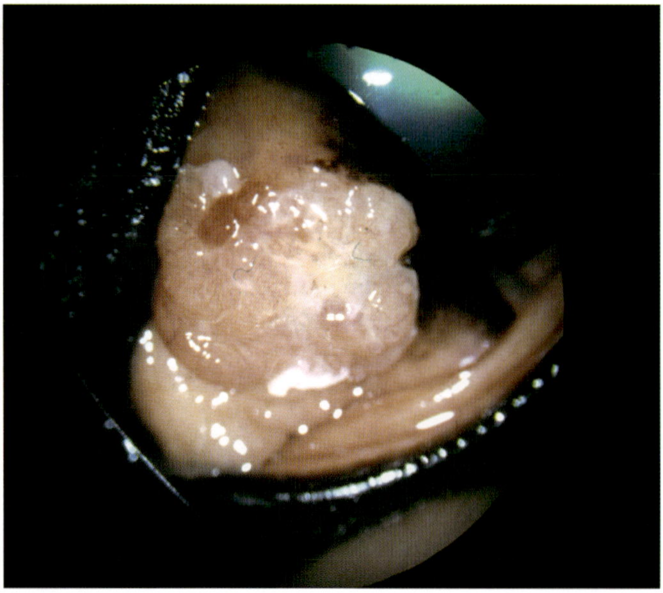

Figure 10.43 Third eyelid squamous cell carcinoma. This salmon pink friable third eyelid mass is consistent in appearance with third eyelid squamous cell carcinoma. Before establishing a treatment plan, a small biopsy should be submitted for light microscopic examination. Squamous cell carcinomas of the third eyelid are best treated by removal of the third eyelid surgically and light microscopic examination of the excised tissue to ensure clean margins. The prognosis for the globe and horse are excellent.

Spindle Cell Sarcoma

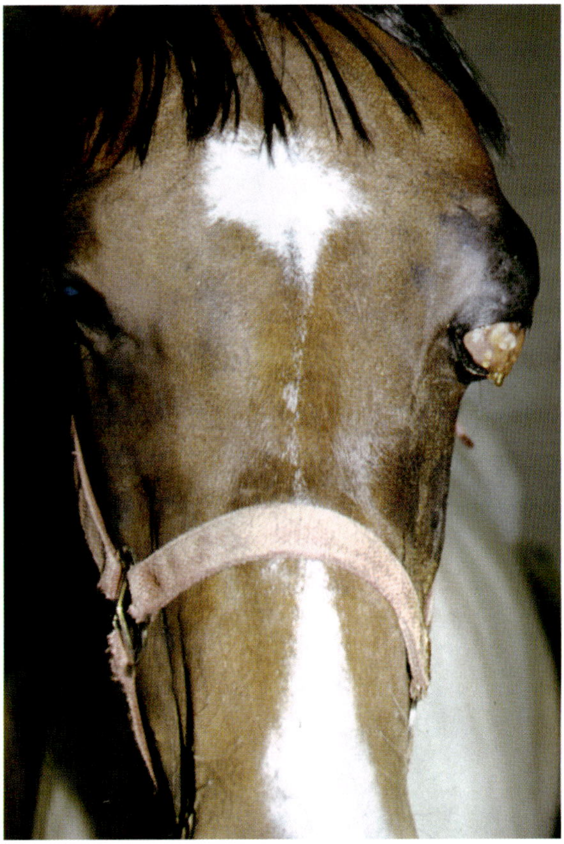

Figure 10.44 Spindle cell sarcoma. A tumor has invaded the left orbit in this horse and has displaced the eye dorsally and temporally. A biopsy has confirmed a spindle cell sarcoma. Most orbital neoplasms in horses have a very poor prognosis for the globe and life as many metastasize despite various surgical, chemotherapeutic, and radiation therapies. Despite local injections of cisplatin this horse succumbed to metastatic disease within weeks.

Sarcoid

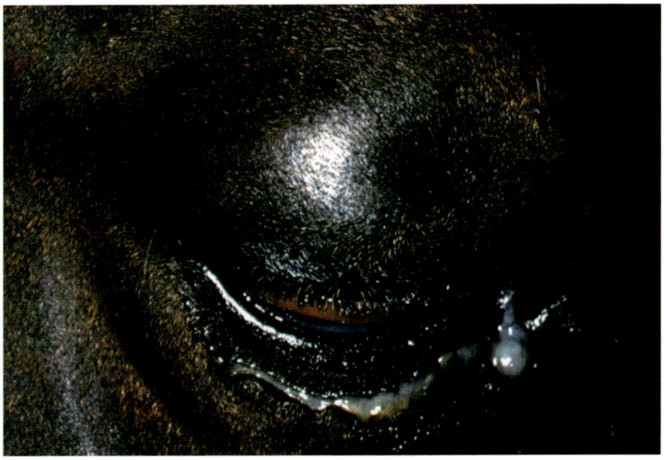

Figure 10.45 Sarcoid. The upper eyelid in this horse is thickened and the mass is firm. A biopsy is warranted to confirm the diagnosis of sarcoid. When eyelid sarcoid is diagnosed, the most common and effective immunotherapy is intralesional bacilli Calmette-Guerin (BCG) injections. Several alternative therapies are also effective including cisplatin injections, cryotherapy, hyperthermia, brachytherapy, and surgical removal.

Granuloma vs Neoplasm

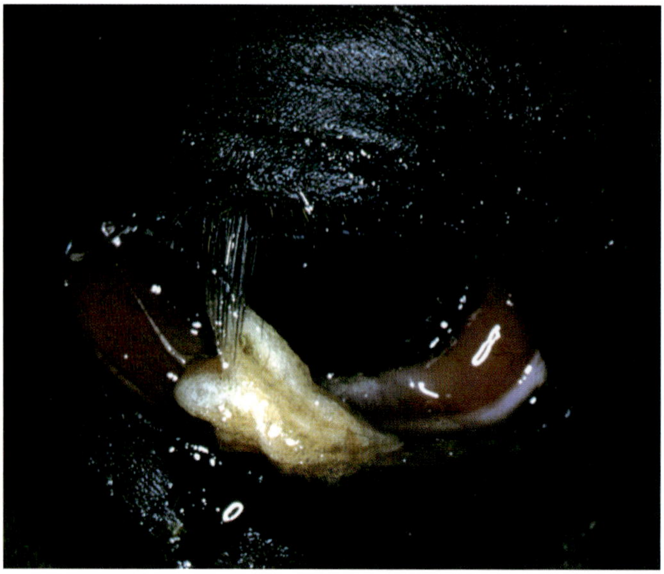

Figure 10.46 Granuloma vs neoplasm. There is a foreign body imbedded in the lower eyelid that was inducing a granulomatous response that could have been mistaken as a neoplasm. A biopsy is important to establish appropriate therapy and prognosis.

Fundic Anomalies

Normal Fundus

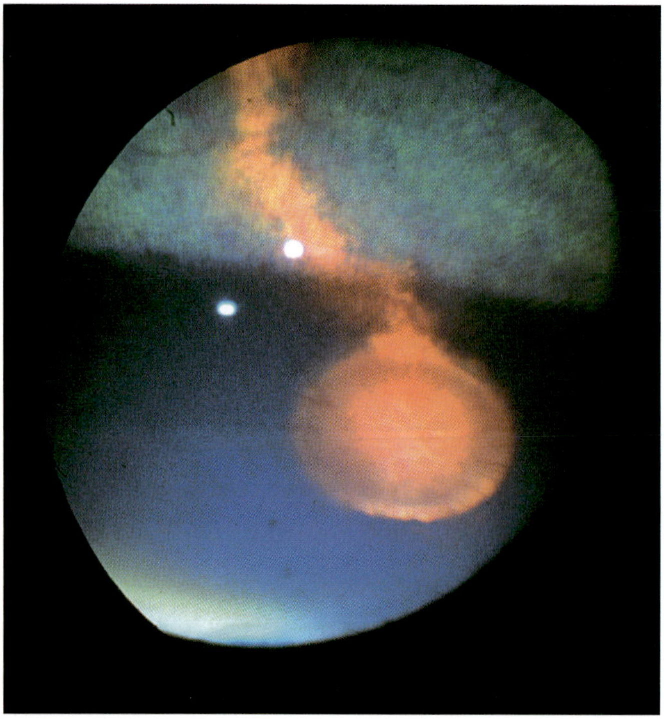

Figure 10.47 Normal fundus. This is a normal fundus from a color dilute pony. Note the orange choroidal streak that extends from the optic disc dorsally. This streak is a region where the tapetum and choroid are poorly developed and pigmented, respectively. These changes allow us to observe the choroidal vascular color.

Optic Nerve Degeneration

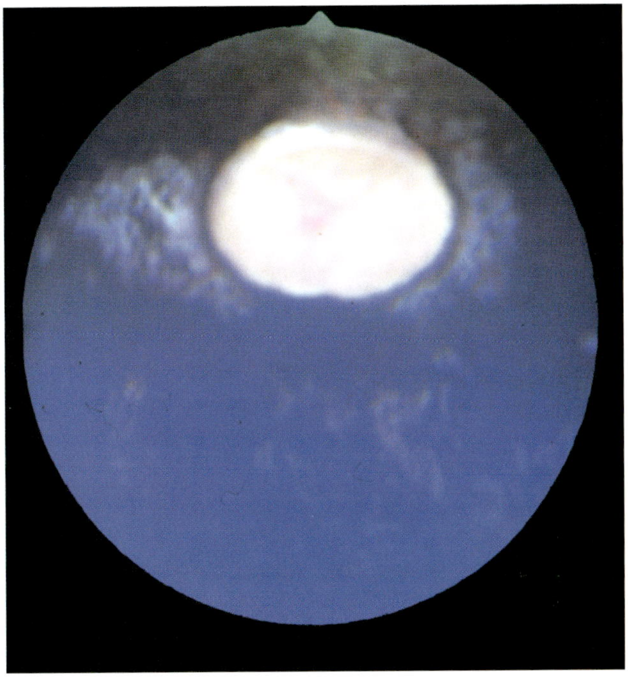

Figure 10.48 Optic nerve degeneration. This optic nerve is degenerate secondary to a previous head trauma that induced optic nerve damage and blindness. Note the pale degenerate optic nerve and loss of peripapillary retinal vessels. See also Chapter 4, Diseases of the Nervous System.

Retinal Degeneration

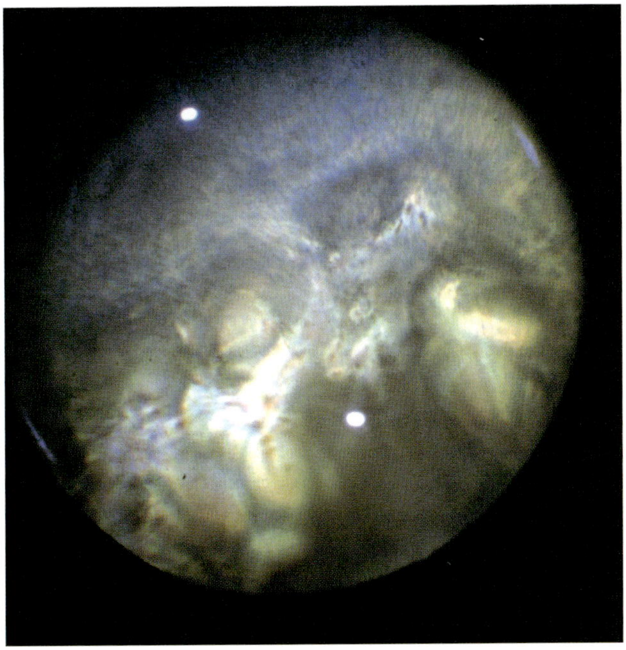

Figure 10.49 Retinal degeneration. There are multiple focal areas of retinal degeneration marked by hyper-reflectivity and focal serous detachments related to an idiopathic choroiditis in this aging Thoroughbred mare.

Peripapillary Butterfly Lesion

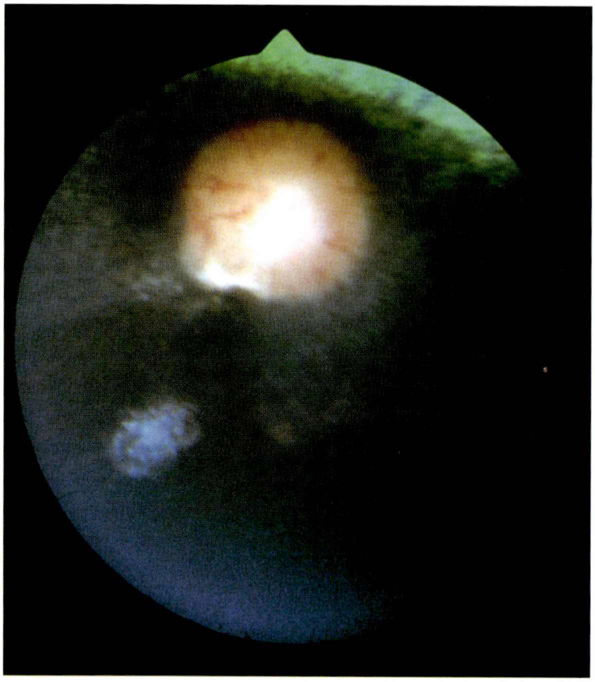

Figure 10.50 Peripapillary butterfly lesion. The classic peripapillary butterfly lesion is seen commonly in horses and has been perhaps in error associated with equine recurrent uveitis. The lesion represents a focal loss of choroidal pigment and the presence of a choroidal scar.

Thin Retina

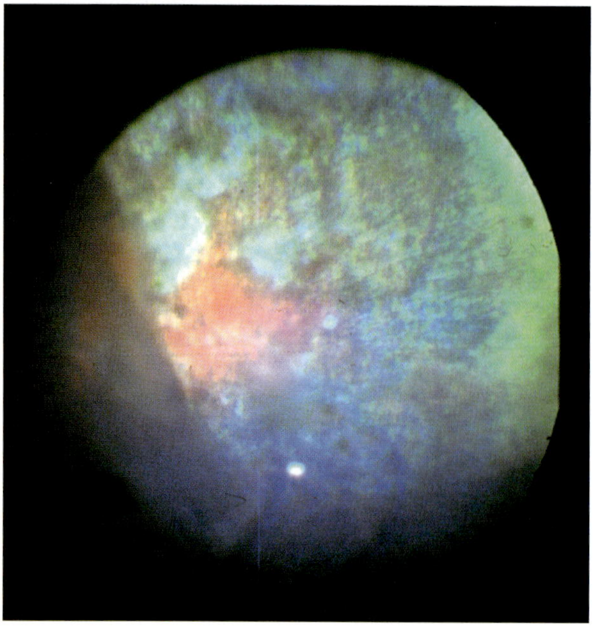

Figure 10.51 Thin retina. Multiple ciliary epithelial cysts are present with multiple semicircular areas of thin retina manifest with mild tapetal hyper-reflectivity. These cysts and curvilinear streaks are common in Rocky Mountain horses with inherited multiple ocular anomalies.

Recommended Reading

Gelatt KN. Veterinary ophthalmology. 4th ed. Ames, IA: Blackwell Publishing, 2007.
Gilger BC. Equine ophthalmology. Philadelphia: WB Saunders, 2005.
Martin C. Ophthalmic disease in veterinary medicine. London: Manson Publishing, 2005.

11

Diseases of the Urinary System

Diseases of the Urinary System
- Psychogenic Polydipsia
- Acute Renal Failure
- Chronic Renal Failure
- Pyelonephritis
- Cystitis
- Verminous Nephritis
- Urethral Rent or Defect
- Urolithiasis (Urethrolithiasis, Cystolithiasis, and Nephrolithiasis)

Psychogenic Polydipsia

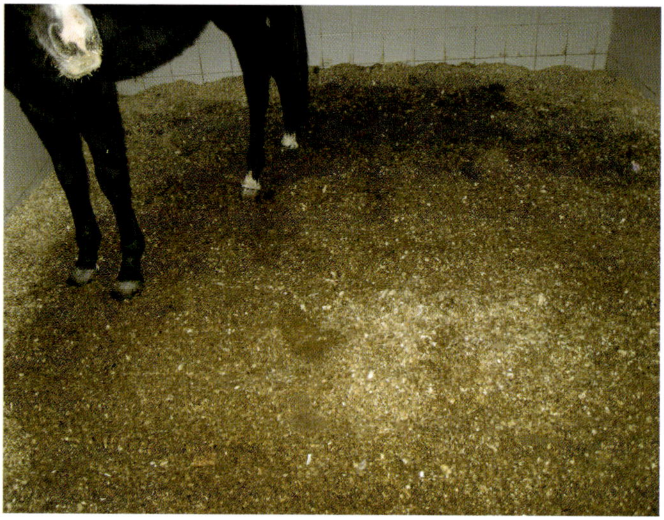

Figure 11.1 Horse affected with psychogenic polydipsia. It is one of the most common causes of PU/PD in mature, young stabled horses and is associated with boredom. Predisposing factors include changes in diet or environment, excessive salt, or dry matter intake. Affected animals are in good body condition, have a very low specific gravity urine (SG < 1.005), and are not azotemic. Owners report that horses with PU/PD drink two to three times more water than their stable mates and their stables are often flooded with urine as in this photo. Water deprivation test is used to confirm this condition. Result will depend on the chronicity of the disease; if polydipsia/polyuria is not long standing (several weeks), affected horses usually concentrate their urine, except in long-standing cases, in which the urine is not concentrated due to renal "medullary wash-out." Horses with medullary wash-out and psychogenic polydipsia usually concentrate their urine in response to the gradual restriction of water as practiced in the modified water deprivation test. Management of this condition is centered on reducing boredom, frequent feeding with increasing the amount of forage, more exercise, and alteration of the management routine. Water availability can be restricted, but should always be sufficient to meet maintenance (50 ml/kg/day), work, and environmental needs of the horse.

Acute Renal Failure

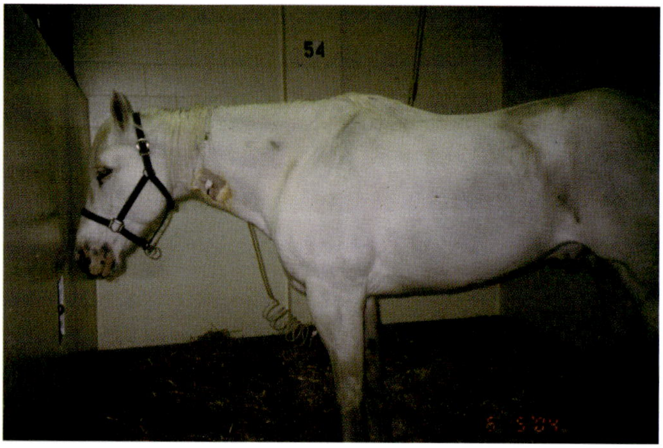

Figure 11.2 A horse affected with acute renal failure, note the severe depression. Renal failure can be caused by exposure to nephrotoxins (aminoglycosides, nonsteroidal anti-inflammatory drugs, myoglobin, and vitamins K_3 or D) or vasomotor nephropathy (hypoperfusion or ischemia). Clinical signs include more marked depression (as seen in this photograph) and anorexia than what is expected for the primary diseases process. Affected horses are usually azotemic with abnormal urinalysis findings. Those include hematuria (fig. 11.3), proteinuria, the presence of casts, and decreased specific gravity. Other clinical findings will depend on the primary disease process. Acute renal failure in horses is initially associated with anuria or oliguria, which could be followed by polyuria if the horse survives.

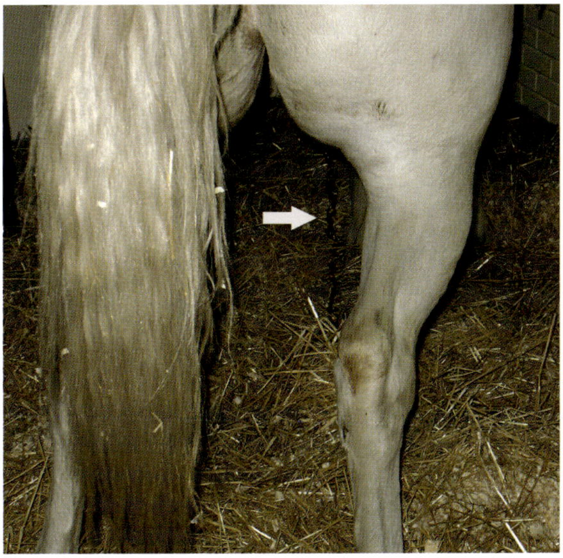

a

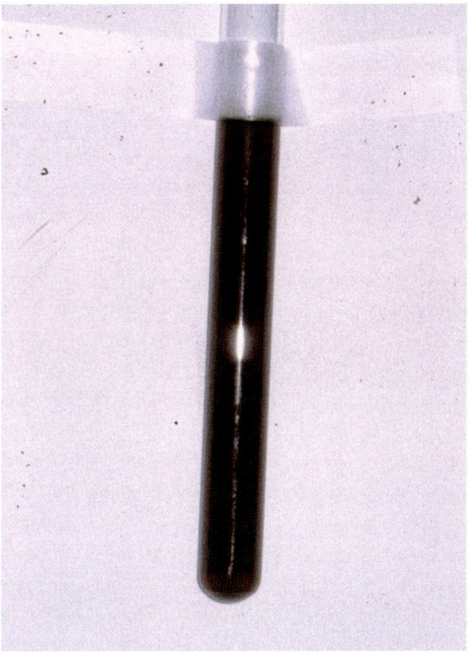

b

Figures 11.3a,b Hematuria (arrow) in a horse affected with acute renal failure (image A). Image B shows the urine collected in a test tube from the same horse shown in image A.

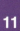

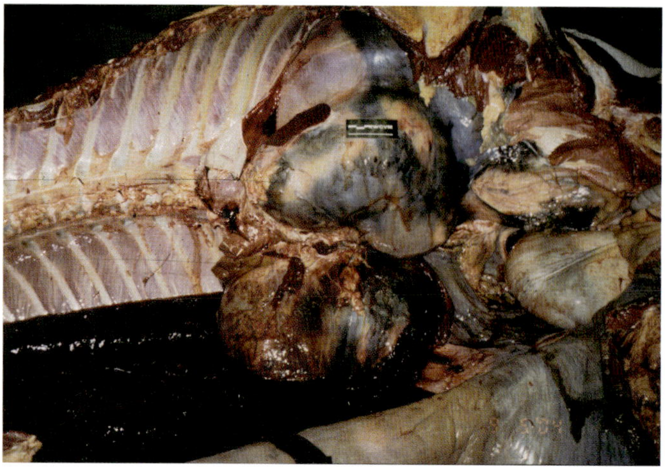

Figure 11.4 Postmortem photograph of a horse affected with acute renal failure; note the severely swollen kidneys.

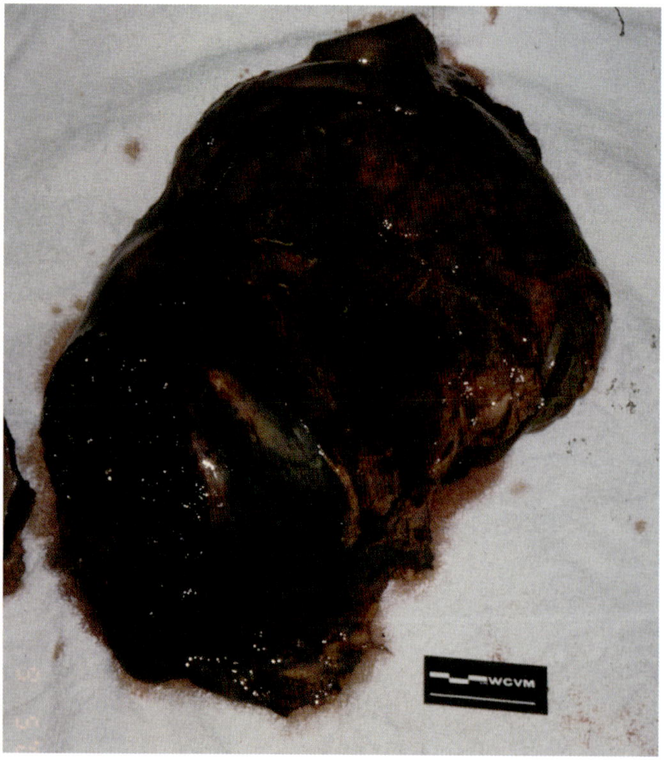

Figure 11.5 Postmortem photograph of a kidney in a horse affected with acute renal failure. Affected kidneys swell as in the previous photograph and may rupture as in this photograph.

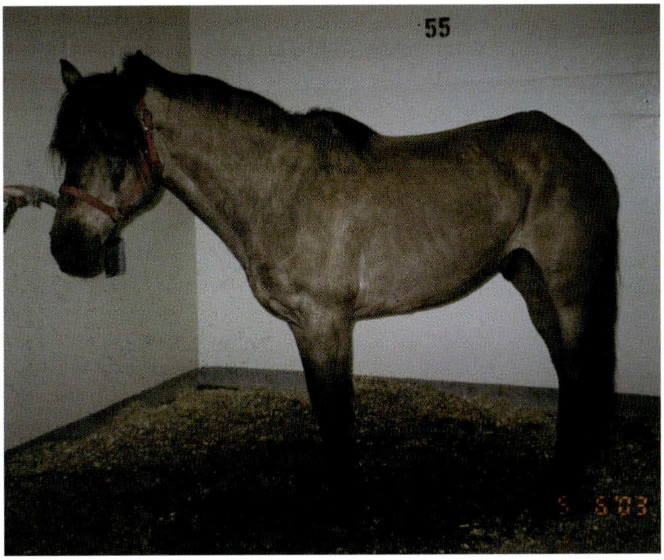

Figure 11.6 Weight loss in a horse affected with chronic renal failure (CRF). CRF can be caused by proliferative glomerulonephritis (immune mediated) (fig. 11.7), chronic interstitial nephritis (consequent to vasomotor nephropathy, exposure to nephrotoxins, renal papillary necrosis, urinary tract obstruction, or renal hypoplasia), or pyelonephritis. Horses with CRF are usually azotemic and have isosthenuria (urine SG 1.008–1.012). Other clinical signs include weight loss, dental tartar (fig. 11.8), decreased appetite, oral ulcers (fig. 11.9), and sometimes ventral (fig. 11.10) and peripheral edema (fig. 11.11) and depression (fig. 11.12). Renal cysts may develop in affected kidneys (figs. 11.13 and 11.14). Urinalysis abnormalities vary according to the primary cause of renal failure. Unless it is caused by pyelonephritis, treatment for CRF is mainly supportive. Water should be available all the time and salt should be offered as long as no edema is present. The forage component of the diet should be changed from legume (alfalfa or clover) to grass to reduce calcium intake and decrease the risk of hypercalcemia. Increasing grain intake and adding fat (corn oil up to 450 ml per day) to the diet can be done to maintain body condition. The dietary protein intake should meet requirements for maintenance and increased urinary protein loss but should not be excessive.

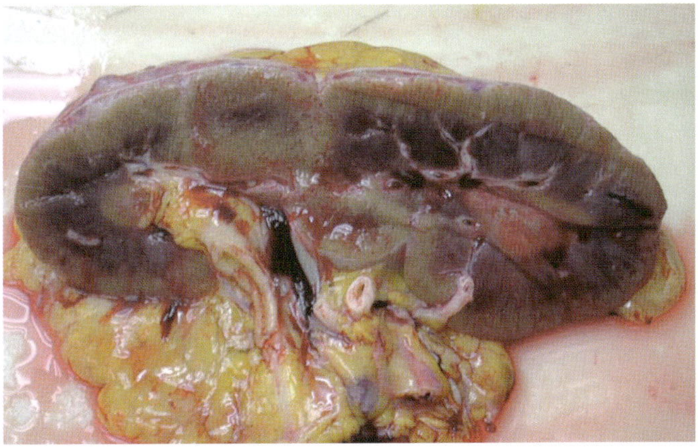

Figure 11.7 Postmortem photograph of a kidney (sagittal section) from a horse affected with glomerulonephritis. Note the fine gross vertical lines on the cortex and medulla.

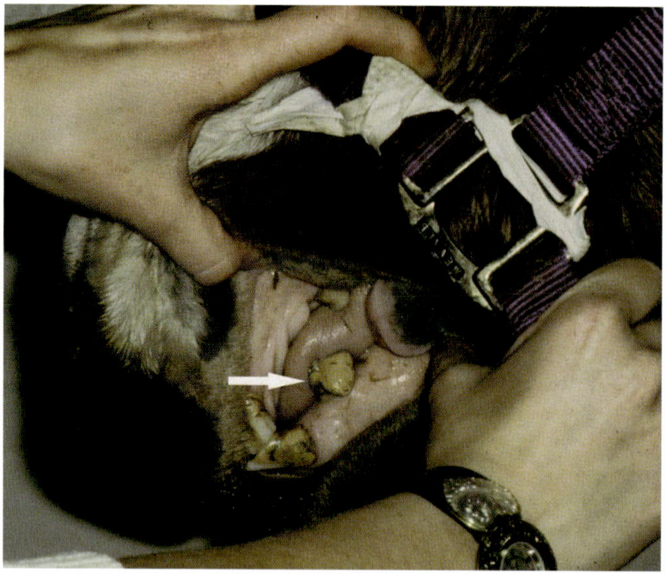

Figure 11.8 Dental tartar in a horse affected with CRF (arrow).

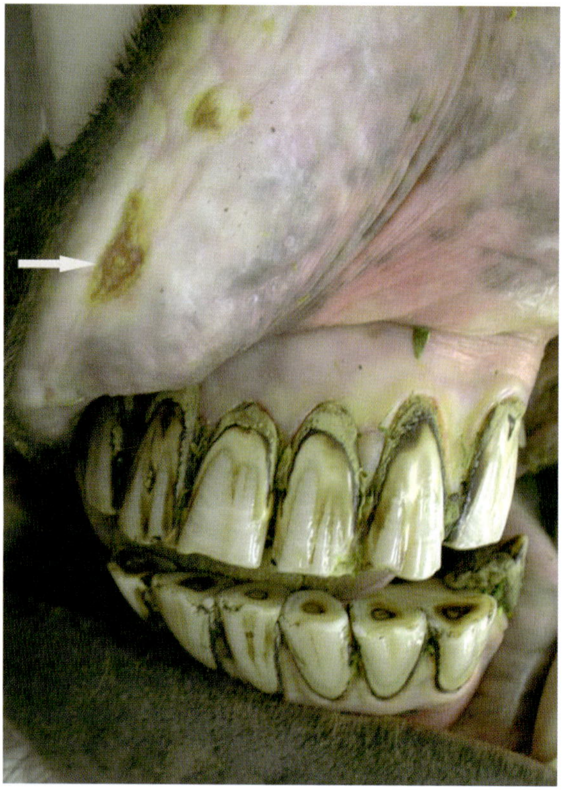

Figure 11.9 Oral ulcers and tartar on the incisors of a horse affected with CRF (arrow).

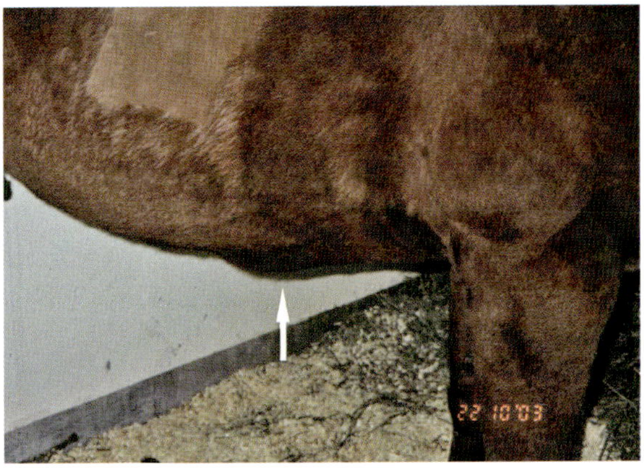

Figure 11.10 Ventral edema in a horse affected with CRF.

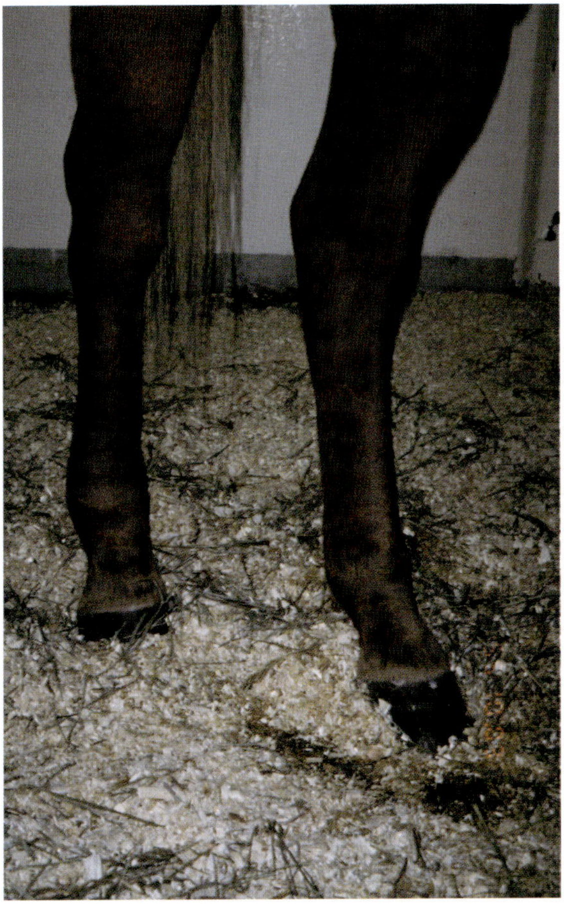

Figure 11.11 Peripheral (limb) edema in a horse affected with CRF.

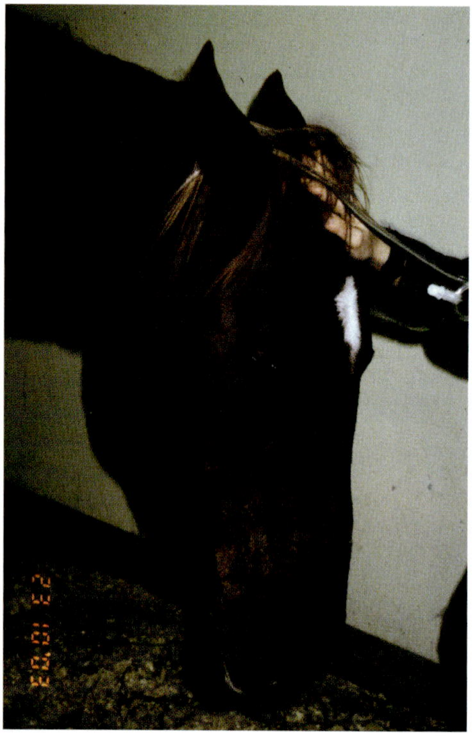

Figure 11.12 Depression in a horse affected with CRF.

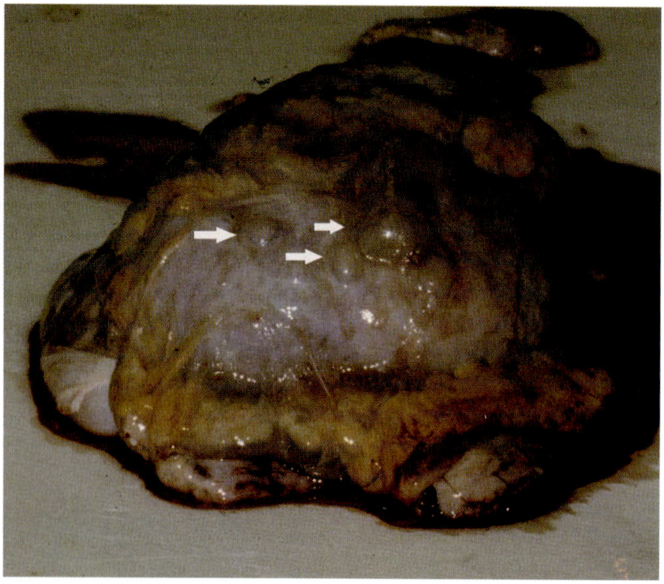

Figure 11.13 A postmortem photograph of a kidney with multiple cysts (arrows) from a horse affected with CRF.

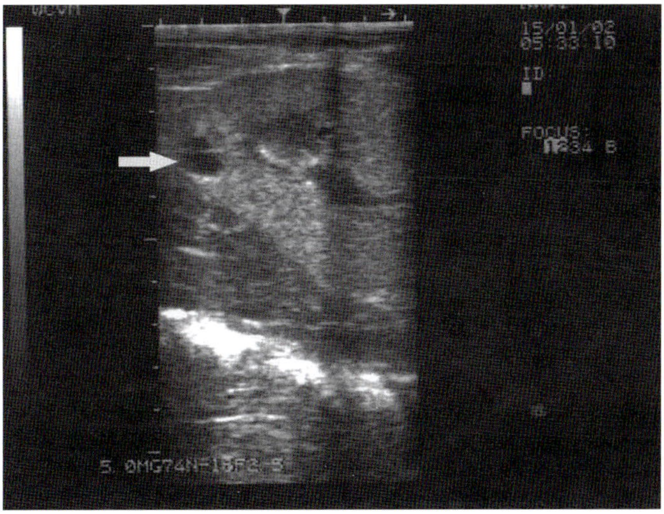

Figure 11.14 Ultrasonographic image of a kidney with cyst (arrow) from a horse affected with CRF.

Pyelonephritis

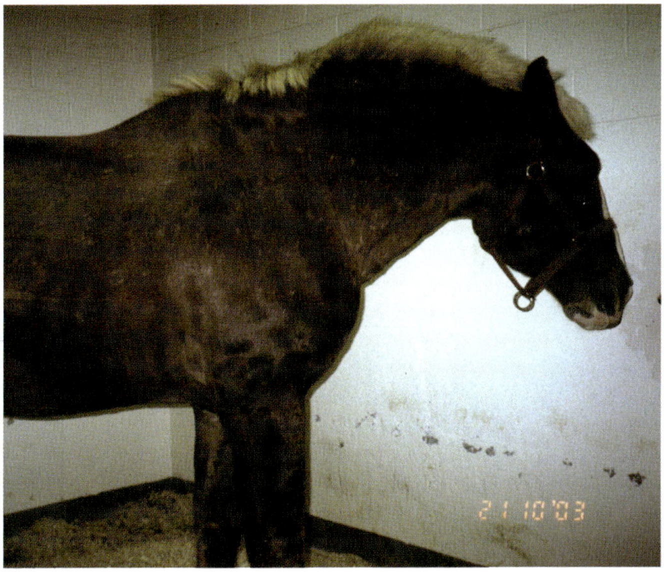

Figure 11.15 A depressed horse affected with pyelonephritis. Pyelonephritis has been associated with urolithiasis, cystitis, and bladder paralysis. Hematuria, dysuria, weight loss, fever, anorexia, or depression are signs of pyelonephritis in horses. Ureteral catheterization can be performed to assess if one or two kidneys are affected. Pyelonephritis is treated with antibiotics based on the urine culture and sensitivity.

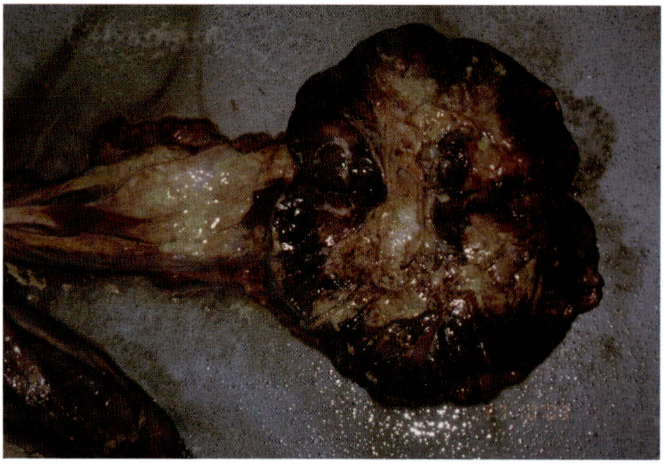

Figure 11.16 A postmortem photograph of a kidney and ureters from a horse affected with pyelonephritis and ureteritis. Note the purulent materials in the renal pelvis and ureters.

Cystitis

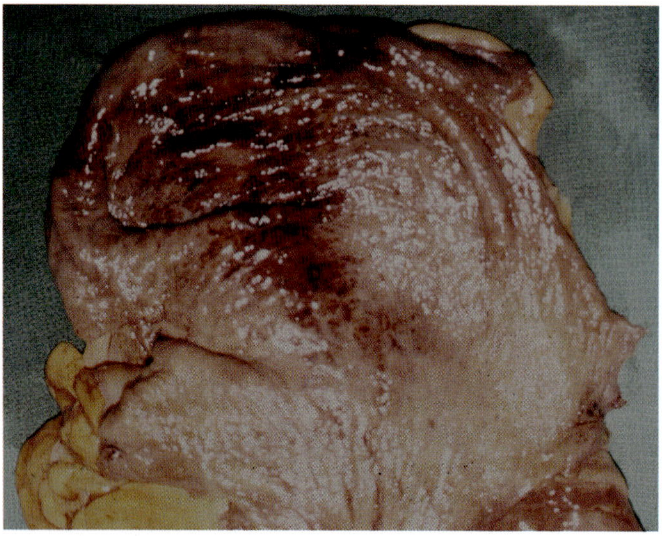

Figure 11.17 Postmortem photograph of a bladder affected with cystitis. Cystitis occurs mostly secondary to urinary flow disturbances caused by urolithiasis, bladder paralysis or tumor, anatomical defect, or iatrogenic trauma (catheterization or endoscopic examination). Vaginitis and repeated urinary catheterization are risk factors. Clinical signs include hematuria, pollakiuria, stranguria, pyuria, or urine scalding of the perineum of mares or the front of the hind limbs of male horses. Pathological perineal urine scalding should be differentiated from urination during normal estrus activities in mares. Diagnosis should be based on physical examination, transrectal palpation, cystoscopy, ultrasonography, urinalysis, and culture. Antibiotics treatment should be based on urine culture and sensitivity, but a trimethoprim-sulfonamide combination is the initial choice. Dietary supplementation with 50–75 g of salt to the diet or administration of a urine acidifying agent such as ammonium chloride 20–40 mg/kg per day by mouth has been recommended as part of the treatment for cystitis.

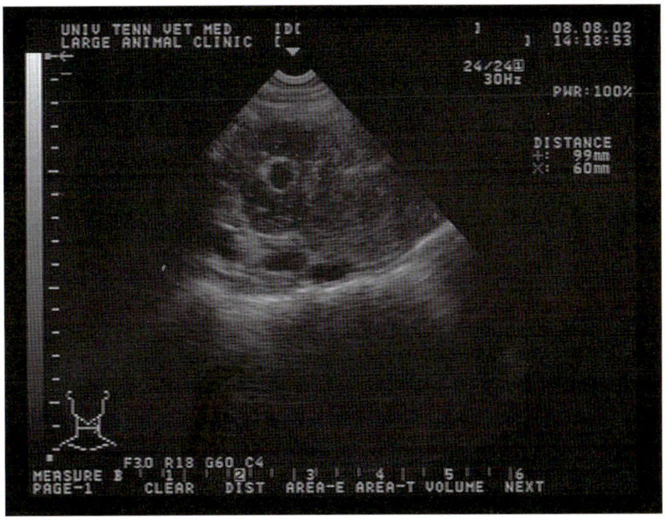

Figure 11.18 Ultrasonographic image of the right kidney of a pony mare affected with verminous nephritis caused by *Halicephalobus* spp. A discrete focal abscess is seen on the cranial pole of the kidney. The mare was presented for anemia and hematuria. *Halicephalobus deletrix* (previously *Micronema deletrix*) can cause nephritis and is often associated with concurrent infection of the nervous system (meningoencephalomyelitis) and bones (maxilla or mandible causing osteomyelitis) (fig. 11.19). The nematode causes granulomas in the affected kidneys and may be found in the urine. Treatment consists of anthelmintics and anti-inflammatory drugs.

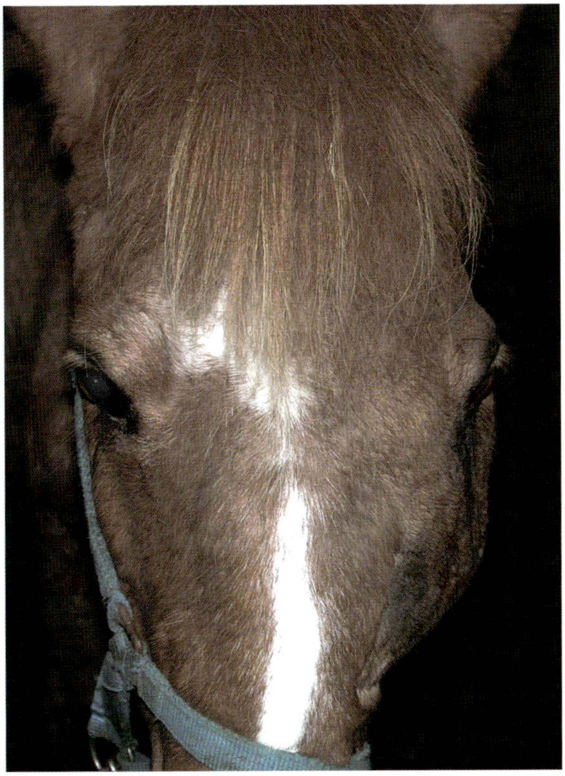

Figure 11.19 Greatly enlarged left sinus of a 10-year-old miniature mare infected with *Halicephalobus* spp.

Urethral Rent or Defect

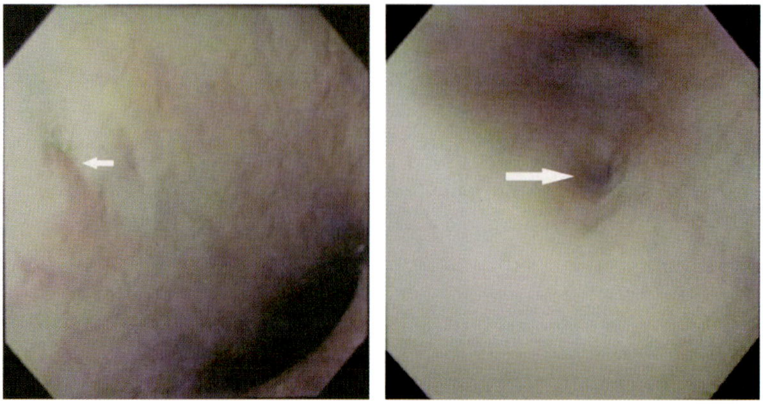

a b

Figures 11.20a,b Endoscopic image of the urethra in a horse affected with urethral rent or defect (arrow). Urethral defect occurs on the convex surface of the urethra at the level of the ischial arch. It causes hematuria in geldings and hemospermia in stallions. Hematuria is typically at the end of urination (fig. 11.21). The exact cause is unknown. Often, urethral rents heal without treatment. However, if hematuria persist more than a month, or the gelding becomes anemic, surgical treatment should be employed. Two surgical approaches have been suggested: temporary ischial urethrotomy or making a vertical incision that extends into the corpus spongiosum of the penis but leaving the urethra intact. Hematuria should resolve in 1 week after the surgical treatment.

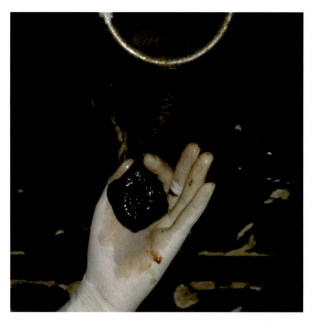

Figure 11.21 Hematuria at the end of urination in a horse affected with a urethral defect.

Urolithiasis (Urethrolithiasis, Cystolithiasis, and Nephrolithiasis)

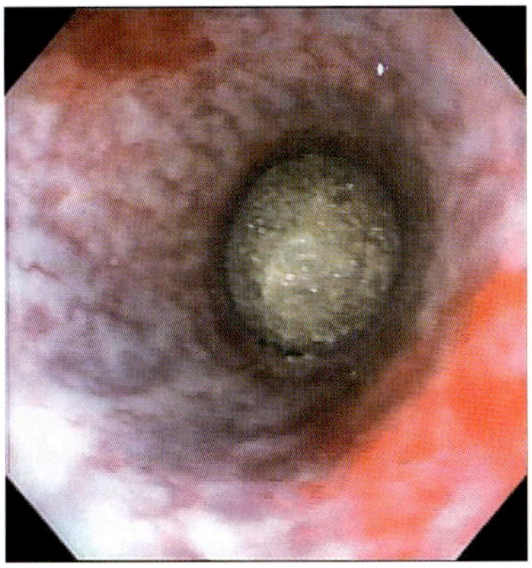

Figure 11.22 Endoscopic image of urethra in a horse with urethrolithiasis. Urethral calculus is mainly a male horse problem. It is usually caused by a small cystolith that passes from the bladder and lodges in the urethra, often in the area of natural narrowing of the urethra at the level of the ischial arch. Affected horses present with signs of colic, frequent posturing to urinate, extension of the penis (fig. 11.23), dribbling of small amounts of urine, and sometimes blood at the end of the urethra. Unresolved complete obstruction can be followed by urinary bladder or urethral rupture (figs. 11.24–26). Diagnosis is based on clinical signs, transrectal palpation findings of a distended bladder and pulsating urethra, and endoscopic examination. Urethral calculi can be removed by urethrotomy, which can be left to heal by second intension (fig. 11.27). (Image from Abutarbush SM and Carmalt JL, Endoscopy and arthroscopy for the equine practitioner. Made Easy Series. Jackson, WY: Teton NewMedia, 2008)

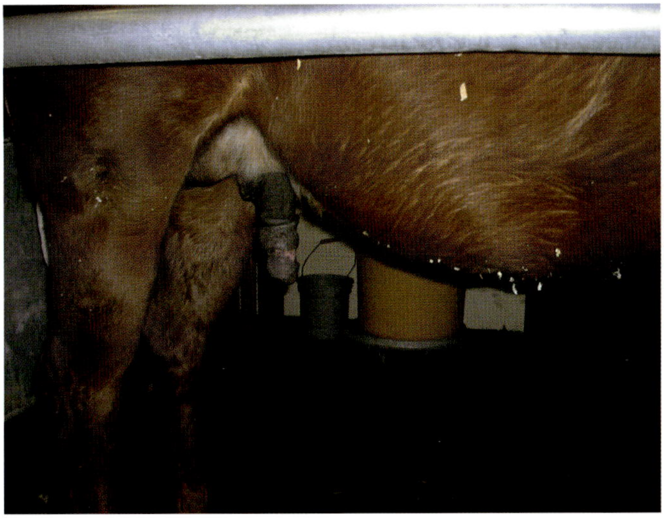

Figure 11.23 A horse affected with urethrolithiasis showing frequent posturing to urinate and extension of the penis.

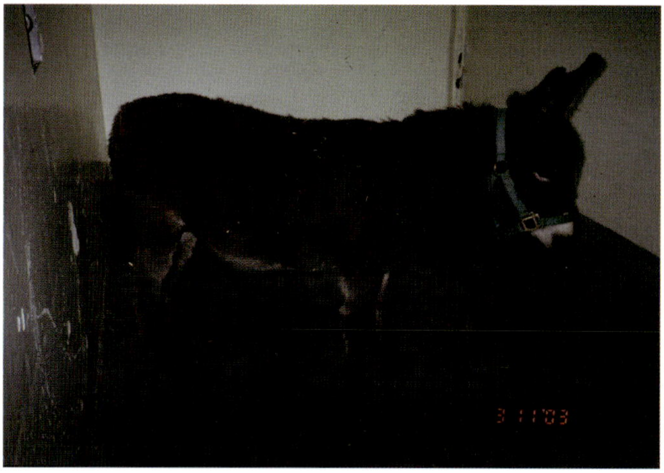

a

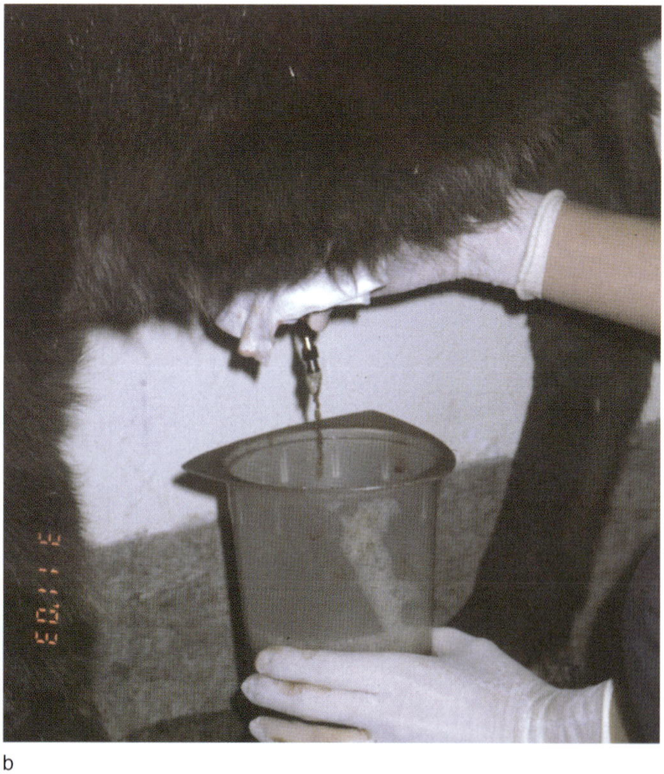

b

Figures 11.24a,b Abdominal distension (a) and abdominocentesis (b) in a male donkey affected with urinary bladder rupture secondary to urethrolithiasis.

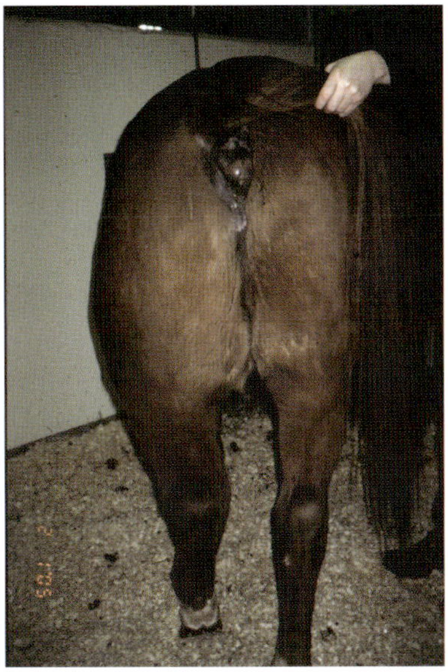

a

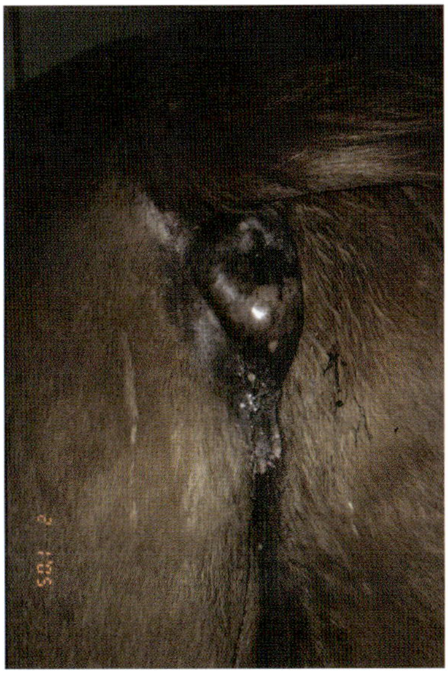

b

Figures 11.25a,b Urethral rupture in a horse secondary to urethrolithiasis. Note the swollen leg (a) and distorted anus (b) due to urine accumulation under the skin and among muscles.

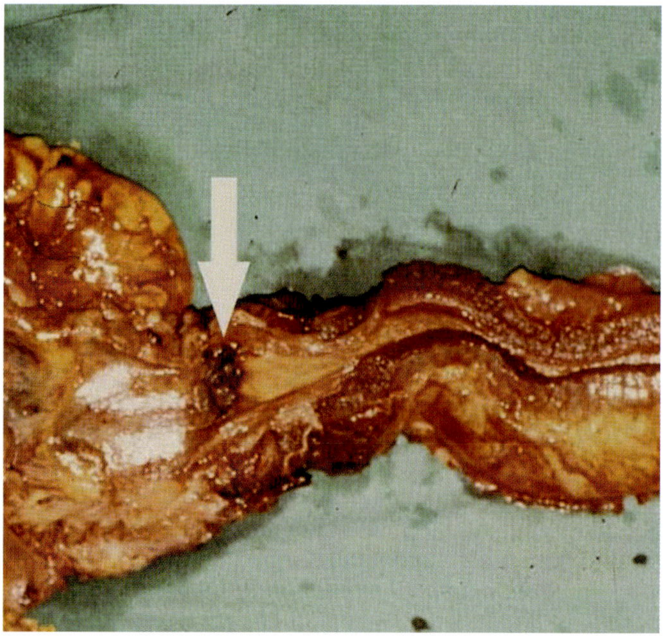

Figure 11.26 Postmortem photograph of the urethra of the horse shown in fig. 11.25. Note the area of rupture in the penis (arrow).

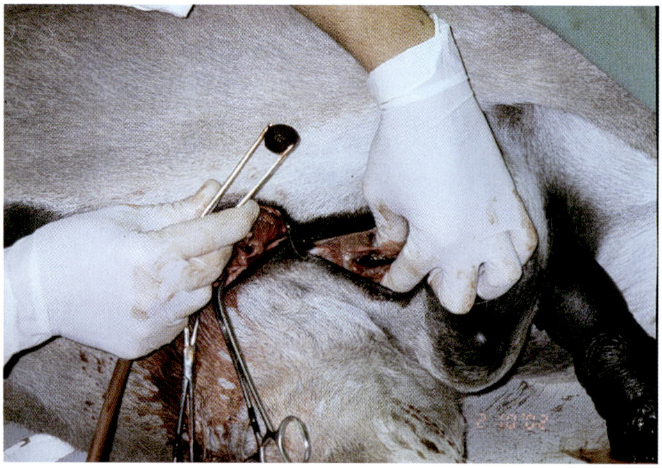

Figure 11.27 Removal of a urethrolith by urethrotomy in a male donkey.

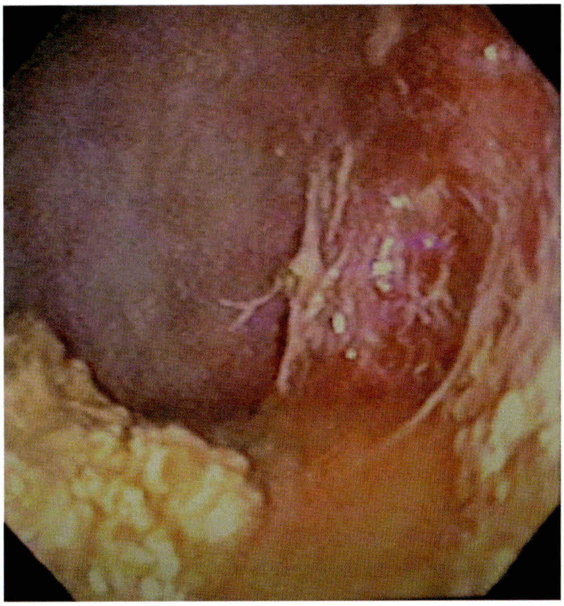

Figure 11.28 Endoscopic image of a bladder with a stone (cystolithiasis). Cystolithiasis is the most common form of urolithiasis in the horse. Clinical signs include hematuria following exercise, pollakiuria, stranguria, urine incontinence, or dysuria. Diagnosis is achieved by transrectal examination, ultrasonography, and endoscopy. Treatment is by surgical removal of the calculus and postoperative systemic antibiotics. In mares, manual distention of the urethra, after sedation and local or epidural anesthesia, allows several fingers or a small hand to pass to the bladder and retrieve the calculus with or without fragmentation. Changing diet from legume to grass or oat hay is recommended to reduce calcium intake and prevent recurrence. Administration of a urine acidifier is unpalatable and should be administered two to three times daily to be effective. More practical is the addition of 60–120 g of salt to the feed daily to increase water intake.

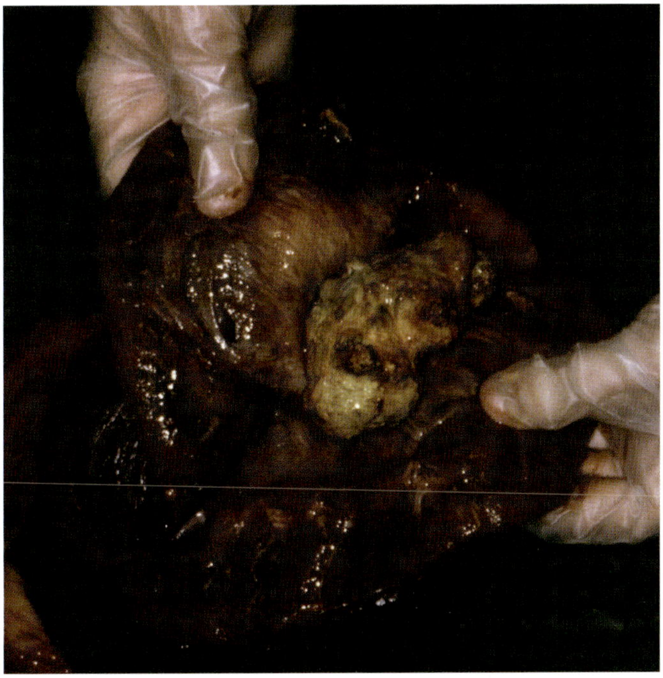

Figure 11.29 Postmortem photograph of a renal calculus in a horse (nephrolithiasis). Nephrolithiasis can be unilateral or bilateral. It occurs usually at the level of the renal pelvis. Nephroliths can lead to hydronephrosis or pass down into the ureters causing blockage. In horses, unlike humans, colic is rarely a clinical sign. Bilateral obstruction of the upper urinary tract leads to chronic renal failure. In such cases, weight loss (fig. 11.30), polyuria, or poor performance are the most common clinical signs. Renal or ureteral calculi are usually associated with microscopic hematuria, unless they are passed to the bladder or urethra. Occasionally they can be associated with intermittent or persistent hematuria.

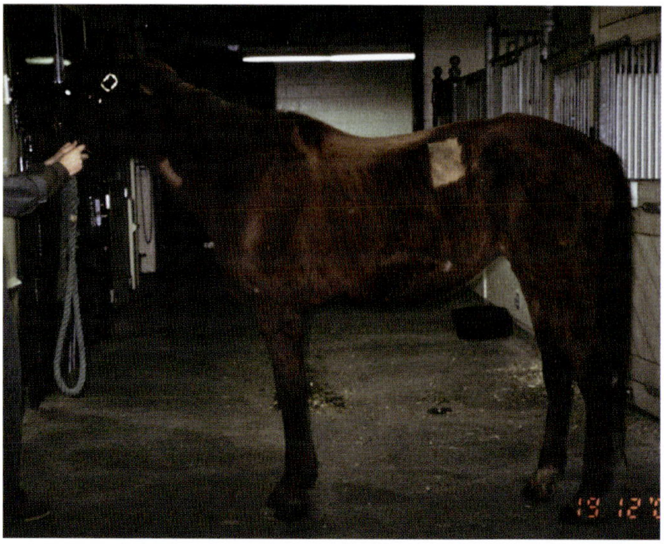

Figure 11.30 Weight loss in a horse with nephrolithiasis.

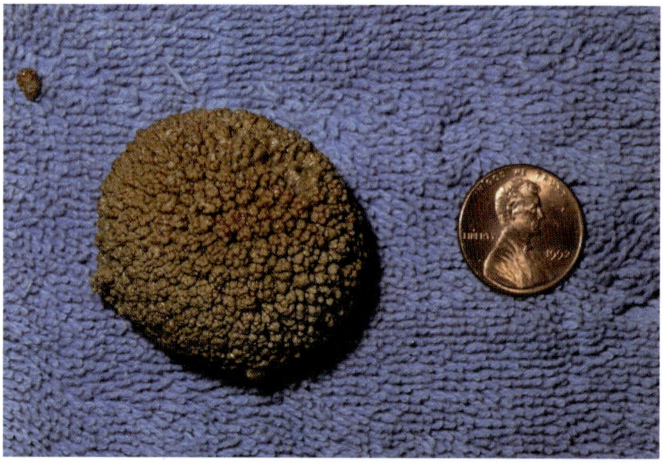

a

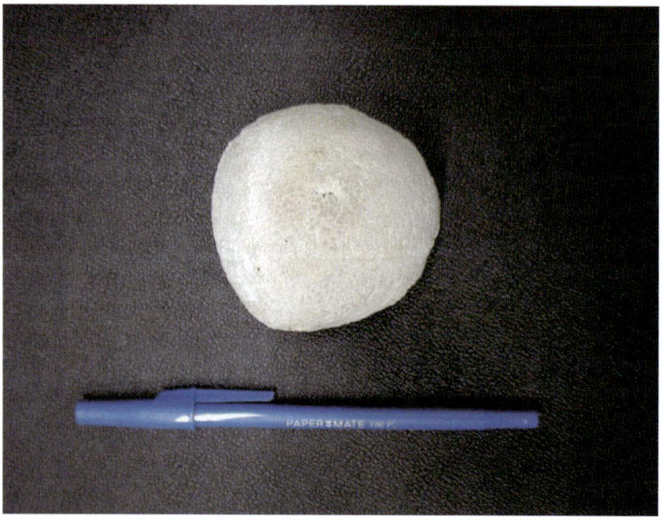

b

Figures 11.31a,b Equine calculi are composed mainly of calcium carbonate and 90% of them are yellow-green in color, spiculated, and easy to fragment (a). Ten percent are gray-white, smooth, and difficult to fragment, and contain phosphate in addition to calcium carbonate (b).

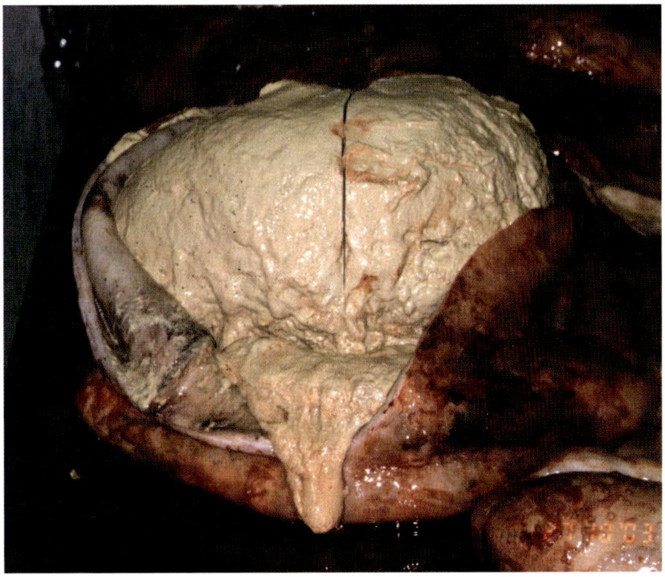

Figure 11.32 Postmortem photograph of the bladder affected with sabulous urolithiasis. Sabulous urolithiasis is an accumulation of large amounts of crystalloid materials in the bladder, usually secondary to bladder atony or paralysis commonly seen in horses with caudal spinal cord lesion. Bladder lavage is particularly important in this form of urolithiasis.

Recommended Reading

Abutarbush SM. Diagnosis of urinary tract disease in the horse. Large Animal Veterinary Rounds. 5(2), 2005.

Abutarbush SM, Carmalt JL. Endoscopy and arthroscopy for the equine practitioner. Made Easy Series. Jackson, WY: Teton NewMedia, 2008.

Ehnen SJ, Divers TJ, Gillette D, Reef VB. Obstructive nephrolithiasis and ureterolithiasis associated with chronic renal failure in horses: eight cases (1981–1987). J Am Vet Med Assoc. 15(197):249–53, 1990.

Johnson PJ, Crenshaw KL. The treatment of cystic and urethral calculi in geldings. Vet Med. 85:891–900, 1990.

Knottenbelt DC. Polyuria-polydipsia in the horse. Equine Vet Educ. 12:179–86, 2000.

Kotebra AM, Coffman JR. Acute and chronic renal disease in the horse. Compend Cont Educ Pract Vet. 3:S461–69, 1981.

Laverty S, Pascoe JR, Ling GV, et al. Urolithiasis in 68 horses. Vet Surg. 21:56–62, 1992.

Reed SM, Bayly WM, Selon D. Equine internal medicine. Philadelphia: WB Saunders, 1253–89, 2004.

Reef VB. Equine diagnostic ultrasound. Philadelphia, WB Saunders, 291–304, 1998.

Ruggles AJ, Beech J, Gillette DM, Midl LT, Reef VB, Freeman DE. Disseminated *Halicephalobus deletrix* infection in a horse. J Am Vet Med Assoc. 203:550–52, 1993.

Schumacher J, Schumacher J, Schmitz D. Macroscopic hematuria of horses Equine Vet Educ. 14:201–10, 2002.

Smith BP. Large animal internal medicine. 3rd ed. St Louis: Mosby, 824–43, 1233–36, 2002.

12 Diseases of the Neonates

Specific Neonatal Diseases
- Hypoxic Ischemic Syndrome
- Sepsis
- Prematurity
- Neonatal Isoerythrolysis

Respiratory System
- Radiography of the Thorax
  - Normal Thorax
  - Acute Pneumonia
  - Chronic Pneumonia (Diffuse Bronchointerstitial Lung Pattern)
  - Pulmonary Abscessation
- *Rhodococcus equi*
- Diaphragmatic Hernia
- Pneumonia

Alimentary System
- Candidiasis
- Cleft Palate
- Inferior Brachygnathism (Parrot Mouth)
- Wry Nose
- Megaesophagus
- Esophageal Stricture
- Gastroduodenal Ulcer Syndrome
- Intussusception
- Ascaridiasis
- Clostridial Enterocolitis
- Rotavirus Diarrhea
- Meconium Impaction
- Intestinal Atresia
- Scrotal Hernia
- Intestinal Aganglionosis (Lethal White Syndrome)
- Functional Ileus

Nervous System
- Hyponatremia
- Brachial Plexus Injury
- Botulism

Ocular System
- Entropion
- Scleral Hemorrhage

Musculoskeletal System
- Bone and Joints
  - Normal Metatarsophalangeal Joint
  - Normal Tarsus

        - Normal Stifle Joint
        - Normal Carpus
        - Physeal Dysplasia (Physitis)
        - Grade 1 Ossification of the Carpal Bones
        - Grade 2 Ossification of the Carpal Bones
        - Angular Limb Deformity—Carpal Valgus
        - Angular Limb Deformity—Tarsal Valgus
        - Angular Limb Deformity—Fetlock Varus
        - Infectious Polyarthritis (Septic Arthritis)
        - Infectious Polyarthritis—S type
        - Infectious Polyarthritis—P type
        - Infectious Polyarthritis—E type
        - Infectious Polyarthritis—T type
        - Salter-Harris Type 2 Fracture of the Proximal Tibia
        - Salter-Harris Type 2 Fracture of the Distal Metacarpus
        - Lateral Luxation of the Patella
        - Avulsion Fracture of the Origin of the Long Digital Extensor Tendon
        - Rib Fracture
    - Tendons, Ligaments, Muscles, and Associated Structures
        - Ruptured Gastrocnemius Muscle/Tendon
        - Ruptured Common Digital Extensor Tendon
        - Flexural Deformities
        - Ventral Abdominal Wall Tear
        - White Muscle Disease

Urinary System

- Urinary Tract Disruption
- Patent Urachus
- Umbilical Remnant Infections
- External Umbilical Swellings

Integumentary System

- Decubital Ulcers
- Ulcerative Dermatitis
- Dermatophilosis

Miscellaneous Conditions

- Alloimmune Thrombocytopenia
- Neonatal Hypothyroidism and Goiter
- Lavender Foal Syndrome
- Congenital Hypothyroidism and Dysmaturity Syndrome

Hypoxic Ischemic Syndrome

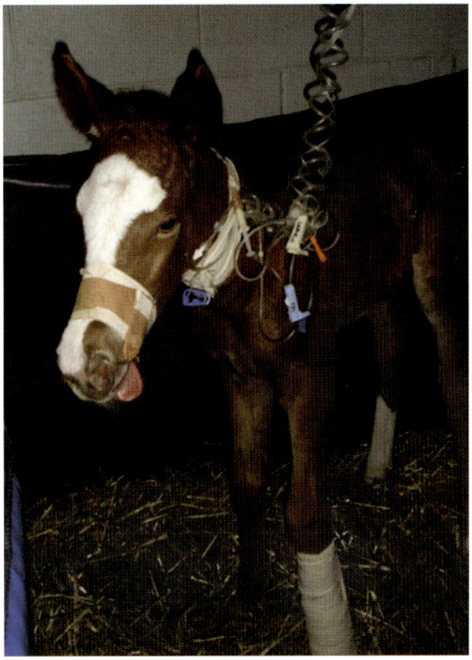

Figure 12.1 A foal recovering from hypoxic ischemic syndrome (HIS) also known as peripartum asphyxia syndrome or neonatal maladjustment syndrome. HIS is a multisystemic disorder resulting from decreased oxygenation and tissue perfusion in the perinatal period. Affected foals present with a variety of clinical signs reflecting the organ or system involved, and duration, severity, and timing of the insult in the perinatal period. The most common systems affected are the central nervous and alimentary systems, and kidneys. Clinical presentation ranges from loss of affinity for the mare and dysphagia to seizurelike activity and grand mal seizures (figs. 12.2–12.6); abnormal gastrointestinal motility and colic to necrotizing enterocolitis (figs. 12.7–12.10); renal dysfunction to anuric renal failure (fig. 12.11); and systematic inflammatory response syndrome (SIRS) if there is severe damage. Differential diagnoses for CNS manifestations include electrolyte and metabolic disorders, meningitis, and trauma; gastrointestinal manifestations include sepsis, meconium impaction, and other causes of colic in neonates; renal manifestations include toxic nephropathy or congenital abnormality. Diagnosis is based on clinical signs and exclusion of other disease processes. HIS often occurs concurrently with sepsis and prematurity. There is no specific treatment for HIS, thus treatment is aimed at systemic support of the neonate while the damaged tissues are healing.

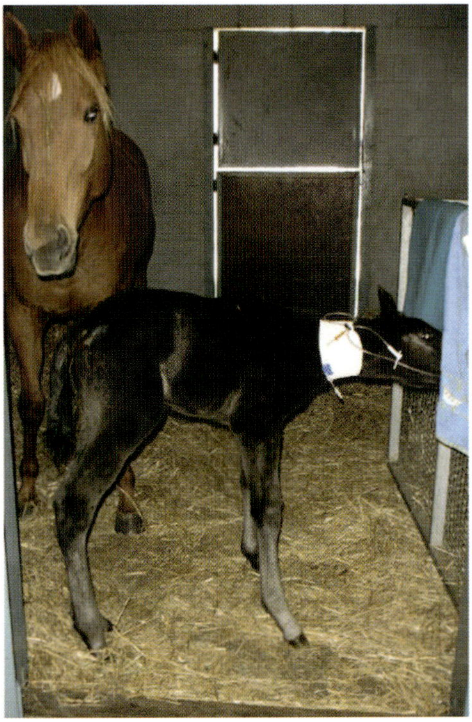

Figure 12.2 Loss of affinity for the mare is one of the common mild CNS manifestations of HIS. The CNS manifestation of HIS is also termed hypoxic ischemic encephalopathy (HIE).

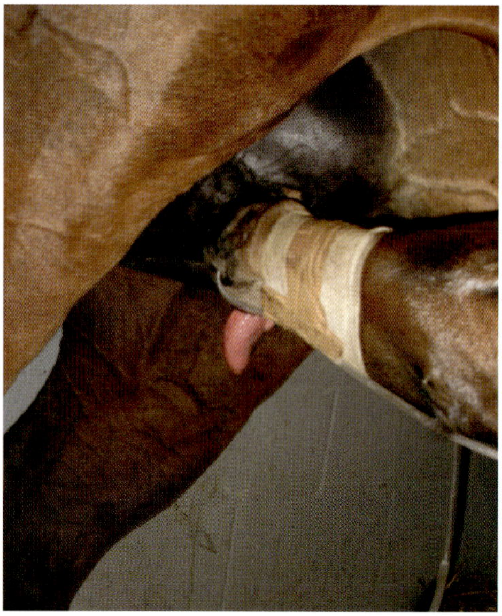

a

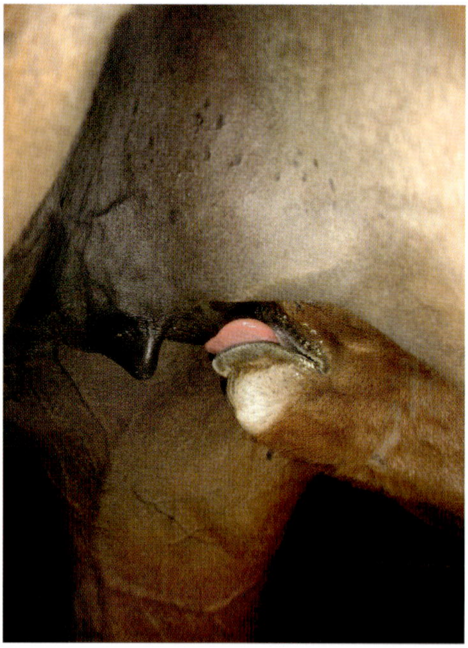

b

Figures 12.3a,b Loss of suckle reflex and tongue control is also a common manifestation of hypoxic ischemic encephalopathy (HIE). B illustrates a normal foal nursing with a good tongue seal.

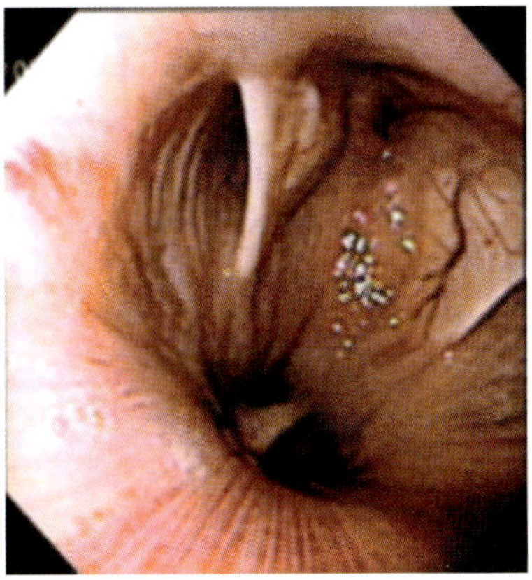

Figure 12.4 Endoscopic view of a collapsed nasopharynx during inspiration. Note the excessive opening of the guttural pouch ostium. The lack of tone of the nasopharyngeal region in foals with hypoxic ischemic encephalopathy (HIE) can result in dysphagia, respiratory noises, and, in more severe cases, respiratory obstruction.

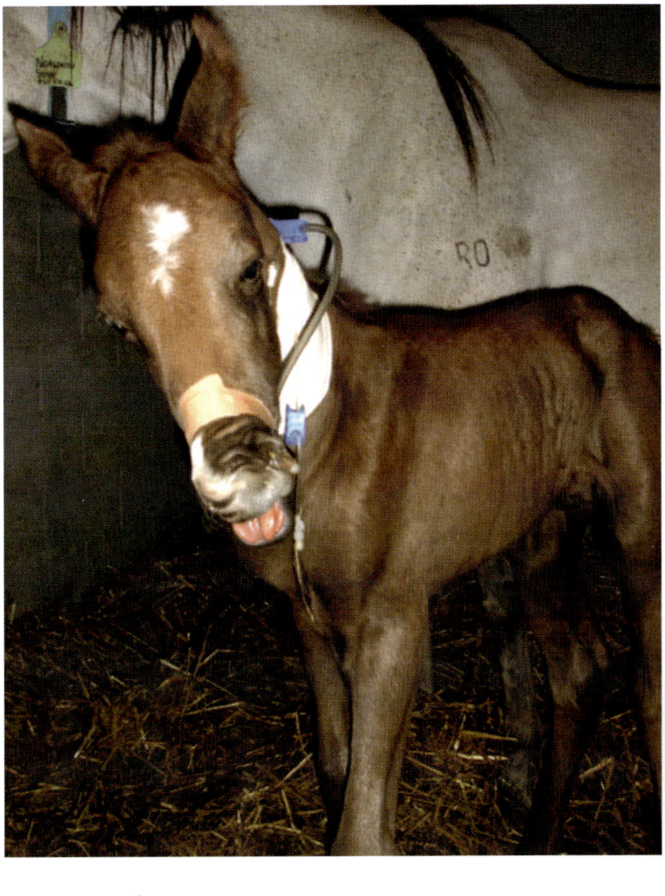

Figure 12.5 Tonic muzzle contractions can be seen as focal seizure activity with hypoxic ischemic encephalopathy (HIE).

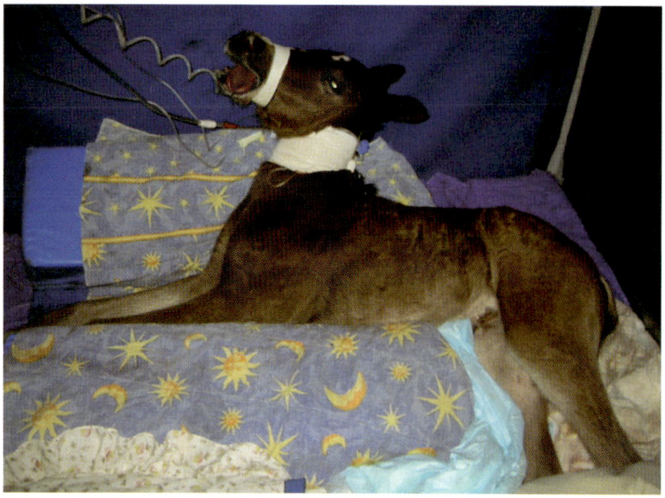

Figure 12.6 A grand mal seizure with extensor rigidity and opisthotonos in a foal with hypoxic ischemic encephalopathy (HIE). This foal also had abnormal vocalization ("Barker").

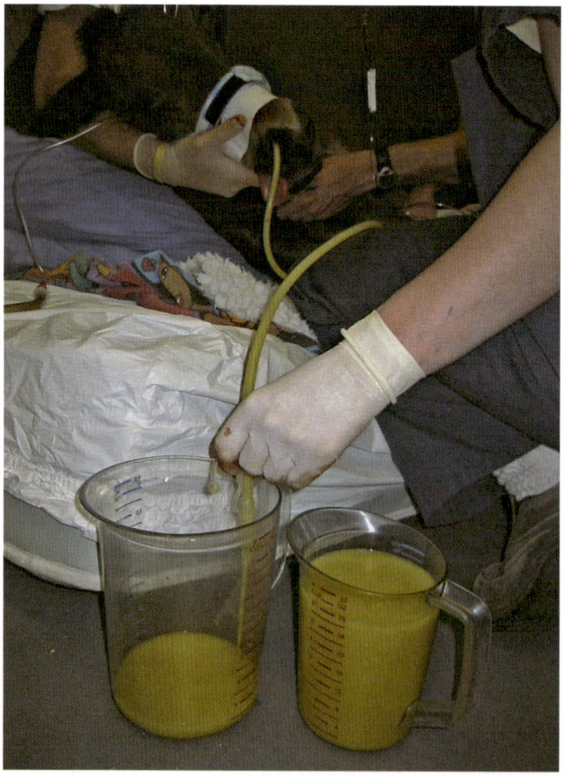

Figure 12.7 Nasogastric reflux due to small intestinal ileus in a foal affected with hypoxic ischemic encephalopathy (HIE).

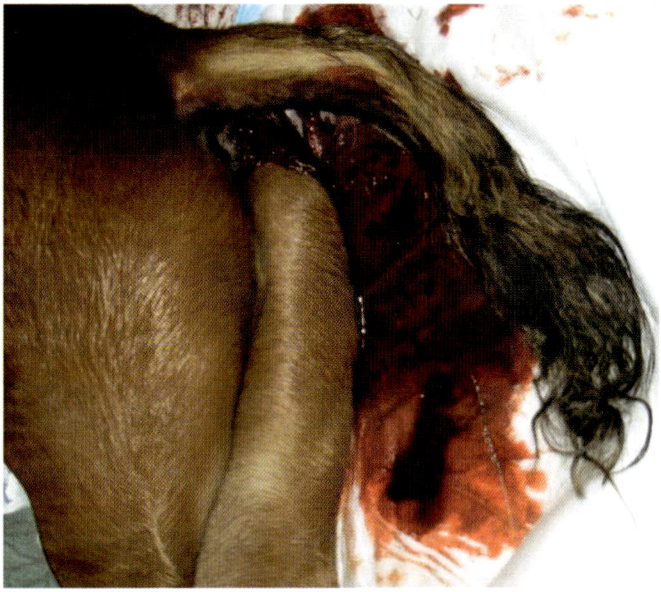

Figure 12.8 Hemorrhagic diarrhea due to necrotizing enterocolitis. This condition should be differentiated from clostridial enterocolitis.

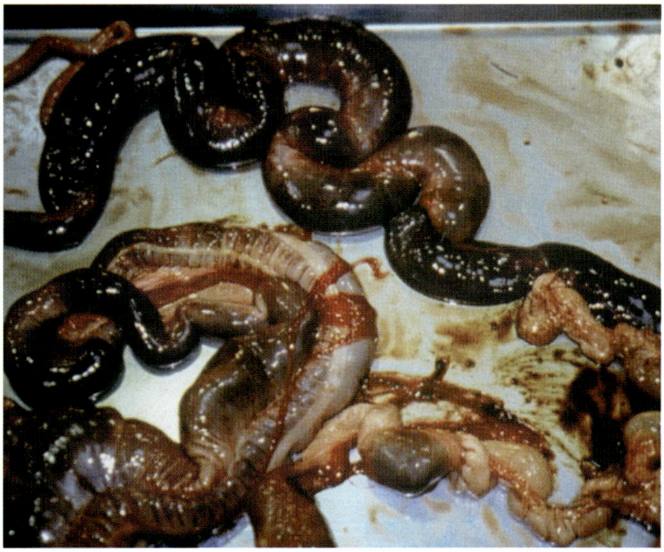

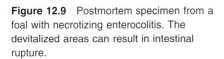

Figure 12.9 Postmortem specimen from a foal with necrotizing enterocolitis. The devitalized areas can result in intestinal rupture.

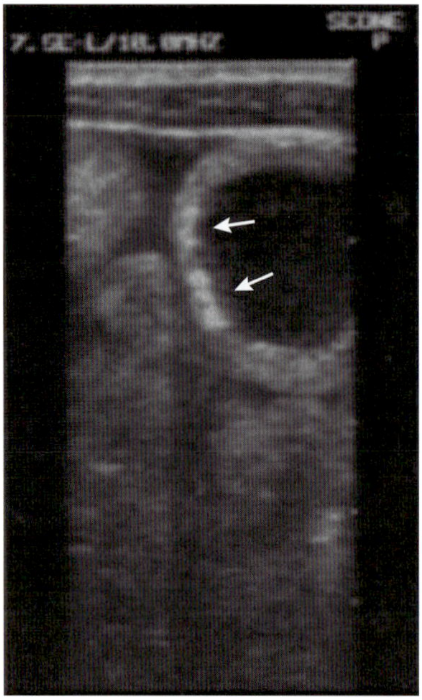

Figure 12.10 Sonogram of a foal's abdomen showing small intestinal loops with pneumatosis intestinalis. This occurs in conjunction with necrotizing enterocolitis when gas-producing bacteria invade the compromised intestinal wall. Note the hyperechoic gas echoes (arrows) within the wall of the intestine.

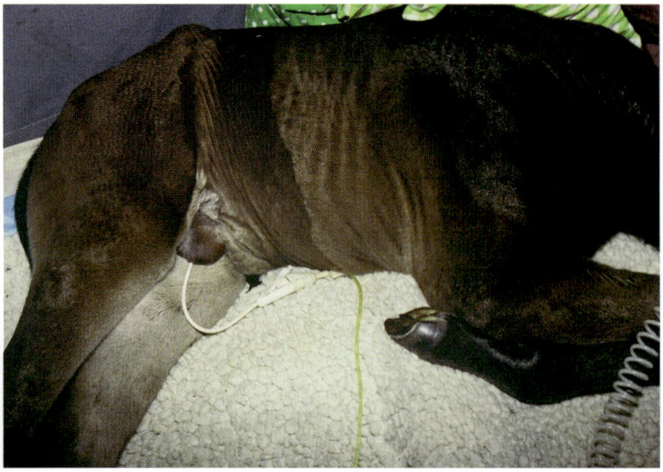

Figure 12.11 Edema formation giving the ventral abdomen of the foal a wrinkled appearance. This is often indicative of fluid overloading associated with altered renal function. A urinary catheter has been placed to assist with monitoring urine production.

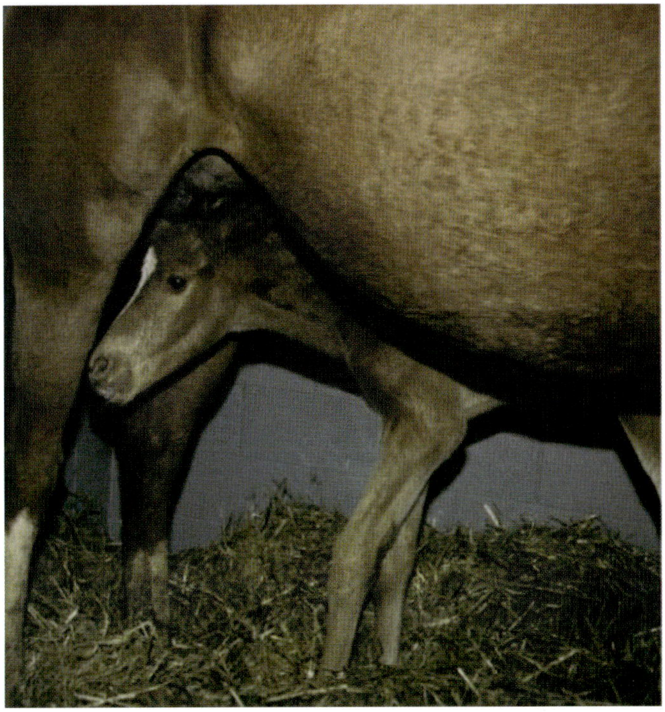

Figure 12.12 A foal standing under the mare and not nursing is often an early nonspecific sign of sepsis. Sepsis is the systemic inflammatory response to an infection. The infection can be acquired in utero or in the perinatal period and most commonly occurs due to placentitis or translocation of bacteria across the intestinal wall. A cascade of reactions is initiated, which results in clinical signs (figs. 12.15–12.21) varying from mild depression to septic shock and multiorgan failure. Microorganisms are disseminated throughout the body and can localize resulting in clinical diseases such as embolic pneumonia (fig. 12.13), embolic nephritis (fig. 12.14), enteritis (fig. 12.22), cellulitis (fig. 12.23), meningitis (fig. 12.24), omphalophlebitis (fig. 12.26), and infectious orthopedic disease (figs. 12.27–12.28 and figs. 12.114–12.119). Differential diagnoses include hypoxic ischemic encephalopathy (HIE), prematurity, and Tyzzers disease. Diagnosis is based on perinatal history, clinical signs, clinicopathologic evaluation, and blood culture or localizing sites of infection. Treatment is aimed at stabilizing the foal, eliminating infection, and treating localized infections.

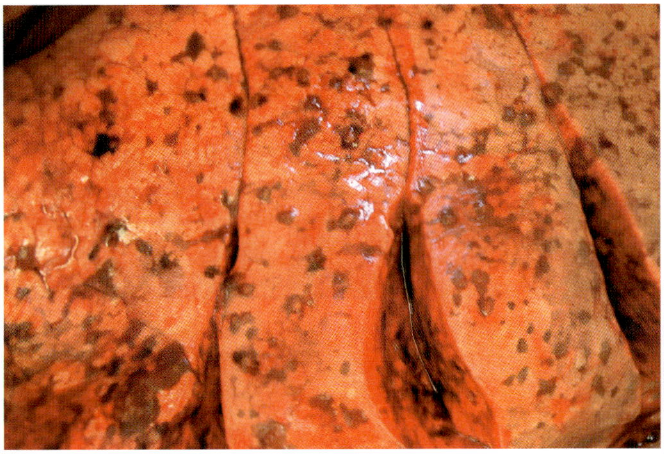

Figure 12.13 Embolic pneumonia in a septicemic neonatal foal.

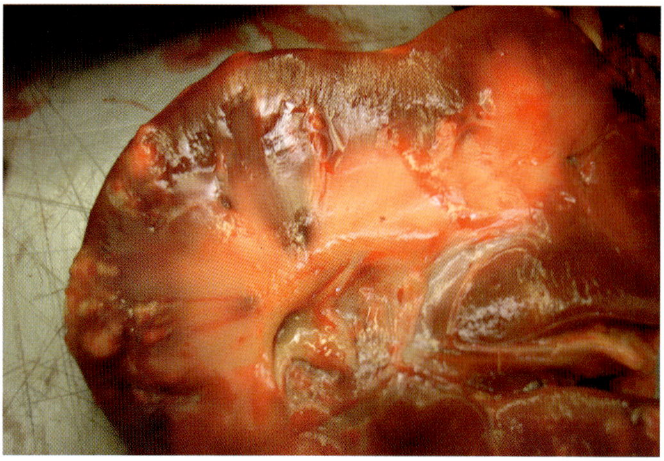

Figure 12.14 Embolic nephritis in a septicemic neonatal foal.

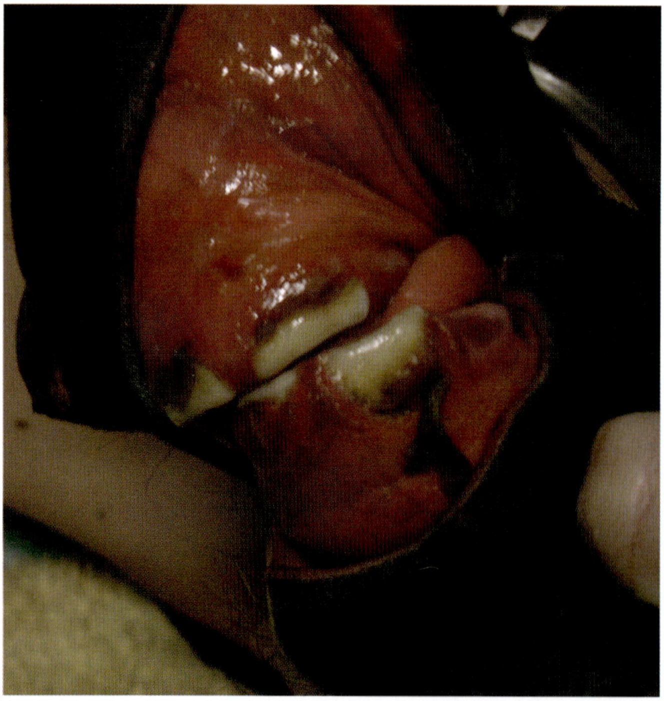

Figure 12.15 Hyperemic mucous membranes seen in a foal with early sepsis. Note slight yellow discoloration, which is often seen with sepsis.

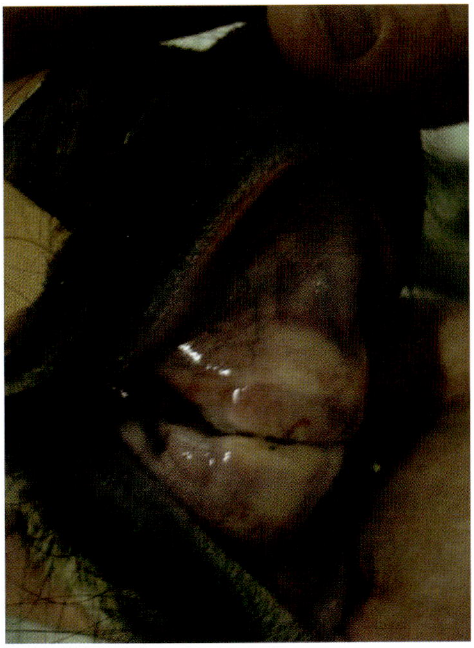

Figure 12.16 Muddy purple discolored mucous membranes in a foal with septic shock.

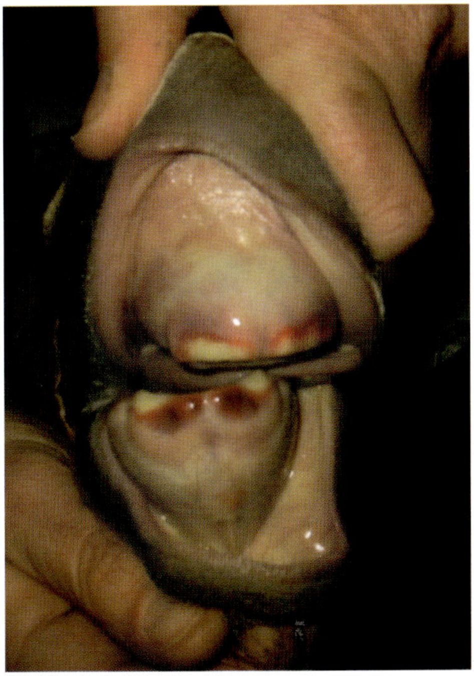

Figure 12.17 Hemorrhagic gingival margins in a foal with disseminated intravascular coagulation, which can be seen in advanced stages of sepsis. Petechiae, ecchymotic hemorrhages, and spontaneous bleeding can also be seen.

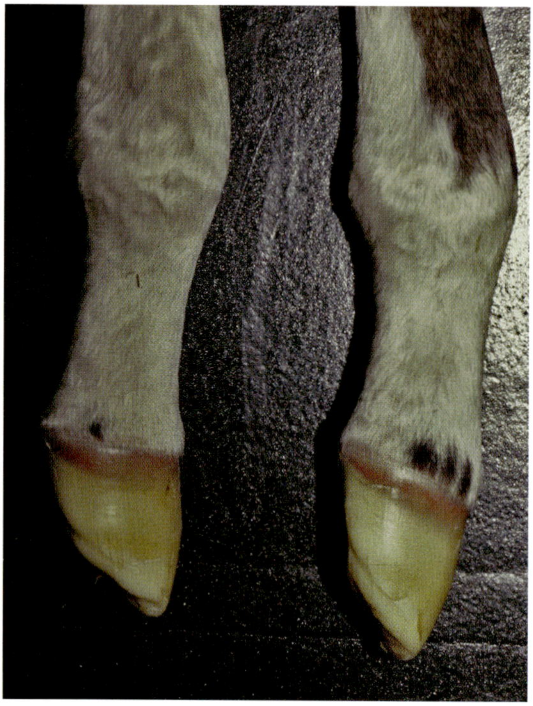

Figure 12.18 Coronitis in a foal with sepsis. This is also seen in foals with pigmented hooves.

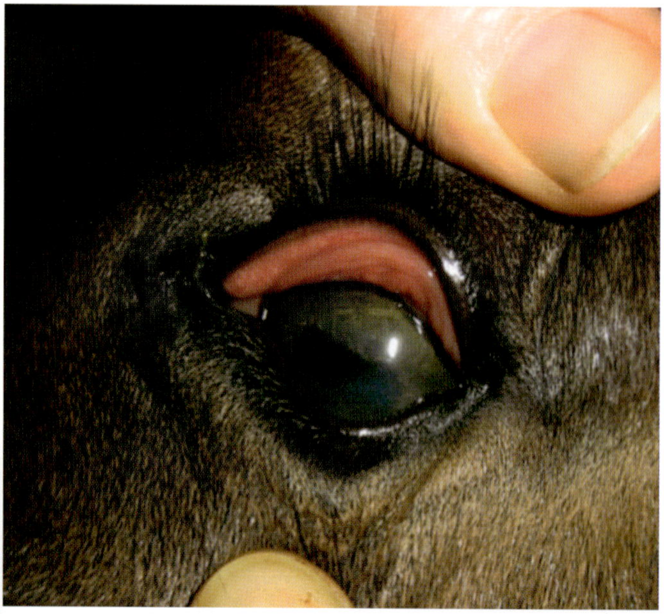

Figure 12.19 Iriditis and anterior uveitis in a newborn foal with sepsis. This is often present in foals that are septicemic at birth. Note the green discoloration of the iris and miotic pupil. The corneal edema was due to an entropion.

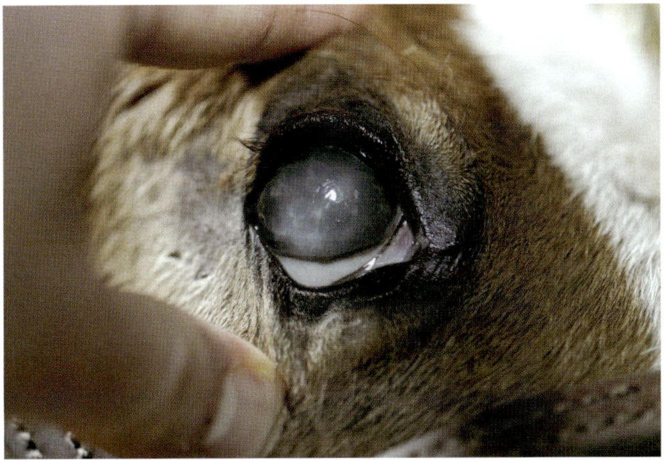

Figure 12.20 Septicemia in a neonatal foal due to *Actinobacillus equuli* manifested as uveitis and hypopyon.

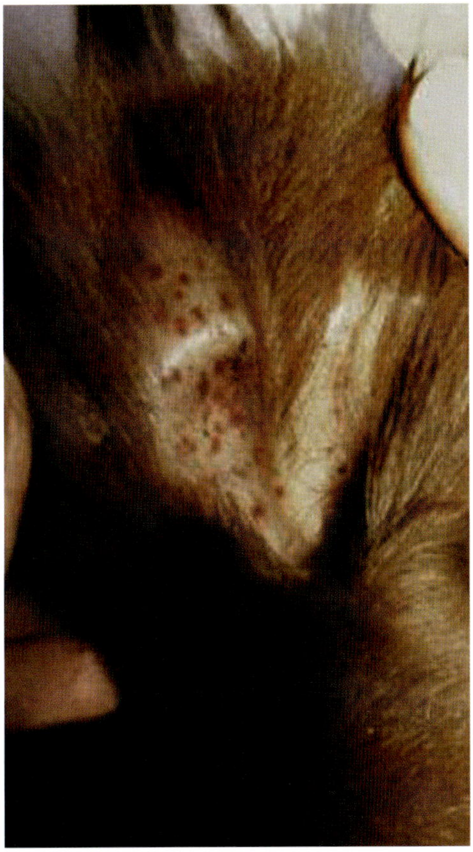

Figure 12.21 Petechiae in the ear of a septicemic foal.

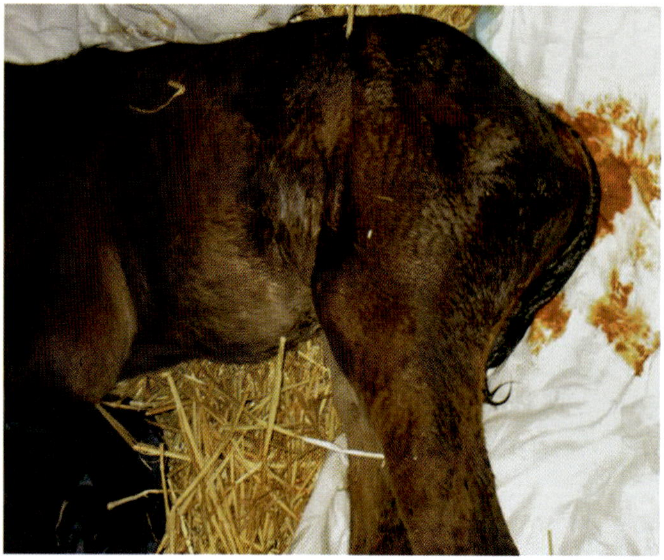

Figure 12.22 Septicemic foal with enterocolitis. Note the mild abdominal distension and diarrhea.

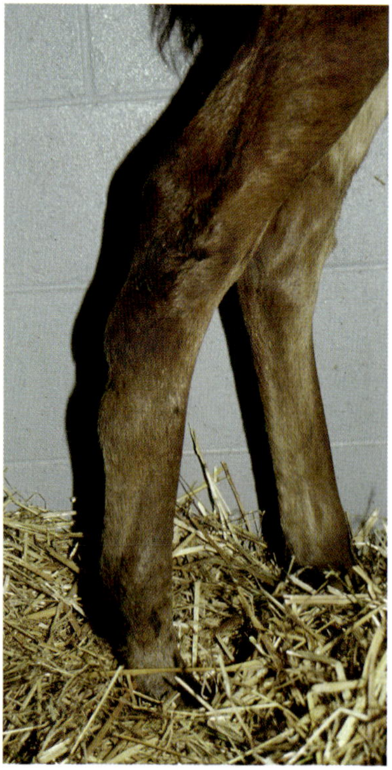

Figure 12.23 Soft fluctuant subcutaneous swellings due to subcutaneous abscess formation in a septicemic foal with localized sepsis.

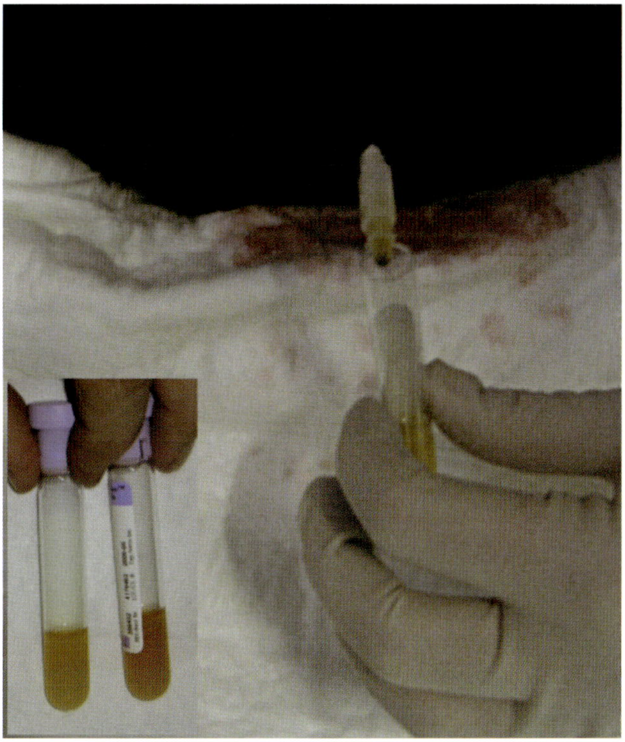

Figure 12.24 Cloudy, xanthochromic, cerebrospinal fluid (CSF) collected from the lumbosacral space of a septicemic foal with meningitis.

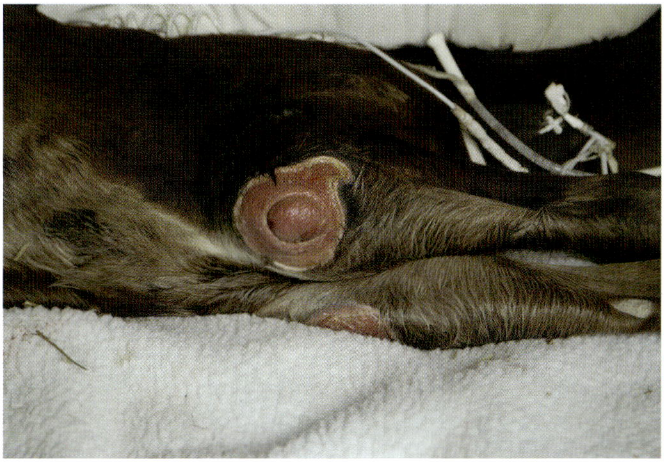

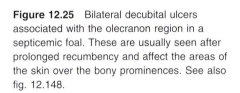

Figure 12.25 Bilateral decubital ulcers associated with the olecranon region in a septicemic foal. These are usually seen after prolonged recumbency and affect the areas of the skin over the bony prominences. See also fig. 12.148.

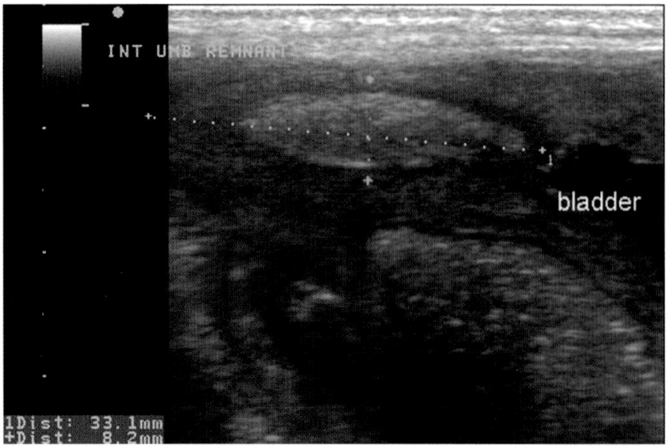

Figure 12.26 Omphalophlebitis with urachal abscessation in a septicemic foal. Sagittal ultrasonographic image of the ventral abdomen of a foal immediately caudal to the external umbilical remnant. Note the hyperechoic content of the urachus, which measures approximately 33.1 × 8.2 mm. Cranial is to the left of the image and the anechoic bladder content is to the right of the abscessed urachus. (Image courtesy of Professor Ann Carstens, Section of Diagnostic Imaging, Faculty of Veterinary Science, University of Pretoria)

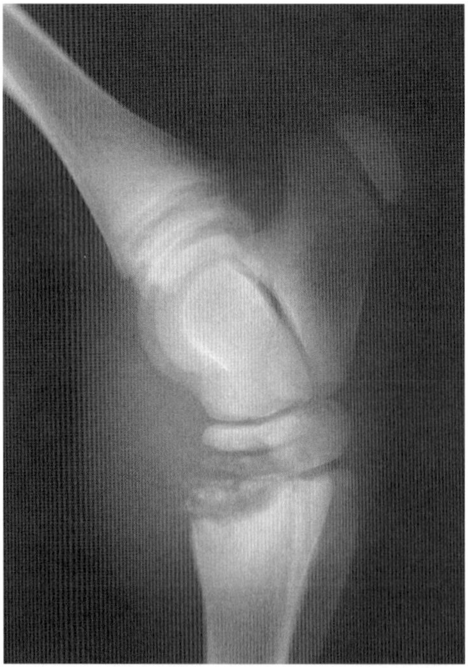

Figure 12.27 Lateral radiograph of the tarsus of a neonatal septicemic foal with type T septic arthritis. Note the severe soft tissue swelling around the tarsus, particularly dorsally, and the bubblelike gas opacities within this fluid. There is marked lysis of the dorsal central tarsal bone and proximodorsal metatarsus III. (Image courtesy of Professor Ann Carstens, Section of Diagnostic Imaging, Faculty of Veterinary Science, University of Pretoria)

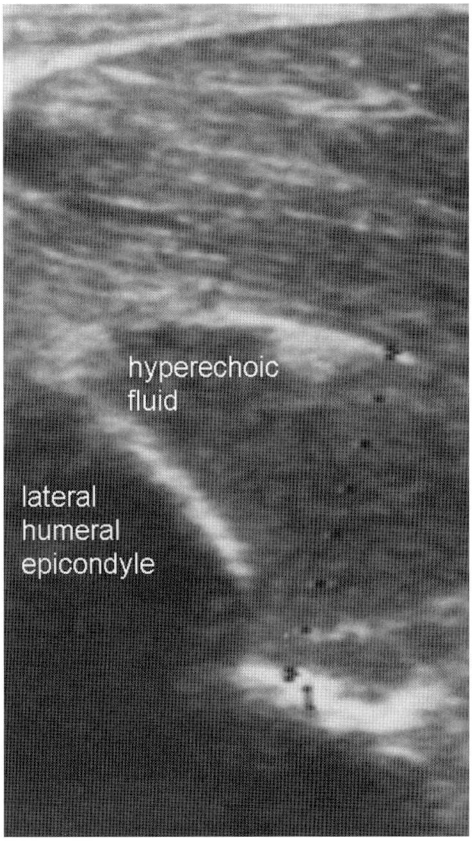

Figure 12.28 Longitudinal ultrasonographic image of the lateral aspect of the elbow of a neonatal septicemic foal showing hyperechoic joint fluid extending between the lateral humeral epicondyle (proximally to the left), the proximal radius (distally to the right of the image), and the lateral collateral ligament more superficially. Note several hyperechoic linear strands within the fluid indicative of fibrin and septic process. (Image courtesy of Professor Ann Carstens, Section of Diagnostic Imaging, Faculty of Veterinary Science, University of Pretoria)

Prematurity

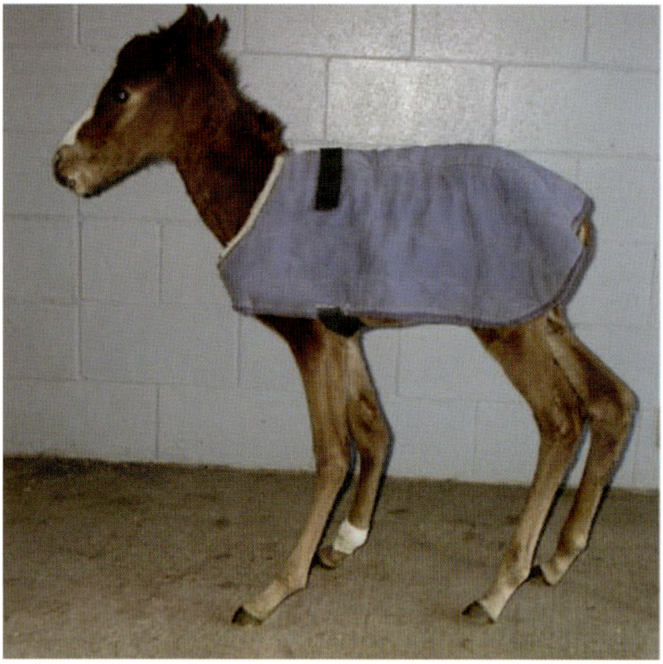

a

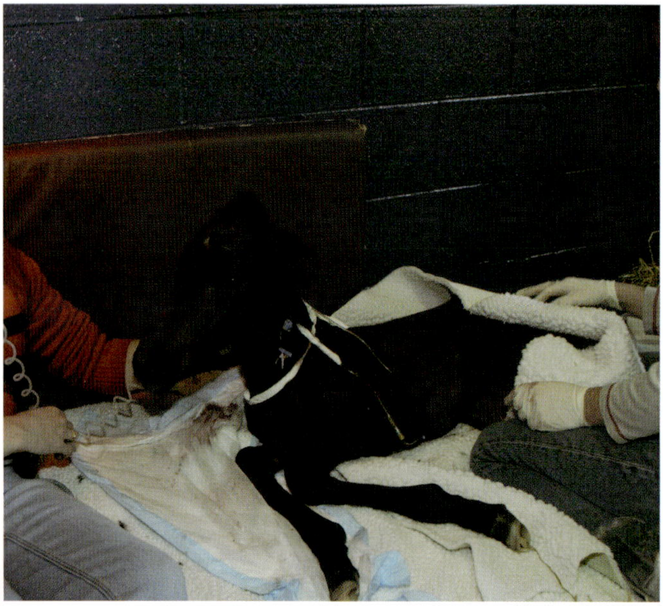

b

Figures 12.29a,b A premature foal. Note small size, domed head, and periarticular laxity. Premature foals have a gestational length less than the normal length for the mare and physical characteristics of prematurity. Causes of prematurity include placental insufficiency (twins, premature placental separation), placentitis, severe maternal illness, conditions requiring premature delivery of the foal, and mistimed parturition. Characteristic clinical signs are small body size and weight, domed forehead, slipper foot, floppy ears, soft silky coat, tendon and periarticular laxity (figs. 12.30–12.33). Foals also have incomplete ossification of the cuboidal bones (figs. 12.34 and 12.35) and may have poor thermoregulation, intolerance to enteral feeding, respiratory failure (fig. 12.36), reversion to fetal circulation, and immature hormonal responses. Differential diagnosis includes sepsis, which often occurs concurrently. Management of a premature foal is difficult and involves multiple organ systems. Premature foals that were exposed to intrauterine stresses such as placentitis have a better chance of survival although still require management of orthopedic problems.

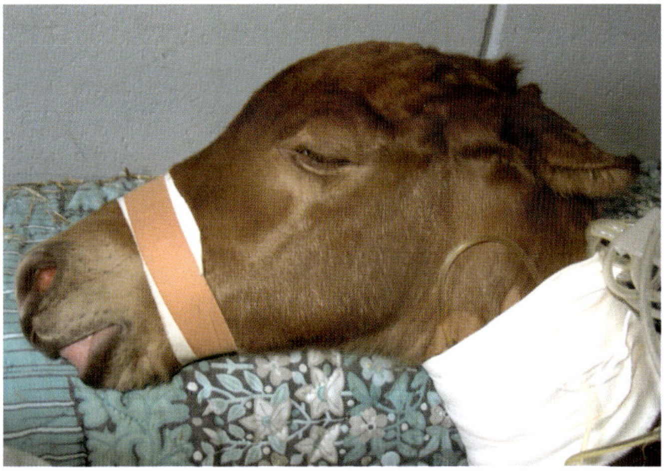

Figure 12.30 The head of a premature foal showing the classic signs of soft silky hair coat, domed forehead, and nonerect ears.

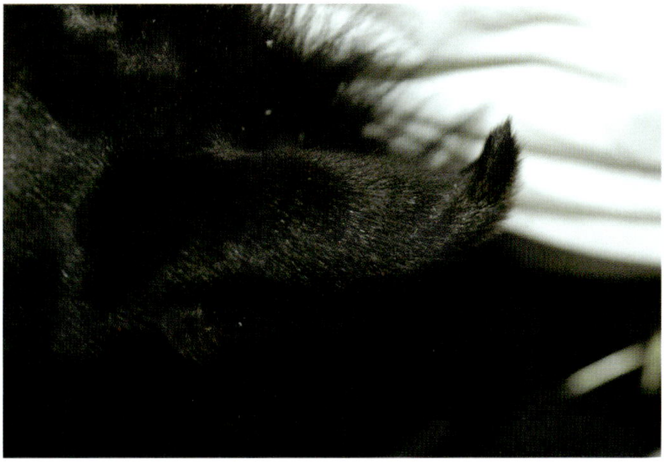

Figure 12.31 A premature foal with curly soft ears.

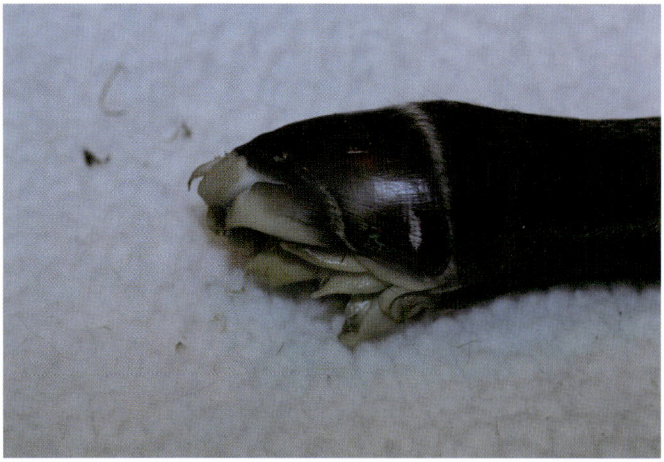

Figure 12.32 A premature foal with slipper foot.

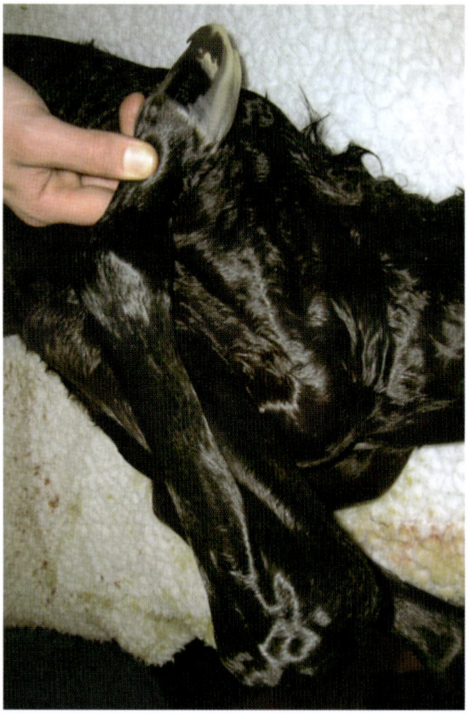

Figure 12.33 Placing the hoof up to the wither's level highlights the increased tendon and periarticular laxity.

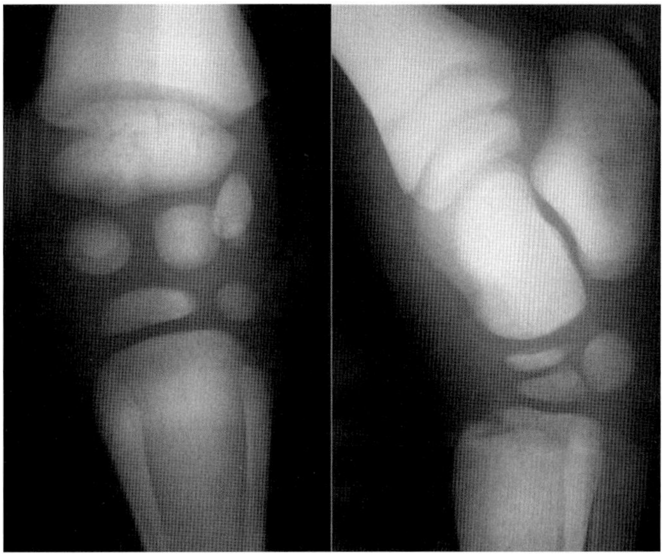

Figure 12.34 Incomplete ossification of the cuboidal bones in the hock and carpus.

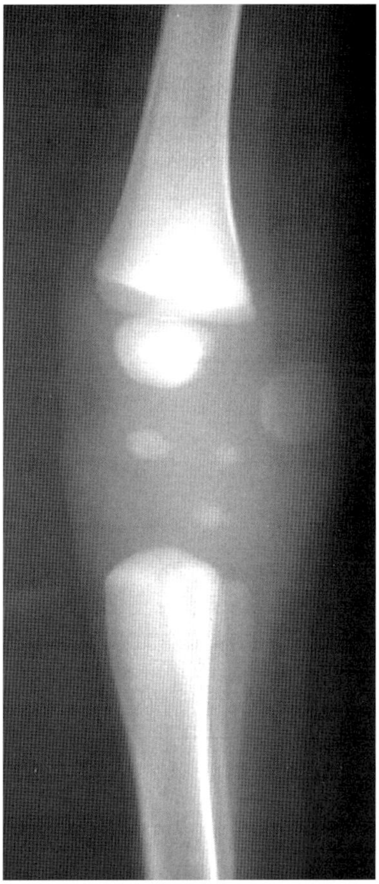

Figure 12.35 Lateral radiograph of a carpus of a premature foal showing incomplete ossification of the carpal bones with only some cuboidal bones showing a degree of ossification—skeletal ossification index = 1. Note that the intermediate carpal bone (CI) is only partially ossified and the third carpal bone that is distal to it shows no ossification. (Image courtesy of Professor Ann Carstens, Section of Diagnostic Imaging, Faculty of Veterinary Science, University of Pretoria)

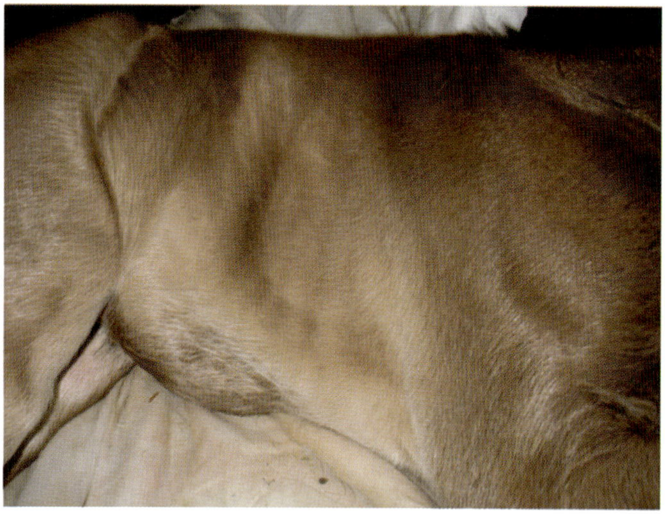

Figure 12.36 Marked paradoxical respiration in a premature foal due to poor lung compliance, weak respiratory muscles, and soft rib cage. Note the inward deviation of the thorax and outward expansion of the abdomen during inspiration.

Neonatal Isoerythrolysis

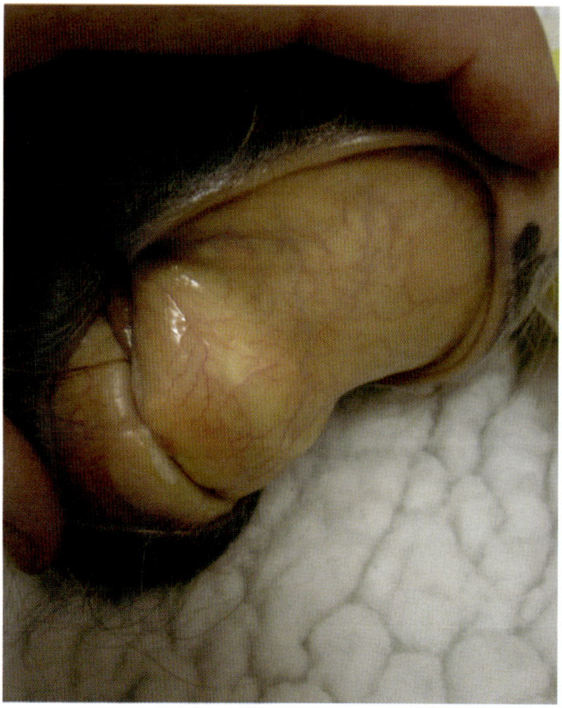

Figure 12.37 A foal with characteristic pale jaundiced mucous membranes due to neonatal isoerythrolysis (NI). NI is an alloimmune hemolytic anemia of neonates caused by antibodies in the mare's colostrum that have been formed against the foal's red blood cells. Clinical signs vary depending on the severity and rate of hemolysis. Diagnosis is based on clinical signs, clinicopathologic evaluation, and demonstration of maternal alloantibodies on the foal's red blood cells. Differential diagnoses include sepsis, internal or external hemorrhage, and liver disease. Treatment is based on the severity of hemolysis and clinical signs and is aimed at improving tissue oxygenation.

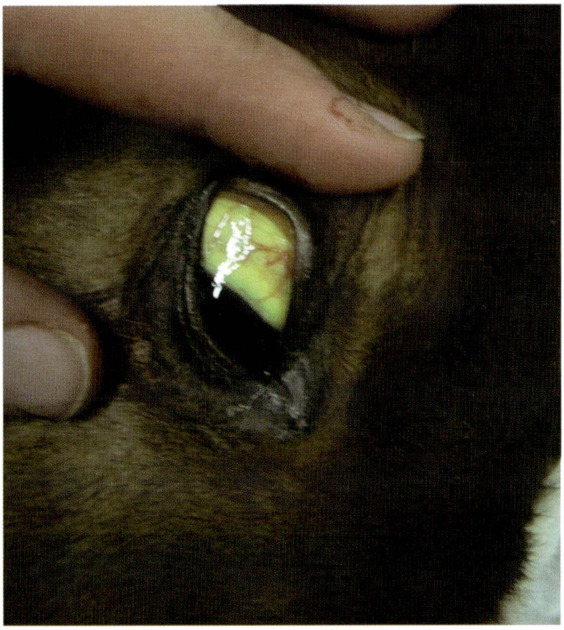

Figure 12.38 Jaundiced sclera in a foal with NI.

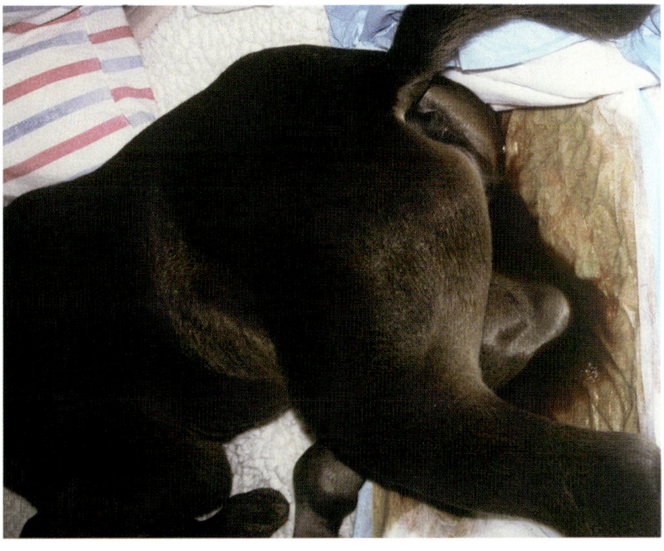

Figure 12.39 Pigmenturia from a foal that had severe acute hemolysis.

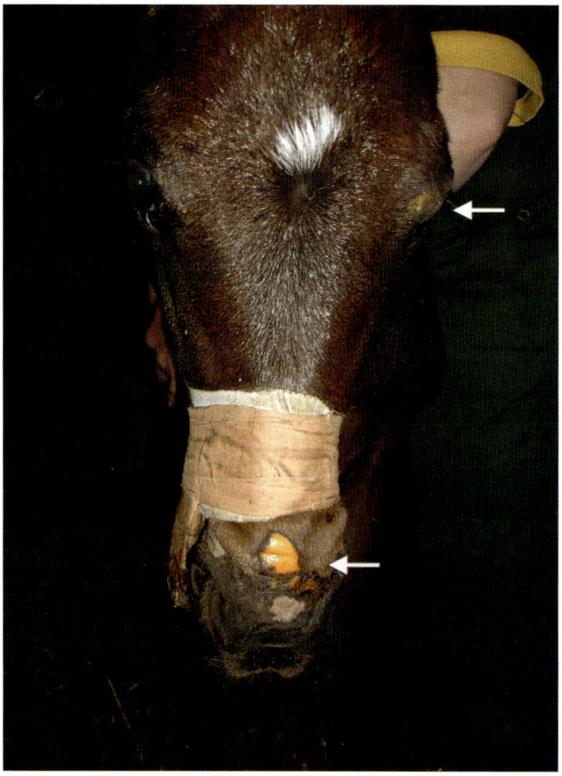

Figure 12.40 Marked jaundice is present throughout the body as highlighted by the yellow discoloration of the skin abrasions (arrows).

Respiratory System

Radiography of the Thorax

Normal Thorax

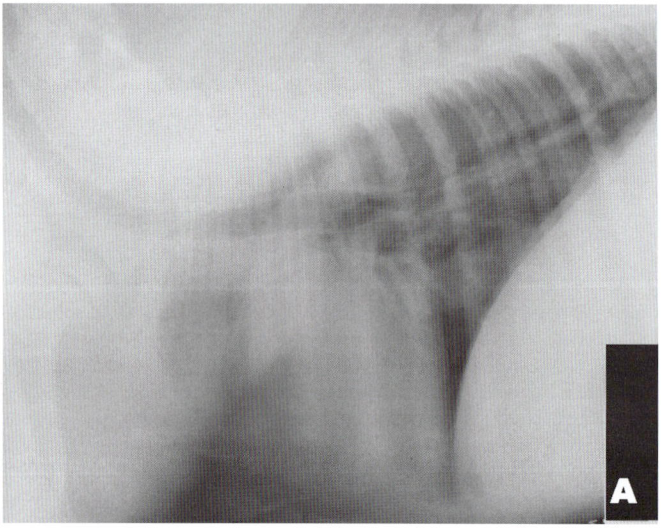

12.41

Figures 12.41–12.42 Lateral radiographic projection of the thoracic cavity in a 12-hour-old Clydesdale (A) and a 3-day-old Welsh pony foal (B). **(A&B) Radiographically normal thorax.** In both radiographs, the cardiac silhouette is within normal limits for size. The craniocaudal dimension of the heart reported to be 5.6–6.3 times the length of a midthoracic vertebra (T7-T11); the apicobasilar dimension is reported to be 6.7–7.8 times the length of a midthoracic vertebra. A subtle and mild increase in interstitial opacity is present in the lung fields of the 12-hour-old foal. This is an expected finding in the newborn. By 12–24 hours following birth, the interstitial opacity should no longer be present. Radiographs of the thorax can be repeated at 24–48 hours after birth to determine if the interstitial opacity has resolved. The lung fields are clear in this normal 3-day-old foal.

Figures 12.41–12.42 *Continued*

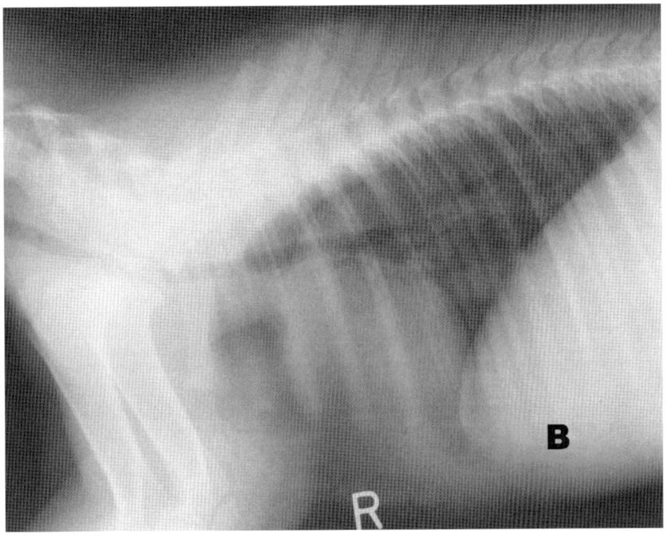

12.42

Acute Pneumonia

Figure 12.43 Lateral radiographic projection of the thoracic cavity in a 9-day-old Standardbred foal. **Alveolar infiltration of the ventral lung fields (acute pneumonia).** There is an impression of increased size of the cardiac silhouette but measurement shows it to be within the normal range for size. Increased opacity of the lung fields is apparent over the caudal margin of the heart (arrow) and extending caudodorsally (arrowheads). Air-bronchograms are faintly visible indicating that the increased opacity is due to infiltration of the air spaces (an alveolar pattern). A minor increase in diffuse interstitial opacity is present in the caudodorsal lung fields. The changes seen are consistent with a diagnosis of bronchopneumonia. Bronchopneumonia may be secondary to aspiration or sepsis in foals of this age.

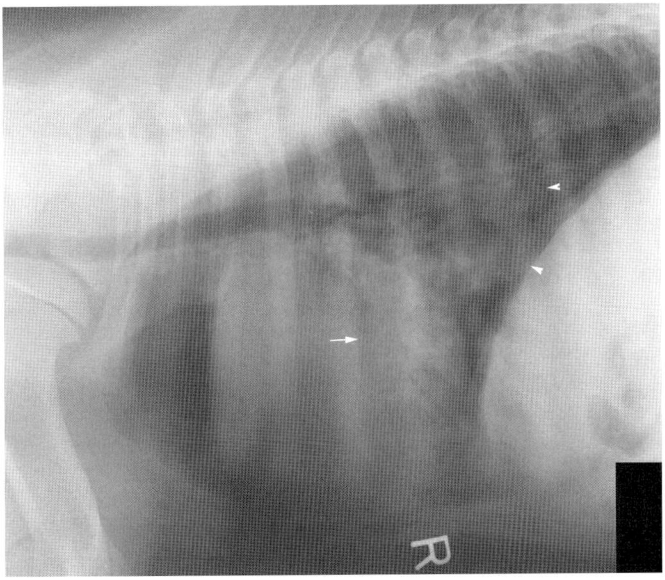

Chronic Pneumonia (Diffuse Bronchointerstitial Lung Pattern)

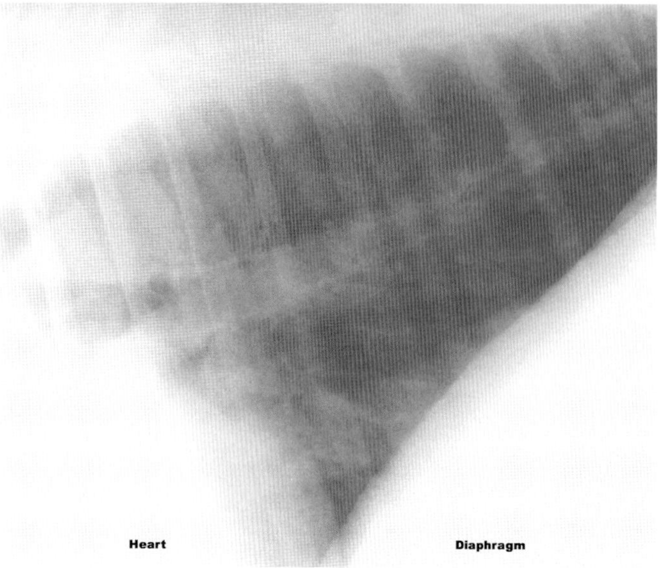

Figure 12.44 Lateral radiographic projection of the caudodorsal lung fields of a 7-month-old Standardbred. **Diffuse bronchointerstitial lung pattern (chronic pneumonia):** There is a diffuse increase in interstitial opacity in the visible lung fields. In addition, the bronchial walls are prominently seen. An interstitial lung pattern is relatively nonspecific but is generally considered evidence of pulmonary inflammation. Thickening of the bronchial walls suggests that a chronic inflammatory process is present. This patient has a 4–5-month history of coughing, nasal discharge, and increased respiratory sounds. The history and radiographic appearance of the pulmonary tissue is consistent with a diagnosis of chronic pneumonia.

Pulmonary abscessation

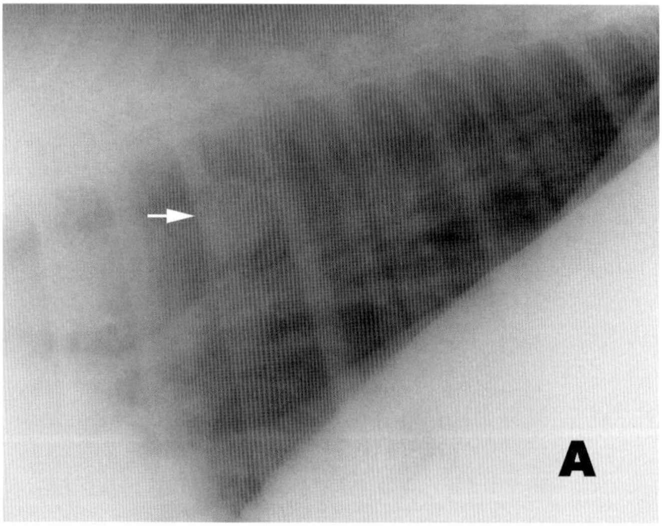

12.45

Figures 12.45–12.46 Right (A) and left (B) lateral radiographic projections of the caudodorsal lung fields of a 4-month-old Standardbred. **(A & B) Pulmonary abscess:** In both views, a mass of soft tissue opacity is visible in the dorsal lung field (arrows). The mass is more clearly seen and smaller in the left lateral radiographic projection. This indicates that the mass is closer to the cassette in the left lateral view and therefore present in the left lung field. In the left lateral view, a lucent area is seen centrally within the mass. This appearance is described as cavitary and is an indication of necrosis of the mass and communication with an airspace. Differential diagnoses for cavitary lung masses include abscess/granuloma and neoplasia. Pulmonary abscessation is most likely the cause in this young individual. Focal lung lesions appear smaller and more sharply defined when closer to the cassette. Since ventrodorsal radiographic projections of the lungs are not possible in horses, with the exception of neonates; right and left lateral views are obtained in an effort to determine the side of focal lung lesions.

Figures 12.45–12.46 *Continued*

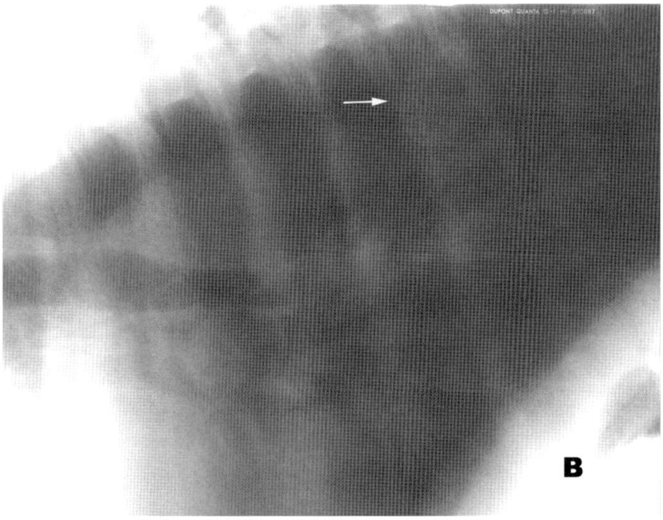

12.46

Figure 12.47 Lateral radiographic projection of the caudal lung fields in a 3-month-old Standardbred. **Pulmonary consolidation, probable pulmonary abscessation, perihilar lymph node enlargement:** The caudal margin of the cardiac silhouette and the caudal vena cava are not visible due to silhouetting with heavily consolidated lung tissue. Focal rounded areas of soft tissue opacity (arrows) are visible within the area of consolidation. The trachea is dorsally deviated as it crosses the heart base (arrowheads). The severe pulmonary consolidation and the presence of pulmonary abscessation are radiographic findings typically present in foals with infection with *Rhodococcus equi*. Elevation of the trachea over the heart base is evidence of enlargement of the perihilar lymph nodes due to the presence of severe pneumonia.

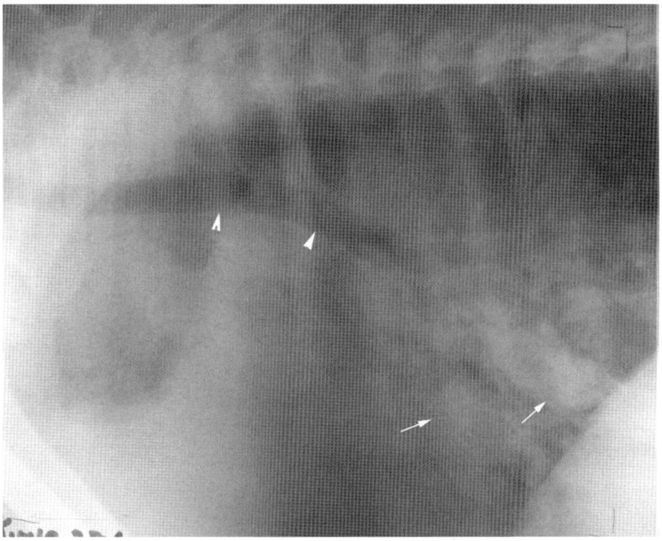

Rhodococcus equi

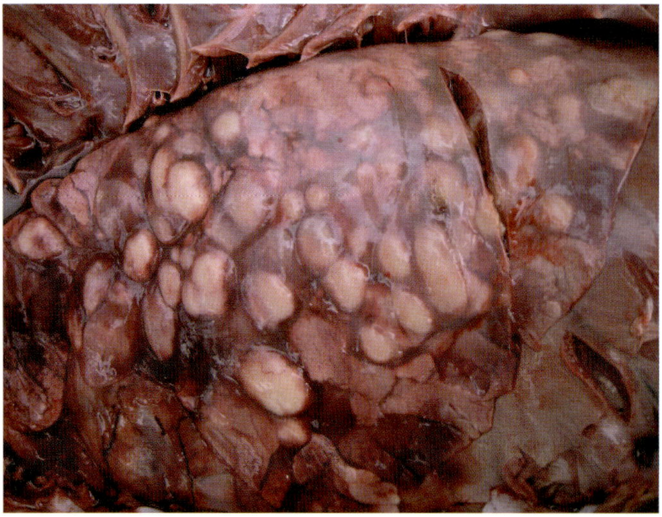

Figure 12.48 Large encapsulated abscesses throughout the lung parenchyma due to *Rhodococcus equi* infection. *R. equi* is a common cause of disease in foals 1–4 months of age. *R. equi* pneumonia (rattles) has an insidious onset and affected foals remain clinically normal until severe disease is present. Clinical signs of *R. equi* pneumonia include increased respiratory rate, abnormal sounds on thoracic auscultation, and acute respiratory distress; nasal discharge or coughing are inconsistent findings. Diagnosis is based on clinical signs, transtracheal aspirate culture and cytology, clinicopathologic evaluation, radiographic (fig. 12.51) and ultrasonographic findings (figs. 12.49 and 12.50). Treatment includes antimicrobial therapy (macrolide and rifampin) and respiratory support. Clinical signs associated with extrapulmonary lesions may also be present (figs. 12.52–12.57).

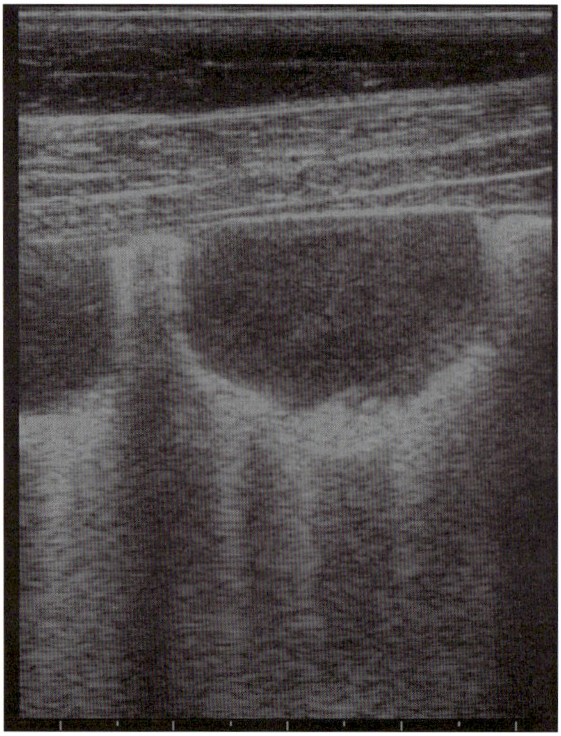

Figure 12.49 Sonogram of a thorax showing discrete superficial abscesses in the lung parenchyma. Ultrasonographic examination is a useful diagnostic tool for screening foals on endemic farms. Transducer is in the intercostal space parallel to the lung surface. Distance mark = 5 mm.

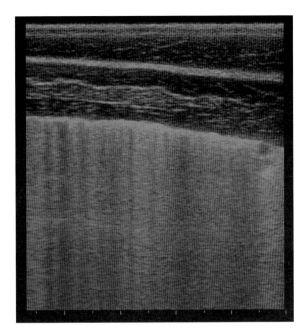

Figure 12.50 Sonogram of a thorax showing "sheets" of comet tail artifacts, which are usually seen with interstitial pneumonia. Foals with this form of the disease present in acute respiratory distress.

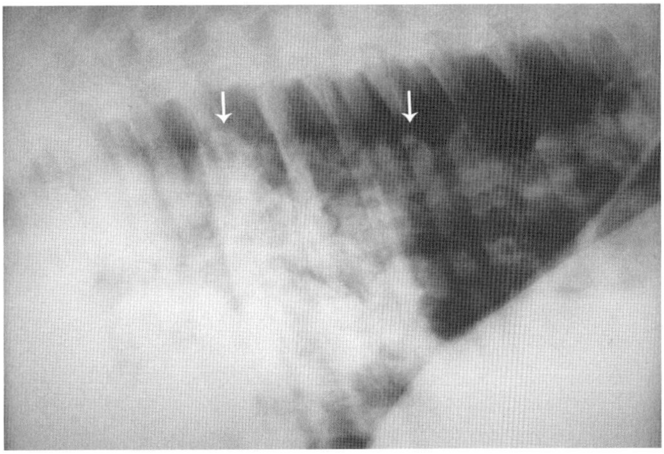

Figure 12.51 Lateral thoracic radiograph of a foal with *R. equi.* Note the cavitary lesions indicative of abscess formation (arrows) and patchy focal alveolar pattern.

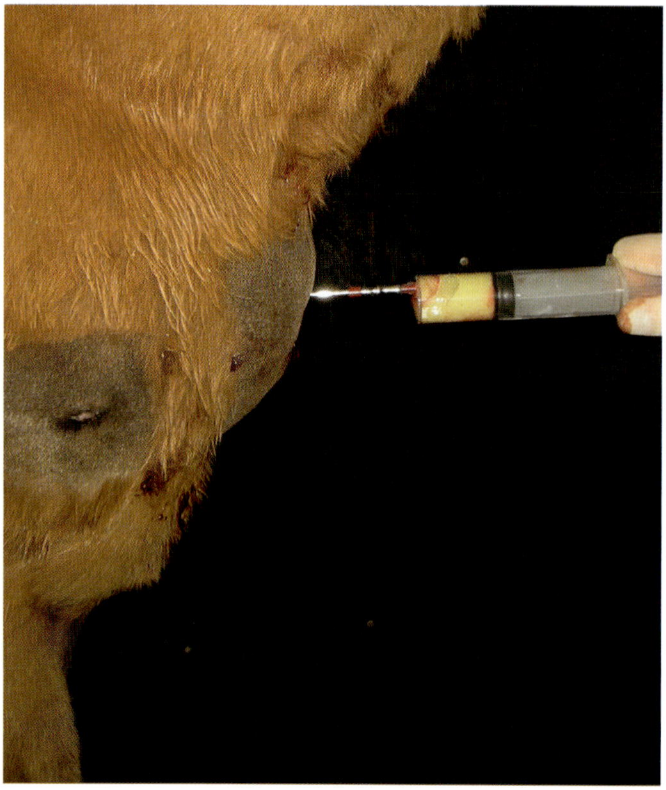

Figure 12.52 Purulent material being removed from an abscessed prescapular lymph node. Suppurative inflammation of lymph nodes due to *R. equi* infection can occur randomly throughout the body.

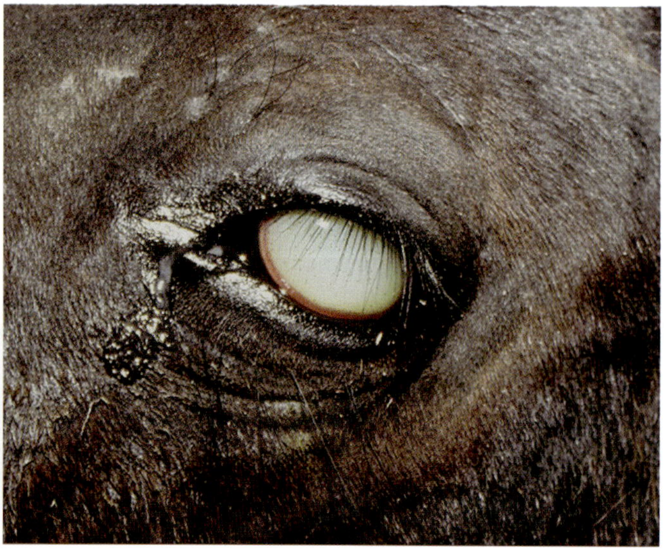

Figure 12.53 Severe keratouveitis due to immune complex deposition associated with *R. equi* infection. This is usually bilateral and resolves with the resolution of the disease.

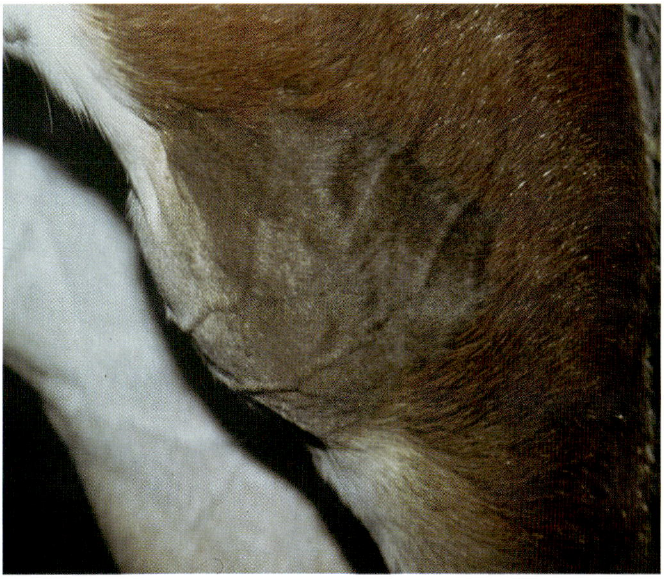

Figure 12.54 Stifle effusion associated with immune complex deposition in synovial structures associated with *R. equi* infection. This results in a polysynovitis with multiple joints and tendon sheaths involved. Foals with the immune mediate polysynovitis have mild lameness, which helps to differentiate from infectious orthopedic disease. The effusion resolves with resolution of the disease.

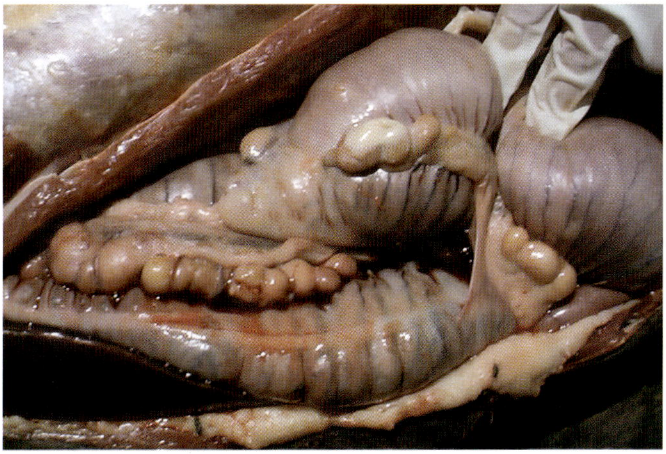

Figure 12.55 Intestinal form of *R. equi*. Suppurative inflammation of lymph nodes of the colon and cecum is seen with an ulcerative enterocolitis. Clinical signs associated with the intestinal form include diarrhea, colic, and ill thrift. (Image courtesy of Dr. A. Gunn)

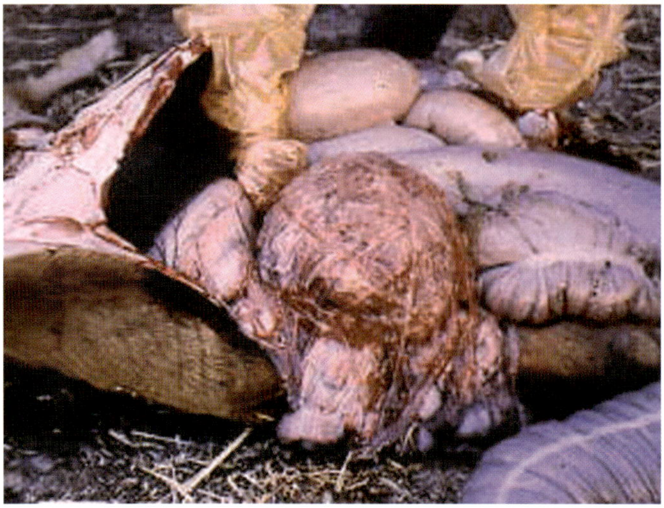

Figure 12.56 A large intra-abdominal abscess due to suppurative inflammation of mesenteric lymph node caused by *R. equi* infection.

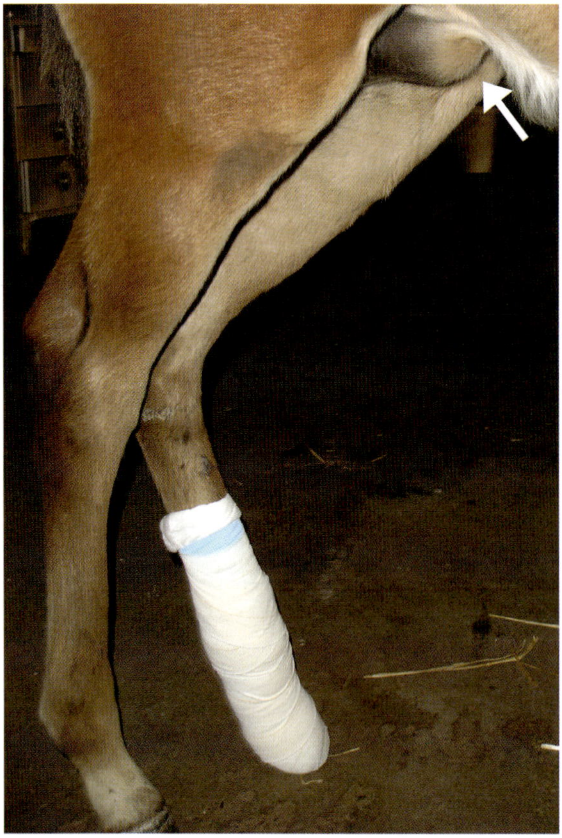

Figure 12.57 A foal with *R. equi* infection causing osteomyelitis of the extensor process of the third phalanx and an inguinal abscess (arrow).

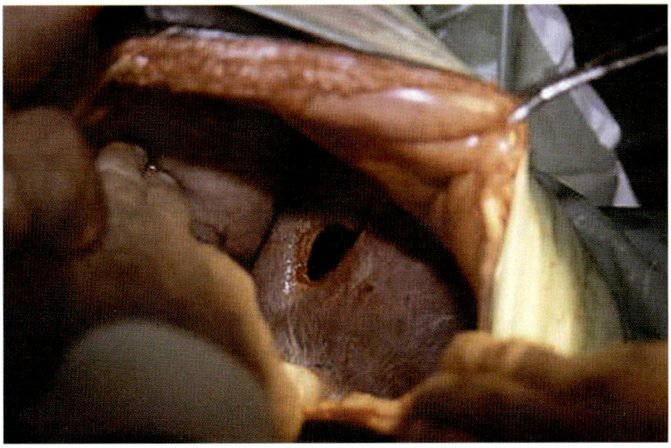

Figure 12.58 A defect in the diaphragm, which resulted in herniation of a portion of the small intestine. Diaphragmatic hernia in foals can be congenital or due to trauma or fractured ribs. Clinical signs include respiratory distress and colic although clinical signs may not be seen until adhesions are formed. Radiographs demonstrate viscera in the thorax (fig. 12.59). An exploratory celiotomy confirms the presence of the defect and assesses potential for repair.

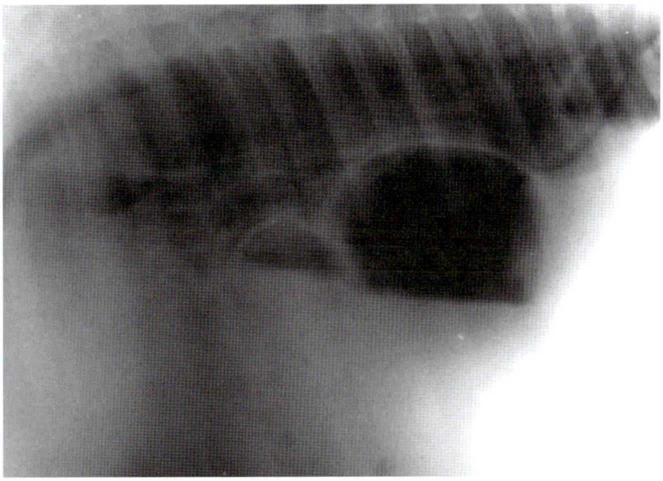

Figure 12.59 Lateral thoracic radiograph demonstrating gas-filled loops of viscera in the thorax.

Pneumonia

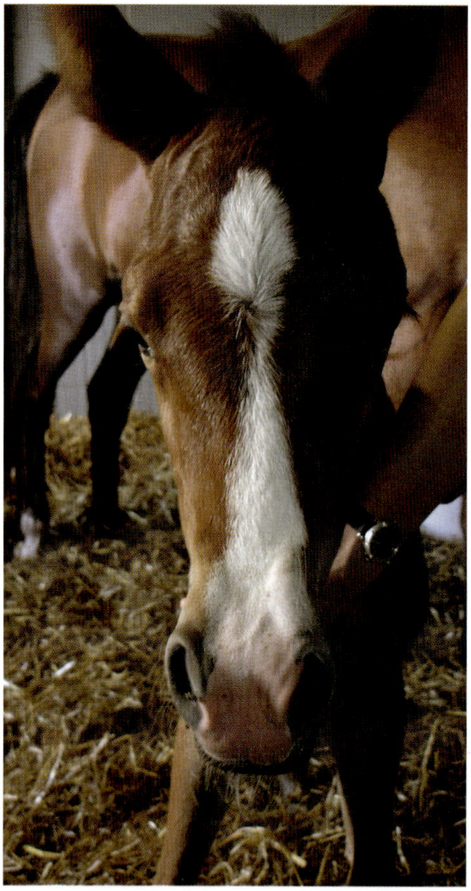

Figure 12.60 A foal with resolving pneumonia exhibiting nostril flaring. Pneumonia in neonates occurs most commonly due to sepsis, aspiration, or recumbency. Clinical signs of pneumonia are usually absent in the early stages of disease. An arterial blood gas analysis will provide information on altered lung function before clinical signs of increased respiratory rate, altered breathing pattern, and nostril flaring are seen. Thoracic auscultation, coughing, and nasal discharge are not reliable indicators of disease. Diagnosis is based on radiographic findings, arterial blood gas analysis, and clinicopathologic evaluation. Treatment involves antimicrobial therapy, respiratory system support, nasogastric tube feeding if aspiration is a concern, and nursing support to improve ventilation (fig. 12.61).

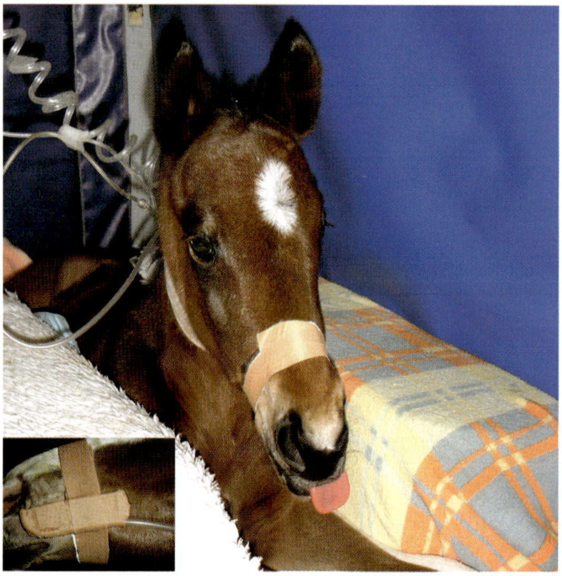

Figure 12.61 A foal recovering from HIS in a sternal support with intranasal oxygen insufflation. Insert shows placement of intranasal oxygen insufflation. Lateral recumbency can reduce the PaO_2 by as much as 30 mmHg. Keeping a foal in sternal recumbency, regular turning, and standing can help improve ventilation.

Candidiasis

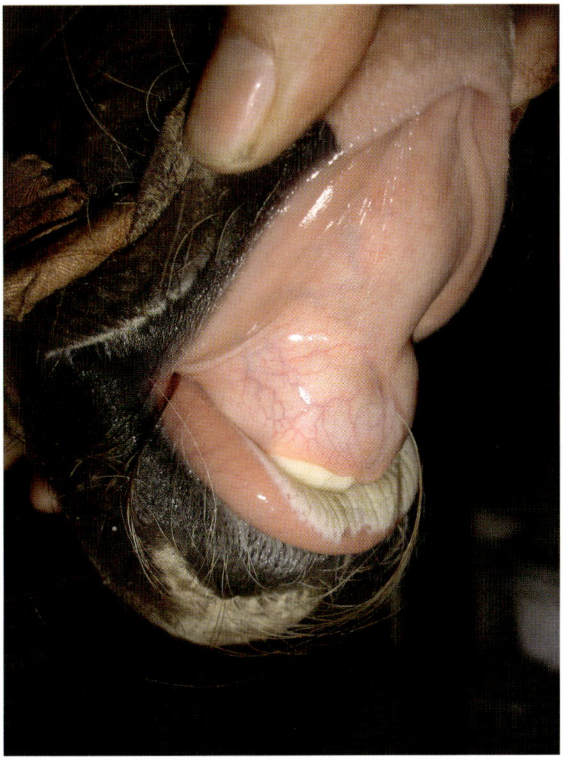

Figure 12.62 Candidiasis on a foal's tongue. This can be an incidental finding in debilitated foals, or associated with inflammation and increased salivation or systemic candidiasis in septicemic neonates. Topical application of dilute potassium permanganate wiped over the tongue with gauze squares is used as treatment for localized candida. Systemic antifungal therapy should be considered if systemic candidiasis is present.

Cleft Palate

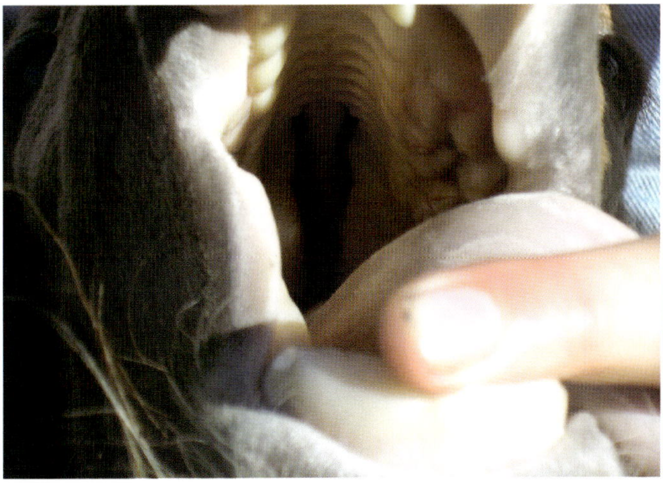

Figure 12.63 Defect in the hard palate of a newborn foal. Defects can involve the soft and hard palate, and can occur with other congenital abnormalities. Clinical signs vary from profuse nasal regurgitation of milk, especially when the hard palate is involved, to no signs of dysphagia and clinically inapparent. Differential diagnoses include subepiglottic cyst, neurologic dysphagia associated with hypoxic ischemic syndrome (HIS), or esophageal disease. Diagnosis of a soft palate defect requires endoscopic examination. (Image courtesy of Dr. S. McKerrow)

Inferior Brachygnathism (Parrot Mouth)

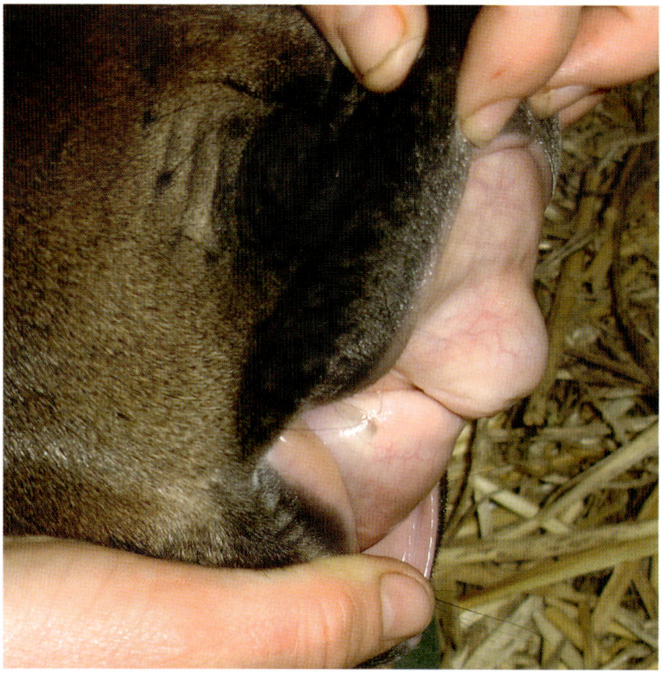

Figure 12.64 Inferior brachygnathism in a foal. This is believed to be a heritable condition. Mild cases may not be noticed until permanent incisors have erupted. Surgery is attempted on more severe cases to slow the growth of the maxilla. The lack of normal occlusion of the incisors results in abnormal wear, which may predispose to oral soft tissue damage.

Wry Nose

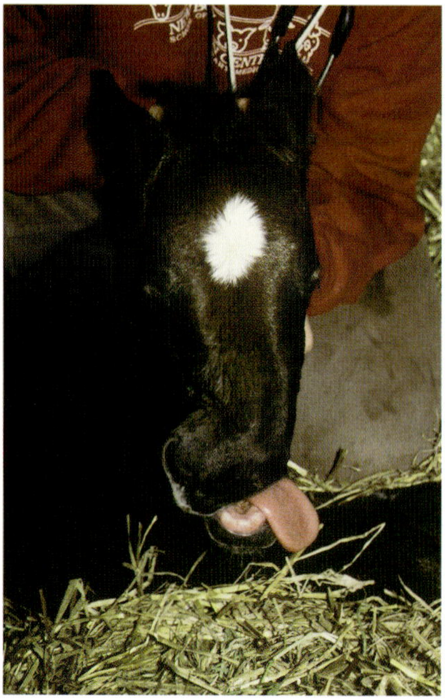

Figure 12.65 Congenital shortening and deviation of the maxillae, premaxillae, nasal bones, and vomer bone known as "wry nose," which results in malocclusion of the incisors. The effect on the foal depends on the degree of malocclusion. Surgery has been performed in an attempt to correct the distortion. Please see Chapter 3, Diseases of the Respiratory System.

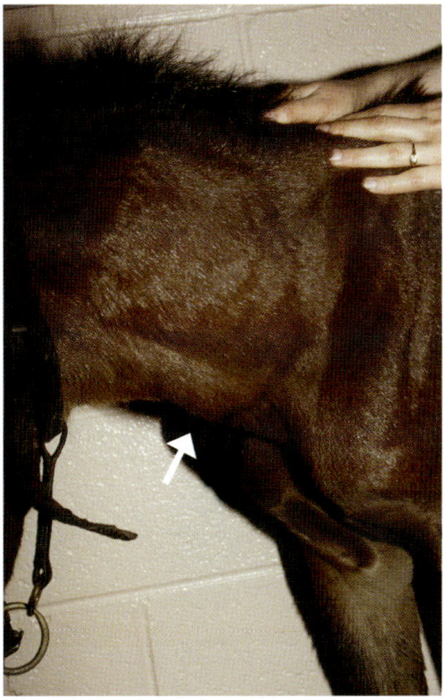

Figure 12.66 Esophageal distension near thoracic inlet (arrow) in a foal with megaesophagus. Etiology is unclear and believed to be related to neurological deficits in the intrinsic nerve plexuses that control esophageal contractions. Dysphagia is often seen and a large amount of milk may be regurgitated if the foal lowers its head after nursing. Dynamic and static contrast radiographic studies can be used to assess the extent of dysfunction.

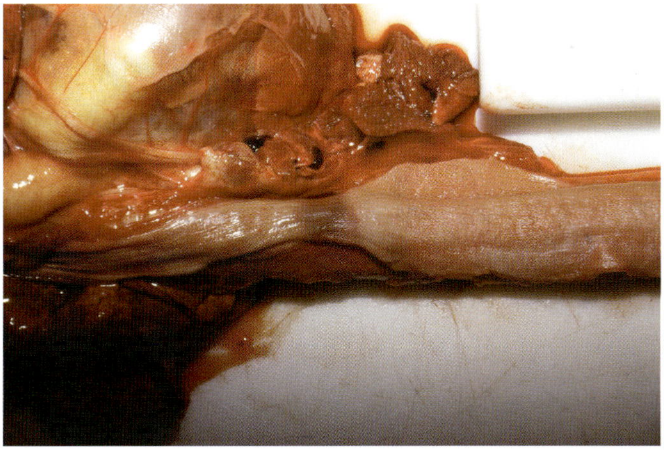

Figure 12.67 Postmortem specimen of the esophagus from the foal in fig. 12.66 showing the distended thin flaccid appearance of the proximal section of esophagus. The hemorrhagic area is iatrogenic.

Esophageal Stricture

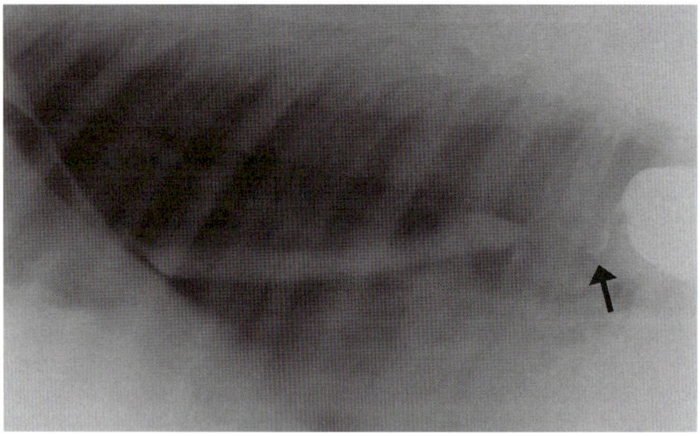

Figure 12.68 A static contrast lateral radiograph of a foal's thorax with an esophageal stricture (arrow). Esophageal strictures vary widely in character from thin superficial strictures, which may resolve with increased dietary fiber intake, to those involving deeper layers of the esophagus, which carry a very poor prognosis. Foals may present with dysphagia or a history of recurrent choke.

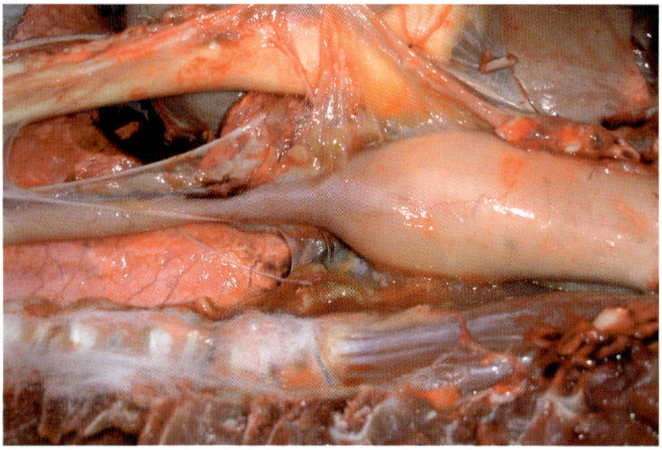

Figure 12.69 Postmortem specimen of foal in fig. 12.68. Histopathological examination of the stricture revealed marked hypertrophy of the muscularis layer of the esophagus.

Figure 12.70 A stomach from a 7-day-old foal with focal ulceration in the squamous and glandular mucosa along the margo plicatus. The foal was a critically ill neonate and had fatal hemorrhage through the ulcer (arrow) (fig. 12.71). Gastroduodenal ulcer syndrome (GDUS) is a well-recognized disease in foals. The cause is unknown and is most likely multifactorial. In neonates, it is believed to be associated with altered tissue perfusion and infection. In older foals, stress, intestinal disturbances, possible infectious organisms, and nonsteroidal anti-inflammatory drugs play a role. Diagnosis is confirmed by gastroscopy. Many foals do not show the classic signs of bruxism or ptyalism and some may be found dead after rupture of the ulcer. In neonates, supportive therapy to maintain tissue perfusion is important. Antiulcer medications are used for treatment and prevention in older foals.

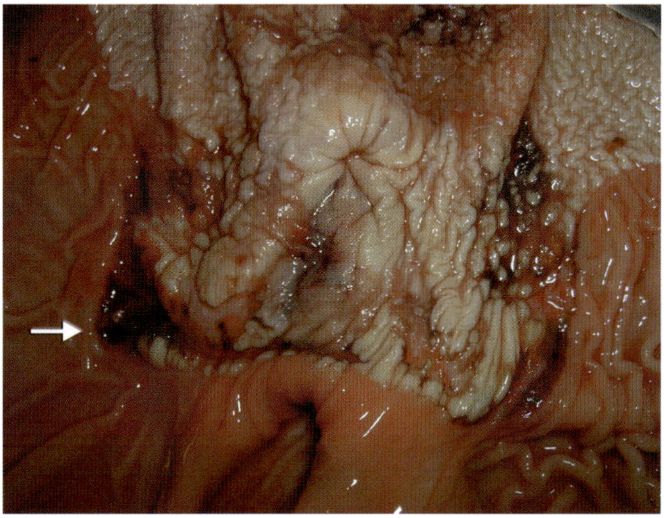

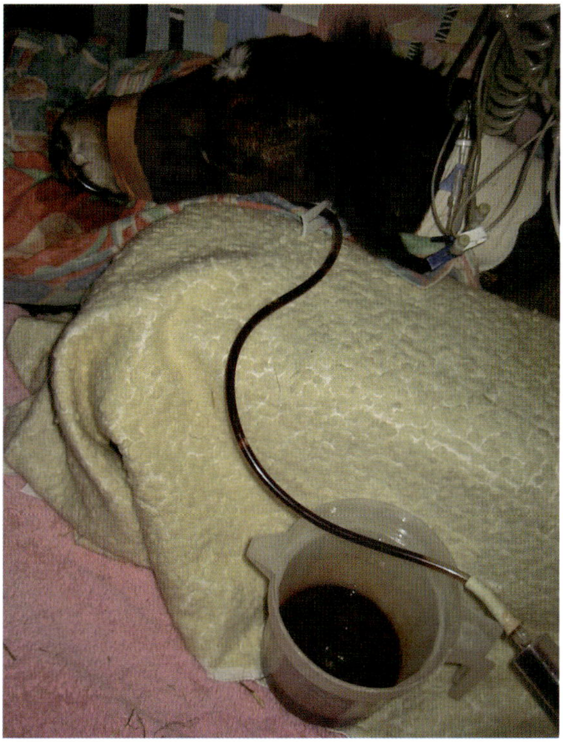

Figure 12.71 Hemorrhagic nasogastric reflux due to erosion of a blood vessel in an ulcer (bleeding gastric ulcer).

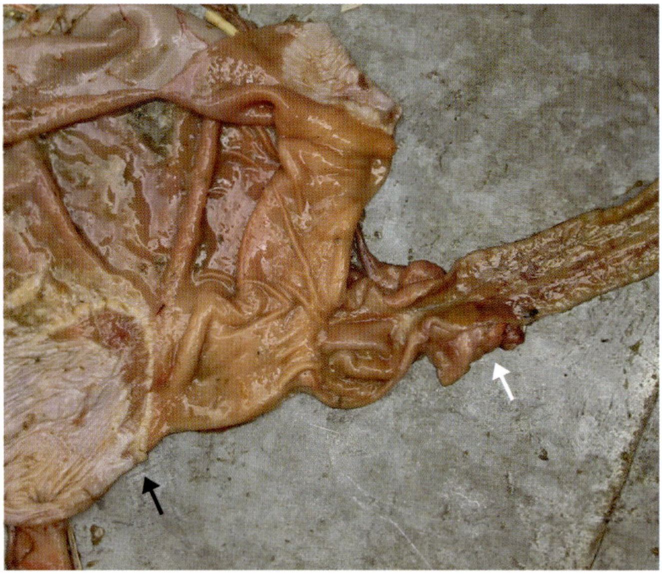

Figure 12.72 Postmortem specimen from a foal with delayed gastric emptying due to a duodenal stricture (white arrow). There is also superficial ulceration in squamous portion of the stomach (black arrow). Duodenal inflammation and ulceration, which can then progress to fibrosis and stricture of duodenum, occurs in older foals (2–6 m) (fig. 12.73). It is difficult to clinically differentiate between the two stages, thus medical treatment is often attempted first. Diagnosis is based on clinical examination findings, contrast studies, ultrasonography, and gastroscopy. Surgery can be performed if medical treatment is not successful.

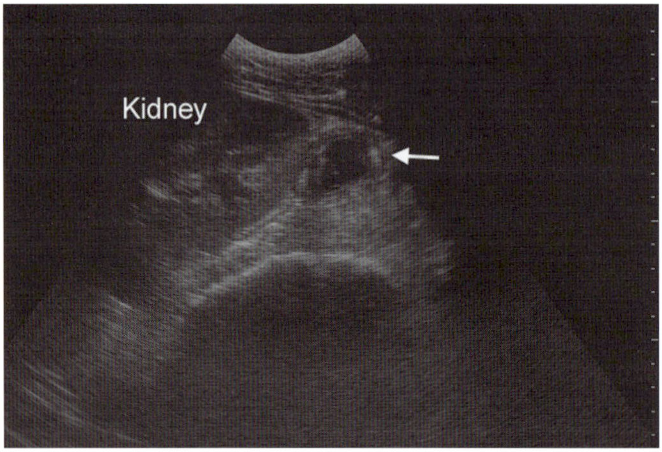

Figure 12.73 Sonogram of the right dorsal abdomen through the 15th intercostal space visualizing a duodenum in a foal that was presented with colic associated with delayed gastric emptying. Note the thickened wall (arrow) of the duodenum. Distance mark = 5 mm.

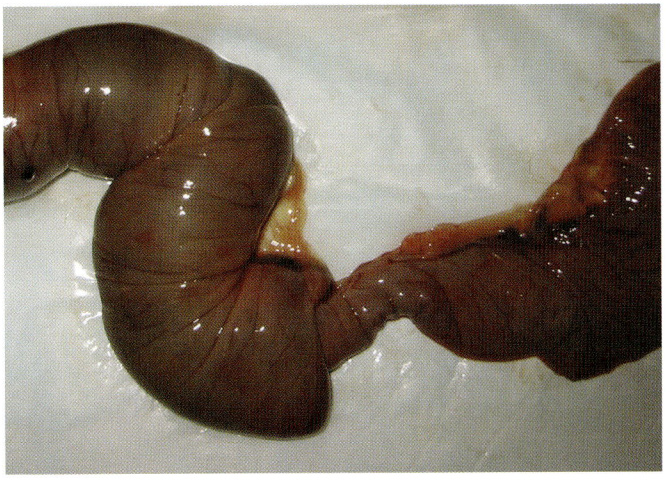

Figure 12.74 Postmortem specimen of a jejunojejunal intussusception in a foal. Affected foals may show signs of acute abdominal pain, however, in compromised neonates, an intussusception is often present without signs of pain and is detected after further investigation of abdominal distension, change in demeanor, or presence of nasogastric reflux.

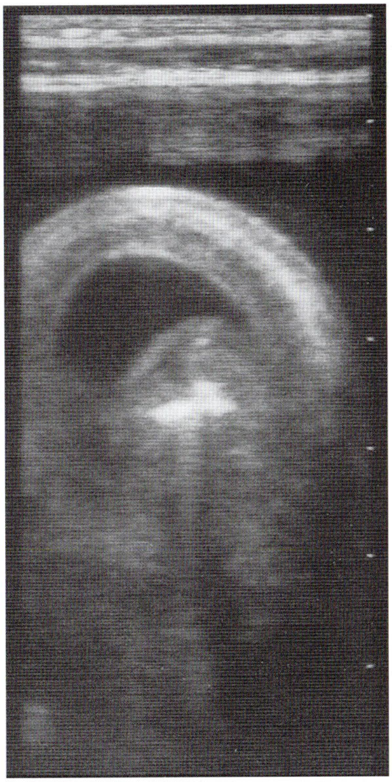

Figure 12.75 An ultrasonographic image of an intussusception in a foal revealing the classic “bull’s-eye” appearance.

Ascaridiasis

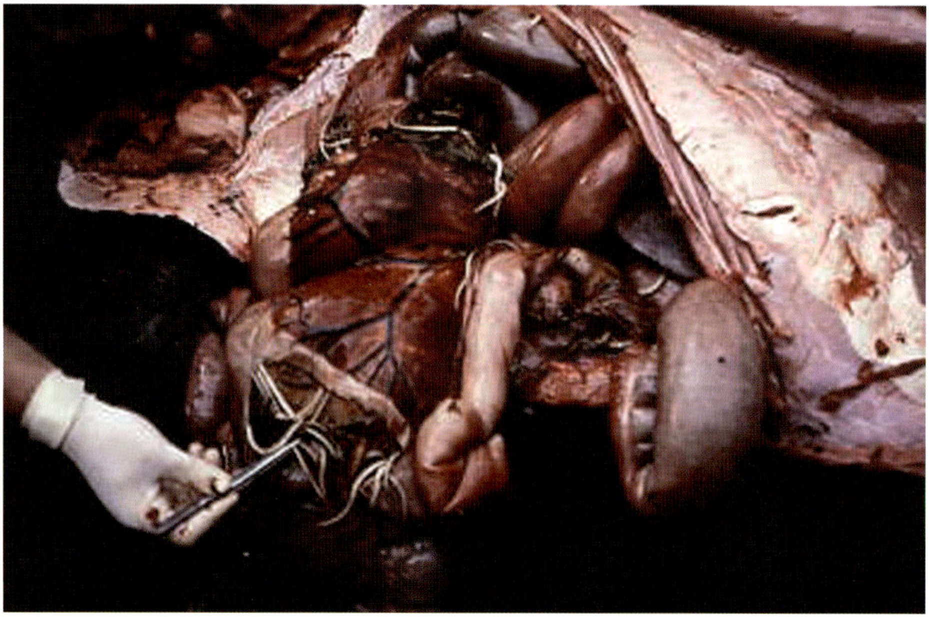

Figure 12.76 Intestinal rupture due to ileal obstruction with *Parascaris equorum*. Clinical signs are consistent with small intestinal obstruction, usually occurring after anthelmintic administration. Coughing may occur with the presence of large numbers of migrating worms in the lungs. Acute intestinal obstruction caused by *Parascaris equorum* is diagnosed based on poor deworming program, small intestinal distension, and ultrasonographic findings.

Clostridial Enterocolitis

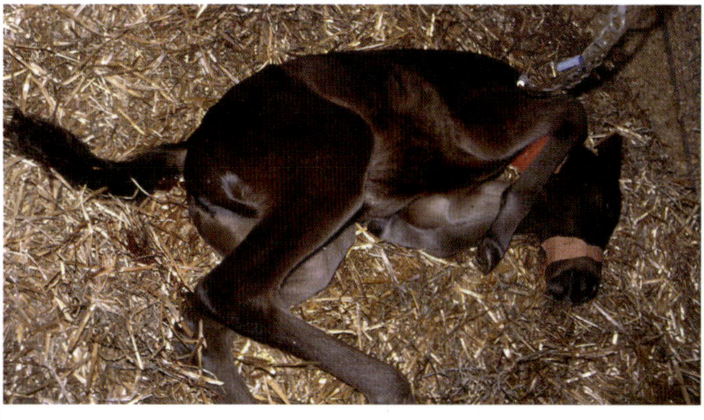

Figure 12.77 Foal with enterocolitis due to *Clostridium perfringens* exhibiting signs of colic and bloody feces. Clostridial enterocolitis is caused by *Clostridium difficile* and *Clostridium perfringens*. Clinical signs vary from watery diarrhea with possible hemorrhage, systemic inflammatory response syndrome (SIRS), to sudden death. Differential diagnoses include other causes of enterocolitis such as salmonellosis, sepsis, necrotizing enterocolitis, and causes of colic in young foals. Diagnosis is based on clinical signs, toxin assays, and fecal smears. Treatment includes systemic supportive therapy and specific antimicrobial therapy.

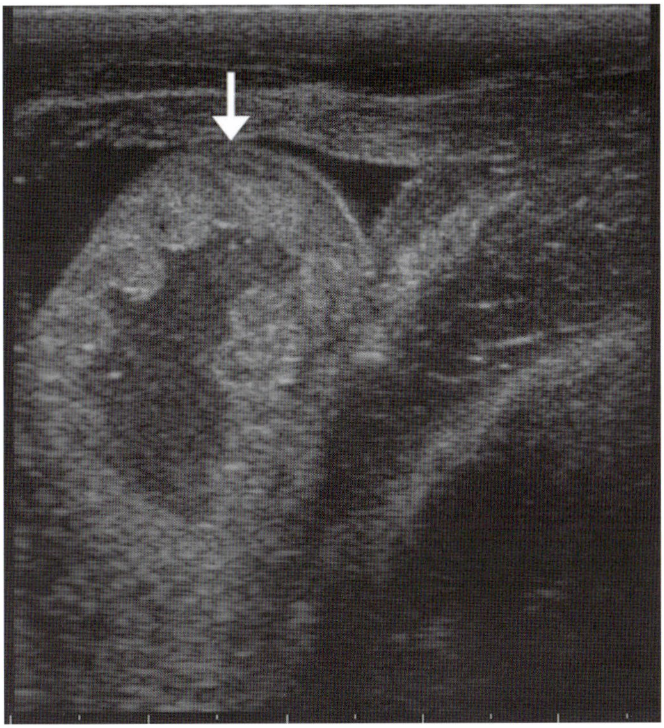

Figure 12.78 Sonogram of the ventral abdomen of a foal with clostridial enterocolitis. Note the moderately distended fluid-filled loops of small intestine with thickened intestinal wall and increased peritoneal fluid. Analysis of the peritoneal fluid is usually consistent with an exudate. These ultrasonographic findings are not specific for clostridial infection.

Rotavirus Diarrhea

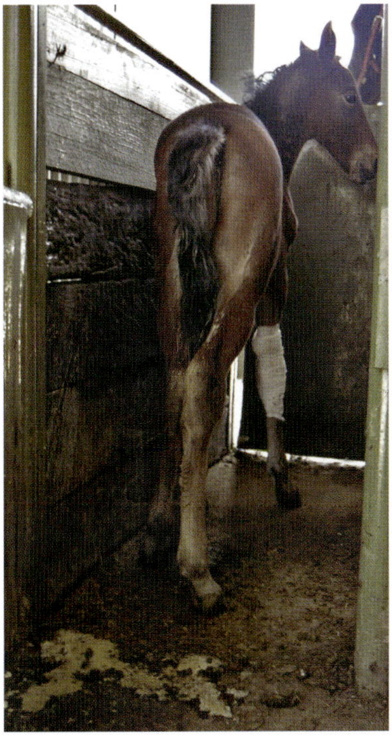

Figure 12.79 Foal with diarrhea due to rotavirus. Rotavirus is the most common cause of viral diarrhea in foals and often occurs in outbreaks. Clinical signs range from mild self-limiting diarrhea to severe watery diarrhea with dehydration and electrolyte abnormalities. Diagnosis is based on clinical signs and demonstration of viral particles in the feces. Differential diagnoses include salmonellosis, gastroduodenal ulcer syndrome (GDUS), *R. equi* infection, other viral causes of diarrhea, and dietary factors. Treatment is supportive.

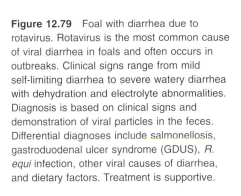

Meconium Impaction

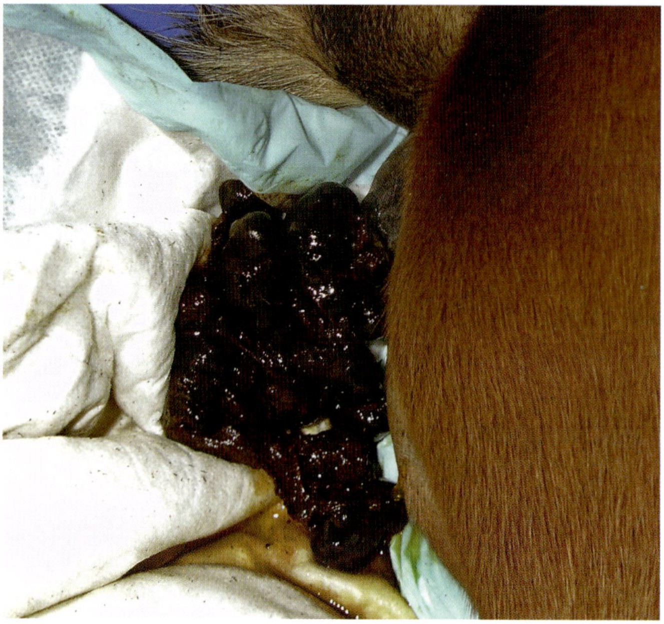

Figure 12.80 Foal passing meconium. Note the dark olive brown fecal balls. Meconium impaction is the most common cause of colic in neonates <3 days of age. Retention of meconium occurs with impaired gastrointestinal motility, failure to ingest colostrum, dehydration, and prolonged recumbency. The impaction can lead to complete intestinal obstruction, gaseous abdominal distension, and signs of colic. Differential diagnoses include intestinal atresia, agangliosis, enterocolitis, and intussusception. Diagnosis is based on ultrasonography, radiography, and digital examination findings. Treatment is aimed at resolving the impaction, providing pain relief, and systemic support.

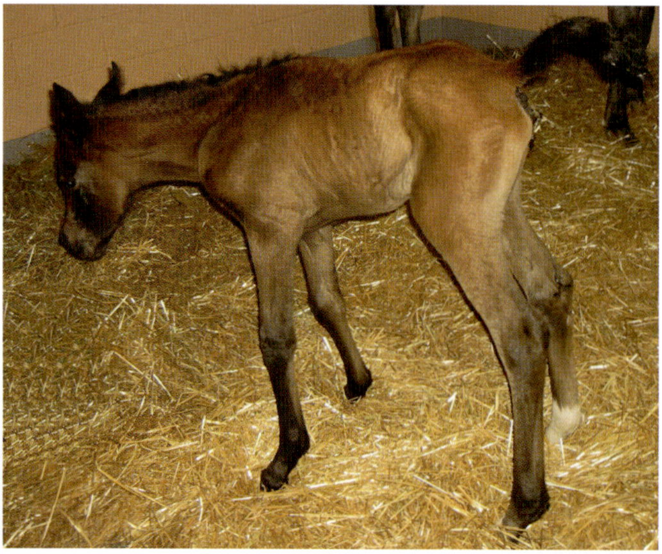

Figure 12.81 Foal straining to pass meconium. Note the arched back and tail position, which is different from the posture for urination.

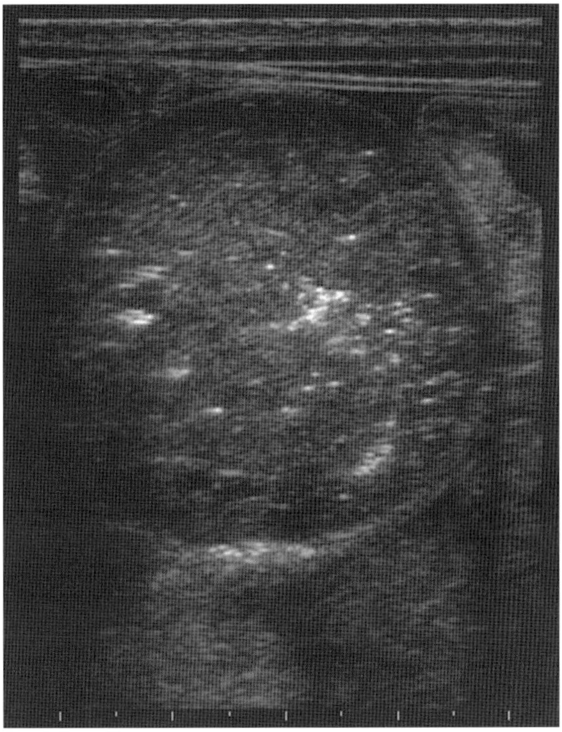

Figure 12.82 Ultrasonographic image of meconium highlighting its "speckled" appearance.

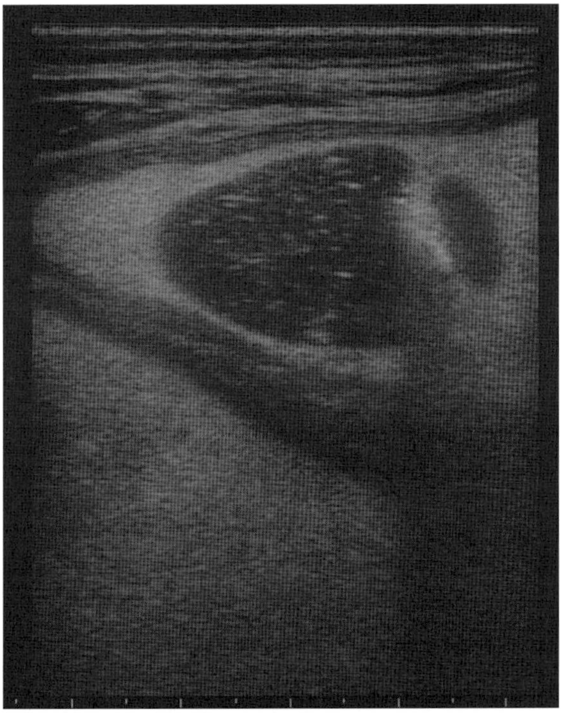

Figure 12.83 Ultrasonographic image of balls of meconium surrounded by mineral oil in the large colon.

Intestinal Atresia

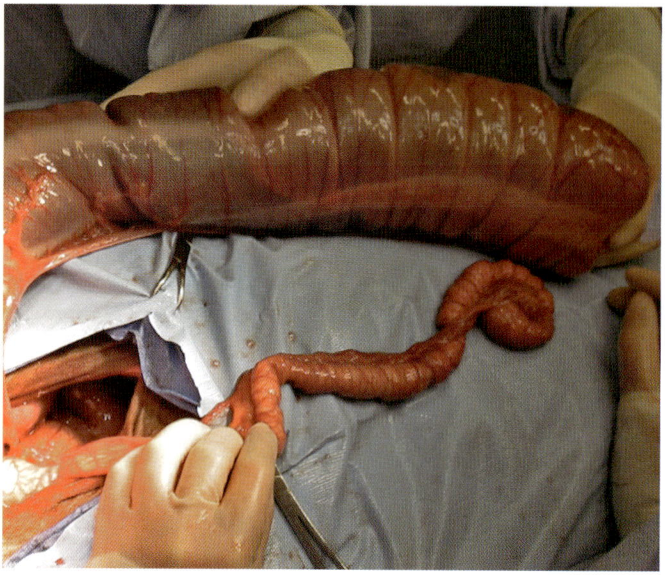

Figure 12.84 Type 3 atresia of the large colon. Intestinal atresia can occur at various locations along the colon, rectum, and anus (fig. 12.85). Clinical signs of abdominal distention and colic occur within the first 2 to 48 hours after birth, depending on the location of the defect. Diagnosis is based on lack of passing meconium (staining) and contrast radiography, however, an exploratory celiotomy may be required for definitive diagnosis.

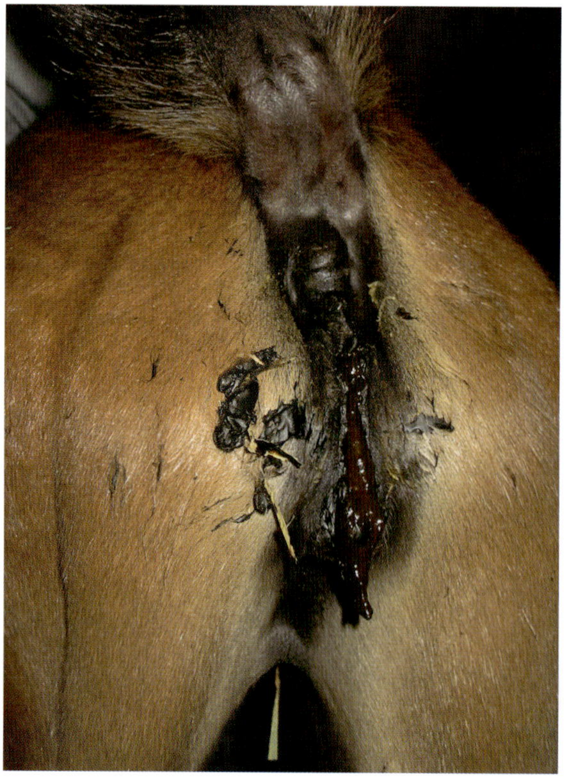

Figure 12.85 Atresia ani in a filly foal. The filly had a congenital malformation resulting in a rectovaginal fistula, which allowed passage of small amounts of meconium.

Scrotal Hernia

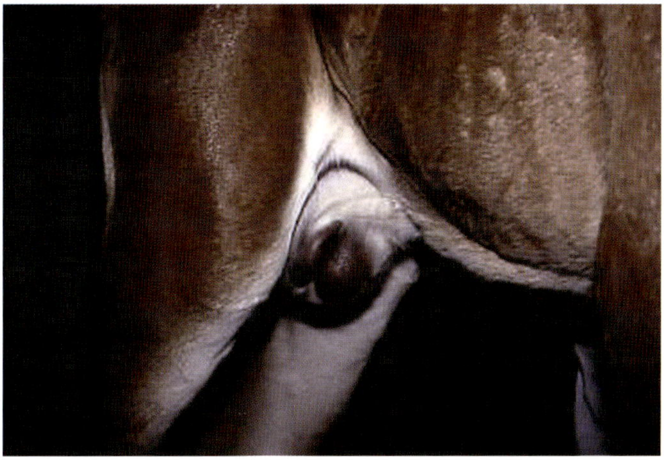

Figure 12.86 A scrotal hernia in a foal. Note the preputial swelling, which is often seen in cases where the intestines have herniated through a tear in the vaginal tunic into subcutaneous tissue of the scrotum. These direct scrotal hernias require surgical intervention. A congenital scrotal hernia where the vaginal tunic is intact is usually asymptomatic and the hernia can be easily reduced. Most of these resolve spontaneously although manual reduction and a truss bandage may be necessary.

Intestinal Aganglionosis (Lethal White Syndrome)

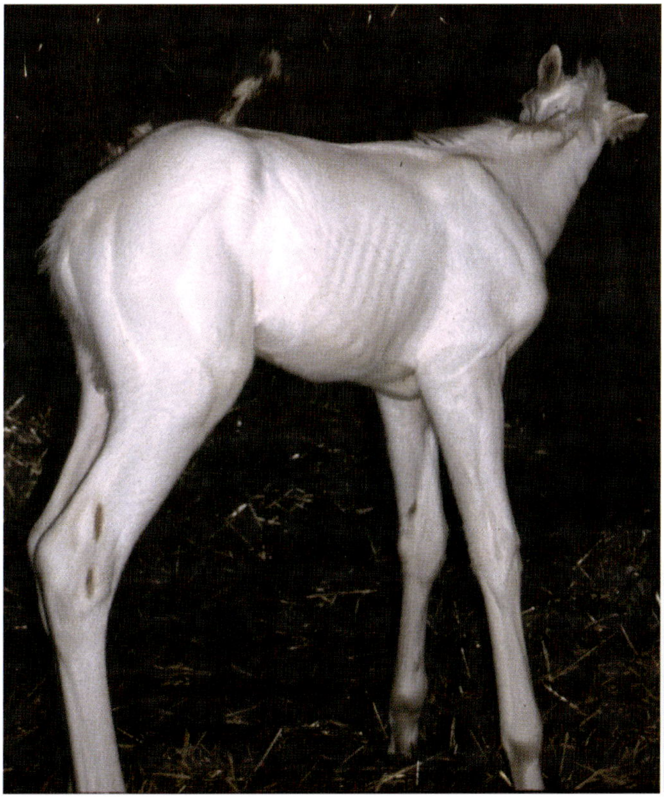

Figure 12.87 A foal with intestinal aganglionosis. This syndrome is an autosomal recessive disease seen in American paint horse foals from overo-overo mating. Affected foals are all or mostly white, however, not all white foals are affected. It has also been reported in other horse breeds. An abnormal configuration in the endothelin-B receptor gene causes submucosal and myenteric aganglionosis of the caudal intestinal tract. Affected foals are normal at birth, pass no meconium, and develop colic shortly after birth. The condition needs to be differentiated from intestinal atresia, meconium impaction, and other forms of colic in the neonatal foal. There is no treatment. See Chapter 5, Diseases of the Integumentary System.

Functional Ileus

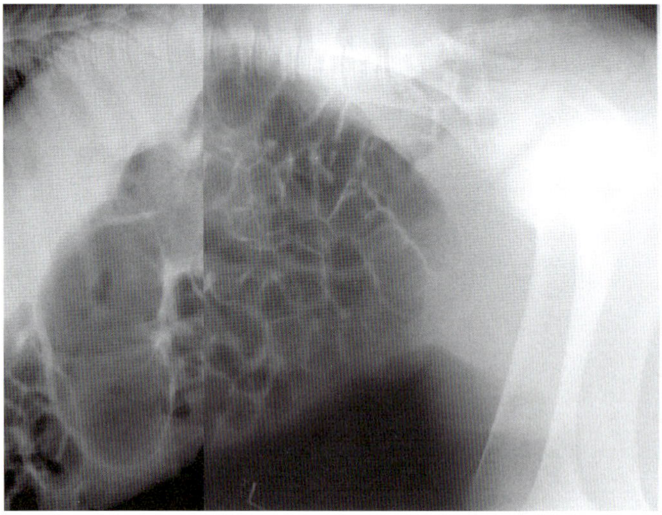

Figure 12.88 Lateral abdominal radiograph of a 9-day-old Standardbred foal. The foal was presented for evaluation of colic. **Functional ileus:** Gas is present in all segments of the intestinal tract. The larger gas-filled viscus structures are large intestinal segments; the smaller are small intestinal segments. Neither portion of the intestinal tract appears to be dilated. An appearance of gas throughout the intestinal tract with no evidence of distension is consistent with a diagnosis of functional ileus. Distension of bowel would be expected with mechanical ileus (obstruction). Note: The vertical line in the cranial abdomen is a film artifact.

Nervous System

Hyponatremia

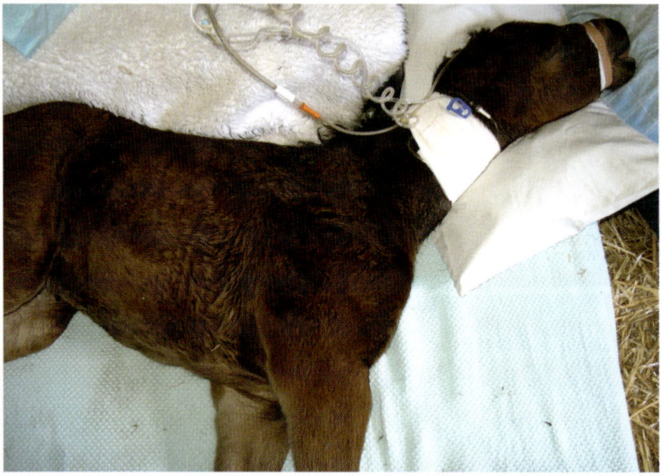

Figure 12.89 Foal with hyponatremia in opisthotonos with seizure activity characterized by rapid chewing and tongue protruding movements. Hyponatremia can be associated with renal failure, iatrogenic water overload, or diarrhea. Neurological signs vary depending on the rate of development and severity of hyponatremia. Signs progress from ataxia, intention tremor, and head-pressing to recumbency with opisthotonos and characteristic rapid chewing and tongue movements. Differential diagnoses include trauma, HIE, and meningitis. The underlying plasma volume disorder determines the treatment options. Sodium concentrations need to be corrected carefully. (Image courtesy of Dr. K. Corley)

Brachial Plexus Injury

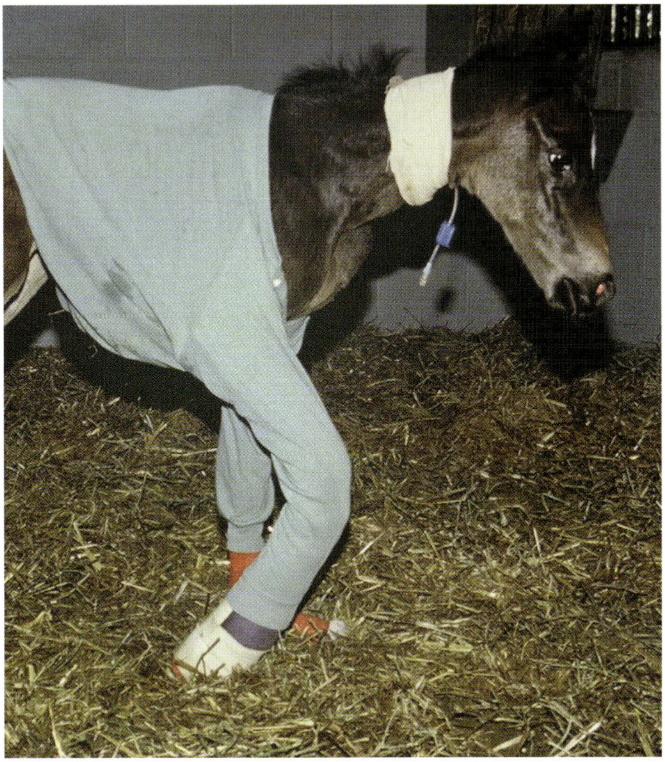

Figure 12.90 A foal with brachial plexus injury following dystocia and manual manipulation. The foal is unable to bear weight on the leg and has a dropped elbow and shoulder. The jumpers are to help prevent decubital ulcer formation.

Botulism

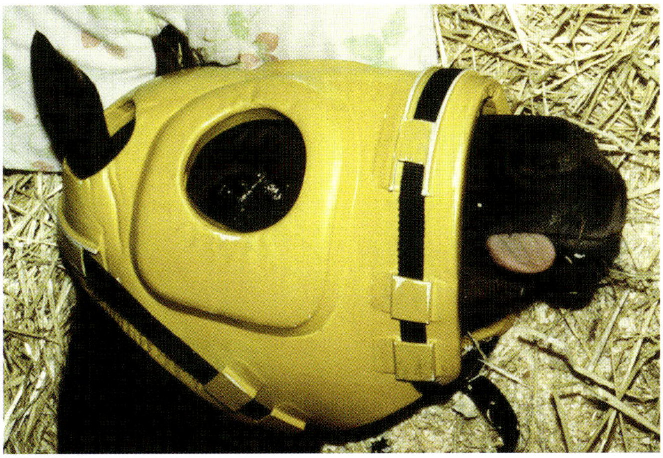

Figure 12.91 Recumbent foal with flaccid paralysis, no tongue withdrawal or eyelid tone due to botulism. Botulism is caused by the neurotoxin of *Clostridium botulinum* and in foals is most commonly due to the toxico-infectious form where the organism multiplies in the gut and the toxin is subsequently absorbed. Clinical signs of the disease range from not keeping up with the mare, lying down more than normal, dysphagia, muscle tremors while standing ("shaker foal") to loss of tongue and eyelid tone, recumbency, and respiratory failure. Diagnosis is based on clinical signs, lack of systemic signs of illness, and demonstration of the toxin in feces or blood. Treatment is aimed at systemic support and preventing aspiration pneumonia. Positive pressure ventilation can be used in foals with respiratory failure. Polyvalent antitoxin can be given if early in the course of disease.

Entropion

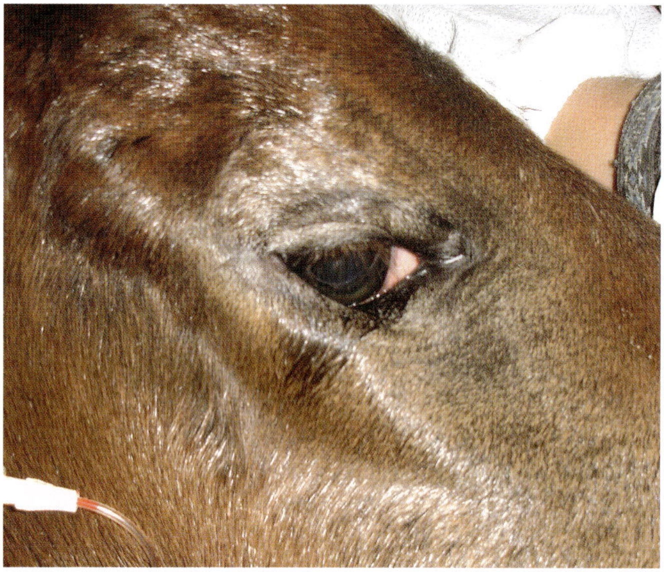

Figure 12.92 Entropion in a dehydrated foal. Entropion is the inward rolling of the eyelid. In this photograph, note tearing around eye, which is an indication that an ulcer may be present. Often with rehydration the lid will return to the normal position. Also, in uncomplicated cases, repeated outward rolling of the affected lid and application of antibiotic ointment might help. In weak debilitated foals, the lid needs to be sutured out until there is increased tone in the surrounding skin. The cornea needs to be monitored for signs of ulceration.

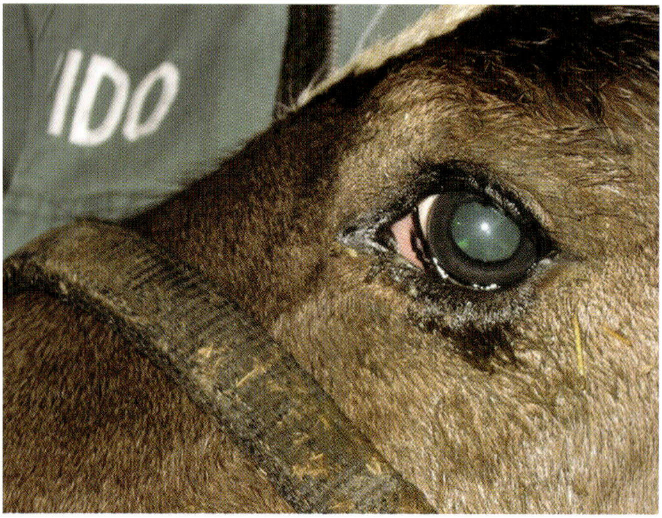

Figure 12.93 A foal with entropion. Severe cases of entropion that are unresponsive to conservative treatment may require surgical treatment by placing vertical mattress sutures along the affected lid.

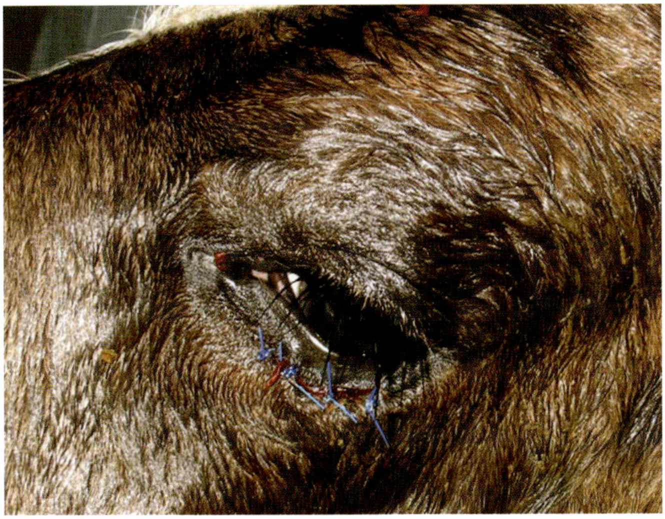

Figure 12.94 The same foal in fig. 12.93 after surgical treatment.

Scleral Hemorrhage

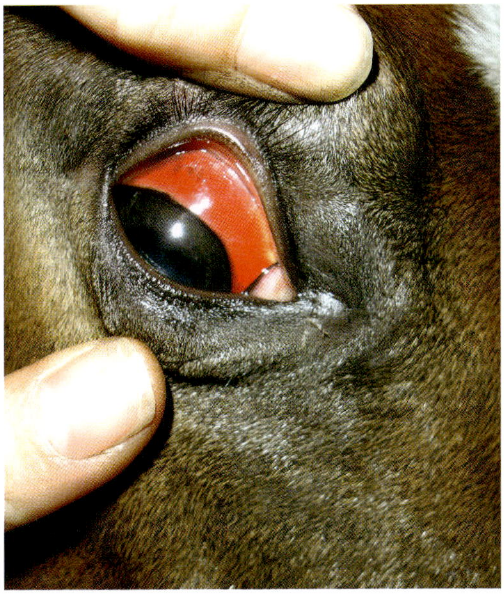

Figure 12.95 Scleral hemorrhage. Although hemorrhages can be seen associated with a traumatic birth, they can also be an incidental finding.

Bone and Joints

Normal Metatarsophalangeal Joint

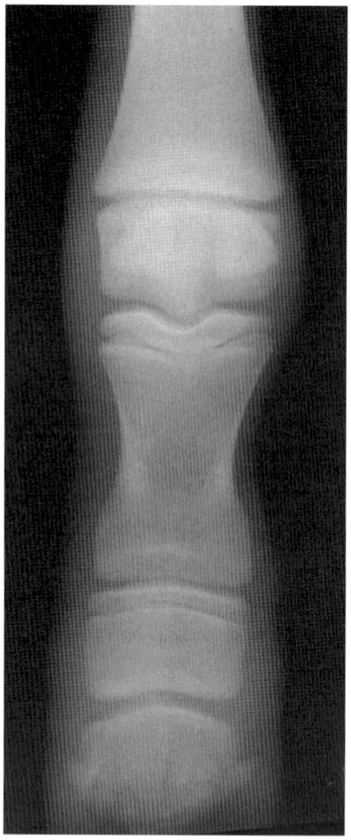

Figure 12.96 Dorsoplantar radiographic projection of the metatarsophalangeal joint of an 8-day-old Thoroughbred foal. **Normal metatarsophalangeal joint:** The distal physis of the third metatarsal bone will fuse at approximately 6 months of age; the proximal physis of the proximal phalanx will fuse at approximately 12 months of age; and the proximal physis of the second phalanx will fuse at 8–12 months of age. Times of physeal closure are the same for the fore- and hind limbs.

Normal Tarsus

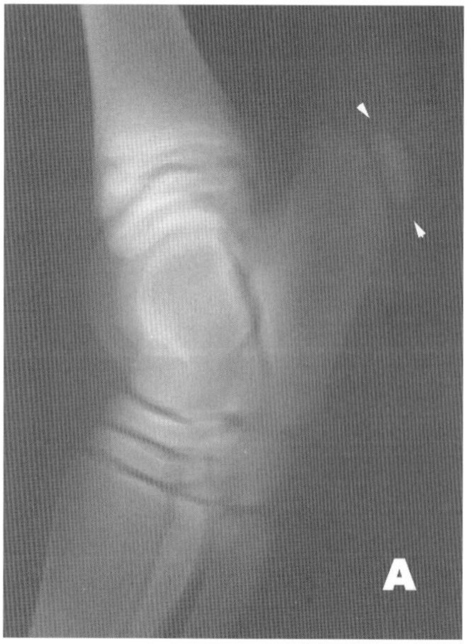

12.97

Figures 12.97–12.98 Lateromedial (A) and dorsoplantar (B) radiographic projections of the tarsus of an 8-day-old Thoroughbred foal. **Normal tarsus:** The tuber calcani (arrowheads—lateral view) is a separate center of ossification. It fuses to the calcaneus between 16 and 24 months of age. The small separate osseous structure on the lateral aspect of the distal tibia (arrow—dorsoplantar view) is the separate center of ossification of the lateral malleolus. This will fuse to the tibia by approximately 3 months of age. The small tarsal bones (central, third, and fourth) are rectangular in shape and are considered to be fully ossified.

Figures 12.97–12.98 *Continued*

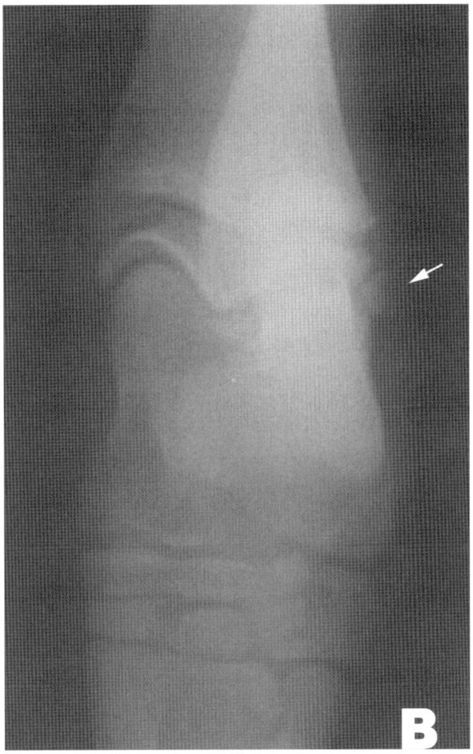

12.98

Normal Stifle Joint

Figure 12.99 Lateromedial radiographic projection of the stifle of an 8-day-old Thoroughbred foal. **Normal stifle joint:** The irregular margins and small size of the patella and trochlear ridges of the femur (arrows) are the result of incomplete ossification of the bones. The tibial tuberosity is very small (arrowhead) due to incomplete ossification. By approximately 4–5 months of age, the radiographic appearance of the stifle will be that of an adult horse except for the presence of open physeal structures.

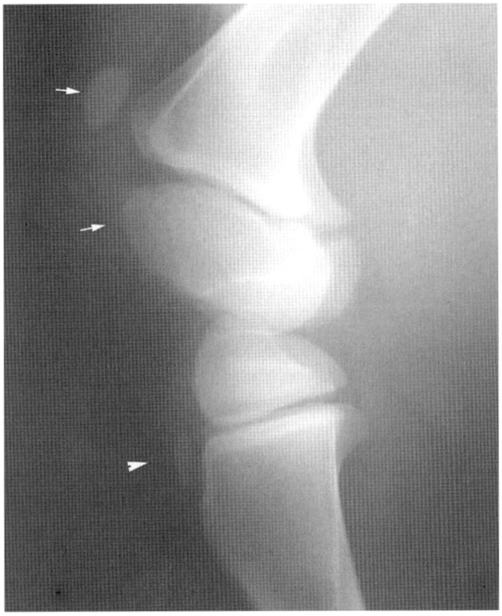

Normal Carpus

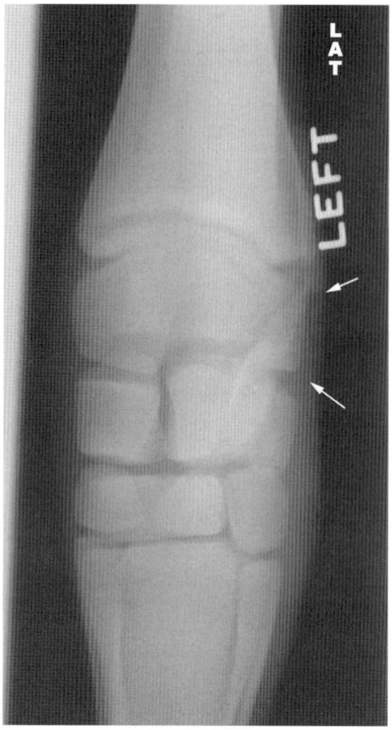

Figure 12.100 Dorsopalmar radiographic projection of the carpus of a 30-day-old Standardbred foal. **Normal carpus:** The separate osseous structure on the lateral aspect of the distal radius (arrows) is the separate center of ossification of the lateral styloid process. This fuses to the radius in the first year of life—usually by 3–4 months of age. The distal radial physis closes by approximately 24 months of age.

Physeal Dysplasia (Physitis)

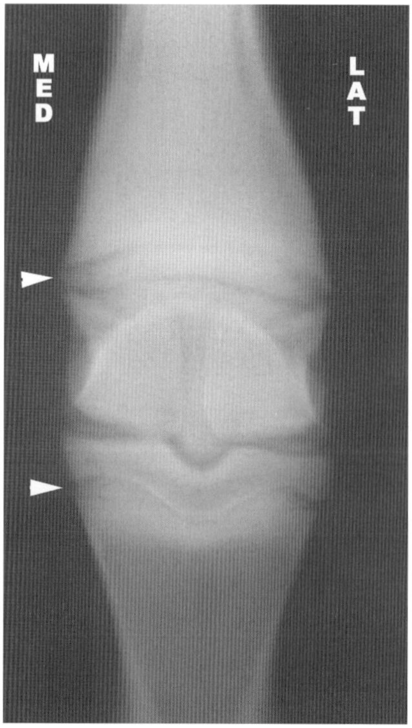

Figure 12.101 Dorsoplantar radiographic projection of the left metatarsophalangeal joint of a 5-month-old quarter horse foal. The foal was stiff and sore in her hind limbs and the fetlocks appeared swollen. **Physeal dysplasia of the distal physis of the third metacarpus and proximal physis of the proximal phalanx:** The distal physis of the third metatarsus is irregular and wider than normal. Similar changes are present in the proximal physis of the proximal phalanx (arrowheads) of the distal third metatarsus. This condition is commonly referred to as physitis but is more properly termed physeal dysplasia. It occurs in rapidly growing foals and is thought to result from nutritional causes (excessive nutrient intake with or without mineral imbalance). In the distal metacarpus and distal metatarsus, physeal dysplasia occurs most commonly in foals of approximately 6 months of age.

Figure 12.102 Dorsopalmar radiographic projection of the left carpal joint of an 11-month-old quarter horse foal. **Physeal dysplasia of the distal physis of the radius:** The medial aspect of the distal physis of radius is irregular and wider than normal and there is flaring of the metaphysis of the distal third metatarsus (arrow). Compare to the normal lateral aspect of the physis. In the distal radius, physeal dysplasia occurs most commonly in foals of approximately 12 months of age.

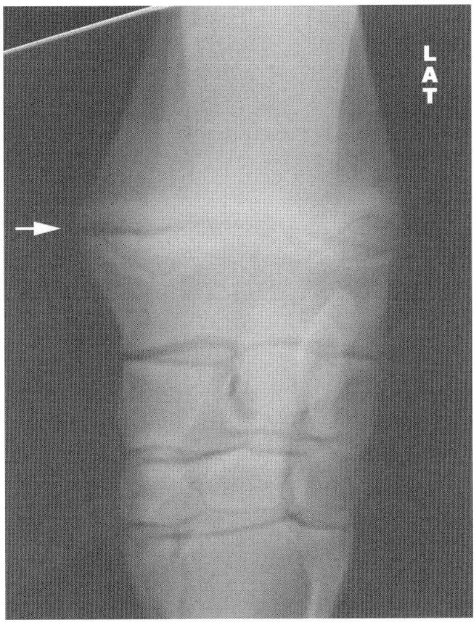

Grade 1 Ossification of the Carpal Bones

Figure 12.103 Dorsopalmar radiographic projection of the left carpal joint of a 4-day-old Thoroughbred foal. The foal was born prematurely. **Grade 1 ossification of the carpal bones:** A grading system has been described for classification of carpal and tarsal bone ossification in foals. Grade 1—some of the bones have some evidence of ossification; grade 2—all of the bones have some evidence of ossification; grade 3—all bones have an evidence for ossification but are small and round in shape; grade 4—the bones are normal in size and shape.

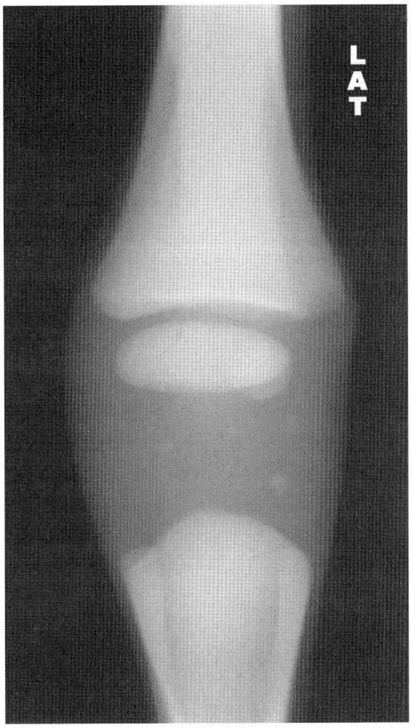

Grade 2 Ossification of the Carpal Bones

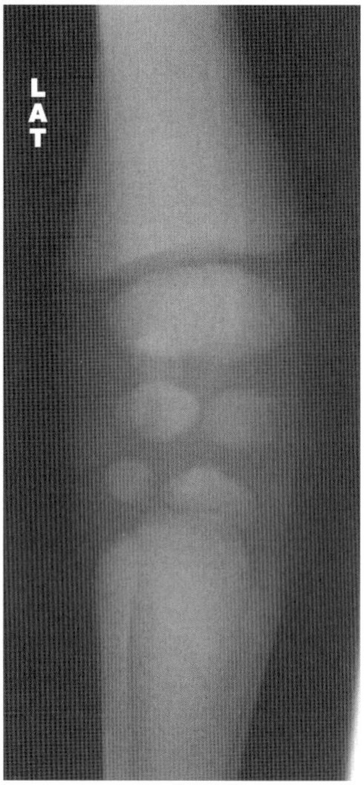

Figure 12.104 Dorsopalmar radiographic projection of the right carpal joint of a 2-day-old quarter horse foal. **Grade 2 ossification of the carpal bones:** There is some ossification of all of the carpal bones. Some of the bones are well-ossified but all are abnormally shaped.

Angular Limb Deformity—Carpal Valgus

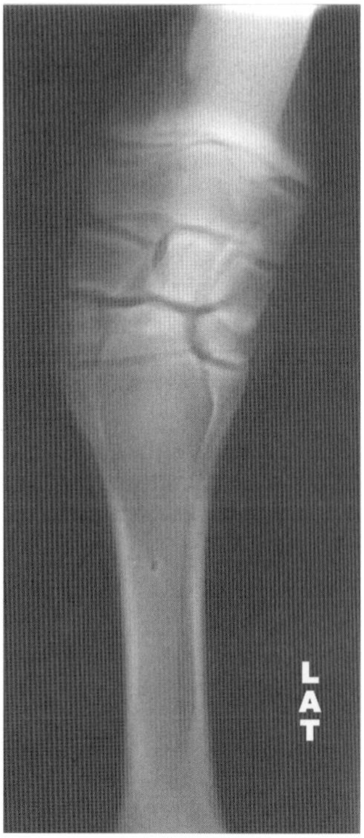

Figure 12.105 Dorsopalmar radiographic projection of the right carpal joint of a 4-week-old quarter horse foal. **Angular limb deformity—carpal valgus:** There is abnormal angulation of the distal limb away from its central axis. The angulation is in a lateral (valgus) direction. The angular limb deformity is named by indicating the joint where the deviation starts and the direction of the deviation (lateral: valgus; medial: varus).

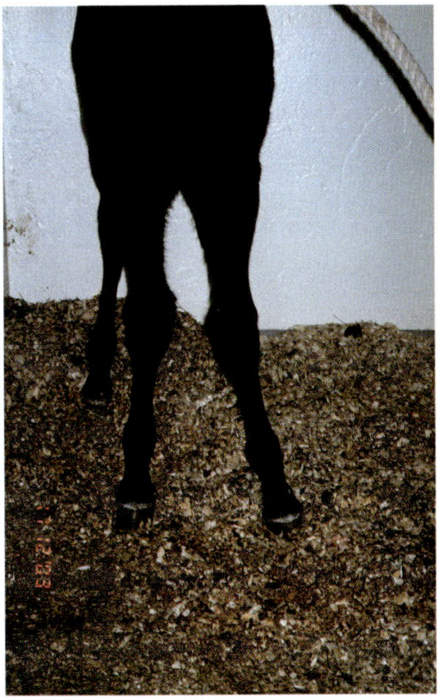

Figure 12.106 A foal with carpal valgus.

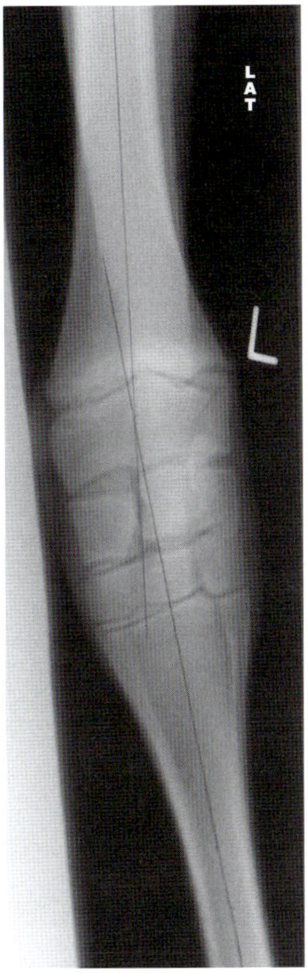

Figure 12.107 Dorsopalmar radiographic projection of the left carpal joint of a 6-week-old quarter horse foal. **Angular limb deformity—carpal valgus:** To determine the cause of the angulation and the degree of angulation that is present, lines are drawn through the central axis of the bones proximal and distal to the affected joint. In this case, the lines intersect in the distal radial epiphysis indicating that the angular deformity is the result of decreased growth at the lateral aspect of the radial physis. This type of angular limb deformity is treated by lateral periosteal release with or without medial growth retardation.

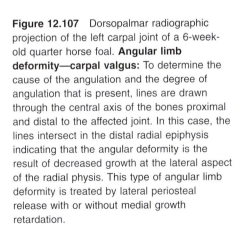

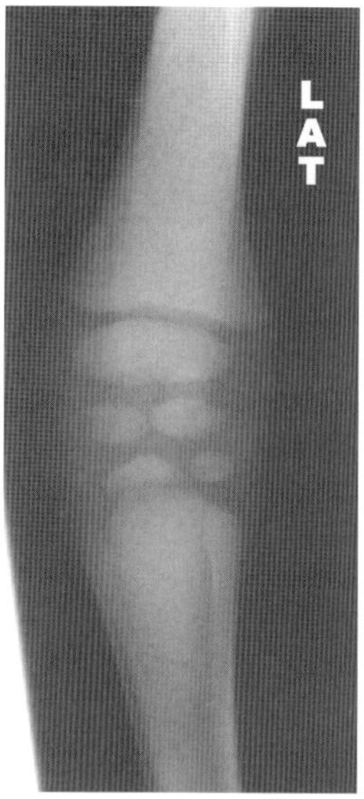

Figure 12.108 Dorsopalmar radiographic projection of the right carpal joint of a 2-day-old quarter horse foal. **Angular limb deformity—carpal valgus:** This foal has grade 2 ossification of the carpal bones and evidence of carpal valgus. The incompletely ossified carpal bones are compressing under the stress of weight-bearing allowing abnormal angulation of the limb. If the limbs are not supported until ossification of the bones occurs, progressive angular limb deformity will result.

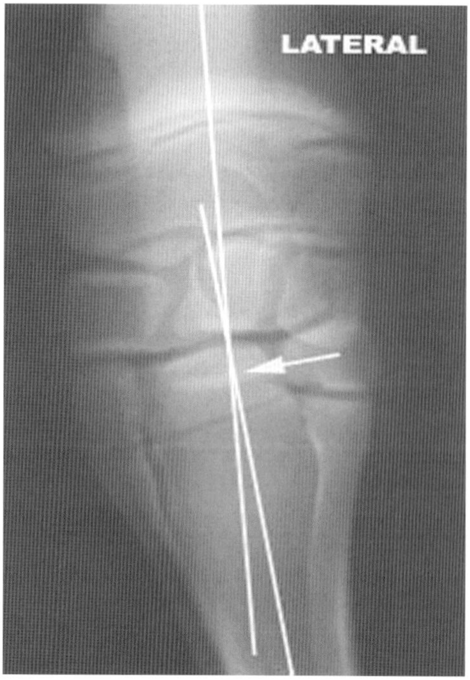

Figure 12.109 Dorsopalmar radiographic projection of the right carpal joint of a 4-week-old quarter horse foal. **Angular limb deformity—carpal valgus:** The lines drawn through the radius and third metacarpus intersect in the distal row of carpal bones. Careful evaluation shows wedging of the lateral aspect of the third carpal bone and the medial aspect of the 4th carpal bone (arrow). Lack of ossification of the carpal bones at birth is suspected to be the cause of angular limb deformity. Compression of the cartilage templates prior to ossification has resulted in abnormal shape of the carpal bones. The abnormal shape of the bones has allowed the carpus to collapse along the lateral aspect.

Figures 12.110–12.111 Dorsoplantar (A) and lateral (B) radiographic projections of the left tarsus in a 5-week-old quarter horse foal. **Angular limb deformity—tarsal valgus:** When tarsal valgus is present, it is usually due to incomplete ossification of the tarsal bones or of ligamentous laxity; uneven growth of the distal tibial physis is uncommon. The lines drawn through the tibia and third metatarsus intersect in the proximal row of tarsal bones. Careful evaluation of the tarsal bones (inset) reveals wedging of the central tarsal bone laterally (arrowhead) and collapse of the middle of the third tarsal bone (arrow) as a result of incomplete ossification. The lateral view shows the effect of incomplete ossification of the tarsal bones (arrow). The dorsal margin of the central tarsal bone is narrow and has an irregular pattern of ossification. The middle of the third tarsal bone is collapsed and the dorsal portion of the bone is displaced dorsally.

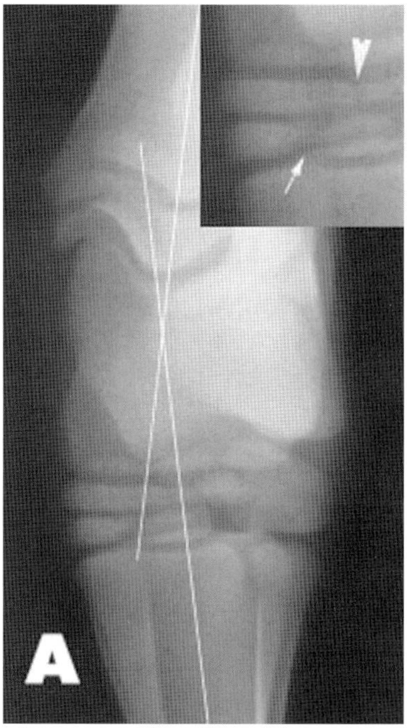

12.110

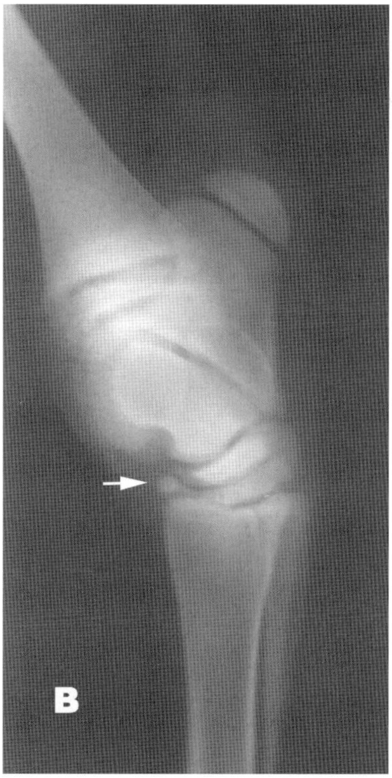

12.111

Angular Limb Deformity—Fetlock Varus

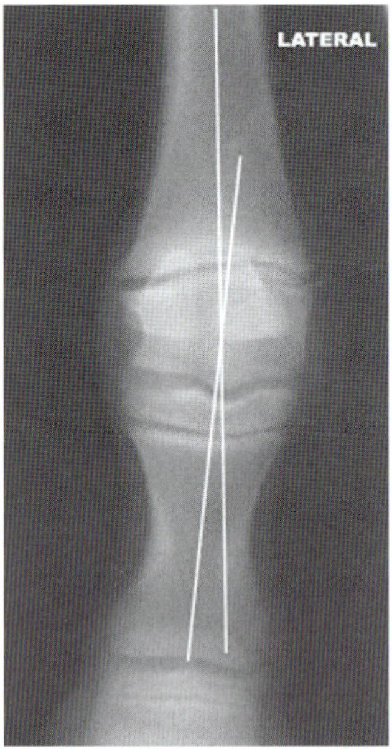

Figure 12.112 Dorsopalmar radiographic projection of the right metacarpophalangeal joint of a 5-week-old Thoroughbred foal. **Angular limb deformity—fetlock varus:** This is an example of a varus deformity (fetlock varus). The axial lines intersect in the distal epiphysis of the 3rd metacarpus and the medial aspect of the metacarpal epiphysis is shorter than the lateral aspect. The cause of the deformity is uneven growth at the distal metacarpal physis. Fetlock varus is rarely a primary abnormality; it is usually seen as in association with carpal valgus or tarsal valgus. This type of angular limb deformity is treated by medial periosteal release with or without lateral growth retardation.

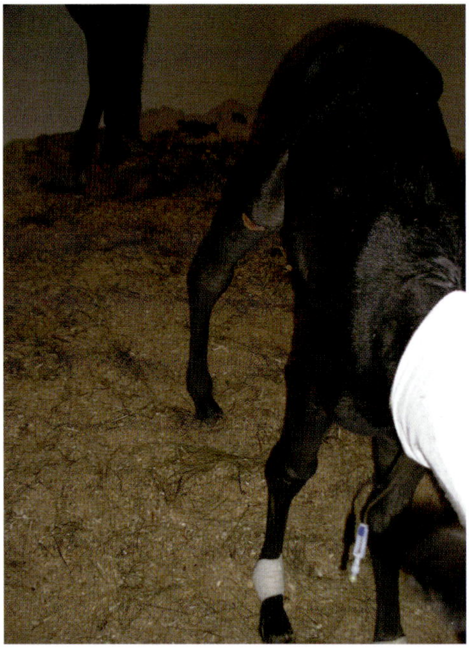

Figure 12.113 A clinical photograph of a foal with fetlock and tarsus varus.

Infectious Polyarthritis (Septic Arthritis)

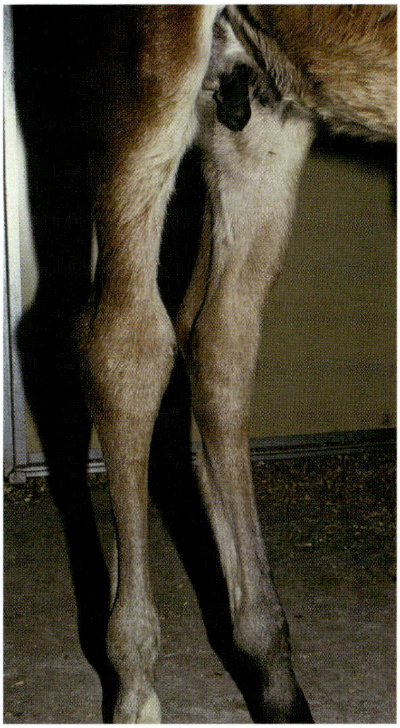

Figure 12.114 Septic arthritis and osteomyelitis are common in foals <4 months of age. Foals can present with single or multiple affected legs or joints. The affected areas are often swollen, warm, and painful on manipulation and the foal is lame (fig. 12.114). Infection occurs via hematogenous spread of bacteria or by direct penetration of the joint. Diagnosis is made by clinical examination, results of imaging, and joint fluid analysis and culture. Infectious orthopedic disease should be excluded before other causes of lameness are considered. Treatment requires aggressive therapy with antimicrobial therapy and joint lavage.

Infectious Polyarthritis—S type

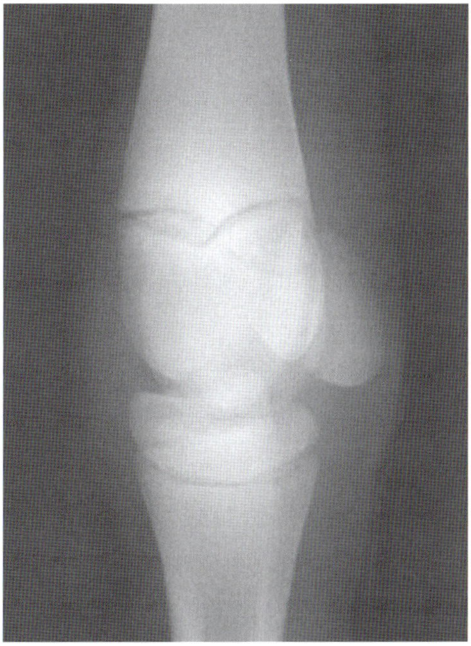

Figure 12.115 Lateral radiographic projection of the right metacarpophalangeal joint of a 4-week-old Standardbred foal. **Infectious polyarthritis—S type (synovial):** The only abnormality present is swelling of the soft tissues surrounding the joint. This is the result of joint effusion and of extracapsular swelling.

Infectious Polyarthritis—P type

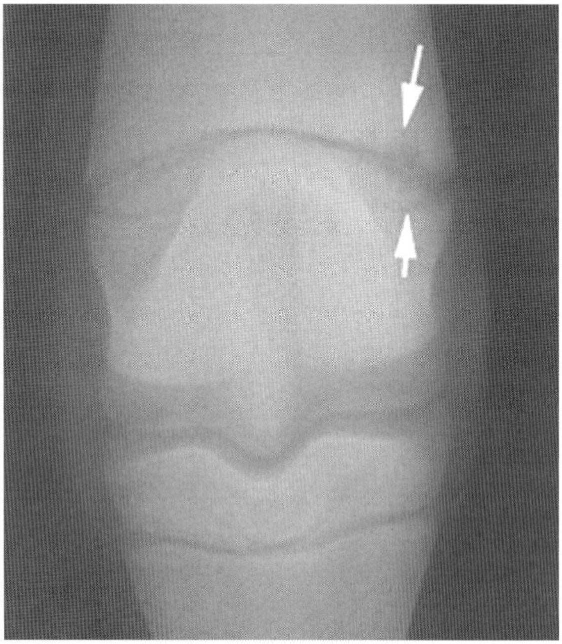

Figure 12.116 Dorsopalmar radiographic projection of the left metacarpophalangeal joint of a 4-week-old Standardbred foal. **Infectious polyarthritis—P type (physeal):** A focal area of lysis is present within the distal physis of the third metacarpus (arrows). Distension of the joint capsule is also present.

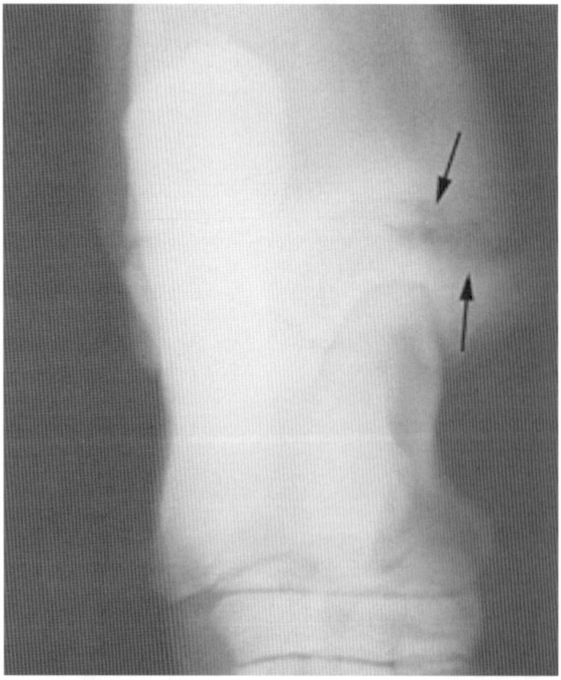

Figure 12.117 Dorsoplantar radiographic projection of the right tarsus of an 8-month-old quarter horse foal. **Infectious polyarthritis—P type (physeal):** There is a lytic and irregular appearance to the medial aspect of the distal tibial physis (arrows). Distension of the tibiotarsal joint capsule was also present (but not visible in the radiograph). This patient has the P type (physeal) of infectious polyarthritis. This case demonstrates that although most infectious polyarthritis occurs in young foals it can also occur in older foals.

Infectious Polyarthritis—E type

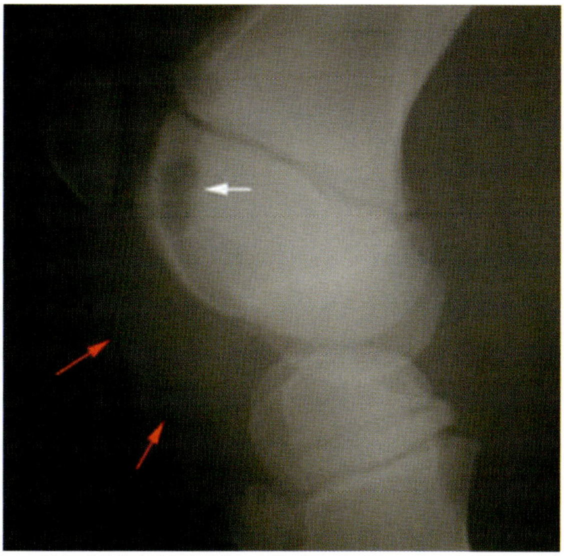

Figure 12.118 Lateral radiographic projection of the left stifle of a 4-week-old quarter horse foal. **Infectious polyarthritis—E type (epiphyseal):** A large focal area of lysis is present in the dorsal aspect of the distal femoral epiphysis (arrow). The joint capsule is massively distended (arrows).

Infectious Polyarthritis—T type

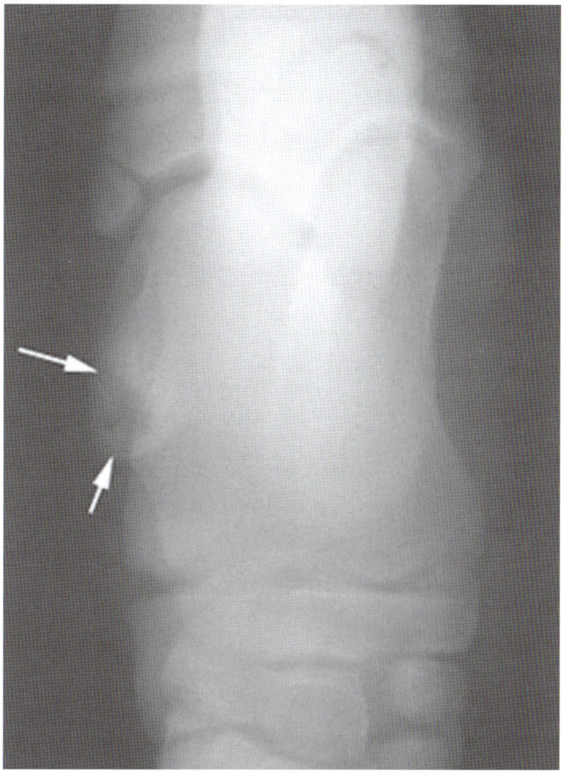

Figure 12.119 Dorsoplantar radiographic projection of the left tarsus of a 4-week-old quarter horse foal. **Infectious polyarthritis—T type (tarsal):** A well-defined focal area of lysis is present in the lateral trochlear ridge of the talus. The area of lysis is surrounded by a sclerotic margin—the bone is attempting to wall off the lesion (arrows). Significant distension of the tibiotarsal joint capsule is present. The final type of infectious polyarthritis is C type (carpal).

Salter-Harris Type 2 Fracture of the Proximal Tibia

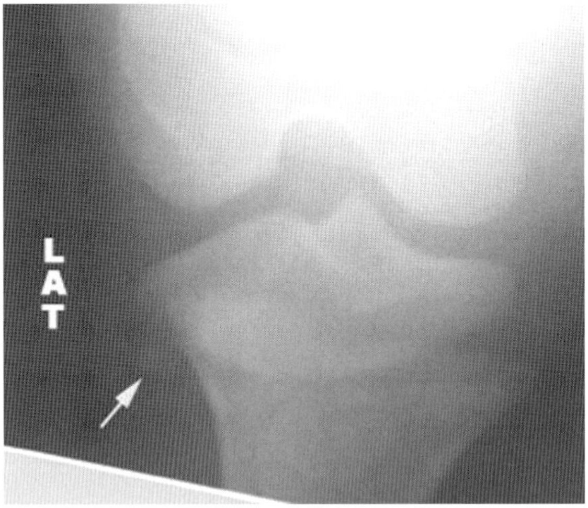

Figure 12.120 Craniocaudal radiographic projection of the stifle in a 4-week-old Standardbred foal. **Salter-Harris type 2 fracture of the proximal tibia:** The proximal tibial epiphysis is displaced laterally. The metaphyseal component of the fracture is small and is located on the lateral aspect of the limb (arrow). This is a relatively common type of Salter-Harris fracture in the foal and occurs when the mare steps on the recumbent foal or when the foal is kicked.

Salter-Harris Type 2 Fracture of the Distal Metacarpus

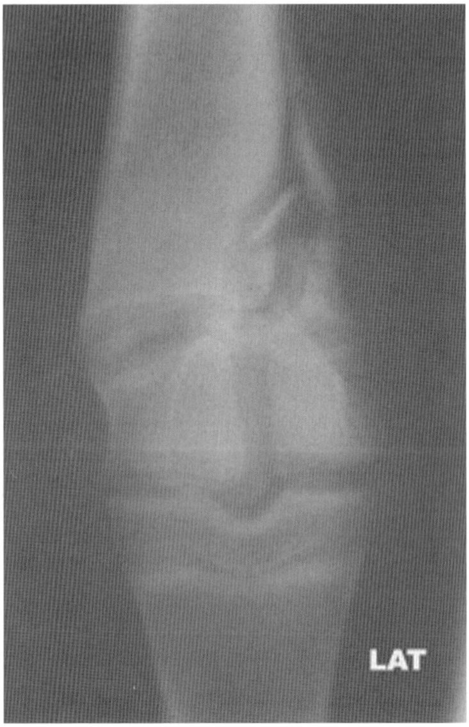

Figure 12.121 Dorsopalmar radiographic projection of the left metacarpophalangeal joint of a 3-month-old pony foal. **Salter-Harris type 2 fracture of the distal metacarpus:** The metaphyseal component is lateral and comminuted. Periosteal response is present along the lateral aspect of the metacarpus. This fracture is 4 days old and in a foal of this age, early radiographic evidence of healing is already present.

Lateral Luxation of the Patella

Figures 12.122–12.123 Lateral and caudocranial radiographic projections of the left stifle of a 4-week-old Standardbred foal. The foal has had a swollen stifle and been lame since birth. **Lateral luxation of the patella:** In the lateral view, the patella overlies the trochlear ridges of the femur indicating that it is luxated from its normal position. With only the lateral view, it is not possible to determine if the luxation is lateral or medial; assessment of the caudocranial view shows the luxation to be lateral. Congenital patellar luxation is more common in miniature horse foals but can occur in other breeds. Malformation of the distal femur (hypoplasia of the femoral condyles with or without shallowness of the trochlear groove) contributes to luxation of the patella.

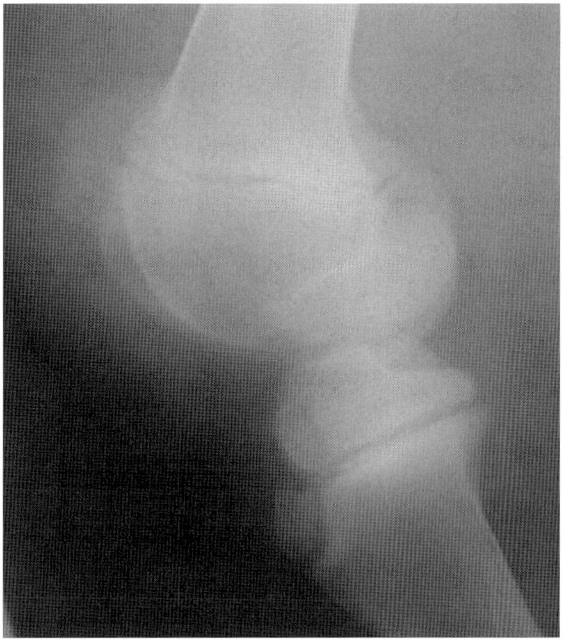

12.122

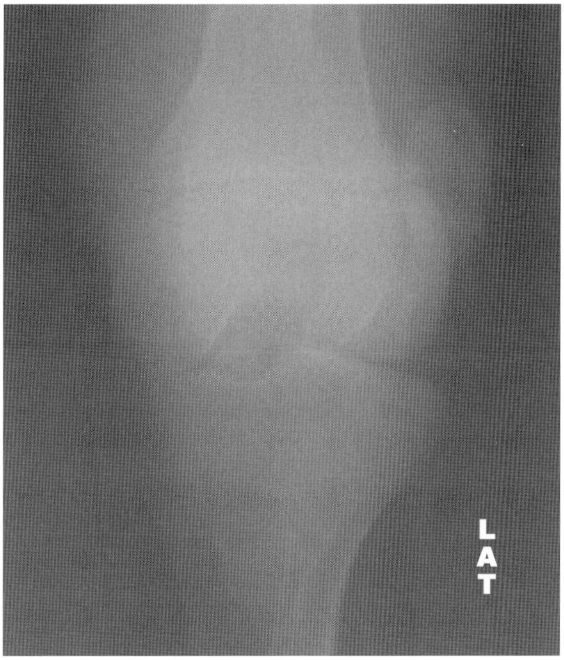

12.123

Avulsion Fracture of the Origin of the Long Digital Extensor Tendon

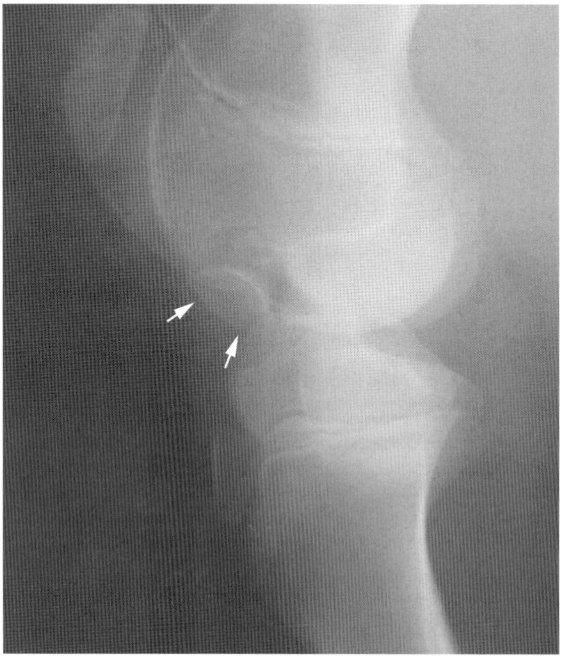

12.124

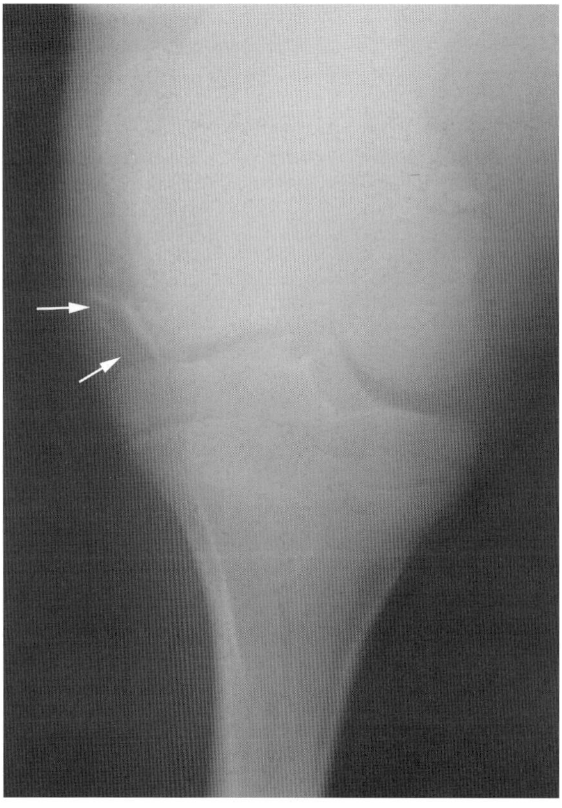

12.125

Figures 12.124–12.125 Lateral and caudocranial radiographic projections of the left stifle of a 2-month-old Thoroughbred foal. The foal has been Grade 4 of 4 lame for 2 weeks. **Avulsion fracture of the origin of the long digital extensor tendon:** In the lateral view, a large bone fragment is seen displaced from the junction of the lateral trochlear ridge and lateral condyle of the femur (arrows). Several smaller bone fragments are faintly visible at the dorsal margin of the fracture bed. In the craniocaudal view, multiple bone fragments are visible lateral to the lateral femoral condyle (arrows). None of these fragments seem as large as the one seen on the lateral view, but this may be due to the orientation of the large fragment (it may be viewed end-on in this projection). The location and appearance of the fracture are consistent with an avulsion fracture at the origin of the long digital extensor tendon.

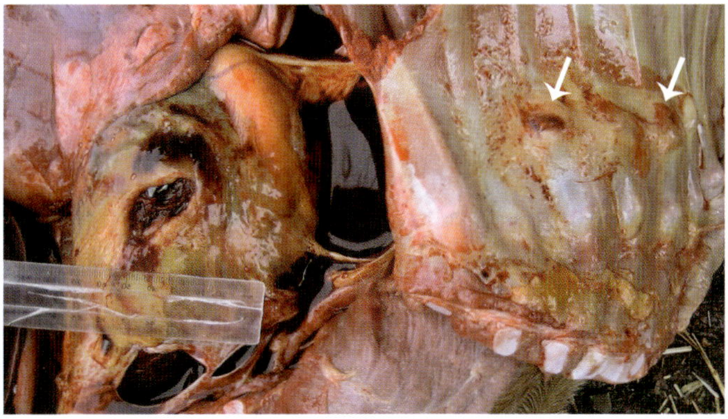

Figure 12.126 Fractured ribs (arrows) that resulted in a fatal puncture of the myocardium. Fractured ribs in newborn foals occur commonly due to trauma during parturition; in older foals they are usually due to external trauma. The resulting fractures or costochondral dislocations are usually multiple and can be subclinical or cause a range of clinical signs including respiratory distress and sudden death. Diagnosis is based on palpation of crepitus, radiographs, or, more reliably, ultrasonographic examination. Conservative management is successful in most cases, however, surgery is utilized in some cases.

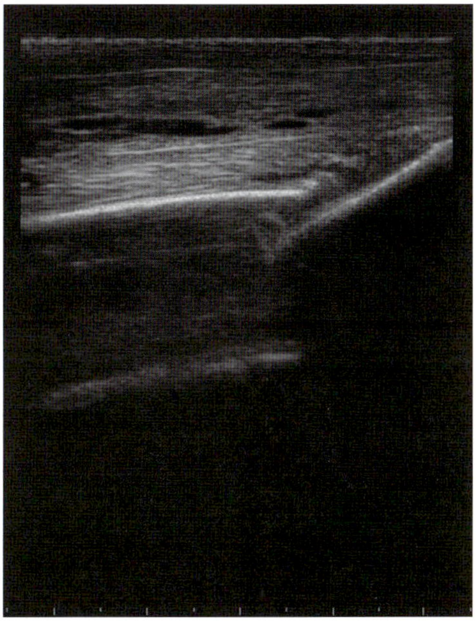

Figure 12.127 Ultrasonographic appearance of a rib fracture. Note the disruption of bone surface and anechoic fluid indicative of edema around the fracture site. Sagittal view. Left is dorsal.

Ruptured Gastrocnemius Muscle/Tendon

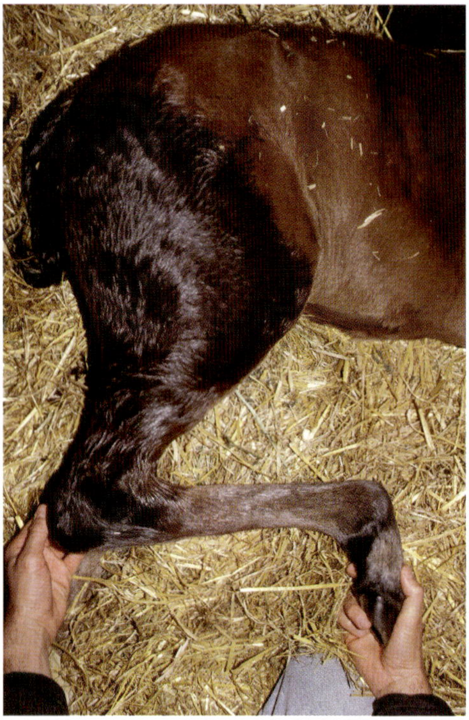

Figure 12.128 Excessive flexion of the hock due to rupture of the gastrocnemius muscle. This can be unilateral or bilateral and is usually associated with dystocia and assisted deliveries, although it has been seen as a result of muscle necrosis from intramuscular injections. The foal is recumbent if bilateral rupture occurs. The affected areas are hot and swollen; ultrasonography can visualize the damaged area. Treatment is supportive and, if severe, judicial splinting can be used to assist with ambulation.

Ruptured Common Digital Extensor Tendon

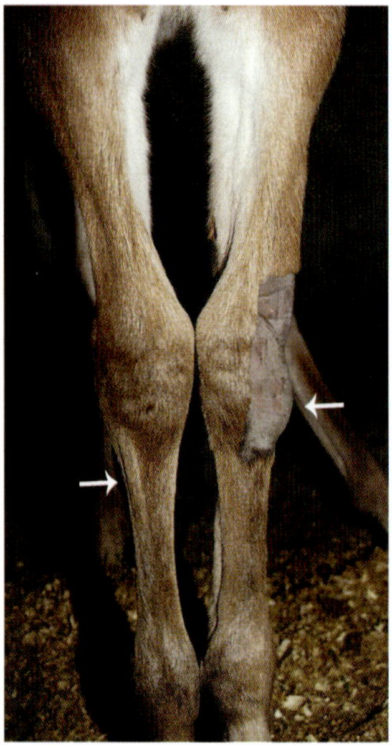

Figure 12.129 Fluctuant swelling over the dorsolateral aspect of the carpus associated with rupture of the common digital tendon within the tendon sheath (upper arrow). The condition can be bilateral and is often seen as a secondary problem in foals with flexural deformities that result in excessive tension on the extensor tendon (lower arrow). Diagnosis is based on physical examination findings and ability to straighten the leg. Treatment is rest, however, a bandage and splint may be required in foals that knuckle forward onto the fetlock when walking.

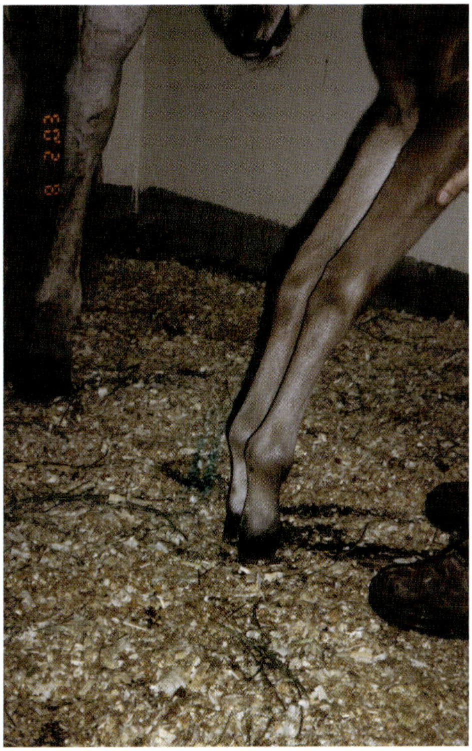

Figure 12.130 Flexural contracture can be congenital or acquired. Intrauterine malposition is thought to cause congenital flexural contracture, however, the exact cause remains unknown. The acquired flexural contracture is seen in growing foals and is related to growth patterns and periods of maximal skeletal growth. This foal has deep digital flexor contraction.

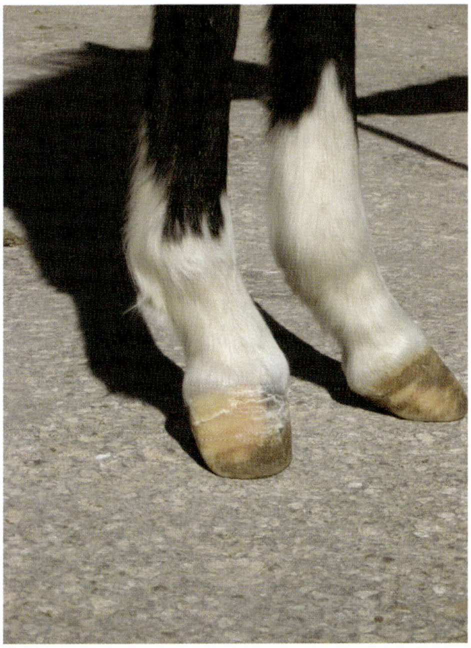

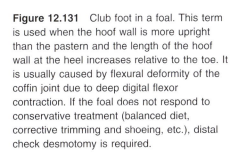

Figure 12.131 Club foot in a foal. This term is used when the hoof wall is more upright than the pastern and the length of the hoof wall at the heel increases relative to the toe. It is usually caused by flexural deformity of the coffin joint due to deep digital flexor contraction. If the foal does not respond to conservative treatment (balanced diet, corrective trimming and shoeing, etc.), distal check desmotomy is required.

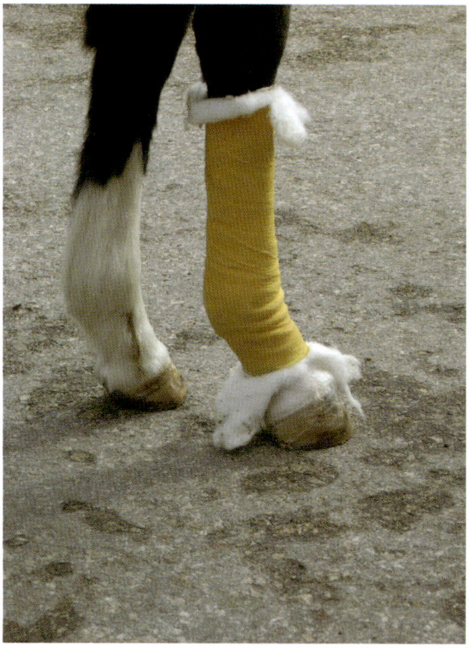

Figure 12.132 The same foal in fig. 12.131 after distal check desmotomy was performed.

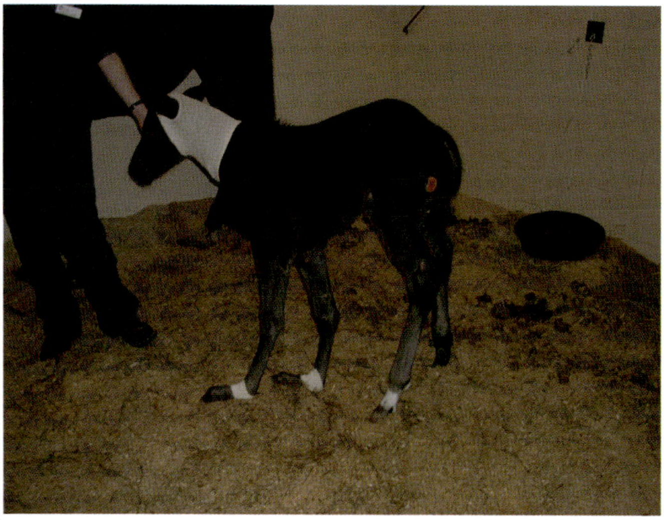

Figure 12.133 Flexural laxity is thought to be caused by abnormal flaccidity of the flexor muscles. It is seen more in premature foals. This foal has digital hyperextension deformity. Note the severe fetlock hyperextension.

Ventral Abdominal Wall Tear

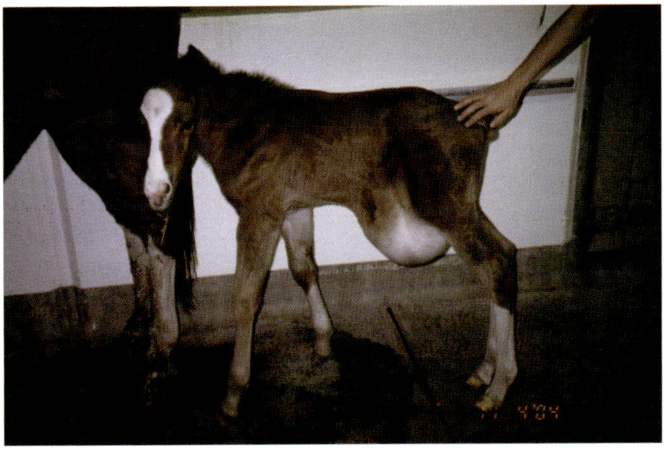

Figure 12.134 An 18-hour-old foal with ventral abdominal wall tear or rupture. The owner has noticed it since birth. The cause is probably dystocia. The tear was repaired surgically and the foal recovered uneventfully.

White Muscle Disease

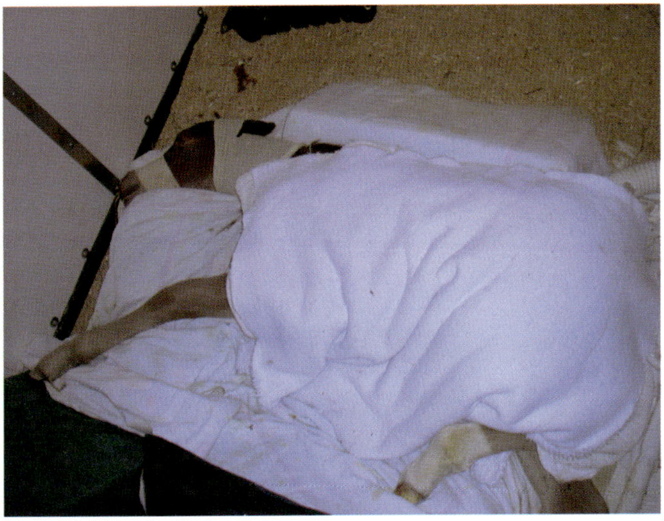

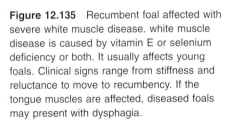

Figure 12.135 Recumbent foal affected with severe white muscle disease. white muscle disease is caused by vitamin E or selenium deficiency or both. It usually affects young foals. Clinical signs range from stiffness and reluctance to move to recumbency. If the tongue muscles are affected, diseased foals may present with dysphagia.

Urinary Tract Disruption

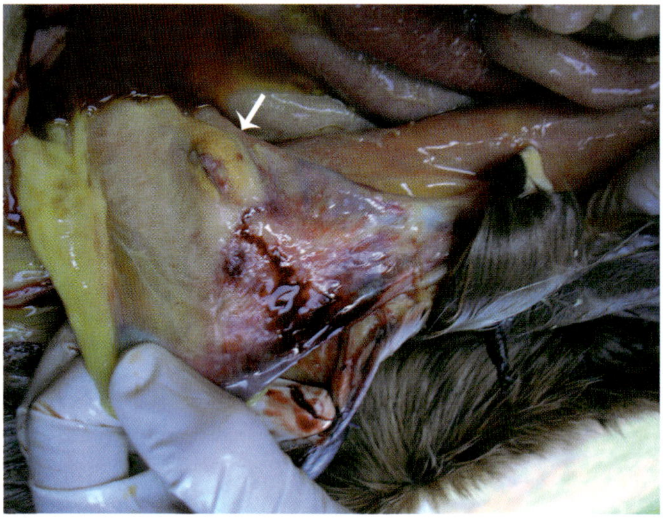

Figure 12.136 Postmortem image of a foal with a rupture in the dorsal wall of the bladder and concurrent peritonitis. Urinary tract disruption can also occur in the urachus (fig. 12.140), ureters, and urethra. Affected foals are usually less than 7 days old. There is no sex predilection. Causes include local ischemia, necrosis, and sepsis. Clinical signs include straining to urinate, dribbling urine, and stretching out frequently followed by abdominal distension and depression. Biochemistry analysis may show hyponatremia, hypochloremia, hyperkalemia, and azotemia, however, these are not consistent findings. Differential diagnoses include renal failure, urachitis, and other causes of colic in neonates. Ultrasonography (fig. 12.138–12.139) and analysis of peritoneal fluid are useful in diagnosis. Contrast radiography may be needed to identify disruption in the urethra or ureters. Treatment is aimed at correction of the electrolyte abnormalities and, once stabilized, surgical repair is undertaken.

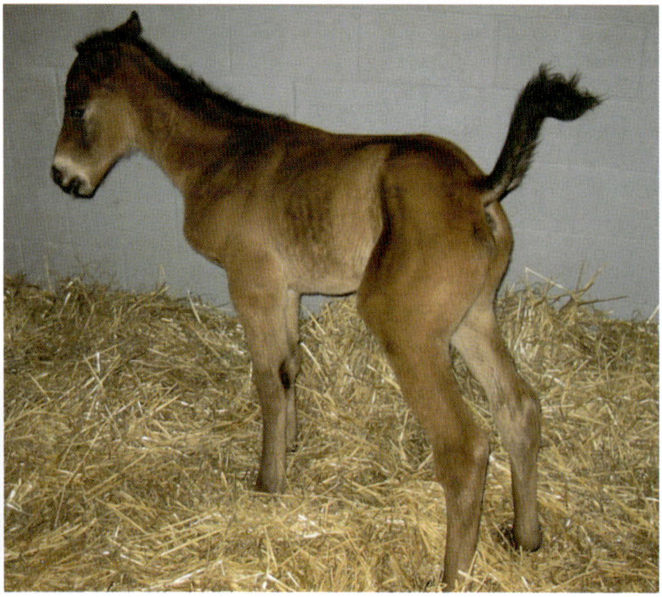

Figure 12.137 Foal straining to urinate. Note the dorsoflexion of back and elevated tail position. Straining to urinate can be a sign of urinary tract disruption, however, it is also seen with abdominal pain and urachitis.

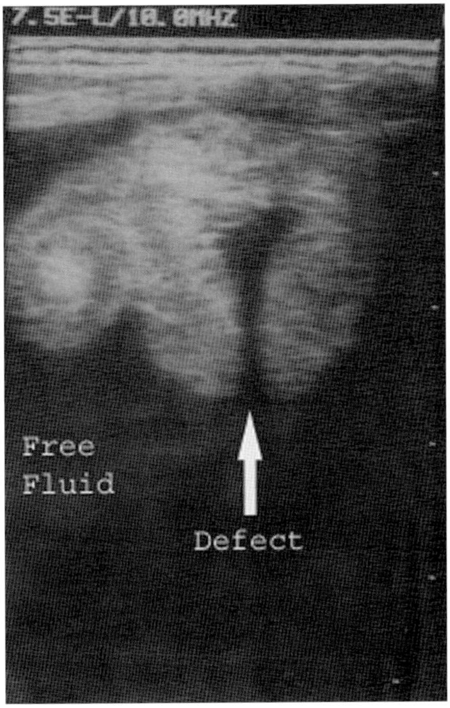

12.138

Figures 12.138–12.139 Ultrasonographic examination of the ventral part of the caudal abdomen of two foals with ruptured bladders. Note the different images of the bladders showing a defect in the wall (arrow) and the increased amount of anechoic fluid in the abdomen.

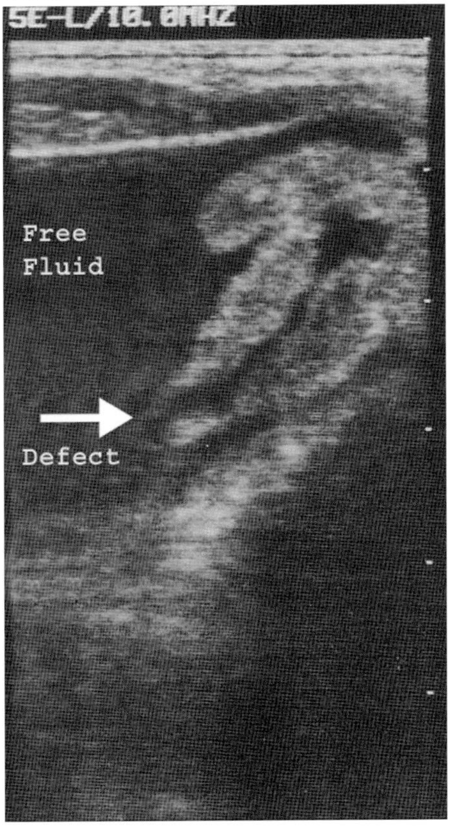

12.139

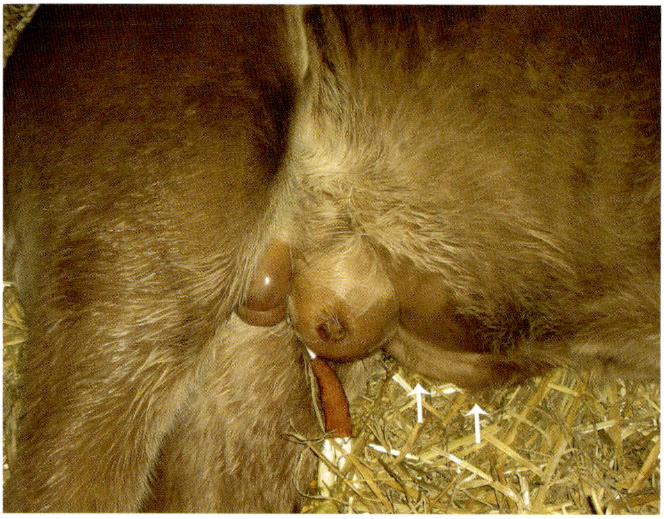

Figure 12.140 Rupture of the urachus in a foal. Swelling of the external umbilicus, prepuce, and surrounding tissue due to urine leakage from the external urachus. A urinary catheter is used to keep the bladder empty and an abdominal bandage can be placed to decrease the swelling prior to surgical removal of the remnant. This may also result in closing of the defect, thus eliminating the need for surgery.

Patent Urachus

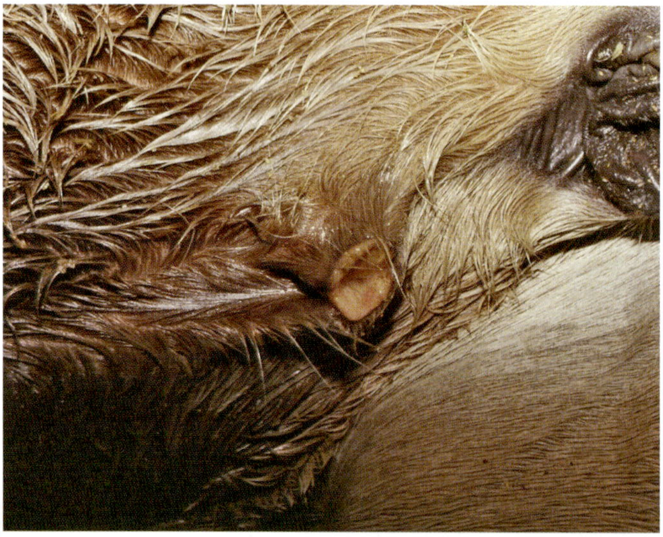

Figure 12.141 A patent urachus. This is a common finding in debilitated recumbent neonates and may also be associated with an umbilical infection. Treatment includes broad-spectrum antimicrobial therapy, keeping the external area around the urachus clean, and keeping the foal in a clean environment. The majority heal with time; rarely is surgery necessary.

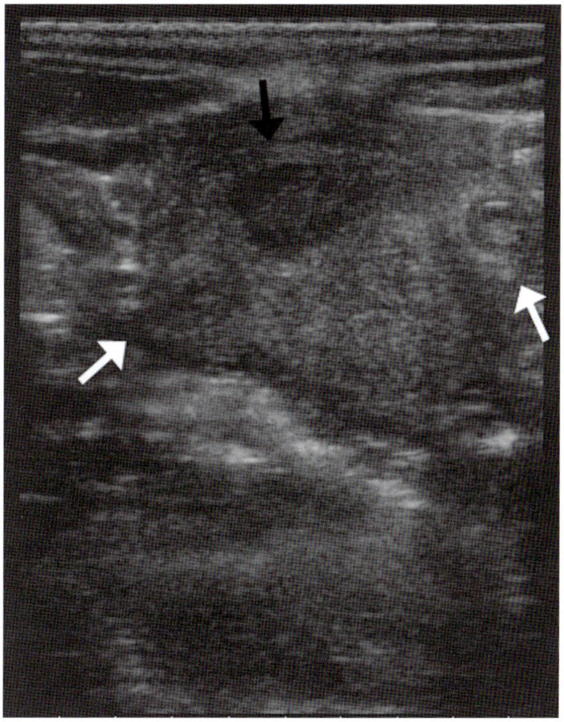

Figure 12.142 Sonogram of the caudal part of the ventral abdomen of a foal, caudal to the external umbilical remnant. The transducer is perpendicular to midline. The two umbilical arteries (white arrows) are seen on each side of the urachus, which is under an abscess (black arrow). Many umbilical remnant infections are not visible externally, thus ultrasonographic examination is necessary for full evaluation of the umbilical remnants. It is important to determine if the fluid seen on ultrasonography is due to an infectious process, or is hemorrhage or urine.

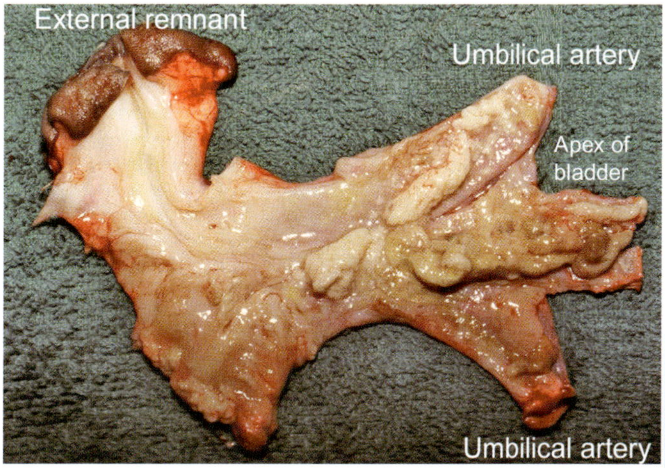

Figure 12.143 An infected umbilical remnant. Note the purulent caseous material in the umbilical arteries and apex of bladder. Surgical resection is not recommended in most cases. Broad-spectrum antimicrobial therapy results in the resolution of the majority of remnant infections. If, however, there is a concurrent localized infection or a large discrete abscess, surgical removal may be warranted.

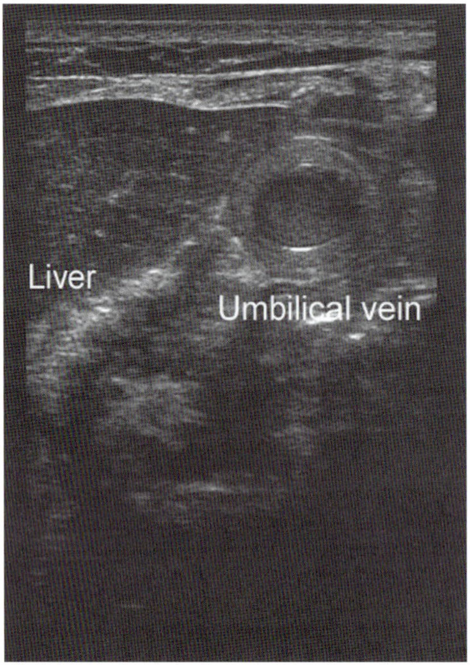

Figure 12.144 Ultrasonographic image of an infected umbilical vein. The normal diameter of the vein is <4 mm. Examination of the vein should extend cranially from the umbilicus to the liver.

External Umbilical Swellings

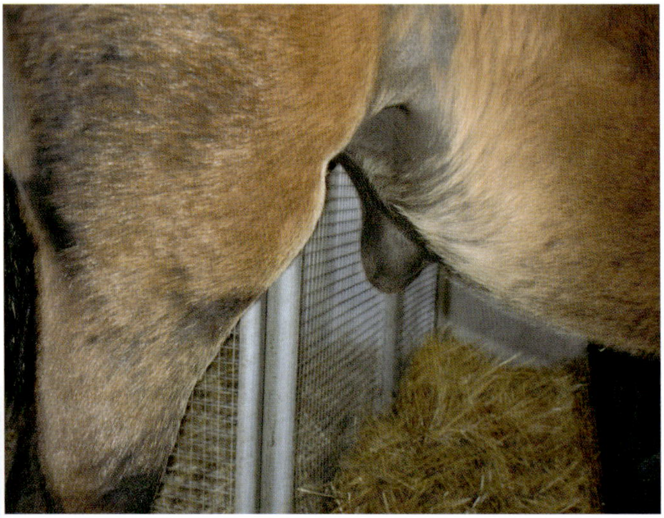

Figure 12.145 An umbilical hernia in a foal. This should be differentiated from a hematoma (fig. 12.146), urine leakage, or an abscess (fig. 12.147).

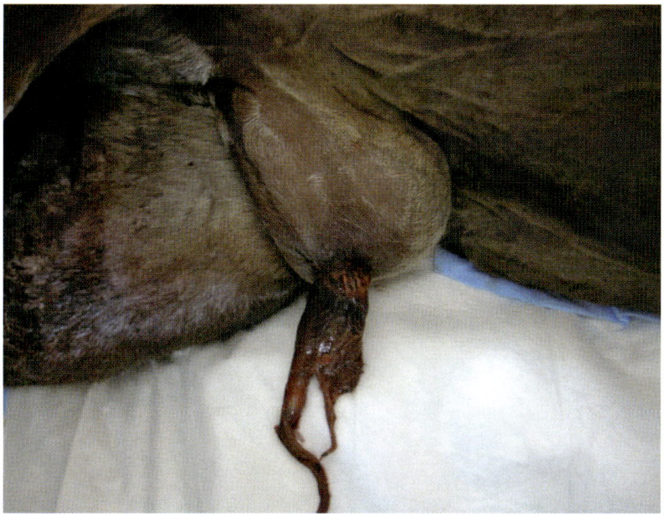

Figure 12.146 An umbilical hematoma due to subcutaneous bleeding from a torn umbilical artery. These are at a high risk of becoming infected and an abscess may subsequently develop.

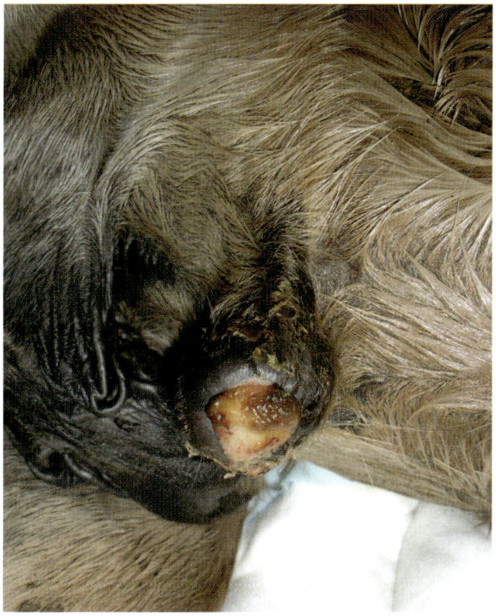

Figure 12.147 An infected external umbilical remnant, which was a localized abscess; it was opened and drained.

Decubital Ulcers

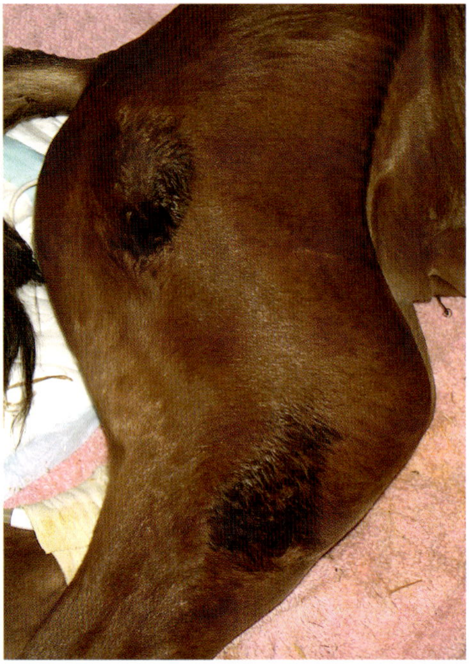

Figure 12.148 Discrete areas of moisture on the hip and stifle, which are indicative of early decubital ulcer formation. These can occur in recumbent compromised neonates and are prevented with adequate clean dry soft bedding and regular turning. If not adequately managed, full thickness skin defects can occur. See fig. 12.25.

Ulcerative Dermatitis

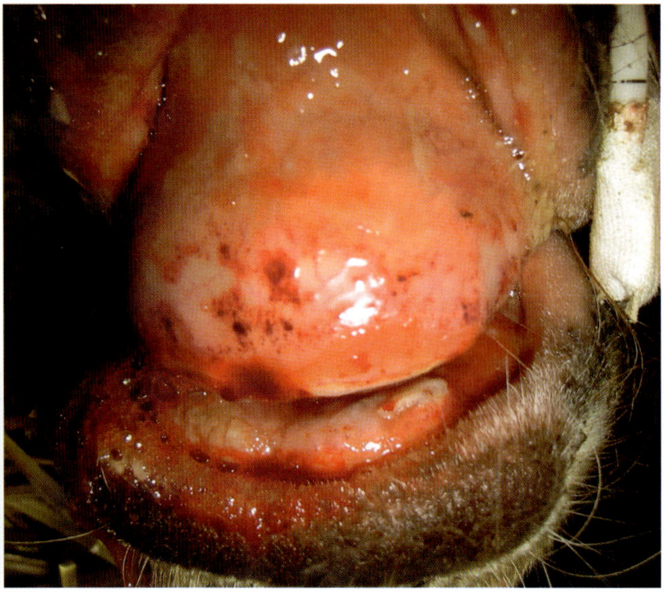

Figure 12.149 Hemorrhagic vesicles, petechiae, and ulceration of the mucosa associated with a syndrome of ulcerative dermatitis, thrombocytopenia, and neutropenia reported in foals <4 days of age. Erythema and crusting around the eyes, perineum, axilla, inguinal region, trunk, and neck are also seen (fig. 12.151). Etiology of the disease is unclear but is believed to have some association with unknown factors in colostrum. The condition is transient, though supportive therapy and various treatments have been reported.

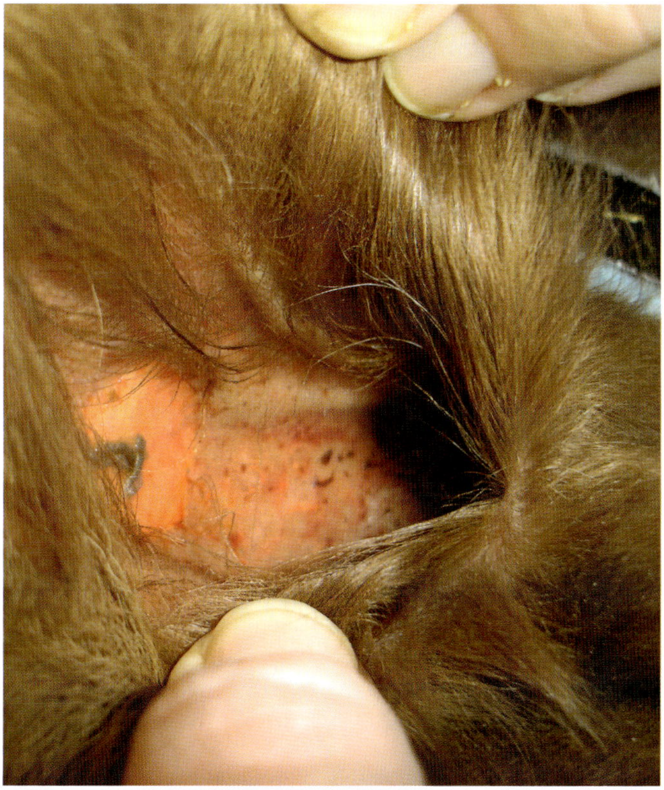

Figure 12.150 Epithelial loss in the ear of a foal affected with ulcerative dermatitis.

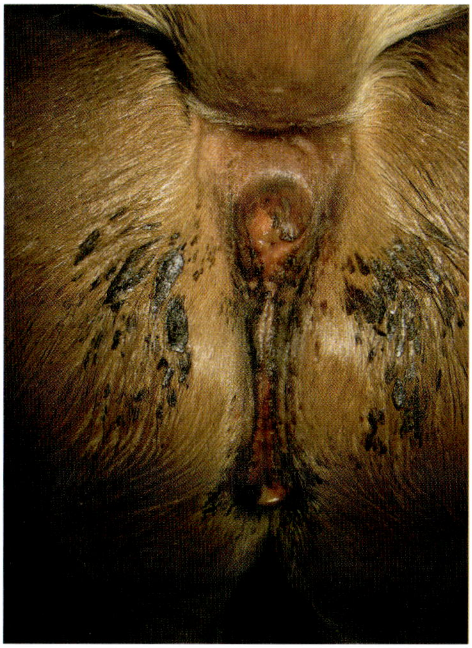

Figure 12.151 Crusting and erythema around anus and vulva.

Dermatophilosis

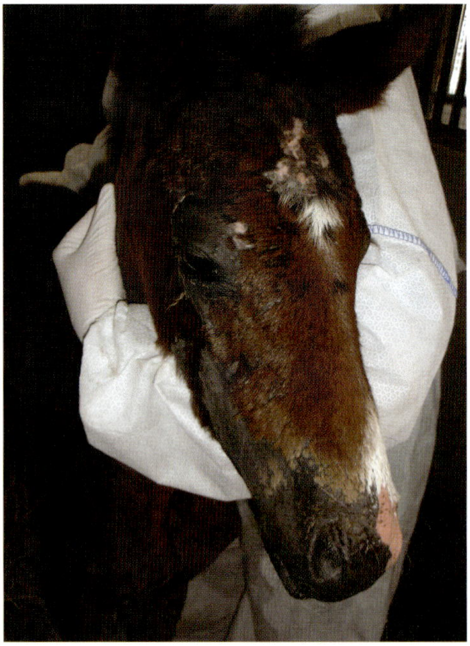

Figure 12.152 *Dermatophilus congolensis* infection in a foal. The clinical appearance of the lesions is similar to adults, though distribution is often more generalized. Diagnosis is based on clinical signs, appearance of the plucked hairs with crusts, and laboratory analysis. Dermatophilosis is self-limiting, however, in debilitated foals, treatment with penicillin and improving the foal's environment is warranted. See Chapter 5, Diseases of the Integumentary System.

Miscellaneous Conditions

Alloimmune Thrombocytopenia

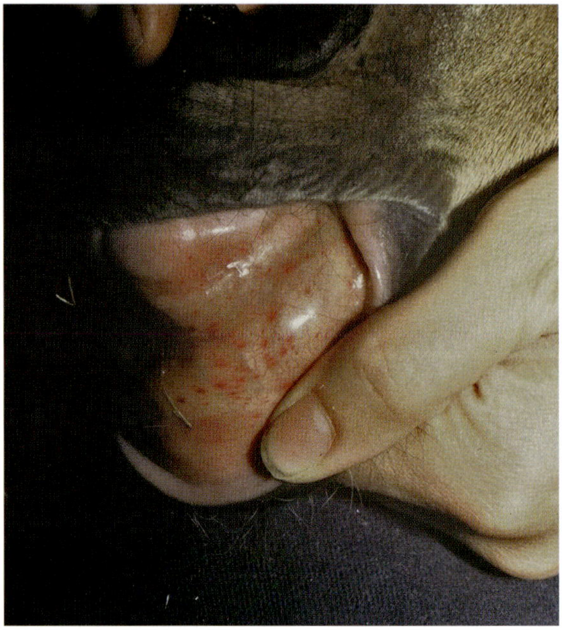

Figure 12.153 Mucous membrane petechiae due to alloimmune mediated thrombocytopenia. The foal absorbs antibodies in the mare's colostrum, which have been formed against the foal's platelets. Clinical signs vary depending on the severity of the thrombocytopenia and include lethargy, petechiae, subcutaneous hematomas, melena, and blood loss anemia. Diagnosis is based on clinical signs, severe thrombocytopenia without sepsis, and positive platelet antibody test. Differential diagnoses include sepsis and congenital bleeding disorders. Treatment is based on clinical signs; platelet-rich plasma or a blood transfusion may be necessary.

Neonatal Hypothyroidism and Goiter

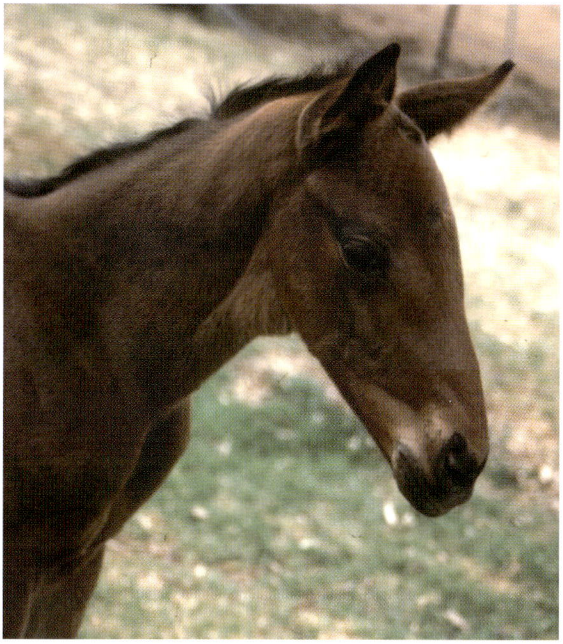

Figure 12.154 Congenital enlarged thyroid glands in a foal due to inadequate iodine intake by the mare. Enlargement can also be associated with excessive iodine intake by the mare. Thyroid function tests need to be performed to confirm hypothyroidism, noting that high thyroid hormone levels are normal in foals. Other clinical signs seen at birth include dysmaturity, muscle weakness, flexural deformities, and mandibular prognathism. (Image courtesy of Dr. D. Racklyeft)

Lavender Foal Syndrome

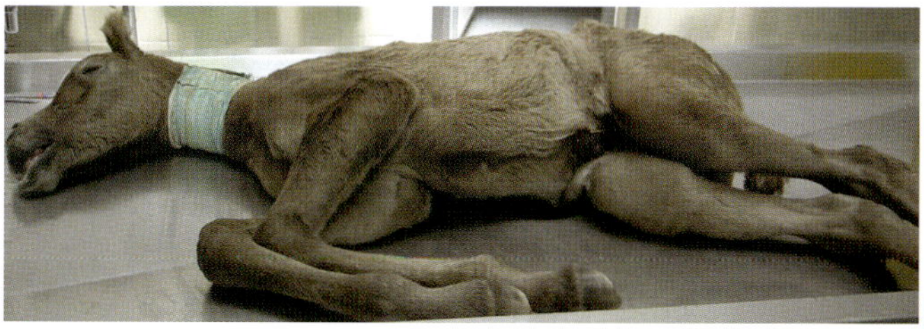

Figure 12.155 A foal affected with lavender foal syndrome showing the characteristic lavender coat color (diluted black/blue, bluish/purple). This is a neurological syndrome of Egyptian Arab foals characterized by neurological signs and dilution of normal hair coat color. Neurological signs include opisthotonos and paddling, and inability to assume sternal recumbency, however, a suckle reflex is present. Differential diagnoses include meningitis, hypoxic ischemic encephalopathy (HIE), and benign epilepsy in Egyptian Arabs. Diagnosis is by the presence of dilute-color coat and tetanic seizures at birth. There is no treatment. (Image courtesy of Dr. J. Neser and Dr. R. Parker)

Congenital Hypothyroidism and Dysmaturity Syndrome

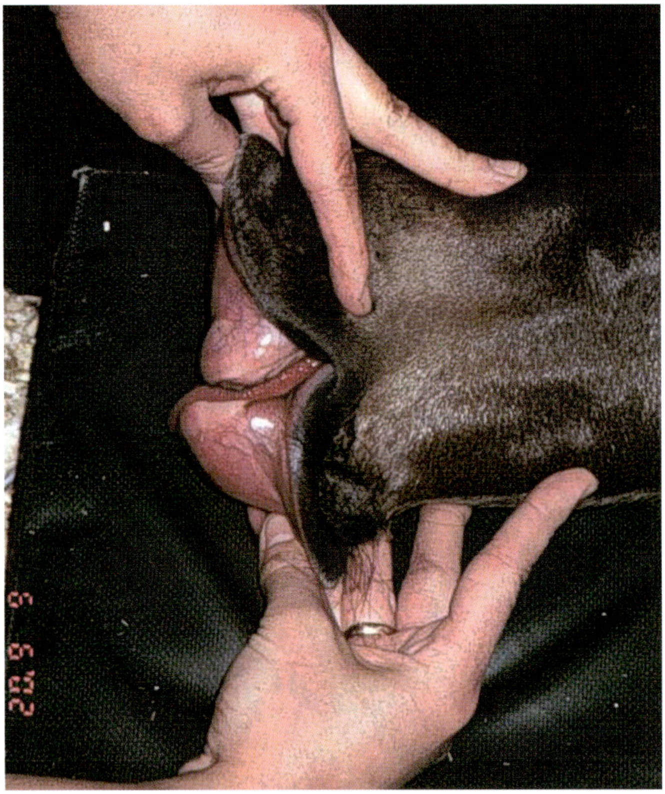

Figure 12.156 A foal with mandibular prognathism, which is seen as part of a syndrome reported in western Canada that is characterized by thyroid hyperplasia and congenital musculoskeletal deformities. Musculoskeletal deformities include angular limb deformities, ruptured common digital extensor tendons, and incomplete ossification of cuboidal bones (fig. 12.157). The syndrome is currently believed to be due to high dietary nitrate concentrations.

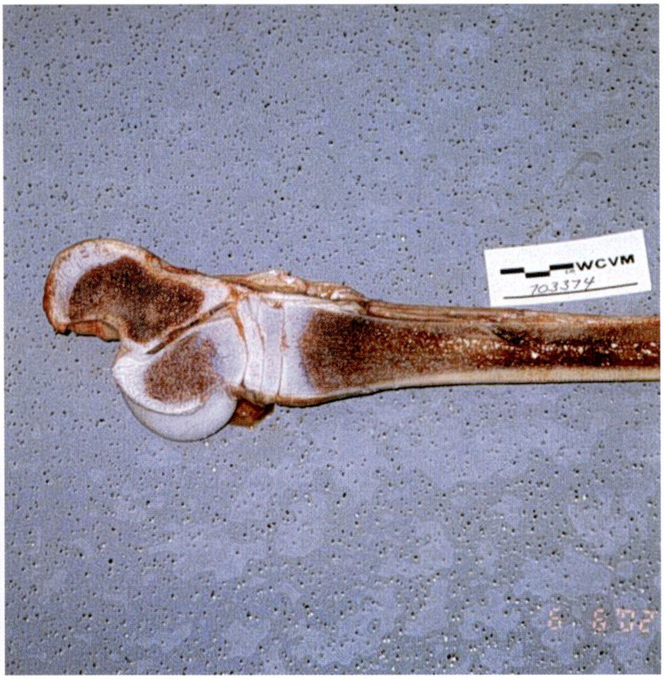

Figure 12.157 Incomplete ossification of cuboidal bones in foal.

Recommended Reading

Bryant JE, Gaughan EM. Abdominal surgery in neonatal foals. Veterinary Clinics of North America: Equine Practice 21:511–35, 2005.

Butler JA, et al. Clinical radiology of the horse. Ames, IA: Blackwell Scientific Publications, 1993.

Clare A, Ryan L, Sanchez C. Nondiarrheal disorders of the gastrointestinal tract in neonatal foal. Veterinary Clinics of North America: Equine Practice 21:313–32, 2005.

Fanelli HH. Coat colour dilution lethal ("Lavender foal syndrome"): a tetany syndrome of Arabian foals. Equine Vet Education, pp. 338–41, 2005.

Giguere S, Polkes AC. Immunologic disorders in neonatal foals. Veterinary Clinics of North America, Equine Practice 21(2):241–72, 2005.

Giguere S, Prescott JF. Clinical manifestations, diagnosis, treatment and prevention of *Rhodococcus equi* infections in foals. Veterinary Microbiology 56:313–34, 1997.

Knottenbelt DC, Madigan JE, Holdstock N. Equine neonatology: medicine and surgery, St. Louis: WB Saunders, 2004.

Lamb CR, O'Callaghan MW, Paradis MR. Thoracic radiography in the neonatal foal: a preliminary report. Vet Rad and US. 31(1):11–16, 1990.

Lester GD. Maturity of the neonatal foal. Veterinary Clinics of North America: Equine Practice 21(2):333–55, 2005.

Magdesian KG. Neonatal foal diarrhea. Veterinary Clinics of North America: Equine Practice 21:295–312, 2005.

Mahew, IW. A handbook of large animal neurology. Philadelphia: Lea and Febiger, 1989.

Sanchez LC. Equine neonatal sepsis. Veterinary Clinics of North America: Equine Practice 21(2):273–93, 2005.

Stashak TS. Adams' Lameness in horses. 4th ed. Philadelphia: Lea & Febiger, 1987.

Thrall DE, ed. Textbook of veterinary diagnostic radiology. 4th ed. St. Louis: WB Saunders.

Toribio RE, Duckett WM. Thyroid gland. In Reed SM, Bayly WM, Sellon, DC, eds. Equine internal medicine, 2nd ed. St Louis: Saunders, pp. 1340–56, 2004.

Trumble TN. Orthopedic disorders in neonatal foal. Veterinary Clinics of North America: Equine Practice 21:357–85, 2005.

Vaala WE. Peripartum asphyxia. Veterinary Clinics of North America, Equine Practice 10(1):187–218, 1994.

White NA, Moore JA. Current practice of equine surgery. Lippincott, 1990.

Wilkins PA. Disorders of foals. In Reed SM, Bayly WM, Sellon DC, eds. Equine internal medicine. 2nd ed. St. Louis: WB Saunders, pp. 1381–431, 2004.

Index

A

Abdominal abscessation, 103–104
  adult horse with, 103
  postmortem examination of horse with, 103
  thickened large colon in horse affected by, 104
Abdominal adhesions, 104–105
  adult horse with, diarrhea and "cow pie" feces related to, 105
  adult horse with severe weight loss caused by, 104
Abdominal pain (colic), 46–52. *See also* Colic
Abdominal region, diseases of, 46–115
  abdominal pain (colic), 46–52
  large intestine diseases, 78–99
  miscellaneous diseases, 103–115
  small colon diseases, 99–102
  small intestine diseases, 59–77
  stomach diseases, 53–59
Abdominal ultrasonography, *105*, 107
Abdominocentesis, in horse affected by peritonitis, *105*, 106
Abnormal tooth wear, 36–37
  at buccal aspect of tooth 406 and 407 in 10-year-old gelding, 36
  severe atypical wear of mandibular incisors, 37
Abortion
  close to term, 502
  long umbilical cord as cause of, 502–503
  mammary gland enlargement prior to, 501
  twinning and, 497–499
Abscesses
  corneal, 534–535
  pulmonary, 604–605
  tooth root, 436–437
Acquired flexural contracture, 647
Acquired leukotrichia, 257–259
  cribbing strap and, 257
  incorrect bandaging and mature quarter horse with, 257
  mature quarter horse with, 257
Actinobacillosis, 259–260
  characteristics and treatment of, *259*
  mare with, after foaling, 260
  mature pregnant mare affected with, serum exudation related to, 259
Actinobacillus equuli, septicemia in neonatal foal due to, manifested as uveitis and hypopyon, 591
Acute pneumonia, 603
Acute renal failure
  hematuria in horse affected with, 561
  horse with severe depression affected with, 560
  postmortem photograph of horse affected with, showing severely swollen kidneys, 562
  postmortem photograph of kidney in horse affected with, 562
Adenocarcinoma, *181*
Adrenal gland, adenoma of, found in horse with clinical signs of PPID, 527
Adrenal tumor
  adenoma, 527
  pheochromocytoma, 527
African horse sickness, 208–209
  clinical signs and diagnosis of, *208*
  pulmonary subserosal petechiae and ecchymoses, 209
  severe intermuscular edema, 209
  subcutaneous edema of supraorbital fossa, 208
  Thoroughbred racehorse with severe conjunctival edema due to, 208
Agitation, colic and, 46, 47–48
AI. *See* Aortic valve insufficiency
Allantoic fluid, normal amount of, *490*
Allergens, recurrent airway obstruction (heaves) and, *190*
Alloimmune thrombocytopenia
  clinical signs, diagnosis, and treatment of, *658*
  mucous membrane petechiae in foal due to, 658
Alopecia
  dermatophilosis and, *279*
  dermatophytosis (ringworm) and, *281*
  onchocerciasis and, 296
  telogen defluxion and, 319
ALS. *See* Amyotrophic lateral sclerosis (Lou Gehrig's disease)
Alternaria, phaeohyphomycosis and, *323*
Altrenogest (Regumate), *498*
American paint horse foals, intestinal aganglionosis (lethal white syndrome) in due to overo-overo mating, *625*
Amiodarone, atrial fibrillation treatment and, *154*
Amputation, penile, 456
Amyotrophic lateral sclerosis (Lou Gehrig's disease), *237*
Anestrus, fetal death followed by, 477
Aneuploidy, intersex and, 473
Angular limb deformity
  carpal valgus, in foal, 634–636
  fetlock varus, in foal, 638
  tarsal valgus, in foal, 637

Anhydrosis, 336–337
clinical signs, diagnosis, and treatment of, *336*
dose-dependent sweating in response to intradermal injection of beta-2 agonist in neck of unaffected horse 20 minutes postinjection, 337
horse evaluated for poor performance due to, 336
intradermal injection of beta-2 agonist using tuberculin syringe, 336
intradermal injection of serial dilutions of beta-2 agonist 3 minutes postinjection, 337
Antebrachiocarpal joint, mild osteoarthritis of, 392
Anti-arrhythmic therapy, for hemodynamically unstable horses, *166*
Antibiogram, 478
Antibiotic induced colitis
horse with watery diarrhea affected with, 102
ultrasonographic image of right dorsal colon of 6-month-old foal with, 102
Anti-inflammatory medications, *191*
Anus, ulcerative dermatitis and crusting and erythema around, 657
Aortic aneurysm, *164*
postmortem photograph of, 166
Aortic insufficiency
characteristics of, *143*
color flow Doppler image of, right parasternal long axis view, 143
electrocardiogram from horse with chronic degenerative valve disease, ventricular premature contraction, aortic insufficiency and, 146
M-mode image of mitral valve from horse with, 144
Aortic regurgitation, continuous wave Doppler evaluation of, 144
Aortic root disease, 164–168
Aortic rupture, uniform ventricular tachycardia secondary to, Holter monitor recording, 166
Aortic valve, bacterial endocarditis of, 145
Aortic valve insufficiency, 143–146
echocardiographic image, right parasternal long axis left ventricular outflow view, 143
phonocardiogram of, 145
Aortocardiac fistula
color flow Doppler image of, 165
echocardiographic image of, 164, 165
postmortem photograph of rupture into right atrium, 167
Aortoiliac thrombus
characteristics of, *168*
sonogram of, 168
APC. *See* Atrial premature contraction
Apical fractures, description of, *385*
Appaloosa breed, equine recurrent uveitis and, 546
Appaloosa gelding, with chronic incisor periodontal disease with cemental hypoplasia, 19
Arabian fading syndrome, horse affected with, 328
Arrhythmogenic right ventricular dysplasia, *137*
Articular facet reaction bone (bone proliferation), 424–425
Articular fracture, of wing of third phalanx, 367–368
Artificial insemination, vaginal examination and, 464
Aryepiglottic fold entrapment, 440–441
Arytenoid chondropathy
cause, signs, and treatment for, *188*
with “kissing” lesion on right arytenoid, 188
Ascaridiasis, intestinal rupture due to ileal obstruction with *Pascaris equorum*, 620
Ascarid impaction, 60
Ascending placentitis, 501
Aspiration pneumonia
causes of, *196*
lateral thoracic radiograph in horse with, secondary to esophageal obstruction, 196
secondary to esophageal obstruction, in a foal, 44
Asynchronous teeth eruption, 27
Ataxia
equine herpes virus 1 (EHV-1) myeloencephalitis and, *229*
equine protozoal myeloencephalitis and, *234*
Atheromas, 260–261
approaching cyst directly from dorsolateral aspect of nostril, 261
weanling Arabian filly with, 260, 261
Atresia ani, in filly foal, 624
Atrial fibrillation, 154–158
base apex surface ECG showing, with delivery of electrical shock, and conversion to normal sinus rhythm, 158
characteristics and treatment of, *154*
ECG from horse with, secondary to mitral regurgitation and left atrial enlargement, 154
exercising heart rates in horses with, *155*
Holter monitor recording of horse converting from, to normal sinus rhythm, 155
lone, exercising ECG from horse with, 155
rapid, in horse with history of weakness during exercise, 154
rapid and chaotic depolarization in intra-atrial ECG consistent with, *157*
Atrial premature contraction
nonconducted, Holter monitor recording, 152
with normal ventricular conduction, 152
Atrial rates, elevated, *152*
Atrial tachycardia
with second degree AV block at rest, 153
during trotting exercise, telemetric recording from horse with atrial tachycardia and second degree AV block, 153
Atrioventricular (AV) block, 151–152
advanced second degree, base apex recording from horse with severe exercise intolerance, 151
second degree at rest, atrial tachycardia with, 153
third degree (complete), base apex recording from neonatal foal with septic myocarditis, 152
Type I second degree, 151
Auditory diverticula, 438
Aural plaques, 262–263
chronic lesions centrally, 262
early lesions peripherally, 262
horse presenting with head-shaking due to, 263
viral basis for, 330
Aureobasidium, phaeohyphomycosis and, *323*
Australian stringhalt, *240*
Avulsion fracture, of origin of long digital extensor tendon in 2-month-old foal, 644

B

Bacterial endocarditis
of aortic valve, 145
tricuspid valve insufficiency and, 146

two-dimensional echocardiographic image, right parasternal long axis view, 141
Bacterial folliculitis, 263–264
of axillae, mature quarter horse with, 263
differential diagnosis of, *263*
extension of lesion over pectoral region, 264
Bacterial pneumonia in adult horses
clinical signs of, *195*
mucupurulent nasal discharge and, 195
"Barker" vocalization, hypoxic ischemic encephalopathy and, *584*
Barn fire, postmortem picture of mature horse caught in, 265
Basilar bones, poll impact and damage to, *215*
Basilar fracture
of medial proximal sesamoid bone, 387
postmortem photograph of horse with, 215
Basilar sesamoid fractures, prognosis for, *387*
Basophilic enterocolitis, *101*
"Bastard strangles," *204*
"Beans," smegma accumulation, in fossa glandis, 461
Bedding, pressure sores and lack of, 272
Belgian/Belgian-cross foals, junctional epidermolysis bullosa in, *339*
Belgium draft mare, unusual case of dystocia in, 483
Belly bandages, penile injuries and use of, 455
Beta hemolysis, 478
Bilateral cryptorchidism, 447
Bilateral soft tissue damage, to interdental spaces of young quarter horse, 32
Biopsies, endometrial, 479–480
Bit pressure, bilateral soft tissue damage to interdental spaces and, 32
Bladder
with cystitis, postmortem photograph of, 568
with cystolithiasis, 575
infected umbilical remnant with purulent caseous material in umbilical arteries and apex of, 653
premature placental separation and prolapse of, 486
ruptured, ultrasonographic examination of ventral part of caudal abdomen of two foals with, 651
sabulous urolithiasis and, 577
Bleeding gastric ulcer, hemorrhagic nasogastric reflux due to erosion of blood vessel in, 617
"Blind" biopsy technique, endometrial biopsy and, *479*
Blindness
leukoencephalomalacia (Moldy Corn Disease) and, *224*
West Nile Virus and, *225*
Blue to white irides, 550
Bone cysts, subchondral, 416
Bone remodeling, mild osteoarthritis of antebrachiocarpal joint and, *392*
Bones, diseases of, 353–443
carpus and metacarpus, 392–407
in foals, 630–645
head, 427–443
metacarpophalangeal and metatarsophalangeal joints, 378–391
navicular bone, 356–362
phalanges, 363–378
spine, 422–427
stifle and tibia, 416–421
tarsus and metatarsus, 407–415
Botulism
cause, clinical signs, diagnosis and treatment of, *627*
recumbent foal with flaccid paralysis due to, 627
Bouin's fluid, endometrial biopsy and, *479*
Bovine papilloma virus, *304*
Brachial plexus injury, foal with, following dystocia and manual manipulation, 627
Brain abscess, 212–214
causes and clinical signs of, 212
close-up view of, 214
head-pressing in horse affected with, 212
horse affected with, showing droopy lip due to cranial nerve VII deficit, 213
mature horse affected with, showing depressed mentation, 212
postmortem photograph of brain in horse with, 213
Bran disease, 525
Breeding accidents, causes of, *464*
"Breeding stitch," poor vulvar conformation and, *474*
Brisket edema, in adult horse affected by nonsteroidal anti-inflammatory drugs toxicity, 97
Broken hoof-pastern axis, osteoarthritis of left distal interphalangeal joint and, 365
Bronchial edema
endoscopy of crina revealing rounded airway bifurcation and hyperemia consistent with, 191
treatment of, *191*
Bronchodilators, *191*
Bronchopneumonia, *603*
Brucellosis, 271
Bruxism, gastric ulcers and, *56*
Buccal mucosal ulcer, sharp enamel point at level of tooth 107 and, 34
"Bucked shin," 403
Bulbar squamous cell carcinoma, invasion of temporal cornea from limbal conjunctiva in 10-year-old paint mare, 552
Bulls, testicular descent in, 447
Burns, 264–269
estimated percentage body surface areas in adult horse, 269
estimated percentage body surface areas in foal, 269
horse healing from, sustained over dorsum of his poll and back when tractor exploded next to his stall, 266–268
postmortem picture of mature horse caught in barn fire, 265
prognosis for and consequences of, *264*
"Burns technique," retained placenta and, 504
Bursitis (shoe boil and fistulous withers), 270–272

C

Calcaneus, sequestration of, 413
Calcinosis circumscripta (tumoral calcinosis), 272–273, 420
characteristics of, *272*
dorsolateral view of horse affected with, 273
lateromedial view of horse affected with, 273
Calculus accumulation, over and around 404, 20
Campylorrhinus lateralis, *176*
Candidiasis, on foal's tongue, 613
Canine tooth, supernumerary, 35
Capture beats, VPCs and, 160
Cardiac arrhythmias, 150–160
atrial fibrillation, 154–158
atrioventricular block, 151–152
sinus rhythm, 150

supraventricular arrhythmias, 152–153
ventricular arrhythmias, 158–160
Cardiac cachexia, mare with, 135
Cardiac tamponade, with pericardial effusion, 129, 132
Cardiomyopathy, 134–136
dilated, two-dimensional echocardiographic image from broodmare in late gestation with congestive heart failure and, 134
Cardiovascular system, diseases of, 119–173
aortic root disease, 164–168
aortic valve insufficiency, 143–146
atrial fibrillation, 154–158
atrioventricular block, 151–152
cardiac arrhythmias, 150–160
cardiomyopathy, 134–136
congenital cardiac defects, 120–128
cor pulmonale, 138
endocardial and valvular diseases, 139–149
endocarditis, 148–149
mitral valve insufficiency, 139–142
myocardial diseases, 134–138
myocarditis, 137–138
neoplasia, 132–133
pericardial diseases, 129–133
pericarditis, 129–132
purpura hemorrhagica, 168–173
sinus rhythm, 150
supraventricular arrhythmias, 152–153
tetralogy of Fallot, 128
thrombosis and thrombophlebitis, 161–164
tricuspid valve insufficiency, 146–147
truncus arteriosus, 126–127
vascular diseases, 161–173
ventricular arrhythmias, 158–160
ventricular septal defect, 120–125
Carpal bone ossification, grading system for, in foals, 633
Carpal bones
grade 1 ossification of, in foals, 633
grade 2 ossification of, in foals, 634, 636
Carpal valgus
angular limb deformity of, in 2-day-old quarter horse foal
angular limb deformity of, in 4-week-old quarter horse foal, 634, 636
angular limb deformity of, in 6-week-old quarter horse foal, 635
foal with, 635
Carpometacarpal joint, severe osteoarthritis of, 394
Carpus
isotope uptake in dorsal aspect of distal carpal row, 396
normal, in 30-day-old Standardbred foal, 632
prematurity and incomplete ossification of cuboidal bones in, 599
sclerosis of radial and intermediate facets of third carpal bone, 396
soft tissue swelling of, 392
Carpus and metacarupus, 392–407
avulsion fracture of origin of suspensory ligament, 405
enchondroma and enthesiophyte formation at attachment of superior check ligament, 402
fractures of
distal radius, 398
fourth metacarpal bone with evidence of osteomyelitis, 407
radial carpal bone, 397
third carpal bone, 398–400
metacarpal periostitis, 403
normal third carpal bone and third carpal bone with mild sclerosis of radial facet, 395
nuclear scintigraphic imaging of carpus, 396
osteoarthritis of, 392–394
periostitis at origin of suspensory ligament, 406
radial cysts, 401
soft tissue swelling of the carpus, 392
splint exostosis of second metacarpal bone, 406
stress fracture of third metacarpus, 404
ulnar carpal bone cyst, 401
Caslick's operation, *474*, *475*
Castration
bilateral, testicular torsion with hydrocele and, 460
scrotal hernia after, 460
Cataract
hypermature, in young quarter horse, 541
immature, in yearling Arabian filly, 540
mature
one month after phacoemulsification, 541
in young Arabian colt, 540
Caudal hooks or ramps, 7
Caudal maxillary sinuses, fluid within, *428*, 430, 431
Caudal vena cava
epiploic foramen entrapment of small intestines bounded dorsally by, 70
normal boundaries of epiploic foramen and, 71
CEM. *See* Contagious equine metritis
Cemental decay, peripheral, at palatal aspect of 210 and 211, 19
Cervical spinal cord compression, *236*
Cervical spine, normal, 422, 427
Cervical tears, 476
Cervical vertebral malformation, *236*
Cervical vertebral malformation instability, *424*, 425–426
Cervical vertebral stenosis/instability, *236*
Chemical scalding
alopecia and scaling due to use of alcohol-based leg wrap in mature horse, 310
axillary serum exudation in mature horse due to failure to remove shampoo after bathing, 310
periaural serum exudation in mature horse due to failure to remove shampoo after bathing, 309
Chemosis
corneal abscess and, 534
with granuloma and periocular calcification, 531
Choke
primary, 40–44
clinical signs of, *41*
secondary, 45–46, 206
Cholesterol granuloma (cholesteatomas)
clinical signs of, *244*
postmortem examination of brain of horse affected with, 244
Chondroids
appearance typical of, 439
chronic empyema and formation of, *184*
Chondroma, *181*
Chorioallantois, 486
Choroid detachment, ultrasonographic examination and, *549*
Chronic incisor periodontal disease, 19
with concurrent cemental hyperplasia, 20

Chronic pneumonia, 604
Chronic proliferative synovitis, of metacarpophalangeal joint, 381–382
Chronic renal failure, 563–567
  bilateral obstruction of upper urinary tract and, *575*
  dental tartar in horse affected with, 564
  depression in horse affected with, 566
  oral ulcers and tartar on incisors of horse affected with, 564
  peripheral limb edema in horse affected with, 565
  postmortem photograph of kidney with multiple cysts from horse affected with, 566
  ultrasonographic image of kidney from horse affected with, 567
  ventral edema in horse affected with, 565
  weight loss in horse affected with, 563
Chronic uveitis, vitreous floaters, collagen clumping, vascularization, and focal dispersion in Appaloosa with, 547
Circumduction, equine protozoal myeloencephalitis and, *234*
Cisplatin injections, sarcoid treatment and, *553*
CL. *See* Corpus luteum
Cladophialophora, phaeohyphomycosis and, *323*
Cleft palate
  clinical signs and diagnosis of, *613*
  in newborn foal, 613
Clitoral sinuses, sampling, 465
Clitoris, anatomy of, 465
Clostridial enterocolitis, 620–621
  clinical signs, diagnosis, and treatment of, *620*
  foal with, due to *Clostridium perfringens*, 620
  necrotizing enterocolitis *vs.*, *585*
  sonogram of ventral abdomen of foal with, 621
Clostridium botulinum, botulism caused by, *627*
Clostridium perfringens, foal with clostridial enterocolitis due to, 620
Clostridium tetani, tetanus caused by, *240*
Club foot, in foal, 647
Coital exanthema ("spots"), 475
  cause of, *475*
Colic, 46–52
  agitation, flank watching with, 46, 47–48
  clinical signs of, *46*
  equine herpes virus 1 (EHV-1) myeloencephalitis and, *229*
  facial nerve trauma following severe episode of, 252
  frequent lying down and, 46, 50
  kicking at the abdomen and, 46, 49
  pawing and, 46, 48
  rolling and, 46, 51–52
  stretching and, 46, 49
  tetanus (lockjaw) and, *240*
Coliforms, pure culture of, 478
Colitis, antibiotic induced, 102
Collagenolysis, melting corneal ulcer and, 532
Comet tail artifacts, coalescing, with ruptured chorda tendinea and congestive heart failure, 141
Common digital extensor tendon, ruptured, in foal, 646
Congenital cardiac defects, 120–128
  tetralogy of Fallot, 128
  truncus arteriorsus, 126–127
  ventricular septal defect, 120–125
Congenital flexural contracture, 647
Congenital glaucoma, buphthalmic globe in 7-day-old Arabian filly, 537
Congenital goiter, from newborn foal, 522
Congenital hypothyroidism and dysmaturity syndrome, foal with, 660
Congestive heart failure
  mare with, 135
  sonographic image of pulmonary edema in horse with ruptured chorda tendinea and, 141
Conjunctival corneal pedicle flap, healed, 535
Conjunctival edema, severe, due to African horse sickness, 208
Conjunctivitis
  corneal abscess and, 534
  with granuloma and periocular calcification, 531
Constrictive pericarditis, 131
Contagious equine metritis, *461*
  culturing clitoral sinuses for, *465*
Cord length, abortion and, *502*
Corneal abscess, 534–535
  nonulcerative, 535
  treatment of, *534*, 535
Corneal degeneration, keratopathy and, 532
Corneal laceration, with iridal prolapse after kick to right facial area, 531
Corneal ulcer
  indolent with fluorescein stain migrating underneath epithelial flaps, 536
  melting, 532
  perforated, 534
Coronary artery thromboemboli, numerous myocardial infarcts caused by, *167*
Coronitis, in foal with sepsis, 590
Corpora nigra laceration, 550
Cor pulmonale, two-dimensional echocardiographic image from horse with, secondary to recurrent airway obstruction, 138
Corpus luteum, formation of, 462
Cotwin embryos, fate of crushed, 498
Cotwin pregnancies, managing, *499*
Cox test (hCG stimulation test), cryptochordism diagnosis and, *448*
Cranial cruciate ligament injury, chronic, osteoarthritis of stifle joint and, 418
Cranial deficits, equine herpes virus 1 (EHV-1) myeloencephalitis and deficits in, *229*
Cranial nerves
  guttural pouch diseases and, *182*
  poll impact and damage to, *215*
  West Nile Virus and deficits in, *225*, *227*
Cresty neck
  insulin resistance and, 516, 517
  pituitary pars intermedia dysfunction and, 509
CRF. *See* Chronic renal failure
"Cribber," 37
Crossing over, equine protozoal myeloencephalitis and, *234*
Crowded teeth, 24
Crown, large amount of excessive, at mesial portion of 106 in 10-year-old quarter horse stallion, 7
Cryptorchidism, 447–449
  bilateral, 447
  comparison of normal and cryptorchid testicles, 448

diagnosis of, *448*
disruption of spermatogenesis and, 449
image of intra-abdominal testicles in 7-year-old quarter horse stallion, 448
C type (carpal), of infectious polyarthritis in foals, *641*
Cubital bursitis, shoe-boil roll in case of, 270
Cuboidal bones
congenital hypothyroidism and dysmaturity syndrome and incomplete ossification of, 660
premature and incomplete ossification of, in hock and carpus, 599
Culicoides hypersensitivity, mature quarter horse gelding with, 288
Culturing instruments, for mares, *478*
Cushing's syndrome, 274
adrenal tumor, *274*
clinical signs of, *274*
matted hair coat of horse with, *274*
Cutaneous drug reactions (drug eruption)
description of, *334*
type IV hypersensitivity reaction in horse, 334
vaccinations and, 334, 335
Cutaneous habronemiasis, 275–276
areas affected by, 276
causes and diagnosis of, *275*
horse after undergoing treatment for, 275
mature quarter horse with extensive case of, 275
preputial, 276
Cutaneous lymphosarcoma, 277–278
"figure 8" shaped lesion caudal to elbow in horse affected with, 278
horse with firm subcutaneous mass on proximomedial aspect of right front leg, 277
mare with multiple, firm nodules on proximomedial aspect of left hind leg, 278
mature gelding with large, firm mass in ventral perineal region, 277
types of, *277*
CVC. *See* Caudal vena cava
CVMI. *See* Cervical vertebral malformation instability
Cyathostomiasis, 93–95
in cecum of horse with strongylosis, causes of, 93
microscopic examination of encysted larvae in intestinal mucosa, 94–95
postmortem photograph of large colon of horse affected with typhlocolitis caused by, 93
Cystitis
clinical signs, diagnosis and treatment of, *568*
postmortem photograph of bladder affected with, 568
Cystolithiasis, 571
clinical signs, diagnosis, and treatment of, *575*
endoscopic image of bladder with, 575
Cysts
endometrial, 471–472
iridal, 549
radial, 401
sinus, 429–430
uveal, 551

D

Dactylaria, phaeohyphomycosis and, *323*
DCM. *See* Dilated cardiomyopathy
DDSP. *See* Dorsal displacement of the soft palate
Decubital ulcers, in foals, 656
Defibrillation, general anesthesia used for, *156*
Degenerative joint disease, 379, 410–412
Dehydrated foal, entropion in, 628
Dental structures
normal, 432–435
lateral view, 432
maxillary in immature horse, 434
maxillary in mature horse, 434
radiographic projections of skull, 433
ventrodorsal view, 433
Dental tartar, chronic renal failure and, 564
Dental tumor, of mandible, 442–443
Dentigerous cyst, 320–321
Depression
acute renal failure and, *560*
chronic renal failure and, 566
pyelonephritis and, 567
Dermatophilosis (rain scald), 279–281
diagnosis of, *658*
epilating hair results in number of hair shafts stuck within crust of dried serum, 280
in foal, 658
lesions on muzzle, 281
seasonal forms of, *279*
severely affected animals with depression, anorexia, and pyrexic condition, 280
Dermatophilus congolensis infection
dermatophilosis and, *279*
foal infected with, 658
photosensitization and, *301*
Dermatophytosis (ringworm), 281–284
clinical signs of, *281*
extensive hair loss in Thoroughbred horse affected with, 281–282
overlying scab that can be easily removed, 283
self-limiting treatment for, 284
Dermoid cyst, 284–285
elevation of skin resulting in obvious bump in top line of horse, 284
in horse, clipped prior to expressing contents, 285
manual expression of contents, 285
Diagonal incisor malocclusion (DGL3), 11
deviation of maxilla and, 26
Diaphragmatic hernia, 72, 611
clinical signs of, *611*
defect in diaphragm resulting in, 611
lateral thoracic radiograph demonstrating gas-filled loops of viscera in abdomen, 611
Diarrhea
hemorrhagic, due to necrotizing enterocolitis, *585*
rotavirus, 621
Diastema, periodontal pocket and, 16
Diet, cystolithiasis treatment and change in, *575*
Diffuse bronchointerstitial lung pattern, 604
Digital hyperextension deformity, *648*
Dilated cardiomyopathy, 134
color flow Doppler evaluation of tricuspid valve in horse with, 135
M-mode echocardiographic image from horse with, 134

Disseminated intravascular coagulation, hemorrhagic gingival margins in foal with, 589
Distal check desmotomy
after foal treated for, 648
club foot in foal and, *647*
Distal femur, malformation of, and luxation of patella, *643*
Distal interphalangeal joint, osteoarthritis of, 364–365
Distal intertarsal joint
mild osteoarthritis of, 410
moderate osteoarthritis of, 410
severe osteoarthritis of, 411
Distal metacarpus, Salter-Harris type 2 fracture of, in foal, 642
Distal radial physis, closure of, *632*
Distal radius, fracture of, 398
DJD. *See* Degenerative joint disease
Dorsal conchal sinuses, *427*
Dorsal displacement of the soft palate
intermittent or persistent, clinical signs and diagnosis of, *186*
as visualized by endoscopy at rest in horse with dysphagia, 186
Dorsal incisor curvature, in juvenile, 11
DPJ. *See* Duodenitis-proximal jejunitis
Draschia megastoma, *275*
Drechslera, phaeohyphomycosis and, *323*
Dumb rabies, *239*
Duodenal stricture
diagnosis of, *618*
postmortem specimen from foal with delayed gastric emptying due to, 618
Duodenitis-proximal jejunitis, 75–76
anterior or proximal enteritis, postmortem photograph of, 75
ultrasonographic image of right caudal abdomen showing distension and thickening of duodenum in case of, 76
Dysmaturity, *487*
Dysphagia
choke and, 206
hypoxic ichemic encephalopathy and, *583*
mega-esophagus and, *615*
Dysplastic teeth, in aged miniature horse with abnormal mastication, 36
Dystocia
foal with brachial plexus injury following, 627
general approaches and forms of, 481–483
general comments about, *481*
hydrocephalus as cause of, 481
mesenteric tear as cause of, 483
ruptured gastrocnemius muscle and, 646
salivary cyst as cause of, 482
severe skeletal malformation as cause of, 482
ventral abdominal wall tear and, *649*

E

Ear, ulcerative dermatitis and epithelial loss in, 657
Ear tooth, 320–321
Ecchymoses in oral mucosa, in horse affected with purpura hemorrhagica, 170
Ecchymoses in vulvar mucosa, in mare affected with purpura hemorrhagica, 171
Ecchymotic hemorrhage, on muzzle of horse affected with purpura hemorrhagica, 171
eCG. *See* Equine chorionic gonadotropin
Edema
chronic renal failure and, 565
of head, in horse with purpura hemorrhagica, 169
Egyptian Arab foals, lavender foal syndrome and, *659*
Ehler Danlos syndrome, 286–287
EHV III. *See* Equine herpes virus III
EIPH. *See* Exercise-induced pulmonary hemorrhage
Electrical cardioversion, intra-atrial ECG obtained from horse undergoing, 157
Electrical cardioversion catheters, horse fitted with, 156
Embolic nephritis, in septicemic neonatal foal, 588
Embolic pneumonia, in septicemic neonatal foal, 587
Embryonic death
at about 55 days of gestation, 496
due to twinning, 497–499
early and later, 496
general characteristics of, *496*
Embryos
heartbeat of, early pregnancy monitoring, 463
tracking during early pregnancy diagnosis, 497
Enamel decay, focal areas of, 18
Encephalomyelitis, West Nile Virus and, *225*
Enchondroma, at attachment of superior check ligament, 402
Endocardial and valvular diseases, 139–149
aortic valve insufficiency, 143–146
endocarditis, 148–149
mitral valve insufficiency, 139–142
tricuspid valve insufficiency, 146–147
Endocarditis, 148–149
atrial
ECG from horse with, involving AV node region, 149
echocardiographic image from horse with history of weakness and near collapse during exercise with, 148
postmortem examination of horse with, showing raised irregular tan areas along right atrial septum, 149
short axis echocardiographic image from horse with, 148
Endocrine system, diseases of, 507–527
adrenal gland diseases, 527
glucose metabolism diseases, 516–517
goiter in newborn foals, 522
hyperparathyroidism, 523–526
pituitary disease, 508–515
thyroid diseases, 518–522
vitamin D toxicity, 523
Endometrial biopsy, 479–480
annotated anatomy of, 480
general comments about, *479*
hemorrhage after, 479
jaws of biopsy instrument, 479
Endometrial cups, 477
Endometrial cysts, 471–472
Endometrium, normal epithelial cells from, *478*
Endophthalmitis, in horse affected by otitis media-interna (temporohyoid osteoarthropathy), 247
Enilconazole, dermatophytosis (ringworm) treatment with, *284*
Enterocolitis, septicemic foal with, 592
Enterocutaneous fistula, in horse as sequela to parietal (Richter's) hernia, 108
Enteroliths
intraluminal obstruction of small colon with, 100
photograph of, diagnosis of, 100

Enthesiophyte formation, at attachment of superior check ligament, 402
Enthesopathy, radiographs of navicular bone cyst with, 359
Enthesophytes, *359*
Entropion, 628–629
 in dehydrated foal, 628
 foal after surgical treatment for, 629
 foal with, 628
 treatment of, *628*
Epididymis, comparison of normal and cryptorchid testicles and tail of, *448*
Epidural anesthesia, in mare, *481*
Epiglottic entrapment
 by aryepiglottic membrane in racehorse, 187
 treatment of, *187*
Epiploic foramen, postmortem photograph of normal abdomen in horse showing normal boundaries of, 71
Epiploic foramen entrapment of small intestines, 69–71
 postmortem photograph of, 70
Epistaxis
 in horse with exercise-induced pulmonary hemorrhage, 192
 progressive ethmoid hematoma and, *178*
Epithelial excoriation, dermatophytosis (ringworm) and, 283
Epitheliotropic lymphosarcoma, clinical signs of, *277*
Epizootic lymphangitis (histoplasmosis), 338–339
 cutaneous, ulcerative nodules along ventral abdomen and preputial sheath of horse with, 338
 description, diagnosis and treatment of, *338*
Equine calculi, composition of, 576
Equine chorionic gonadotropin, 477
Equine Cushing's disease, 508
Equine dysautonomia, 109–115
Equine herpes virus 1 (EHV-1) myeloencephalitis, 229–233
 adult horse with, with more involvement in hind limbs than in front limbs, 231
 atlanto-occipital centesis of cerebrospinal fluid in horse affected with, 232
 causes, clinical signs and treatment of, *229*
 cerebrospinal fluid from horse affected with, showing xanthochromia, 233
 flaccid anus and tail in horse affected with, 231
 mare with, showing wide-based forelimb stance and knuckling of hind limb, 229
 patchy sweating in horse affected with, 232
 photomicrograph of cerebrospinal fluid from horse affected with, showing mononuclear pleocytosis, 233
 tetraplegia in horse affected with, 230
 urinary incontinence and urine scalding in horse affected with, 230
Equine herpes virus III, coital exanthema ("spots") caused by, *475*
Equine motor neuron disease, 237–239
 adult horse affected by, 237
 biopsy of spinal accessory nerve or sacrocaudalis dorsalis muscle and diagnosis of, 238
 clinical signs of, *237*
 diagnosis of, *238*
 fundus of normal horse, 239
 lipofuscinlike pigment in tapetal fundus of retina and, 238
Equine mummies, *500*
Equine placentation, practical anatomy and nature of, 504
Equine protozoal myeloencephalitis, 234–235
 adult horse affected with, shown with droopy lips due to damaged facial nerve, 235
 adult horse affected with, which previously had tetraparesis, 234
 adult horse suspected to be affected with, showing atrophy of gluteal muscles, 234
 adult horse with tongue paralysis due to, 235
 clinical signs of, *234*
Equine recurrent uveitis, with corneal stromal vascularization, 546
Equine stud medicine, common diagnostic techniques used in, 478
Equine wobbler syndrome, 236–237
 adult horse affected with, showing wide-base stance, 236
 adult horse affected with, with failure to replace limbs to normal position when limb is placed in abnormal position, 237
 clinical signs and diagnosis of, *236*
 toe scuffing in adult horse affected with, 236
Erection, persistent, *456*
Esophageal diverticulae, secondary choke and, 45
Esophageal lavage, 43
Esophageal obstruction
 aspiration pneumonia secondary to, in a foal, 44
 choke, primary, 40–44
 endoscopic image of, 42
 endoscopic image of esophagus after resolution of, 42
 esophageal laceration and peri-esophageal cellulitis in foal secondary to, 41
 esophageal lavage and, 43
 long-standing, postmortem image of circumferential esophageal ulceration in horse secondary to, 43
 postmortem photograph of megaesophagus in foal secondary to, 44
 radiological examination of cervical and thoracic esophagus, equipment for, 42
Esophageal stricture
 postmortem specimen of foal with, 616
 static contrast lateral radiograph of foal's thorax with, 616
Esophagus, diseases of, 40–46
 esophageal obstruction (choke), primary, 40–44
 esophageal obstruction (choke), secondary, 45–46
Estrone sulphate test, cryptochordism diagnosis and, *448*
Estrous cycle, following, 462
Ethmoid hematoma, 431–432
 treatment of, *178*
E type (epiphyseal), of infectious polyarthritis, in 4-week-old quarter horse foal, 641
Exercise-induced pulmonary hemorrhage, 192–195
 chronic, lateral radiograph of racehorse with, 195
 clinical signs and diagnosis of, *192*
 epistaxis postexercise in horse with, 192
 grade 1, racehorse with, as detected by tracheobronchoscopy, 193
 grade 2, racehorse with, as detected by tracheobronchoscopy, 193
 grade 3, racehorse with, as detected by tracheobronchoscopy, 193
 grade 4, racehorse with, as detected by tracheobronchoscopy, 194

photomicrograph of bronchoalveolar lavage fluid showing hemosiderophages in racehorse with, 194
Thoroughbred racehorse with epistaxis and, 192
Exophiala, phaeohyphomycosis and, *323*
Exserohilum, phaeohyphomycosis and, *323*
External umbilical remnant, infected, 655
External umbilical swellings, diagnostic differentiations for, *654*
Extrathoracic airways, diseases of, 176–189
arytenoid chondropathy, 188
dorsal displacement of the soft palate, 186
epiglottic entrapment, 187
guttaral pouch diseases, 181–184
guttural pouch empyema, 182–184
guttural pouch mycosis, 185
guttural pouch tympany, 184–185
laryngeal diseases, 187–188
laryngeal hemiplegia, 188
nasal passages, 176
pharyngeal diseases, 186
pharyngitis, 186
progressive ethmoid hematoma, 178
sinonasal neoplasia and polyps, 181
sinus cyst, 180–181
sinusitis, 179–180
subepiglottic cyst, 187
tracheal collapse, 189
wry nose, 176–178
Eye diseases, 529–556
corneal disorders, 531–536
glaucoma, 537–539
lenticular disorders, 540–543
ocular tumors, 552–556
uveal disorders, 543–551
Eyelid tone, botulism and loss of, *627*

F

Face lesions, with pemphigus foliaceus, *299*
Facial nerve trauma
horse affected with, during episode of severe colic, 252
horse with, after lateral recumbency, 252
False nostril cysts, *260*
Fat pads, displacement and/or compression of and distension of middle carpal joint, *392*
Fecaliths, intraluminal obstruction of small colon with, 100
Feed impaction, fractured tooth and, 27
Female fetus, transrectal scan of, 485
Female reproductive system diseases. *See* Reproductive system diseases, female
Fetal death
followed by anestrus, 477
followed by mummification, 500
Fetal sexing, 484–485
early and late gestation, 484
fetal gender diagnosed during advanced gestation, 485
general comments about, *484*
Fetlock hyperextension, severe, *648*
Fetlock joint capsule, setpic arthritis in and massive distension of, 384
Fetlock varus
angular limb deformity of, in 5-week-old Thoroughbred foal, 638
foal with, clinical photograph of, 638
Fetus, aging of, 464
Fibroblastic lesions, sarcoids and, *304*
Fibrofatty metaplasia, cut section of, from adult horse, 137
Fibroma, *181*
Fibrous osteodystrophy, 524
First phalanx
complete fracture of, 374–375
dorsoproximal, fracture of, 389
osseous fragment arising from plantar margin of, 391
osseous fragmentation of lateral plantar process of, 390
proximal, fracture of, 388
subchondral cystic lesion of, 372
Fistulous withers, 270–272
old horse with, showing purulent debris and rim of granulation tissue, 271
Flank watching, colic and, 46, 47–48
Flecainide, atrial fibrillation treatment and, *154*
Flexural deformities
club foot in foals, 647
in foals, 647–648
Flexural laxity, in foals, 648
Fly control, habronemiasis control and, *450*
Fly infestations, sarcoids and, *304*
Foaling
cervical tears and, *476*
impending, estimating time of, 486
Foaling injuries, 491–495
intra-abdominal hemorrhage, 493
normal contusion of the vagina, 491
rectal, vaginal, and perineal tears and lacerations, 493–495
rectal prolapse, 492
severe vaginal contusions and pelvic subluxation, 492
uterine hemorrhage, 493
vulvar injuries, *475*
Foals. *See also* Neonates, diseases of
newborn, goiter in, 522
Fonsecaea, phaeohyphomycosis and, *323*
Food hypersensitivity
clinical signs of, *335*
mature horse with perineal pruritus caused by feed hypersensitivity, 335
Forehead trauma, injuries related to, *220*
Foreign bodies
intraluminal obstruction of small colon with, 100
postmortem photographs of horse with small colon rupture as result of, 100
Foreign body, oral, 38
Fossa glandis (urethral diverticulum), smegma accumulation "beans" in, 461
"Founder rings," formation of, *376*
Fourth metatarsal bone
comminuted fracture and osteomyelitis of, 414
comminuted fracture of, 414
Fractured tooth, 27–31
appearance of tooth 308 following removal of buccal fragment, 30
8-year-old warmblood gelding with sagittal fracture of tooth 308, 29
extraction of, 29
multiple sequestrae fragments removed from tooth 408 alveolus, 31

object visible within alveolus 8 weeks postextraction of fractured tooth 408, 30
sagittal, of tooth 206 in middle-aged quarter horse mare, 28
Fractures
articular, of wing of third phalanx, 367–368
avulsion, of origin of long digital extensor tendon in foal, 644
avulsion, of suspensory ligament, 405
basilar, of medial proximal sesamoid bone, 387
complete, of first phalanx in 3-year-old Standardbred, 374–375
of distal radius, 398
possible cause of, *398*
of dorsoproximal first phalanx, 389
of extensor process of third phalanx, 365–366
of fourth metacarpal bone with evidence of osteomyelitis, 407
of fourth metatarsal bone, 414
incomplete sagittal, of proximal first phalanx, 388
midbody, of medial proximal sesamoid bone, 366
of navicular bone, 361
nonarticular, of wing of third phalanx, 366–367
of palmar process of third phalanx, 369
of patella, 419
of proximal sesamoid bone, 385–387
of radial carpal bone, 396
of ribs, in foals, 645
sagittal, of third phalanx, 366
Salter-Harris type 2, of distal metacarpus, in foal, 642
Salter-Harris type 2, of proximal tibia, in foal, 642
of sphenoid bone and guttural pouch hemorrhage, 441–442
stress, of third metacarpus, 404
of talus, 412–413
of third carpal bone, 398–400
of third metacarpus, 389
tibial stress, 421
Frontal/parietal impact, head trauma and, *214*
Frontal sinuses, *427*
fluid within, *428*
Froth at the mouth, gastric ulcers and, *56*, 57
Fumonisin B1 toxin, Moldy Corn Disease and, *224*
Functional ileus, lateral abdominal radiograph of 9-day-old Standardbred foal with, 626
Functional obstruction of small intestine, 75–77
duodenitis-proximal jejunitis (anterior or proximal enteretis), 75–76
proliferative enteropathy *(Lawsonia intracellularis)*, 76–77
Fundus, normal, from color dilute pony, 554
Fungal endophthalmitis, *543*
Fusarium moniliforme
liquefactive necrosis and degeneration of white matter of right cerebral hemisphere due to, 224
moldy corn infected with, 225
Fusions beats, VPCs and, 160

G

Gastric dilatation
in horse, with small intestinal obstruction, 53
postmortem photograph of stomach rupture in horse secondary to, 54
Gastric emptying, delayed, sonogram of right dorsal abdomen through 15th intercostal space of duodenum in foal presenting with colic related to, 618
Gastric impaction
postmortem photograph of gastric rupture in horse secondary to, 55
postmortem photographs of, 54
Gastric ulcers, 56–59
in foals
dorsal recumbency and, 58
frothing at the mouth and, 57
showing signs of colic, 58
of glandular part of stomach, postmortem photograph of, 56
on margo plicatus in foal, postmortem photograph of, 57
of nonglandular part of stomach
endoscopic image of, 59
postmortem photograph of, 56
Gastrocnemius muscle, ruptured, in foal, 646
Gastroduodenal ulcer syndrome, 617–618
diagnosis of, *617*
rotavirus diarrhea and, *621*
stomach from 7-day-old foal with focal ulceration in squamous and glandular mucosa along margo plicatus, 617
Gastrointestinal colic, causes of, *46*
Gastrosplenic ligament
postmortem photograph of incarceration of small intestine through, 73
postmortem photograph of rent in, through which small intestines have gotten strangulated, 74
GCTs. *See* Granulosa cell tumors
GDUS. *See* Gastroduodenal ulcer syndrome
Geldings, nephrosplenic entrapment of large colon in, *83*
Genital squamous cell carcinoma, preputial habronemiasis distinguished from, *276*
Geriatric wear, 21
Gestation
advanced, fetal gender diagnosed during, 485
late, ventral abdominal rupture in, 488
late, ventral edema in, 488
Gingival ulceration, of systemic origin, 34
Glaucoma, 537–539
clinical diagnosis for, *538*
congenital, 537
ocular trauma *vs.*, 538
primary (idiopathic), 537
secondary, 539
Glomerulonephritis, postmortem photograph of kidney from horse affected with, 563
Glossitis
in adult horse suspected to be secondary to accidental ingestion of irritant chemical agent, 39
severe traumatic, in adult horse, 38
site of trauma (penetrating) leading to, 39
Goiter, 518
neonatal, 659
in newborn foals, 522
GPM. *See* Guttural pouch mycosis
Grain (carbohydrate) overload, 98–99
adult horse with laminitis due to, 99
adult horse with severe diarrhea due to, 98
clinical signs of, *98*
Grand mal seizure, with extensor rigidity and opisthotonos in foal with hypoxic ischemic encephalopathy, 584
Grand Prix-level jumpers, atrial fibrillation and, *155*

Granuloma
neoplasm *vs.*, 554
periocular calcification and, 531
Granulomatous enteritis, *101*
Granulosa cell tumors, 466–467
monocystic, 467
solid, 466
Grass sickness (equine dysautonomia), 109–115
abdominal pain (colic) in horse affected with, 111
adult horse affected with, 109
clinical forms, clinical signs and diagnosis of, *109*
drooling of saliva and dysphagia in horse affected with, 110
large colon impaction found during postmortem examination of horse affected with, 111
narrow base stance and leaning against walls in horse affected with, 114
patchy sweating in horse affected with, 112
penile prolapse and paralysis in horse affected with, 115
piloerection in horse affected with, 112
pstosis in horse affected with, 114
rhinitis sicca in horse affected with, showing mucupurulent material in nasal passages, 113
"tucked up" appearance and weight loss in horse affected by, 110
Greasy heel, 311–313
Gubernaculum, testicular descent and, 447
"Guided" biopsy technique, endometrial biopsy and, *479*
Guttural pouch diseases, 182–185
neurological deficits or hemorrhage related to, *182*
Guttural pouch empyema, 182–184, 438–439
causes of, *182*
endoscopic view of, secondary to streptococcal infection, 182
Guttural pouches, *182*
anatomy and, 438
chondroid located in lateral compartment of, 184
chondroids and fluid (empyema), 439–440
endoscopic examination revealing purulent exudate draining from swollen retropharyngeal node inside medial compartment of, 182
poll impact and bleeding into, *215*
swelling of, symptoms associated with, *184*
Guttural pouch hemorrhage, fracture of sphenoid bone of, 441–442
Guttural pouch mycosis
clinical signs and diagnosis of, *185*
fungal plaque on wall of right guttural pouch in case of, 185
Guttural pouch openings, purulent discharge draining from, 183
Guttural pouch tympany, 184–185
guttural pouch mycosis, 185
lateral radiograph of foal with, 185
marked distension of throat latch region in foal with, 184

H

Habronema muscae, *275*
Habronema spp., *450*
Habronemiasis
causes and diagnosis of, *450*
hemosemen due to, 450
on penis of quarter horse stallion, 450
Haematopinus asini, *291*
Halicephalobus spp.
greatly enlarged left sinus of 10-year-old mare infected with, 569
ultrasonographic image of right kidney of pony mare affected with verminous nephritis caused by, 569
Hard fixative, endometrial biopsy and, *479*
HCM. *See* Hypertrophic cardiomyopathy
Head, 427–443
anatomy and guttural pouches, 438
anatomy of skull, 427–428
dental tumor of mandible, 442–443
ethmoid hematoma, 431–432
fracture of sphenoid bone and guttural pouch hemorrhage, 441–442
guttural pouches empyema, 438–440
mandibular osteomyelitis, 443
normal dental structures, 432–435
normal larynx and aryepiglottic fold entrapment, 440–441
sinus cyst, 429–431
sinusitis, 428–429
tooth root abscess, 436–437
Head-pressing
brain abscessation and, 212
hepatoencephalopathy and, *223*
leukoencephalomalacia (Moldy Corn Disease) and, *224*
verminous meningoencephalomyelitis and, 228
Head tilt, in horse affected by otitis media-interna (temporohyoid osteoarthropathy), 246
Head trauma, 214–222
adult horses affected with
due to poll impact, 215, 216
due to poll impact, showing bloody discharge from ear, 217
due to poll impact, with wide-base stance, 219
showing abnormal wide-base stance, 214
adult horse with recumbency caused by, due to poll impact, 217
cerebrospinal fluid sample from horse affected with, showing presence of frank blood due to acute hemorrhage, 221
cerebrospinal fluid sample from horse affected with, showing xanthochromia characteristic of longer cases of head trauma, 223
close-up view of fracture, 216
cytological examination of cerebrospinal fluid sample from horse affected with, 223
donkey foal affected with, blindness and paralysis due to, 220
in foal, blindness and optic nerve dysfunction due to, 218
permanent dilatation of pupils in foal with, 220
postmortem photograph in foal with, showing severe intracranial hemorrhage, 221
postmortem photograph of eyeball and optic nerve from foal with, 218
postmortem photograph of skull from horse affected by, and fracture of occipital condyles, 219
Heaves
accumulation of mucopurulent respiratory secretions in trachea of horse with, 190
horse flaring its nostrils during attack of, 190
Helminth infection, cutaneous habronemiasis and, 275
Hematomas, estrous cycle and, *462*

Hematuria, *570*
  at end of urination in horse affected with urethral defect, 570
  in horse affected with acute renal failure, 561
  renal or ureteral calculi and, *575*
Hemolysis, severe acute, pigmenturia from foal with, 601
Hemosemen, 449–450
  habronemiasis and, 450
  habronemiasis on penis of quarter horse stallion, 450
  trauma and, 449
  unknown etiology of, *450*
Hemosiderin deposition, progressive ethmoid hematoma and, *178*
Hepatoencephalopathy, 223–224
  adult horses affected with
    as result of diffuse hepatitis, 223
    as result of diffuse hepatitis, showing signs of photodermatitis, 223
    showing icteric sclera, 224
  clinical signs of, *223*
Hernias
  diaphragmatic, 72, 611
  omental, 109
  parietal (Richter's), 108
  scrotal, 457–460
    in foal, 625
  umbilical, 108
Heterotrophic polydontia, 320–321
HIE. *See* Hypoxic ischemic encephalopathy
High ringbone, osteoarthritis of, 363
Hirsutism
  Cushing's syndrome and, *274*
  pituitary pars intermedia dysfunction and, 508, 509, 510, 512, 513
HIS. *See* Hypoxic ischemic syndrome
Histoplasma capsulatum var. *farciminosum*, in ulcerated nodule showing yeast organisms surrounded by clear halos, 339
Histoplasmosis, 338–339
Hock
  excessive flexion of, due to rupture of gastrocnemius muscle, 646
  prematurity and incomplete ossification of cuboidal bones in, 599
Hock joint, stringhalt and hyperflexion of, 240
Holosystolic crescendo decrescendo murmur, *120*
Holter monitor recordings
  of horse receiving reserpine, 151
  uses for, *150*
Hooks or ramps, 9
Horner's syndrome
  adult horses affected with
    droopy left eyelid (ptosis) and, 245
    sweating at base of ear and, 245
  clinical signs of, *245*
Horses, testicular descent in, 447
Hydrocele, right-sided, testicular torsion and, 460–461
Hydrocephalus, as cause of dystocia, 481
Hydrops allantois, 490
Hymen
  intact, bulging through vulvar lips of mare, 464
  persistent, breeding accidents and, *464*
Hyperadrenocorticism (Cushing's syndrome), 274
Hyperechoic linear strands, within fluid indicative of fibrin and septic process, 595
Hyperelastosis cutis (Ehler Danlos syndrome)
  hyperelasticity of skin in horse with, 287
  prolonged skin tent time in horse with, 287
  in 3-year-old cutting horse, showing region of reduced pigmentation, 286–287
Hyperhydrosis, *274*
Hyperkalemic periodic paralysis, 344–345
  clinical signs of and breeds affected by, *344*
  prolapsed third eyelid in horse affected with, 344
  quarter horse affected with, showing sweating and muscle cramping, 344
  respiratory distress and flaring of nostrils in horse affected with, 345
Hyperlipemia and hyperlipidemia, 115–117
  clinical signs of, *115*
  fatty and swollen liver obtained during postmortem examination from pony affected with, 117
  icteric mucous membranes of pony affected with, 116
  milky plasma in pony affected with, 116
  in pony, 115
Hypermature cataract, 541
Hyperparathyroidism, 523–526
  primary, 523–525
  secondary, 525–526
Hypertrophic cardiomyopathy
  M-mode echocardiographic image of left ventricle from horse with, 136
  two-dimensional echocardiographic image showing markedly thickened left ventricular free wall and interventricular septum, 136
Hypodema spp., verminous meningoencephalomyelitis and, *228*
Hyponatremia
  foal with, in opisthotonos with seizure activity characterized by rapid chewing and tongue protruding movements, 626
  nervous signs and differential diagnosis of, *626*
Hypotensive horses, recognizing signs of, *156*
Hypothyroidism, neonatal, 659
Hypoxic ischemic encephalopathy, *581*
  grand mal seizure with extensor rigidity and opisthotonos in foal with, 584
  lack of tone of nasopharyngeal region in foals with, 583
  lavender foal syndrome differentiated from, *659*
  loss of suckle reflex and tongue control with, 582
  nasogastric reflux due to small intestinal ileus in foal with, 584
  tonic muzzle contractions as focal seizure activity with, 583
Hypoxic ischemic syndrome, 581–586
  description, clinical signs and diagnosis of, *581*
  foal recovering from, 581
  loss of affinity for mare in foal with, 581

I

IAD. *See* Inflammatory airway disease
Icteric sclera, hepatoencephalopathy and, 224
Idiopathic eosinophilic enterocolitis, *101*

Idiopathic immune mediated keratouveitis, 546
Idiopathic inflammatory bowel disease
  loose feces associated with, 101
  severe weight loss associated with, 101
Ileal hypertrophy, 60
Ileal impaction, 59
Ileocecal intussusception, 74
Immature cataract, 540
Immune-mediated vasculitis, *326*
Incisors
  curvature of, 11–12
    dorsal, in juvenile, 11
    ventral, in aged horse, 12
  irregular malocclusion of, 12
  permanent, large area of enamel decay and involvement of, 18
  supernumerary, 13
  third, overlong distal portion of, 10
Indolent corneal ulcer, treatment of, *536*
Infections, burn-related, *264*
Infectious polyarthritis (septic arthritis)
  C type (carpal), in foals, *641*
  diagnosis and treatment of, *639*
  E type (epiphyseal), in 4-week-old quarter horse foal, 641
  in foals, 639
  P type (physeal), in older foals, 640
  P type (physeal), in 4-week-old Standardbred foal, 640
  S type (synovial), in 4-week-old Standardbred foal, 639
  T type (tarsal), in 4-week-old quarter horse foal, 641
Infectious pulmonary diseases, 195–203
  aspiration pneumonia, 196
  bacterial pneumonia in adult horse, 195
  interstitial pneumonia in adult horses, 201–203
  pleuropneumonia, 196–201
Inferior brachygnathism (parrot mouth), in foal, 614
Infertility, 469–480
  aneuploidy and intersex, 473
  coital exanthema, 475–476
  endometrial biopsy, 479–480
  fetal death followed by anestrus, 477
  lymphatic lacunae or cyst, 471–472
  periovarian adhesions, 476
  poor vulvar conformation, 474
  pyometra, 470
  routine culture and cytology to investigate infertility, 478
  transitional state, 469
  transluminal adhesions, 471
  vulvar injuries, 475
Inflammatory airway disease, mucupurulent exudates visible by endoscopic examination of trachea of racehorse with, 191
Inhibin, *466*
  granulosa cell tumor, *466*, *467*
Insect bite hypersensitivity, 288–289
  clinical signs and differential diagnoses of, *288*
  mature quarter horse gelding with, 288
  tail head of mature horse with, 288
Insulin resistance, 516–517
  close-up of neck of horse suffering from, 517
  in horse with normal to low condition score, 516
  typical phenotype of horse with, 516
Integumentary system, diseases of, 255–341
  acquired leukotrichia, 257–259
  actinobacillosis, 259–260
  anhydrosis, 336–337
  Arabian fading syndrome, 328
  atheroma, 260–261
  aural plaques, 262–263
  bacterial folliculitis, 263–264
  burns, 264–269
  bursitis and pressure sores, 270–272
  calcinosis circumscripta (tumoral calcinosis), 272–273
  Cushing's syndrome, 274
  cutaneous drug reactions, 334–335
  cutaneous habronemiasis, 275–276
  cutaneous lymphosarcoma, 277–278
  dermatophilosis (rain scald), 279–281
  dermatophytosis (ringworm), 281–284
  dermoid cyst, 284–285
  epizootic lymphangitis (histoplasmosis), 338–339
  food hypersensitivity, 335
  hyperelastosis cutis (Ehler Danlos syndrome), 286–287
  insect bite hypersensitivity, 288–289
  junctional epidermolysis bullosa, 339–341
  lethal white syndrome, 289–290
  lice (pediculosis), 291–292
  melanoma, 293–294
  nodular necrobiosis (eosinophilic collagen necrosis), 294–295
  onchocerciasis, 295–296
  pemphigus, 297–301
  phaeohyphomycosis, 323
  photosensitization, 301–303
  sarcoidosis, 306–307
  sarcoids, 304–306
  scalding (urine, serum, chemical), 307–311
  scratches (greasy heel, pastern dermatitis), 311–313
  sporotrichosis, 313–315
  squamous cell carcinoma, 316–317
  stud crud (idiopathic cannon keratosis), 318
  sunburn, 318
  telogen defluxion, 319–320
  temporal teratoma, 320–322
  tick infestation, 324–325
  urticaria, 325–326
  vasculitis (immune-mediated or photoactive), 326–327
  vitiligo, 329
  warts (papillomatosis), 330–332
  winter atopy, 333
Interdental spaces, bilateral soft tissue damage to, in young quarter horse, 32
Intermittent dorsal displacement of the soft palate, *186*
Intersex
  aneuploidy and, 473
  description of condition, *473*
Interstitial pneumonia
  in adult horses, 201–203
    causes, clinical signs, and diagnosis of, *201*
    lateral thoracic radiograph of horse with, 202
    postmortem photograph of lung with, 202, 203
    showing signs of, 201
  sonogram of thorax showing "sheets" of comet tail artifacts seen with, *607*

Intestinal aganglionosis (lethal white syndrome)
description of, *625*
foal with, 625
Intestinal atresia
clinical signs and diagnosis of, *624*
type 3, of large colon, 624
Intestinal obstruction, caused by *Pascaris equorum*, diagnosis of, 620
Intra-abdominal hemorrhage, 493
Intralesional bacilli Calmette-Guerin, sarcoid treatment and, *553*
Intrascleral prosthesis, 551
Intrathoracic airways, diseases of, 190–203
African horse sickness, 208–209
aspiration pneumonia, 196
bacterial pneumonia in adult horses, 195
exercise-induced pulmonary hemorrhage, 192–195
infectious pulmonary diseases, 195–203
inflammatory airway disease, 191
interstitial pneumonia in adult horses, 201–203
noninfectious pulmonary diseases, 190–195
pleuropneumonia, 196–201
pneumothorax, 203–204
recurrent airway obstruction (RAO, heaves), 190–191
strangles, 204–207
thoracic wall and pleural diseases, 203–204
Intravitreous hemorrhage, uveitis and, 545
Intussusception, 619
jejunojenunal, postmortem specimen of, in foal, 619
large intestinal, 87
small intestinal, 74
target lesion seen on ultrasonography diagnostic for, 75
ultrasonographic image of, in foal revealing classic "bull's-eye" appearance, 619
Iridal cysts, behavioral anomalies related to, *549*
Iridal prolapse
treatment of, *548*
yellow-tan colored fibrin within anterior chamber of eye of young filly, 548
Irregular incisor malocclusion, 12
Ivermectin
deworming with, and avoidance of cutaneous habronemiasis, 276
habronemiasis treatment and, *450*

J

Jaundice, marked, throughout body due to neonatal isoerythrolysis, 602
JEB. *See* Junctional epidermolysis bullosa
Jejunojejunal intussusception, signs of, *619*
Jennys (or "jennets"), gestations of, 487
Jet lesion, 142
Joints, neonatal diseases in, 630–645
Joint sepsis, severe osteoarthritis of carpometacarpal joint and, *394*
Jugular vein
postsurgical removal, 163
sonogram of septic thrombophlebitis of, 161
Jugular vein thrombophlebitis
postoperative appearance of horse previously affected with, 164
surgical removal and, *163*
Jumpers, decubital ulcer formation prevention in, *627*
Junctional epidermolysis bullosa, 339–341
blistering of gums and mucocutaneous junction of mouth, 339
blistering of perineal area, 340
characteristics of, *339*
pressure sores developing over bony protruberances, 341
sloughing of hoof, or "red foot," 340

K

Keratitis
chronic uveitis and, 548
in horse affected by otitis media-interna (temporohyoid osteoarthropathy), 247
Keratomas
description of, *370*
lateral and dorsoproximal-palmarodistal oblique radiographic projections of right hind foot of 10-year-old Appaloosa, 370
Keratomycosis
clinical manifestations and diagnosis of, *533*
large, 533
Keratopathy, aged mare with band keratopathy, 532
Keratouveitis
idiopathic immune-mediated, 546
severe, *Rhodococcus equi* infection and, 608
Kicking at the abdomen, colic and, 46, 49–50
Kicking injuries, 453–455
breeding, hydrotherapy and, *453*
by other horses
comminuted fractures of fourth metatarsal bone and, 414
sequestration of calcaneus and, 413
penile injury and hematoma, in 3-year-old Appaloosa stallion, 454
plexus damage during mounting, 454
suspensory choices for penile injuries, 455
Kidneys
of horse affected with acute renal failure, 562
with multiple cysts from horse affected with chronic renal failure, 566
sagittal section, from horse affected with glomerulonephritis, 563
ultrasonographic image of, in horse with chronic renal failure, 567
Knuckling, equine protozoal myeloencephalitis and, *234*

L

Laceration, of oral mucosa caused by sharp enamel point on distal aspect of 211 as it occludes with 311, 33
Lameness, fracture chip of dorsoproximal first phalanx and, *389*
Laminar thickening, laminitis with rotation and laminar separation and, *375*
Laminitis
chronic
in left forefoot of 12-year-old pony, 376
in 10-year-old pony, 377
grain (carbohydrate) overload and, in adult horse, 99
insulin resistance and, 516
pituitary pars intermedia dysfunction and, 508, 511
with rotation, 375
with rotation and laminar separation, 376

Large colon displacement, 82–85
left and right, *82*
Large colon impaction, 86–87
long-standing, adult horse who has developed colitis and diarrhea with, 86
postmortem photograph of horse with, 86, 87
risk factors with, *86*
Large colon volvulus, 78–82
cross and sagittal section diagram of location of left large colon in normal horses and horses with degrees of, 79
horse with abdominal distension due to, 78
postmortem photograph of, in horse showing site of rotation between strangulated and nonstrangulated parts of large colon, 79
postmortem photograph of, in horse with severely thickened large colon, 79
postmortem photograph of horse with, 78
ultrasonographic image of left ventral abdomen in horse with, showing thickened large colon in cases of, 82
ultrasonographic images of abdomen in normal horse, 80
ultrasonographic images of left ventral abdomen in horse with 540° of, 81
ultrasonography and diagnosis of, landmarks for ventral colon, 80
Large intestinal intussusception, ultrasonographic image of right paralumbar fossa showing classic target lesion (bull's eye) of, 87
Large intestines, diseases of, 78–99
grain (carbohydrate) overload, 98–99
large colon displacement, 82–85
large colon impaction, 86–87
large colon volvulus, 78–82
nonsteroidal anti-inflammatory drugs toxicity, 95–98
salmonellosis, 88–91
strongylosis, 92–95
Laryngeal diseases, 187–188
arytenoid chondropathy, 188
epiglottic entrapment, 187
laryngeal hemiplegia, 188
subepiglottic cyst, 187
Laryngeal hemiplegia
cause and treatment of, *188*
left, in horse with complaint of exercise intolerance, 188
Larynx, normal, 440
Lateral plantar process of first phalanx, osseous fragmentation of, 390
Lateral styloid process, ossification of, *632*
Lavender foal syndrome
foal affected with, showing characteristic lavender coat color, 659
neurological signs and diagnosis of, *659*
LCD. *See* Large colon displacement
LCI. *See* Large colon impaction
LCV. *See* Large colon volvulus
LDLC. *See* Left dorsal displacement of large colon
Lead poisoning, 243–244
acute, tongue paralysis and dysphagia in horse affected with, 243
clinical sign, diagnosis, and treatment of, *243*
horse with, following oral ingestion of lead solders, 243
lead pellets found in stomach of horse with acute cerebral dysfunction, 244
Left dorsal displacement of large colon, 83–85
cross-section diagrams of abdomen of horse with
advanced stage of, 84
early stage of, 83
and its treatment by rolling, 84–85
Left large colon displacement, 82
Leiomyosarcoma, 467
Lens, subluxated, 542
Lens rupture
acute corneal and anterior lens capsule perforations in Thoroughbred gelding, 542
inflamed eye of adult Percheron mare with penetrating corneal injury one month previous to presentation, 543
treatment of, *543*
Lethal white syndrome, 289–290
autosomal recessive condition resulting from breeding two overo-paint horses, 289
foal with, 625
gastrointestinal tract of white foal, 290
postmortem photograph of 4-day-old foal presenting for colic with, 290
Leucocoria, white, mature cataract and, 540
Leukoencephalomalacia (Moldy Corn Disease), 224–225
clinical signs and therapy for, *224*
postmortem examination of brain in horse affected with, 224
Leydig cells
cryptorchidism and, *448*
disruption of spermatogenesis due to cryptorchidism and, *449*
tumors of, 451
Lice (pediculosis), 291–292
causes and diagnosis of, *291*
diagnosis by identification of eggs attached to hair shafts, 292
Ligament injuries, in foals, 646–649
Lighting program, transitional mares and, *469*
Limb edema, in horse affected with purpura hemorrhagica, 169
Lingual laceration or ulceration
chronic, due to sharp enamel points on lingual aspects of mandibular cheek teeth, 33
of systemic origin, 34
in 13-year-old Thoroughbred gelding, 31
Lipoma, 64, 66
with long stalk, strangling loop(s) of small intestines, 65, 68
serving as point where intestines rotated, 68
Live mount, semen collection and, *453*
Lockjaw. *See* Tetanus (lockjaw)
"Lollipop" lesions, *358*
Long digital extensor tendon, avulsion fracture of origin of, in foal, 644
Long-stalk lipoma, 65, 68
Long umbilical cord, as cause of abortion, 502–503
Longus muscles, poll impact and damage to, *215*
Luminal epithelium, 480
Lymphatic lacunae or cyst (endometrial cysts), 471–472
appearance of, 471
large, 472
mapping, pathogenesis and treatment of, *471*
recognition of pregnancy affected by, 472
Lymph nodes, retropharyngeal, enlarged in horse with strangles, 183

Lymphocytic-plasmocytic enterocolitis, *101*
Lymphosarcoma, 452

M

Male fetus, transrectal scan of, 485
Male pseudohemaphrodites, *473*
Male reproductive system diseases. *See* Reproductive system diseases, male
Malevolent lesions, sarcoids and, *304*
mal seco, *109*
Mammary gland
- enlargement of, prior to abortion, 501
- impending foaling and filling of, *486*

Mandible, dental tumor of, 442–443
Mandibular dental structures
- normal, in an immature horse, 435
- normal, in mature horse, 435

Mandibular incisors, severe atypical wear of, 37
Mandibular osteomyelitis, 443
Mandibular prognathism, foal with, 660
Manic behavior, leukoencephalomalacia (Moldy Corn Disease) and, *224*
Mare immunopregnancy test, *477*
Mares
- maceration of advanced age fetus in, 500
- poor vulvar conformation in, 474
- pyometra in, 470
- retained placenta in, 504
- routine monitoring of early pregnancy and, 463
- transitional, *469*

Masseter muscle atrophy, in 2-year-old quarter horse stallion, 346
Masturbation, hemosemen and, 449
Mature cataract, 540–541
Maxilla, deviation of, 26
Maxillary dental structures, normal, in aged horse, 432
Maxillary sinuses, anatomy of, 428
Meckel's diverticulum, 61
Meconium
- balls of, ultrasonographic image of, surrounded by mineral oil in large colon, 623
- foal passing, 622
- foal straining to pass, showing arched back and tail position, 622
- impaction, 622–623
- retention and diagnosis of, *622*
- ultrasonographic image of, highlighting "speckled" appearance of, 623

Megaesophagus
- esophageal distension near thoracic inlet in foal with, 615
- postmortem photograph of, in foal secondary to esophageal obstruction, 44
- postmortem specimen of esophagus from foal, 615

Melanoma, 293–294
- in Arab mare, 468
- older grey horses with, 293
- other regions of, in old grey mare, 294
- in parotid region of aged grey mare, 293
- perianal, 293

Melting corneal ulcer, 532
Membranous ventricular septal defect, murmurs associated with, *120*
Meningitis
- causes of, *253*
- cloudy, xanthochromic, cerebrospinal fluid collected from lumbosacral space of septicemic foal with, 593
- recumbent adult horse affected with, 253

Mesenteric tear, as cause of dystocia, 483
Mesenteric torsion, 62
- partial, postmortem photograph of, in adult horse, 62–63
- peritoneal fluid from horse affected with, 63

Mesodiverticular band, small loop of small intestine strangulated by, 61
Mesorchium, testicular torsion and, *460*
Metacarpal periostitis, nuclear scintigraphic image and dorsolateral-palmaromedial oblique radiographic projection of left metacarpal region of 2-year-old Standardbred, 403
Metacarpophalangeal and metatarsophalangeal joints (fetlock joint), 378–391
- chronic proliferative synovitis of, 381–382
- fracture (chip) of dorsoproximal first phalanx, 389
- fracture of proximal first phalanx, 388
- fracture of proximal sesamoid bone, 385–387
- fracture of third metacarpus, 389
- mild osteoarthritis of, 379–380
- moderate osteoarthritis of, 379
- osseous fragment arising from plantar margin of first phalanx, 391
- osseous fragmentation of lateral plantar process of first phalanx, 390
- osteoarthritis of, 378–382
- osteochondritis dissecans and, 382
- septic arthritis and osteomyelitis of, 384
- sesamoiditis and, 383
- severe osteoarthritis of, 380–381

Metatarsophalangeal joint, normal, in foal, 630
Methylprednisolone, nodular necrobiosis (eosinophilic collagen necrosis) treatment with, *295*
Microsporum equinum, dermatophytosis (ringworm) and, *281*
Midbody sesamoid fractures, prognosis for, *386*
Middle carple joint, moderate osteoarthritis of, 393
Midsagittal fracture of third phalanx (type 3 fracture), *368*
Milk electrolyte assays, scoring, impending foaling and, *486*
Miller, M. A., pituitary pars intermedia dysfunction and grading system developed by, 515
Miniature horses
- congenital patellar luxation in foals, *643*
- tracheal collapse in, *189*

Miosis, with granuloma and periocular calcification, 531
MIP test. *See* Mare immunopregnancy test
Mitral regurgitation
- atrial fibrillation secondary to, 142
- mitral valve insufficiency and, 139

Mitral valve insufficiency, 139–142
- color flow Doppler image from right parasternal long axis view showing small eccentric jet of mitral regurgitation, 139
- severe, color flow Doppler image from right parasternal long axis view showing large jet of mitral regurgitation, 139

Mitral valve regurgitation, jet lesion, postmortem image of localized areas of subendocardial fibrosis in left atrium secondary to jet of, 142

Mixed sarcoid lesions, *304*
Moldy corn, *Fusarium moniliforme* infection of, 225
Moldy Corn Disease, 224–225
Monkey mouth (underbite), 15
Monocystic granulosa cell tumor, 467
Mount mare, semen collection and, *453*
Mouth, diseases of, 37–39
glossitis, 38–39
oral foreign body, 38
squamous cell carcinoma, 37
Mullerian system, remnants of, breeding accidents and, *464*
Multifocal vasculitis, *326*
Multisystemic eosinophilic epitheliotropic disease, *101*
Mummification, fetal death followed by, 500
Murmurs, with aortic valve insufficiency, *145*
Muscle atrophy
masseter muscle, in 2-year-old quarter horse stallion, 346
Streptococcus equi infection-associated myopathies and, 345
Muscle injuries, in foals, 646–649
Muscles, diseases of, 343–350
hyperkalemic periodic paralysis, 344–345
muscle atrophy (masseter muscle), 346
myopathies associated with *Streptococcus equi* infection, 345
polysaccharide storage myopathy, 347–349
recurrent exertional rhabdomyolysis, 350
sporadic exertional rhabdomyolysis, 346
Muscle wasting, Cushing's syndrome and, *274*
Muscular ventricular septal defect, *120*, 121
Muzzle papillomas, 330
Myocardial diseases, 134–138
cardiomyopathy, 134–136
cor pulmonale, 138
myocarditis, 137–138
Myocarditis, 137–138
in adult horse, postmortem photograph of heart with ventricular dysrhythmia, 137
Holter recording from horse with, 138
signs of, *138*
Myocardium, rib fracture and fatal puncture of, 645
Myopathies, *Streptococcus equi* infection-associated, 345

N

Nasal cavity, fluid opacity throughout, 429
Nasal discharge, with primary choke, 40
Nasogastric tube, passing, 53
Nasopharyngeal region, hypoxic ichemic encephalopathy and lack of tone in, 583
Natural breeding, vaginal examination and, 464
Natural service, for semen collection, *453*
Navicular bone, 356–362
cysts of
description of, *358*
enlarged and abnormally shaped synovial invaginations, and enthesopathy, 358–359
degenerative change in, 360–361, *361*
dorsoproximal-palmarodistal oblique radiographic projections of, for two horses, 356, 358
fracture of, 361
lateral and solar views from bone phase of scintigraphic study of 7-year-old quarter horse, 362
normal radiographic appearance of, 356–357, *357*, 360
palmaroproximal-palmarodistal oblique radiographic projections of, in two horses, 357
Navicular degeneration, evidence of, 358
NCC. *See* Noncoronary cusp
Necrotizing enterocolitis
hemorrhagic diarrhea due to, 585
postmortem specimen from foal with, *585*
sonogram of foal's abdomen showing small intestinal loops with pneumatosis intestinalis in conjunction with, 586
Neonatal hypothyroidism, 522
Neonatal hypothyroidism and goiter, 659
clinical signs and diagnosis of, *659*
Neonatal isoerythrolysis, 600–602
clinical signs, diagnosis, and treatment of, *600*
foal with characteristic pale jaundiced mucous membranes due to, 600
jaundiced sclera in foal with, 601
marked jaundice throughout body and, 602
pigmenturia from foal with severe acute hemolysis, 601
Neonatal maladjustment syndrome, *581*
Neonates, diseases of, 579–660
alimentary system, 613–626
alloimmune thrombocytopenia, 658
congenital hypothyroidism and dysmaturity syndrome, 660
hypoxic ischemic syndrome, 581–586
integument system, 656–658
lavender foal syndrome, 659
musculoskeletal system, 630–649
neonatal hypothyroidism and goiter, 659
neonatal isoerythrolysis, 600–602
nervous system, 626–627
ocular system, 628–629
prematurity, 596–600
respiratory system, 602–612
sepsis, 587–595
urinary system, 650–655
Neoplasia, 132–133, 451–452
granulosa cell tumors, 466–468
leiomyosarcoma, 467
lymphosarcoma, 452
melanoma, 468
monocystic granulosa cell tumors, 467
precancerous lesions, 451
seminoma, 451
squamous cell carcinoma, 468
squamous cell carcinoma on penis of horse, 452
Neoplasm, granuloma *vs.*, 554
Nephrolithiasis, 571
postmortem photograph of renal calculus in horse with, 575
weight loss in horse with, 576
Nephroliths, *575*
Nephrosplenic entrapment of large colon, *83*
Nervous system, diseases of, 211–253
brain abscess, 212–214
cholesterol granuloma (cholesteatomas), 244
equine herpes virus myeloencephalitis, 229–233
equine motor neuron disease, 237–239
equine protozoal myeloencephalitis, 234–235
equine wobbler syndrome, 236–237
facial nerve trauma, 252
head trauma, 214–222

hepatoencephalopathy, 223–224
Horner's syndrome, 245
lead poisoning, 243–244
leukoencephalomalacia (Moldy Corn Disease), 224–225
meningitis, 253
otitis media-interna (temporohyoid osteoarthropathy), 246–251
rabies, 239
radial nerve paralysis, 251
stringhalt, 240
tetanus (lockjaw), 240–242
verminous meningoencephalomyelitis, 228–229
West Nile Virus, 225–227
Neurological deficits, guttural pouch diseases and, *182*
NI. *See* Neonatal isoerythrolysis
Nitrate concentrations in diet, congenital hypothyroidism and dysmaturity syndrome due to, *660*
Nodular lesions, sarcoids and, *304*
Nodular necrobiosis (eosinophilic collagen necrosis), 294–295
low-grade discomfort to horse "under-saddle," 295
slight melanotrichosis in chestnut horse, 294
Nonarticular fracture of wing of third phalanx, 366–367
Noncoronary cusp, echocardiographic image of ventricular septal defect and, 122
Nonepitheliotropic lymphosarcoma, clinical signs of, *277*
Nongastrointestinal colic, causes of, 46
Noninfectious pulmonary diseases, 190–195
exercise-induced pulmonary hemorrhage, 192–195
inflammatory airway disease, 191
recurrent airway obstruction (RAO, heaves), 190–191
Nonsteroidal anti-inflammatory drugs toxicity, 95–98
adult horse with oral ulcers affected by, 96
adult horse with weight loss and ventral edema caused by, 95
brisket edema in adult horse with, 97
clinical signs and diagnosis of, *95*
postmortem examination of adult horse with severe necrotic right dorsal colon affected by, 96
prepuptial edema in horse with, 97
ultrasonographic image showing thickened wall of right dorsal colon in adult horse affected with, 98
NSAID toxicity. *See* Nonsteroidal anti-inflammatory drugs toxicity
NSELC. *See* Nephrosplenic entrapment of large colon
Nutritional hyperparathyroidism, 525
Nutritional secondary hyperparathyroidism
postmortem photograph of one side of mandible from horse with, 526
sagittal section of long bone from horse with, 526

O

Occipital condyles, poll impact and fracture of, 219
Occipital cortex dysfunction, poll impact and, *215*
Occult lesions, sarcoids and, *304*
OCD. *See* Osteochondritis dissecans
Ocular trauma, blunt, corneal laceration and, 531
Omental hernia, in foal, 109
Omphalophlebitis, with urachal abscessation in septicemic foal, 594
Onchocerca cervicalis, 295
Onchocerciasis, 295–296
lesions associated with, 295
patchy alopecia, crusting, and depigmentation of ventral midline, 296
Optic nerve degeneration, secondary to previous head trauma that induced optic nerve damage and blindness, 555
Optic nerve dysfunction
in foal, resulting from frontal/parietal impact, 220
head trauma and, *218*
Oral foreign body, 38
Oral ulcers, chronic renal failure and, 564
Orbital neoplasms, prognosis for, *553*
Ossification
of accessory cartilages of third phalanx (sidebone), 371
of accessory cartilages of third phalanx (sidebone), causes of, *371*
grade 1, of carpal bones in foal, 633
grade 2, of carpal bones in foal, 634, 636
incomplete, of cuboidal bones due to congenital hypothyroidism and dysmaturity syndrome, 660
Osteoarthritis, 392–394, 410–412
of distal interphalangeal joint, 364–365
of left distal interphalangeal joint of 10-year-old Thoroughbred, 365
mild
of distal intertarsal and tarsometatarsal joint, 410
of metacarpophalangeal joint in 4-year-old Standardbred, 378–379
mild, of antebrachiocarpal joint, 392
moderate
of distal intertarsal joint, 410
of metacarpophalangeal joint, of 6-year-old Standardbred, 379
of middle carpal joint, 393
of proximal interphalangeal joint (high ringbone) in 13-year-old Appaloosa, 363
severe
of carpometacarpal joint, 394
of distal intertarsal joint, 411
of metacarpophalangeal joint of 2-year-old Standardbred, 380–381
of proximal intertarsal joiont, distal intertarsal joint, and tarsometatarsal joint, 411
of stifle joint, 417
chronic cranial cruciate ligament injury and, 418
Osteochondritis dissecans, 407–409
bilateral, of lateral trochlear ridge, lateral radiographic projections of left and right stifles of 1.5-year-old Standardbred, 416–417
of distal intermediate ridge of tibia, 407
of lateral trochlear ridge of talus, 408
of medial malleolus of tibia, dorsolateral-plantaromedial oblique projection, 409
of medial malleolus of tibia, dorsoplantar radiographic projection, 408
of medial trochlear ridge of talus, 409
of median sagittal ridge of third metatarsal bone, 382
Osteochondrosis, *391*
lesions, *401*
subchondral bone cysts and, *372*
Osteodystrophia fibrosa, 525
Osteoma, *181*

Osteomyelitis
of fourth metatarsal bone, 414
fracture of fourth metacarpal bone with evidence of, 407
hematogenous spread of bacterial infection as cause of, *426*
mandibular, 443
septic arthritis and, in foals, 639
of third cervical vertebra, 426–427
of third phalanx
causes of, *369*
in 9-year-old Hunter, 369
Osteophytes, *378*, *379*
moderate osteoarthritis of middle carple joint and formation of, 393
Otitis media-interna (temporohyoid osteoarthropathy), 246–251
clinical signs and diagnosis of, *246*
computed tomography in horse affected with, 250
endoscopic view of guttural pouch in horse affected by, showing thickened stylohyoid bone, 248
head tilt in horse affected with, 246
keratitis and severe endophthalmis in horse affected with, 247
postmortem examination of stylohyoid bones in horse affected with, 250–251
ptosis in horse affected with, 247
transtympanic lavage in horse affected with, 249
unilateral facial paralysis in horse affected with, 246
ventrodorsal skull radiograph of horse affected with, 248
Ovarian suppression, granulosa cell tumors and, *466*
Ovary, transitional, from a mare, 469
Overbite (parrot mouth), 13–14
Overlong tooth 109, in 4-year-old horse, 27
Overlong tooth 309, due to fractured tooth 209, 28
Overo-overo mating, intestinal aganglionosis (lethal white syndrome) and, *625*
Over-paint horses, lethal white syndrome resulting from breeding of, 289
Ovulating follicle, 462

P

PA. *See* Pulmonary artery
"Paint-brush" tufts, dermatophilosis (rain scald) and, *280*
Pampiniform plexus, systemic body temperature increases, disruption of spermatogenesis due to cryptorchidism and, *449*
Pancreas, normal boundaries of epiploic foramen and, 71
Pansystolic band shaped murmur, phonocardiogram from horse with, 120
Papillomas (wart), photomicrograph of papilloma showing squamous epithelium, stratum corneum, and connective tissue stalk, 332
Paralytic rabies, *239*
Paramastoid processes, poll impact and fracture of, 219
Paranasal sinuses, *427*
fluid opacity throughout, 429
Parascaris equorum
impaction with, 60
intestinal rupture due to ileal obstruction with, 620
Parietal (Richter's) hernia, enterocutaneous fistula in horse as sequela to, 108
Parietal vaginal tunic, scrotal hernia and, 458
Paroxysmal ventricular tachycardia, 160
Parrot mouth (overbite), 13–14, 614
large amount of excessive crown at mesial portion of 106 in 10-year-old quarter horse stallion, 7
rostral hook and, 6
Pastern dermatitis, 311–313
Patella
chronic fracture of, 419
lateral luxation of, in 4-week-old Standardbred foal, 643
Patellar luxation, congenital, in miniature horse foals, *643*
Patent urachus, in debilitated recumbent neonates, 652
Pawing, colic and, 46, 48
PE. *See* Pericardial effusion
Pedunculated lipoma
intraoperative photograph of small intestinal strangulation caused by, 65
postmortem photographs of, 64–65
Pemphigus, 297–301
types and signs of, *297*
Pemphigus foliaceus, *297*
alopecia on inside of proximal hind limb and inguinal region in horse with, 298
characteristic round acantholytic cells on histological section, 301
close-up of flank region in horse with, 297
early, transient blister formation with, 300
face lesions with, *299*
hind limb lesions with, 300
histological section showing separation of epidermis, 301
horse of unknown age with alopecia and oozing due to, 297
in horse with lesions on face, coronary bands, and ventrum, 299
left upper forelimb of quarter horse with alopecia, crusting, and secondary excoriation, 298
Penile prolapse, grass sickness and, 115
Penis
kicking injuries to, 453, 454
paralysis and amputation of, 456
squamous cell carcinomas on, 451
suspensory choices for injuries to, 455
Perforated corneal ulcer, with iridal prolapse, 534
Pergolide administration, pituitary pars intermedia dysfunction treatment and, 513
Pericardial catheter, placement of, 131
Pericardial diseases, 129–133
neoplasia, 132–133
pericarditis, 129–132
Pericardial effusion, 129
cardiac tamponade with, 129
electrocardiograms obtained prior to and immediately after drainage of large amount of, 130
large, ultrasonographic image of ascites and pleural effusion in pony with, 132
M-mode echocardiographic image demonstrating small amount of, 130
Pericardial mesothelioma
clinical signs of, *132*
echocardiographic images of
right parasternal long axis, 132
right parasternal short axis view of ventricles, 133
postmortem examination showing parietal pleura, parietal pericardium and mediastinum covered with coalescing cobblestone nodules, 133
Pericardiocentesis, *131*

Pericarditis, 129–132
  constrictive, postmortem photograph from 3-year-old colt with, showing thickened pericardium peeled back off epicardium, 131
  fibrinoeffusive, two-dimensional echocardiographic image from horse with large pericardial effusion and fibrin on epicardial surface, 129
  physical examination findings and diagnosis of, *129*
Perineal tears and lacerations
  surgical repair of, 495
  third-degree, 494
Periocular calcification, granuloma and, 531
Periocular papillomatosis, 330
Periodontal disease
  chronic incisor, with cemental hypoplasia, 19
  feed trapped at lingual aspect of interproximal space, 17
  in 2-year-old Thoroughbred, 15
Periodontal pocket, 16
  packed feed visible in both views, lingual and buccal aspects, 17
Periostitis
  at origin of suspensory ligament, 406
  stress fractures and, *404*
Periovarian adhesions, 476
Peripapillary butterfly lesion, 556
Peripartum asphyxia syndrome, *581*
Peritoneal fluid, from horse affected with mesenteric torsion, 63
Peritonitis, 105–107
  adult horse affected with, 105
  causes and clinical signs of, *105*
  diffuse, microscopic examination of smear made from peritoneal fluid of horse with, secondary to intestinal rupture, 106
  ultrasonographic image of abdomen in horse affected with, showing cellular fluid and fibrin tag, 107
  ultrasonographic image of abdomen in horse affected with, showing thickened small intestine, surrounded by cellular fluid, 107
Persistent dorsal displacement of the soft palate, *186*
Peruvian Paso mare, with supernumerary and displaced incisors, 13
Petechiae
  alloimmune thrombocytopenia in foal with, 658
  in ear of septicemic foal, 591
  in nasal mucosa of horse affected with purpura hemorrhagica, 170
Petrous temporal bone, hemorrhage into inner/middle ear from fractures of, *217*
Phacoclastic uveitis, clinical diagnosis and prognosis for, *543*
Phaeohyphomycosis
  causes, clinical signs, diagnosis, and treatment of, *323*
  nodular granulomatous dermatitis in horse with, 323
  photomicrograph of, showing pigment-producing yeast organisms, 323
Phalanges, 363–378
  articular fracture of wing of third phalanx, 367–368
  assessment of third phalanx rotation, 377–378
  chronic laminitis, 376–377
  complete fracture of first phalanx, 374–375
  fracture of extensor of third phalanx, 365–366
  fracture of palmar process of third phalanx, 369
  keratoma, 370
  laminitis with rotation and laminar separation, 375–376
  nonarticular fracture of wing of third phalanx, 366–367
  ossification of accessory cartilages of third phalanx, 371
  osteoarthritis of distal interphalangeal joint, 364–365
  osteoarthritis of proximal interphalangeal joint, 363
  osteomyelitis of third phalanx, 369
  sagittal fracture of third phalanx, 368
  subchondral cystic lesions of, 373–374
    distomedial first phalanx, 372
    proximomedial second phalanx, 373
Phallectomy, 452
Phantom mare, semen collection and, 453
Pharangeal region, lateral radiographic projections of, 440
Pharyngeal anatomy, normal, and guttural pouches, 438
Pharyngeal compression, fluid within guttural pouches and, 438
Pharyngeal diseases
  dorsal displacement of the soft palate, 186
  pharyngitis, 186
Pharyngitis, grade 4/4 pharyngeal lymphoid hyperplasia in 2-year-old racehorse, 186
Phenothiazine tranquilizers, penile paralysis and, *456*
Pheochromocytoma, postmortem photograph of, in adrenal medulla of horse, 527
Phialophora, phaeohyphomycosis and, *323*
Photoactive dermatitis, 327
Photodermatitis, hepatoencephalopathy and, 223
Photosensitization, 301–303
  classification of, *301*
  head of mature quarter horse exhibiting signs of, 302
  lateral and medial aspects of left front leg in horse with, 303
Phthisis bulbi, choroid detachment and, *549*
Physeal closure, normal metatarsophalangeal joint and, *630*
Physeal dysplasia (physitis)
  of distal physis of radius in foal, 633
  of distal physis of third metacarpus and proximal physis of proximal phalanx in foal, 632
Physitis, causes of, *632*
Pinky syndrome (Arabian fading syndrome), 328
Pituitary pars intermedia dysfunction, 508–515
  beginning of classical clinical signs in, *509*
  bulging of supraorbital fossa in horse with, 511
  grading system by M. Miller et al. for, 515
  hirsutism and, 508, 509, 510, 512, 513
  horse with, responding to oral pergolide therapy, 513
  inappropriate lactation in horse with, 512
  lack of muscle tone and poor top line conformation characteristic of, 510
  pituitary gland, cut lengthwise showing thickening of pars intermedia, 514
  pituitary gland cut lengthwise, 515
  pony with classic clinical signs of, 508
  pony with cresty neck and, 509
  postmortem photograph of brain and extremely enlarged pituitary gland in horse with, 513
  postmortem photograph of enlarged pituitary gland in situ on bottom of cranial vault, 514
  severe chronic laminitis in pony with, 511
Placenta, retained, 504
Placental insufficiency, prematurity and, *596*
Placental separation, premature, and prolapse of bladder, 486

Placentation, variations in twin pregnancies, *499*
Placentitis, prematurity and, *596*
Pleura, diseases of, 203–204
Pleural fluid, drainage from indwelling chest tube, 199
Pleuropneumonia
acute
intercostal transverse ultrasonographic image of ventral midthorax of racehorse with, 197
lateral radiograph of cranioventral thorax of racehorse with, 197
racehorse with, after long-distance transportation, 196
gross examination of chest cavity in horse with, 201
lateral thoracic radiograph of horse with, 198
photomicrograph of pleural fluid showing degenerate white blood cells and mixed bacteria in racehorse with, 198
risk factors, diagnosis and treatment of, *196*
severe pyogranulomatous pleuritis and pyothorax in horse with, 200
severe pyrogranulomatous pericarditis in horse with, 200
Pneumonia
acute, lateral radiographic projection of thoracic activity in 9-day-old Standardbred, 603
chronic, lateral radiographic projection of caudodorsal lung fields in 7-month-old Standardbred, 604
clinical signs, diagnosis and treatment of, *612*
foal recovering from HIS and, in sternal support with intranasal oxygen insufflation, 612
foal with nostril flaring due to, 612
interstitial, sonogram of thorax showing "sheets" of comet tail artifacts seen with, *607*
Pneumothorax
Heimlich valve attached to indwelling chest tube to allow drainage of pleural fluid while preventing development of, 199
lateral thoracic radiograph of horse with, secondary to pneumonia, 203
pleural exudate draining from chest of horse injured in trailer accident resulting in pleuritis and, 204
Polanski speculum, failure to demonstrate cervical tears and, *476*
Poll impact
adult horse affected with, showing wide-base stance, 219
adult horse with head trauma due to, showing head tilt and facial asymmetry, 216
adult horse with recumbency caused by head trauma due to, 217
adult horse with recumbency caused by head trauma due to, showing bloody discharge from ear, 217
head trauma and, *214*, 215, 216, 217
types of muscular and cranial nerve damage due to, *215*
Polydontia, 5-year-old draft mare with, 35
Polyps, sinonasal, 181
Polysaccharide storage myopathy, 347–349
adult horse affected with, 347
breeds affected by and diagnosis of, *347*
periodic acid-Schiff stained slides for glycogen of muscles from normal horse and horse affected with, 349
semitendinosus/semimembranous muscle biopsy obtained from horse affected with, 347–348
Porphyria, *301*
Portal vein, normal boundaries of epiploic foramen and, 71
PPID. *See* Pituitary pars intermedia dysfunction
Precancerous lesions, 451
Pregnancy
early, routine monitoring of, 463
endometrial cyst affecting recognition of, 472
Prematurity, 487, 596–600
causes, clinical signs and management of, *596*
flexural laxity and, *648*
foal with curly soft ears, 597
foal with slipper foot, 598
head of premature foal showing classic signs of, 597
incomplete ossification of cuboidal bones in hock and carpus, 599
lateral radiograph of carpus of premature foal showing incomplete ossification of carpal bones with some cuboidal bones showing degree of ossification, 599
marked paradoxical respiration in premature foal, 600
placing hoof up to wither's level highlights increased tendon and periarticular laxity, 598
small size, domed head, and periarticular laxity in foal, 596
Preovulatory follicle, ultrasound image of, 462
Prepuptial edema, in adult horse, nonsteroidal anti-inflammatory drugs toxicity and, 97
Pressure sores, 270–272
lack of bedding and, 272
Priapism, *456*
Primary choke
anatomical areas for occurrence of, 40
causes of, *40*
Primary hyperparathyroidism, 523–525
causes of, *524*
close-up of horse with, revealing increased bone growth in skull, 524
side view of horse with, showing fibrous osteodystrophy of skull, 523
side view of skull of horse with, 525
Primary (idiopathic) glaucoma
corneal striae, aphakic crescent, and mild buphthalmia in quarter horse, 537
diagnosis of, *538*
ocular trauma *vs*., 538
Primary photosensitization, *301*
Progressive ethmoid hematoma, endoscopy of caudal nasal passage revealing red, smooth, glistening hematoma protruding from ethmoid region, 178
Proliferative bone at articular facets of C 5-6, 424
Proliferative enteropathy *(Lawsonia intracellularis)*, 76–77
foal with chemosis developed secondary to severe hypoproteinemia, 77
foal with diarrhea and rectal prolapse, 77
foal with intermandibular edema, 76
postmortem photograph of intestine of foal affected with, 77
Proximal interphalangeal joint (high ringbone), osteoarthritis of, 363
Proximal intertarsal joint, severe osteoarthritis of, 411
Proximal sesamoid bone
apical fracture of, 385
fracture of, 385–387
Proximal tibia, Salter-Harris type 2 fracture of, in 4-week-old Standardbred foal, 642
PSSM. *See* Polysaccharide storage myopathy

Psychogenic polydipsia
horse with, 560
predisposing factors for and management of, *560*
PTH secreting tumor, primary hyperparathyroidism and, *524*
Ptosis
Horner's syndrome and, 245
in horse affected by otitis media-interna (temporohyoid osteoarthropathy), 247
in horse with grass sickness, 114
Ptyalism, gastric ulcers and, *56*
P type (physeal) of infectious polyarthritis
in older foals, 640
in 4-week-old Standardbred foal, 640
Pulmonary abscessation, 604–605
lateral radiographic projections of caudodorsal lung fields of 4-month-old Standardbred, 604–605
perihilar lymph node enlargement and, 605
Pulmonary artery
poststenotic dilatation of, 124
radiographic image of radiopaque electrical cardioversion catheter in, 157
Pulsion diverticulum, 45
Purkinje cells, rabies and brown-staining Negris bodies in, 239
Purpura hemorrhagica, 168–173
adult horse with, 168
clinical signs and treatment for, *168*
ecchymoses in oral mucosa in horse affected with, 170
ecchymoses in vulvar mucosa in mare affected with, 171
ecchymotic hemorrhage on muzzle of horse affected with, 171
edema of head in horse affected with, 169
limb edema in horse affected with, 169
petechiae in nasal mucosa in horse affected with, 170
serum exudation and limb edema in horse affected with, 172
skin crusting in horse affected with, 172
skin sloughing in horse affected with, 173
strangles and, *204*
Streptococcus equi-associated, *326*
Pururitis, pemphigus foliaceus and, *299*
Pyelonephritis, 567–568
depressed horse with, 567
postmortem photograph of kidney and ureters from horse affected with ureteritis and, 568
Pyogranulomatous pericarditis, in horse with pleuropneumonia, 200
Pyometra, 470, *500*
causes and treatment of, *470*
endoscopy and ultrasonography of, 470
mare with, discharging pus from vulva, 470

Q

QRS complexes
atrial tachycardia during trotting exercise, telemetric recording from horse with atrial tachycardia and second degree AV block, 153
atrial tachycardia with second degree AV block at rest, 153
in ECG from horse with atrial fibrillation, secondary to mitral regurgitation and left atrial enlargement, 154
in electrocardiogram from horse with aortic valve insufficiency, 146
in Holter recording from horse with myocarditis, 138
multiform ventricular tachycardia, 160
normal, atrial fibrillation secondary to mitral regurgitation and left atrial enlargement, 142
normal resting sinus rhythm, 150
supraventricular arrhythmias and, 152
sustained unifocal ventricular tachycardia, 159
third degree (complete), base apex recording from neonatal foal with septic myocarditis, 152
Type I second degree atrioventricular (AV) block, 151
ventricular premature depolarization, 158
QRS waves, in ECG from horse with atrial endocarditis, 149
Quinidine administration, idiosyncratic and toxic reactions with, *156*
Quinidine gluconate, atrial fibrillation treatment and, *154*
Quinidine sulfate treatment
atrial fibrillation treatment and, *154*
horse fitted with telemetry during, 156

R

Rabies
clinical signs and diagnosis of, *239*
histological examination with immunoperoxidase stain of cerebellum of animal affected with, 239
Racehorses, atrial fibrillation and, *155*
Radial carpal bone, fracture of distal margin of, 396
Radial cysts, 401
Radial facet, third carpal bone with mild sclerosis of, 395
Radial nerve paralysis, foal with dropped elbow and flexion of all distal limb joints due to, 251
Rain scald, 279–281
Ramps, 9
RAO. *See* Recurrent airway obstruction
RCC. *See* Right coronary cusp
RCT. *See* Ruptured chorda tendinea
RDLC. *See* Right displacement of left large colon
Rectal prolapse, 492
Rectal tears and lacerations, 494
Rectovaginal fistula, 495
Rectus capitis muscles, poll impact and damage to, *215*
Recurrent airway obstruction, 190–191
accumulation of mucopurulent respiratory secretions in trachea of horse with, 190
nostril flaring during, 190
Recurrent exertional rhabdomyolysis
breeds affected by and diagnosis of, *350*
hematoxylin and eosin stained slides of muscles obtained from normal horse and horse affected with, 350
"Red foot," junctional epidermolysis bullosa and, 340
Renal failure
acute, hematuria in horse affected with, 561
acute, horse with severe depression and, 560
causes and clinical signs of, *560*
chronic, 563–567
weight loss in horse affected with, 563
Renal function, altered, edema formation giving ventral abdomen of foal a wrinkled appearance, 586
Reproductive system diseases
female, 462–504
aging of fetus, 464
aneuploidy and intersex, 473
ascending placentitis, 501
cervical tears, 476
clitoral anatomy and sampling of clitoral sinuses, 465

coital exanthema, 475
early and late gestation fetal sexing, 484–485
early and later embryonic death, 496
embryonic death and abortion due to twinning, 497–499
endometrial biopsy, 479–480
enlargement of mammary gland prior to abortion, 501
fetal death followed by anestrus, 477
fetal death followed by mummification, 500
general approaches and forms of dystocia, 481–483
granulosa cell tumors, 466–468
hydrops allantois, 490
intra-abdominal hemorrhage, 493
long umbilical cord as cause of abortion, 502–503
lymphatic lacunae or cyst, 471–472
nature of equine placentation, 504
normal contusion of vagina, 491
periovarian adhesions, 476
poor vulvar conformation, 474
premature placental separation and prolapse of bladder, 486
prematurity, 487
pyometra, 470
rectal, vaginal, and perineal tears and lacerations, 494–495
rectal prolapse, 492
routine culture and cytology to investigate infertility, 478
routine diagnostics of estrous cycle, 462
routine monitoring of early pregnancy, 463
severe vaginal contusions and pelvic subluxation, 492
stillbirth or abortion close to term, 501
transitional state, 469
transluminal adhesions, 471
uterine hemorrhage, 493
uterine rupture, 489
vaginal examination, 464
ventral abdominal rupture, 488
ventral edema in late gestation, 488
vulvar injuries, 475
male, 447–461
cryptorchidism, 447–449
hemosemen, 449–450
kicking injuries, 453–455
neoplasia, 451–452
penile paralysis and amputation, 456
scrotal hernias, 457–460
smegma accumulation "beans" in fossa glandis, 461
testicular hypoplasia, 455
testicular torsion and hydrocele, 460–461
RER. *See* Recurrent exertional rhabdomyolysis
Reserpine
Holter monitor recording of horse receiving, 151
side effects with, *151*
Respiratory distress, hyperkalemic periodic paralysis and, 345
Respiratory obstruction, hypoxic ischemic encephalopathy and, *583*
Respiratory system, diseases of, 175–209
African horse sickness, 208–209
diseases of extrathoracic airways, 176–189
diseases of intrathoracic airways, 190–203
diseases of thoracic wall and pleura, 203–204
strangles, 204–207
Retained deciduous teeth "cap," 23
Retained placenta, treatment of, 504
Reticulated leukotrichia
characteristics of and breeds affected by, *258*
in young quarter horse, 258, 259
Retina
degeneration of, 555
tapetal fundus of, lipofuscinlike pigment in, equine motor neuron disease and, 238
thin, 556
Rhinitis sicca, grass sickness and, 113
Rhodococcus equi, 606–610
clinical signs associated with intestinal form of infection with, *609*
foal infected with, causing osteomyelitis of extensor process of third phalanx and inguinal abscess, 610
intestinal form of, 609
large encapsulated abscesses throughout lung parenchyma due to, 606
large intra-abdominal abscess due to suppurative inflammation of mesenteric lymph node caused by infection with, 610
lateral thoracic radiograph of foal with, 607
pulmonary abscessation in foals infected with, 605
purulent material being removed from abscessed precapsular lymph node, 608
rotavirus diarrhea and, *621*
severe keratouveitis due to immune complex deposition associated with, 608
sonogram of thorax showing discrete superficial abscesses in lung parenchyma, 606
sonogram of thorax showing "sheets" of comet tail artifacts, seen with interstitial pneumonia, 607
stifle effusion associated with immune complex deposition in synovial structures associated with infection by, 608
Rhodococcus equi pneumonia, clinical signs, diagnosis, and treatment of, *606*
Rib fracture
fatal puncture of myocardium as result of, 645
ultrasonographic appearance of, 645
Right coronary cusp, echocardiographic image of ventricular septal defect and, 122
Right displacement of left large colon, 82
pelvic flexure in right side of abdomen lateral to cecum, 83
postmortem photograph of horse with, 82
Rocky Mountain horses, thin retina in, *556*
Rolling
colic and, 46, 51–52
treatment for left dorsal displacement of large colon with, 84–85
Rostral hook, 6–7
Rostral maxillary sinuses, *427*
fluid within, *428*
Rostral sinuses, fluid lines in, 430
Rotavirus diarrhea
clinical signs, diagnosis and treatment of, *621*
foal with, 621
Rubbing, hair loss and damage over croup and tail due to, 289
Ruptured bladders, ultrasonographic examination of ventral part of caudal abdomen of two foals with, 651
Ruptured chorda tendinea
postmortem photograph of, 140

postmortem photograph showing splitting of atrial epicardium secondary to, and acute mitral valve regurgitation, 140
sonographic image of pulmonary edema in horse with congestive heart failure and, 141
Ruptured common digital extensor tendon
diagnosis and treatment of, *646*
in foal, 646
Ruptured gastrocnemius muscle/tendon, in foal, 646

S

Sabulous urolithiasis, postmortem photograph of bladder affected with, 577
Salivary cyst, as cause of dystocia, 482
Salmonella typhimurium, salmonellosis and, *88*
Salmonellosis, 88–91
acute, postmortem photograph showing severe enterocolitis in horse affected with, 89
dark red and tacky gum, plus endotoxemia in horse affected with, 91
horse with watery diarrhea affected with, 88
inflamed large colon and, 89–90
rotavirus diarrhea and, *621*
severe dehydration and skin tenting in horse affected with, 91
small intestines affected with, 90
Salter-Harris type 2 fracture
of distal metacarpus in foal, 642
of proximal tibia in foal, 642
Sarcocystis neurona, equine protozoal myeloencephalitis and, *234*
Sarcoidosis, 306–307
clinical signs of, *306*
mature horse with generalized scaling and alopecia due to, 306
progression of clinical signs in horse with, 307
Sarcoids, 304–306
classification, diagnosis and treatment of, *304*
fibroblastic, in dorsolateral aspect of left front fetlock, 305
fibroelastic, on upper lip, 306
flat, with alopecia at base of mane, 304
mature horse with, 304
nodular, dorsal and caudal to commissure of lip in mature horse, 305
treatment for, *553*
of upper eyelid, 553
"Sawhorse" stance, tetanus (lockjaw) and, *240*
Scalding, 307–311
chemical, 309–310
serum, 307–309
urine, 311
SCC. *See* Squamous cell carcinoma
Sclera, jaundiced in foal with neonatal isoerythrolysis, 601
Scleral hemorrhage, foal with, 629
Scratches (greasy heel, pastern dermatitis), 311–313
description of, *311*
in horse with deep horizontal fissures in midpastern region and beginning of photoactive dermatitis, 312
photoactive dermatitis and, 327
photoactive vasculitis originating from pastern dermatitis, 313
photosensitization and, *301*
yearling horse with, 311, 312
Scrotal hernia, 457–460
anatomy of, 458
castration and, 460
congenital
surgery for, 459
30-day-old foal with severe right-sided scrotal hernia, 459
in foal, showing preputial swelling, 625
ultrasonography of, 458
Scrotum, equine, average size of, *455*
Secondary choke, 45–46
esophageal diverticulae and, 45
postmortem photograph of vascular ring anomalies in foal, 46
Secondary glaucoma, 539
aphakic crescent, cataract, and posterior synechiae in ageing polo pony, 539
peripheral corneal edema, miosis, and corneal stromal vascularization in middle-aged horse, 539
treatment of, *539*
Secondary hyperparathyroidism, 525–526
clinical signs and causes of, *525*
horse's head with distorted facial bones due to replacement with fibrous connective tissue, 525
postmortem photograph of one side of mandible from horse with, 526
Secondary photosensitization, *301*
Second metacarpal bone, splint exostosis of, 406
Second phalanx, subchondral cystic lesion of, 373
Seizures
focal, hypoxic ischemic encephalopathy, tonic muzzle contractions and, 583
grand mal, with extensor rigidity and opisthotonos in foal with hypoxic ischemic encephalopathy, 584
Selenium deficiency, white muscle disease in foal and, *649*
Self-excoriation, epidermal damage as result of, *288*
Semen collection, safe, 453
Seminoma, 451
Sepsis, 587–595
bilateral decubital ulcers associated with olecranon region in septicemic foal, 593
clinical signs, diagnosis and treatment of, *587*
coronitis in foal with, 590
early, hyperemic mucous membranes seen in foal with, 588
embolic nephritis and, 588
embolic pneumonia and, 587
foal standing under mare and not nursing as early sign of, 587
foal with enterocolitis and, 592
hemorrhagic gingival margins in foal with, 589
iriditis and anterior uveitis in newborn foal with, 590
localized, soft fluctuant subcutaneous swellings due to subcutaneous abscess formation in foal with, 592
longitudinal ultrasonographic image of lateral aspect of elbow of neonatal septicemic foal, 595
petechiae in ear of foal with, 591
ultrasonographic image of ventral abdomen of foal with omphalophlebitis with urachal abscessation, 594
Septic arthritis
in foals, 639
osteomyelitis with, of lateral proximal sesamoid bone, 384
type T, lateral radiograph of tarsus of neonatal septicemic foal with, 594

Septicemia
multifocal vasculitis and, *326*
in neonatal foal due to *Actinobacillus equuli* manifested as uveitis and hypopyon, 591
Septic jugular vein thrombophlebitis, tricuspid valve insufficiency and, *146*
Septic shock, muddy purple discolored mucous membranes in foal with, 589
Septic thrombophlebitis
of jugular vein, 161
complications and treatment of, *161*
multiocculated, cavitated thrombus in jugular vein consistent with, 162
Sequestration of the calcaneus, 413
Sequestrum formation, on dorsal cortex of third metatarsal bone, 415
SER. *See* Sporadic exertional rhabdomyolysis
Sertoli cells
disruption of spermatogenesis due to cryptorchidism and, *449*
tumors of, 451
Serum scalding
alopecia along drainage pathway in case of proximal hind-limb wound, 309
healing from, alopecia shown along drainage pathway, 308
horse after treatment for, 308
signs of, *307*
in 10-year-old mare, 307
Sesamoiditis
classification of, *383*
type 2 of medial proximal sesamoid bone, 383
type 3 of medial proximal sesamoid bone, 383
Sesamoid osteomyelitis, guarded prognosis for, *384*
Setaria spp., verminous meningoencephalomyelitis and, *228*
"Shaker foal," botulism and, *627*
Shear mouth, 9
Shetland ponies, tracheal collapse in, *189*
Shirodkar-like suture, cervical tears and, *476*
Shoe boil, 270–272
Shoe-boil roll, in case of cubital bursitis, 270
Simulium spp., insect bite hypersensitivity and, *288*
Sinonasal neoplasia and polyps, 181
clinical signs of, *181*
Sinus cyst, 180–181, 429–430
deformation of face over right maxillary region in horse with, 180
fluid within rostral and caudal maxillary sinuses, 430–431
skull radiograph revealing rounded, well-demarcated opacity indicative of, 181
Sinusitis, 179–180, 426–427
chronic
deformation of face over left maxillary region in horse with, 179
unilateral purulent nasal discharge in horse with, 179
clinical signs of, *428*
lateral skull radiograph showing parallel fluid-air interfaces in frontal and maxillary sinuses in horse with, 180
Sinus rhythm, normal, resting, 150
Sinus tachycardia, during exercise, 150
Skeletal growth, acquired flexural contracture related to, *647*
Skeletal malformation, severe, as cause of dystocia, 482
Skin disorders, in foals, 656–658. *See also* Integumentary system, diseases of
Skin sloughing, in horse affected with purpura hermorrhagica, 173
Skin tenting, hyperelastosis cutis (Ehler Danlos syndrome) and, 287
Skull
anatomy of, 427
primary hyperparathyroidism and fibrous osteodystrophy of, 523
primary hyperparathyroidism and increased bone growth in, 524
Slab fracture
defined, *399*
of third carpal bone, 399–400
of third carpal bone, sagittal, 400
Slipper foot, premature foal with, 598
Small colon, diseases of, 99–102
antibiotic induced colitis, 102
idiopathic inflammatory bowel disease, 101
intraluminal obstruction of small colon with enteroliths, fecaliths, or foreign bodies, 100
small colon impaction, 99
Small colon impaction, postmortem photographs of horse with, 99
Small intestinal volvulus (mesenteric torsion), 62
Small intestines
diseases of, 59–77
functional obstruction of, 75–77
simple obstruction of, 59–61
strangulating obstruction of, 62–75
epiploic foramen entrapment of, 69–71
intussusception of, 74
postmortem photograph of incarceration of, through gastrosplenic ligament, 73
simple obstruction of, 59–61
Small intestine strangulation, diaphragmatic hernia and, 72
Small muscular ventricular septal defects, *121*
Smegma
accumulation of
"beans" in fossa glandis, 461
precancerous lesions and, 451
clitoral, 465
"Smooth" tear, geriatric wear and, 21
Soft tissue swelling, of carpus, 392
Sow mouth (underbite), 15
"Spavin," 410–412
Speculum examination, failure to demonstrate cervical tears and, *476*
Spermatogenesis, cryptorchidism and suppression of, *448*, 449
Sphenoid bone, fracture of, 441–422
Spinal canal, malalignment of spinal canal at C 3-4 and compression of at C 3-4, 423
Spinal cord, subtle compression of, at C 5-6, 424–425
Spindle cell carcinoma, invasion of left eye orbit by, 553
Spine, 422–427
articular facet reaction, 424–425
cervical vertebral malformation instability, 425–426
misalignment and compression of spinal canal, 423
normal cervical spine, 422
osteomyelitis of third cervical vertebra, 426–427
Splint exostosis, of second metacarpal bone, 406

Splinting, for ruptured gastrocnemius muscle, 646
Sporadic exertional rhabdomyolysis, myoblobinuria in horse affected with, 346
Sporothrix schenckii
excised fungal granuloma due to, 315
photomicrograph of
in infected nodule showing multinucleated giant cells, 315
in infected nodule showing yeastlike organisms following fine needle aspiration, 315
sporotrichosis caused by, *313*
Sporotrichosis, 313–315
diagnosis of, *314*
excised fungal granuloma due to *Sporothrix schenckii*, 315
horse with cutaneolymphatic form of, 313
photomicrograph of *Sporothrix schenckii* in infected nodule showing multinucleated giant cells, 315
photomicrograph of *Sporothrix schenckii* in infected nodule showing yeastlike organisms following needle aspiration, 315
Squamous cell carcinoma, 37, *181*, 316–317
bilateral, epiphora in horse presenting for, in nictating membranes, 317
on penis of horse, 451, 452
preputial and penile, in mature horse, 316
signs of, *316*
treatment for, *468*
SR-y gene, aneuploidy and, *473*
Stallions
kicking injury to penis of, 453
masturbation, hemosemen and, 449
semen collection and injury to, *453*
testicular descent in, 447
testicular hypoplasia in, 455
Standardbreds, osseous fragments in large proportion of, *391*
Step mouth, 8
"Stepped tooth," 8, 28
Stifle and tibia, 416–421
calcinosis circumscripta, 420
cranial cruciate ligament injury, 418
fracture of patella, 419
osteoarthritis of stifle joint, 417
osteochondritis dissecans, 416–417
subchondral bone cyst, 416
tibial stress fracture, 421
Stifle effusion, in foals infected with *Rhodococcus equi*, 608
Stifle joint
normal, in 8-day-old Thoroughbred, 631
osteoarthritis of, 417
Stillbirth, close to term, 502
Stomach, diseases of, 53–59
gastric dilatation, 53–54
gastric impaction, 54–55
gastric ulcers, 56–59
Strangles, *182*, 204–207
causes and clinical signs of, *204*
choke and signs of dysphagia in adult horse, 206
emergency temporary tracheostomy needed for horses with, *206*
endoscopy of nasopharynx of horse with, showing purulent discharge draining from guttural pouch openings, 183
enlarged lymph node compressing esophagus and causing choke in adult horse, 206
enlarged lymph nodes compressing pharynx and impeding respiration, 206
enlarged retropharyngeal lymph nodes in horse affected with, 183, 205
enlarged submandibular lymph nodes in foal with, 205
enlarged submandibular lymph nodes in horse with, 204
healed tracheostomy site in horse recovering from, 207
mucupurulent nasal discharge in horses with, originating from ruptured abscessed retropharyngeal lymph nodes in medial compartment of guttural pouch, 207
Strangulating obstruction, of small intestine, 62–75
Stratum compactum, 480
Stratum spongiosum, 480
Streptococcal infection, endoscopic view of guttural pouch empyema secondary to, 182
Streptococcus equi infection
brain abscess and, *212*
myopathies associated with, 345, *345*
purpura hemorrhagica associated with, *168*, *326*
Streptococcus zooepidemicus, *478*
brain abscess and, *212*
pyometra and, *470*
Stress fracture, of third metacarpus, 404
Stretching, colic and, 46, 49
Stringhalt
adult horse affected with, showing hyperflexion of hock joint, 240
clinical signs of, *240*
Strongylosis, 92
postmortem photograph of cecum of horse with, showing cyathostomiasis, 93
postmortem photograph of horse with, showing presence of firbrous tags on spleen, 92
postmortem photograph of small intestine of horse with, showing heamomalasma ilii, 92
Strongylus edentatus, *92*
Strongylus equinuus, *92*
Strongylus vulgaris, *92*
verminous meningoencephalomyelitis and, *228*
Stud crud (idiopathic cannon keratosis)
description of, *318*
scaling and crusting with, 318
Stylohyoid bone, unilateral thickening of, otitis media-interna (temporohyoid osteoarthropathy) and, 248
S type infectious polyarthritis, in foal, 639
Subchondral bone, lysis of, *396*
Subchondral bone cyst, of medial condyle, 416
Subchondral cystic lesion
of first phalanx, 372
of phalanx, 373–374
of second phalanx, dorsoplantar horizontal beam radiographic projection of right rear foot of 2-year-old Standardbred, 373
Subchondral sclerosis, *380*
Subcutaneous bursa, of elbow region, inflammation of, 270
Subepiglottic cyst
treatment of, *187*
in 4-year-old racehorse, 187
Subluxated lens, aphakic crescent, cataract, in middle-aged polo pony, 542
Sucking louse, *291*
Suckle reflex, hypoxic ischemic encephalopathy and loss of, 582

Summer solstice, twinning rate in mares and, *497*
Sunblock, *318*
Sunburn, differential diagnoses for, *318*
Sun damage, squamous cell carcinoma and, *316*
Superior check ligament, enchondroma and enthesiophyte formation at attachment of, 402
Supernumerary canine tooth, in aged horse, 35
Supernumerary incisor, 13
Suppurative endometritis, severe, 480
Supraventricular arrhythmias, 152–153
Suspensory ligament
  avulsion fracture at origin of, nuclear scintagraphic images of, 405
  periostitis at origin of, 406
"Swiss cheese septum," muscular ventricular septal defects and, *121*
Synovial invaginations, enlarged and abnormally shaped, 358

T

Talus
  comminuted fracture of, 412–413
  osteochondritis dissecans of medial trochlear ridge of, 409
Tarsal bone ossification, grading system for, in foals, 633
Tarsal valgus
  angular limb deformity of, in 5-week-old quarter horse foal, 637
  causes and evaluation of, *637*
Tarsometatarsal joint
  mild osteoarthritis of, 410
  severe osteoarthritis of, 411
Tarsus, normal, in 8-day-old Thoroughbred foal, 630–631
Tarsus and metatarsus, 407–415
  fracture and osteomyelitis of fourth metartarsal bone, 414
  fracture of fourth metatarsal bone, 414
  fracture of talus, 412–413
  osteoarthritis, 410–412
  osteochondritis dissecans, 407–409
  sequestration of calcaneus, 413
  sequestrum formation on third metartarsal bone, 415
Tarsus varus, foal with, clinical photograph, 638
Taylorella equigenitalis
  contagious equine metritis and, 461
    sampling of clitoral sinuses, 465
Teeth, diseases of, 5–37
  abnormal tooth wear, 36–37
  asynchronous teeth eruption, 27
  caudal hooks or ramps, 7
  deviation of maxilla, 26
  diagonal incisor malocculsion, 11
  dysplastic teeth, 36
  fractured tooth, 27–31
  geriatric wear, 21
  gingival and lingual ulceration of systemic origin, 34
  hooks or ramps, 9
  incisor curvature, 11–12
  irregular incisor malocclusion, 12
  lingual and buccal laceration and bit pressure (injury), 31–34
  overbite (parrot mouth), 13–14
  overlong distal portion of third incisor, 10
  periodontal disease, diastema, enamel and cemental decay, 15–20
  polydontia, 35
  rostral hood, 6–7
  shear mouth, 9
  step mouth, 8
  stepped tooth, 8
  supernumerary canine tooth, 35
  supernumerary incisor, 13
  teeth eruption and retained deciduous teeth "cap," 22–24
  underbite (sow or monkey mouth), 15
  wave malocclusion, 5–6
  wolf teeth, 24–25
Teeth eruption
  retained 803 in 5 and 1/2 year-old, 22
  in 3-year-old patient, 22
Telogen defluxion, 319–320
  description of, *319*
  hair coat of horse treated for, 320
  head of old gelding with, 319
  huge areas of hair loss in old gelding with, 319
Temporal muscle atrophy, in 2-year-old quarter horse stallion, 346
Temporal teratoma, 320–322
  description of, *320*
  large draining mass at base of left ear in mature Thoroughbred mare, 320
  surgical removal of, 321–322
Temporohyoid osteoarthropathy, 246–251
Tendon injuries, in foals, 646–649
Testicles
  cryptorchid, image illustrating testicular echo and its homogeneity, *448*
  of male pseudohemaphrodites, *473*
  normal and cryptorchid, 448
  seminoma on, 451
Testicular descent, species comparison between horses and cattle, 447
Testicular hypoplasia, 455
Testicular torsion
  congenital, in 4-year-old paint stallion, 461
  hydrocele and, 460–461
Testosterone
  disruption of spermatogenesis due to cryptorchidism and, *449*
  granulosa cell tumors and, *466*
Tetanus (lockjaw), 240–242
  adult horses affected with
    showing profuse frothy salivation, 242
    showing prolapsed third eyelid, 241
    showing stiff posture of horse with head and neck extended, 240
    showing trismus, 241
  clinical signs of, *240*
  recumbent adult horse unresponsive to treatment, and subsequent death of, 242
Tetralogy of Fallot
  right parasternal short axis image of horse with, 128
  in 3-year-old Thoroughbred gelding, 128
Tetraparesis, equine protozoal myeloencephalitis and, *234*
Tetraplagia, equine herpes virus 1 (EHV-1) myeloencephalitis and, 230
Thin retina, 556
Third carpal bone
  fracture of, 398–400

fracture of proximal dorsomedial margin of, 398
with mild sclerosis of radial facet, 395
normal, 395
sclerosis of radial and intermediate facets of, 396
Third cervical vertebra, osteomyelitis of, 426–427
Third eyelid
prolapsed, hyperkalemic periodic paralysis and, 344
prolapsed, tetanus (lockjaw) and, 241
Third eyelid squamous cell carcinoma, salmon pink friable third eyelid mass and, 552
Third incisor, overlong distal portion of, 10
Third metacarpus
lateral condylar fracture of, 389
stress fracture of, nuclear scintigraphic images of, 404
Third metatarsal bone, sequestrum formation on, 415
Third phalanx
articular fracture of wing of, 367–368
fracture of extensor process of, 365–366
fracture of palmar process of, 369
nonarticular fracture of wing of, 366–367
ossification of accessory cartilages of, 371
osteomyelitis of, 369
sagittal fracture of, in 10-year-old Morgan, 368
Third phalanx rotation, two methods for assessment of, 377–378
Thoracic wall, diseases of, 203–204
Thorax
normal, lateral radiographic projection of thoracic cavity in 12-year-old Clydesdale, 602
radiography of, 602–603
Thoroughbred gelding, 4-year-old, retained tooth 802 in, and extraction of same tooth, 23
Throat latch region, marked distension of, in foal with guttural pouch tympany, 184
Thrombophlebitis, 161–164
acute, horse with venous distension of head and neck secondary to, 162
septic, sonogram of, 161
Thrombosis, 161–164
bilateral jugular, edema of head and tongue of horse affected with, 163
multiocculated, cavitated, in jugular vein consistent with septic thrombophlebitis, 162
at previous catheter site with no sign of infection, 161
Thyroid adenoma, 518–522
postoperative picture of horse after removal of, 520
surgical removal of, 520
ultrasound image of, 519
unilateral enlargement of thyroid gland due to, 519
Thyroid gland
brachial cysts attached to, found on postmortem examination, 522
enlarged, 518
close-up of, 518
left and right lobes of, removed at postmortem, 521
with two adenomas after surgical removal, 521
Tibia
osteochondritis dissecans of distal intermediate ridge of, 407
osteochondritis dissecans of medial malleolus of, 408
Tibial stress fracture, 421
Tick infestation, 324–325
multiple hard-bodied ticks, 324
number of ticks easily appreciated with use of tick comb, 325
severe, in mature horse, 324
Toe scuffing, equine wobbler syndrome and, 236
Tongue, foal's, candidiasis on, 613
Tongue control, hypoxic ischemic encephalopathy and loss of, 582
Tongue paralysis, lead poisoning and, 243
Tongue seal, good, in foal, 582
Tongue tone, botulism and loss of, *627*
Tooth roots, 434, 435
abscesses of
clinical findings on, *437*
of left first maxillary molar, 436
of left third mandibular premolar, 437
Tooth wear, abnormal, 36–37
Toxicity, nonsteroidal anti-inflammatory drugs, 95–98
Tracheal collapse, 189
endoscopic view of, in miniature foal with complaint of respiratory stridor and exercise intolerance, 189
lateral cervical and thoracic radiograph of miniature foal with, at level of thoracic inlet, 189
Traction diverticulum, 45
Training at fast speeds, metacarpal periostitis and, 403
Transition, *469*
Transitional ovary, ultrasonographic image from mare, 469
Transluminal adhesions, 471
evaluation of, 471
preventing, *471*
purulent discharge seen on floor behind mare, 471
Transtympanic lavage, otitis media-interna (temporohyoid osteoarthropathy) diagnosis and, 249
Trauma, hemosemen and, 449
Triadan numbering system, for equine dentition, 5
Trichophyton equinum var equi, dermatophytosis (ringworm) and, *281*
Tricuspid valve, postmortem photograph of horse with massive proliferative lesions on three cusps of, 147
Tricuspid valve insufficiency, 146–147
bacterial endocarditis and, 146
M-mode echocardiographic image from horse with, showing marked thickening of tricuspid valve leaflets, 147
Trismus, 241
Trophoblast, 463
Truncus arteriosus, 126–127
cause of, *127*
characteristics of, *126*
cyanotic mucous membranes in foal with, 127
in neonatal foal, 126
postmortem photograph of, 127
right parasternal right ventricular outflow tract view, 126
Trusses, penile injuries and use of, 455
T type (tarsal) of infectious polyarthritis, in 4-week-old quarter horse foal, 641
Tuber calcani, normal tarsus and ossification of, 630
Tubular speculum, failure to demonstrate cervical tears and, *476*
"Tucked up" appearance, grass sickness and, 109, 110
Tumoral calcinosis, 272–273, 420
Turner's-like syndrome, *473*
T waves, normal resting sinus rhythm, *150*
Twinning, embryonic death and abortion due to, 497–499
Twin pregnancies
poor management of and related consequences, 499

proper management of, early pregnancy, *463*
variations in placentation in, 499
Twin preovulatory follicles, as seen on ultrasound, 497
Twin reduction, with use of transvaginal ultrasound guided aspiration, 498
Type III hypersensitivity reaction, immune-mediated vasculitis and, *326*
Typhlocolitis, postmortem photograph of large colon of horse affected with, caused by cyathostomes, 93–94

U

Ulceration, of oral mucosa caused by sharp enamel point on distal aspect of 211 as it occludes with 311, 33
Ulcerative dermatitis
crusting and erythema around anus and vulva, 657
description of, *656*
epithelial loss in ear due to, 657
in foals, 656
Ulcers, decubital, in foals, 656
Ulnar carpal bone cyst, 401
Ultrasonography, tracking estrous cycle and, *462*
Umbilical cord
long, as cause of abortion, 502–503
variation in normal length of, 503
yolk sac remnants on, 503
Umbilical hematoma, cause of, 655
Umbilical hernia, in foal, 108
Umbilical remnant infections, 653–654
with purulent caseous material in umbilical arteries and apex of bladder, 653
sonogram of caudal part of ventral abdomen of foal, caudal to external umbilical remnant, 653
treatment of, *653*
Umbilical swellings, external, in foal, 654
Umbilical vein, infected, ultrasonographic image of, in foal, 654
Underbite (sow or monkey mouth), 15
Urachus
bullous dilations of, long umbilical cord as cause of abortion and, 502
rupture of, in foal, and treatment of, *652*
Urethra, endoscopic image of, in horse with urethrolithiasis, 571
Urethral rent or defect, endoscopic image of urethra in horse affected with, 570
Urethrolith, removal of, by urethrotomy in male donkey, 574
Urethrolithiasis, 571
abdominal distension in male donkey affected with urinary bladder rupture secondary to, 572
postmortem photograph of urethra with, showing rupture in penis, 574
urethral rupture in horse secondary to, 573
Urinary incontinence, equine herpes virus 1 (EHV-1) myeloencephalitis and, 230
Urinary system diseases, 559–577
acute renal failure, 560–562
chronic renal failure, 563–567
cystitis, 568
psychogenic polydipsia, 560
pyelonephritis, 567–568
urethral rent or defect, 570
urolithiasis, 571–577
verminous nephritis, 569
Urinary tract disruption
foal straining to urinate, shown with dorsoflexion of back and tail position, 650
postmortem image of foal with rupture in dorsal wall of bladder and concurrent peritonitis, 650
Urine scalding
alopecia, erythema, and crusting in mare due to, 311
equine herpes virus 1 (EHV-1) myeloencephalitis and, 230
Urolithiasis, 571
clinical signs and diagnosis of, *571*
horse affected with, showing frequent posturing to urinate and extension of penis, 571
Urticaria, 325–326
conventional, in Thoroughbred, 326
drug eruption in horse after vaccination and severe dependent chest edema, 334, 335
factors related to, *325*
multifocal wheals on mature Thoroughbred, 325
Urticarial type of lesion, cutaneous lymphosarcoma and, *278*
Uterine hemorrhage, ultrasonographic appearance of, 493
Uterine rupture, 489
Uterine torsion, nonsurgical correction of, 487
Uterine wall, characteristic thickening of, early pregnancy, 463
Uterus, pyometra and physical drainage of, *470*
Uveal cyst, 551
Uveitis, 543–545
acute, leptospirosis and, 547
chronic, 547
chronic, keratitis and, 548
clinical diagnosis and treatment for, *544*
corneal edema, dorsal corneal stromal vascularization, hypopyon, and yellow exudates extending over miotic pupil in horse with, 543
corneal foreign body, misosis and subtle ventral hypopyon with, 544
corneal stromal abscess and secondary anterior uveitis in 2-year-old quarter horse mare, 545
equine recurrent, 546
intravitreous hemorrhage and, 545
perforated corneal abscess with septic endophthalmitis and phthisis bulbi, 544

V

Vaccinations, cutaneous drug reactions (drug eruption) after, 334, 335
Vaginal contusions
normal, 491
severe, and pelvic subluxation, 492
Vaginal examination, 464
Vaginal tears and lacerations, 494
Valvular insufficiency, consequences of, *139*
Varicose veins, mass of, in everted portion of cranial vagina of aged mare, 464
Vascular diseases, 161–173
aortic root disease, 164–168
purpura hemorrhagica, 168–173
thrombosis and thrombophlebitis, 161–164
Vascular ring anomalies, in foal, postmortem photograph of, 46
Vasculitis, 326–327
purpura hemorrhagica in which forelimbs were severely affected, 327
Venipuncture, jugular vein thrombophlebitis secondary to, *161*
Ventral abdominal rupture, 488

Ventral abdominal wall tear, in 18-hour-old foal, 649
Ventral edema, in late gestation, 488
Ventral incisor curvature, in aged horse, 12
Ventral septal defect, 120–125
Ventricular arrhythmias, 158–160
  in horses with aortic insufficiency, *146*
Ventricular bigeminy, Holter recording, 159
Ventricular premature depolarization, 158
Ventricular septal defects
  color flow Doppler image of, showing turbulent flow through septal defect, 123
  continuous wave Doppler image of flow through, 123
  echocardiographic image of, from right parasternal short axis view of aorta, 122
  membranous
    echocardiographic image of, 122
    echocardiographic image of 2-year-old Thoroughbred gelding with history of poor racing performance, 120
    large, echocardiographic image of Welsh pony with, 124
    large, postmortem image of, 125
  outflow, color flow Doppler image of, 121
  radiographic image of pulmonary edema in pony with heart failure due to, 125
  tetralogy of Fallot and, *128*
Ventricular tachycardia
  multiform, Holter recording, 160
  paroxysmal, 160
  sustained unifocal, 159
Verminous arteritis, postmortem photograph of, 167
Verminous meningoencephalomyelitis, 228–229
  adult horse affected by, showing clinical signs of, 228
  ataxia and limb weakness in horse affected with, 229
  clinical signs of, *228*
  head-pressing in horse with, 228
Verminous nephritis, 569
Verrucous (warty) lesions, sarcoids and, *304*
Vestibular cortex dysfunction, poll impact and, *215*
Vet-wrap, penis wrapped in, after kicking injury, 454
Viral diarrhea, rotavirus and, *621*
Viral skin diseases, 330
Visceral vaginal tunic, scrotal hernia and, 458
Vitamin D toxicity, 523
Vitamin E deficiency, white muscle disease in foal and, *649*
Vitiligo
  acquired, of unknown origin in mature quarter horse, 329
  periocular depigmentation in young paint horse, 329
VPD. *See* Ventricular premature depolarization
VSD. *See* Ventricular septal defects
Vulva
  injuries to, 475
  poor conformation of, 474
  ulcerative dermatitis with crusting and erythema around, 657

W

Warts (papillomatosis), 330–332
  congenital, on heel bulb of quarter horse foal, clipped prior to surgical removal, 332
  congenital, on tongue of neonatal quarter horse foal before and after surgical removal, 331
Wave malocclusion, 5–6
  involving 200 and 300 arcades in middle-aged patient, 5
  300 “wave” abnormality, 6
Weanlings, chronic gastric ulceration in, 56, *56*
Weight loss
  chronic renal failure and, 563
  Cushing’s syndrome and, *274*
  grass sickness and, 109, 110
  nephrolithiasis and, 576
  peritonitis and, 105
  severe
    abdominal abscessation and, 103
    abdominal adhesions and, 104
    in horse affected with idiopathic inflammatory bowel disease, 101
Welsh ponies, ventricular septal defects in, *124*
West Nile Virus, 225–227
  adult horses affected with, 226
    depression and, 226
    droopy lips and, 227
    twitching and, 227
    wide-base stance and, 225
  clinical signs of, *225*
Wheals, with urticaria, *325*
White corneal plaques, with granuloma and periocular calcification, 531
White foal, with abnormalities in ileum, caecum, and colons, 290
“White lacing,” *258*
White muscle disease
  clinical signs of, *649*
  recumbent foal affected with, 649
“Wind sucking”
  poor vulvar conformation and, *474*
  vulvar injuries and, *475*
Winter atopy
  causes of, *333*
  early lesion in mature horse with, 333
  horse with healed lesion and remaining alopecic region, 333
Withers skin, burns and protection of from trauma when horse rolls, 266
WNV. *See* West Nile Virus
Wobbler’s syndrome, *424*, 425–426
Wolf teeth, 24–25
  atypical palatal location of, in a yearling, 25
  fragments, 25
  very large, in 2-year-old Thoroughbred, 24
Wryneck, *482*
Wry nose, 176–178
  description of, *176*
  foal born with, 176
  malocclusion of incisors in foal with, 614
  radiograph of maxilla of foal after surgical correction, 177–178
  radiograph of maxilla of foal with, 177
  in 2-year-old Thoroughbred, 26

X

XX karyotypes, aneuploidy and, *473*

Y

Yearling, class 2 malocclusion (“parrot mouth” or “overbite”) in, 14
Yolk sac remnants on umbilical cord, 503